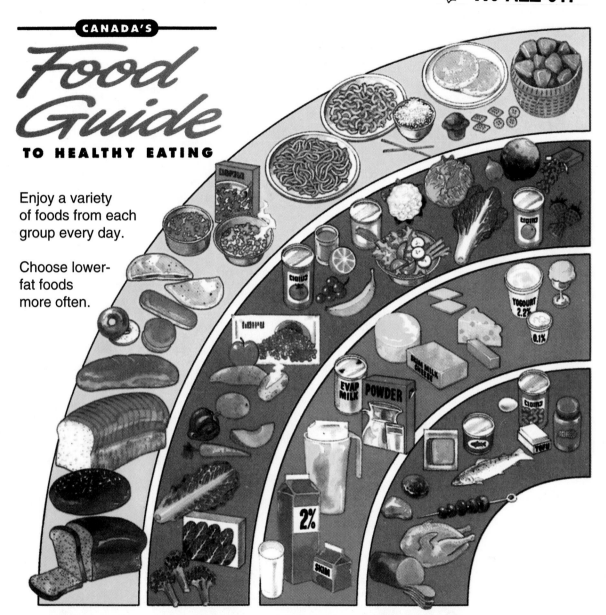

Health Canada **Santé Canada**

W9-AEZ-917

CANADA'S
Food Guide
TO HEALTHY EATING

Enjoy a variety
of foods from each
group every day.

Choose lower-
fat foods
more often.

Grain Products
Choose whole grain
and enriched
products more
often.

Vegetables & Fruit
Choose dark green and
orange vegetables and
orange fruit more often.

Milk Products
Choose lower-fat
milk products more
often.

Meat & Alternatives
Choose leaner meats,
poultry, and fish, as
well as dried peas,
beans, and lentils
more often.

Canada

NUTRITION ESSENTIALS

and Diet Therapy

CONGRATULATIONS

You now have access to a Bonus Online Package!

visit us at:

http://www.wbsaunders.com/MERLIN/peckenpaugh

A website just for you as you learn nutrition with the new 9th edition of
Nutrition Essentials and Diet Therapy

for students:

WebLinks   An exciting resource that lets you link to hundreds of websites carefully chosen to supplement the content of your textbook. The WebLinks are regularly updated, with new ones added as they develop.

for instructors:

State-of-the-art security protects valuable online teaching tools. A unique passcode (available from your sales representative) is your key to a complete web-based **Instructor's Manual** that includes:

• Critical Thinking Discussion Tips
• Answers to Chapter Study Questions and Classroom Activities
• Sample Test Questions and Answers
• PowerPoint Presentations
• 40 Electronic Images

These same instructor resources are available on CD-ROM (ISBN 0-7216-0165-0) from your sales representative.

Free NutriTrac Nutrition Analysis CD-ROM
with every copy of Nutrition Essentials and Diet Therapy, 9th Edition

plus:

The new version of this valuable CD-ROM features:
• Expanded Food Database of over 3000 items in 18 different food categories
• Expanded Activities Database of over 150 items in activity categories such as daily/common, sporting, recreational, and occupational
• Personal Profile Screen (includes user height, weight, age, etc., and a **new** Body Mass Index calculator)
• User Food Intake Record (tracks daily food intake)
• Detailed Energy Expenditure Log (tracks daily activities)
• Weight Management Planner
• Comprehensive Nutritional Evaluation (nutrient summary, Food Guide Pyramid, calorie source pie chart, fat composition pie chart, DRI/RNI graphs, etc.)

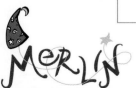

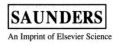

SAUNDERS
An Imprint of Elsevier Science

NUTRITION ESSENTIALS

and Diet Therapy

Ninth Edition

Nancy J. Peckenpaugh

MSEd, RD, CDN, CDE

Dietitian in Private Practice, Lifetime Nutrition Services

Dietitian, Offices of Dr. Adam Law and Dryden Family Medicine

**Nutrition Consultant, Tompkins Community Action Head Start,
Franziska Racker Centers (formerly The Special Children's Center),
Early Intervention Program (EIP) of Tompkins County,
Lakeside Nursing Home,
and Medicaid Obstetrical and Maternal Services (MOMS) of Tompkins County**

**Lecturer, Department of Health,
State University of New York College at Cortland,
Ithaca, New York**

Saunders

An Imprint of Elsevier Science

Philadelphia   London   Toronto   Montreal   Sydney   Tokyo

Saunders

An Imprint of Elsevier Science

11830 Westline Industrial Drive
St. Louis, Missouri 63146

NUTRITION ESSENTIALS AND DIET THERAPY, Ninth Edition   ISBN 0-7216-9532-9
Copyright © 2003, Elsevier Science (USA). All rights reserved.

NOTICE

Nutrition is an ever-changing field. Standard safety precautions must be followed, but as new research and clinical experience broaden our knowledge, changes in treatment and drug therapy may become necessary or appropriate. Readers are advised to check the most current product information provided by the manufacturer of each drug to be administered to verify the recommended dose, the method and duration of administration, and contraindications. It is the responsibility of the licensed prescriber, relying on experience and knowledge of the patient, to determine dosages and the best treatment for each individual patient. Neither the publisher nor the author assumes any liability for any injury and/or damage to persons or property arising from this publication.

Previous editions copyrighted 1999, 1995, 1991, 1984, 1979, 1972, 1966, 1960

International Standard Book Number 0-7216-9532-9

Vice President and Publishing Director, Nursing: Sally Schrefer
Editor: Yvonne Alexopoulos
Associate Developmental Editor: Danielle Frazier
Publishing Services Manager: Catherine Jackson
Project Manager: Mary Stueck
Designer: Amy Buxton

GW/RDC

Printed in the United States of America

Last digit is the print number: 9   8   7   6   5   4   3   2   1

To my former co-author,

Charlotte Mallery Poleman, RD, CDN,

a wonderful professional mentor and personal friend.

May retirement be long, healthy, and happy.

Nancy J. Peckenpaugh

Preface

Every year we learn something significantly new about nutrition. Ongoing research at every level, from the biochemical to the sociocultural, expands our knowledge base in this important discipline. This new knowledge increases our potential for improving the care we bring to our patients and it makes the teaching and learning of nutrition more complex and difficult, particularly given the limited class time devoted to nutrition in the education of health care professionals. In writing the Ninth Edition of *Nutrition Essentials and Diet Therapy*, the objective has been to provide an updated, concise, focused, and practical approach to basic health care nutrition.

In providing a better focus, we concentrate on what is most important for the health care provider to know about the nutrition basics and the application of nutrition knowledge. The current edition has been rigorously reviewed and revised with the following goals:

The earlier groupings of the macronutrients carbohydrate, protein, and fat remain in one chapter. This best allows for discussion of the application of this information to food choices as food typically contains more than one macronutrient. The chapter on vitamins, minerals, phytochemicals, and water also takes this same approach. These two chapters are subdivided for instructors who prefer to teach these nutrients separately.

Popular features of the book have been retained, including full-color text, Facts & Fallacies, Critical Thinking Case Studies, Teaching Pearls for promotion of positive nutrition counseling, question format for the major headings within the text, and basic readability.

FEATURES IN THE NEW EDITION

The former four sections have been condensed into three sections.

Section One: The Art and Science of Nutrition in Health and Disease focuses on the basic nutritional science and application within a total health care system.

Section Two: Chronic and Acute Illness leads with a new chapter on the insulin resistance syndrome, otherwise called the Metabolic Syndrome or Syndrome X. This new chapter outlines the current knowledge base of this syndrome as it relates to common health conditions. The chapters that follow in the second section expand on the health conditions related to this syndrome. The chapter on weight management was moved to this section with the recognition that obesity is a common condition found with the insulin resistance syndrome.

Section Three: Lifespan and Wellness Concerns in Promoting Health and Managing Illness covers nutritional issues over the life cycle with an overview of nutrition programs that promote health nationally and internationally.

The former 22 chapters have been condensed into 15 chapters to better allow integration within a standard one-semester course. This reorganization helps reduce repetition of information that is impractical in a one-semester course.

NUTRITIONAL ANALYSIS SOFTWARE

The latest version of NUTRITRAC CD-ROM (Version III) will be packaged **FREE** with each copy of the text. The nutrition software program allows students to perform complete nutritional analyses on the computer.

INSTRUCTOR'S RESOURCES

New to this edition are instructor's resources, available online at:

www.wbsaunders.com/MERLIN/peckenpaugh/

and on CD-ROM. This ancillary is designed to help instructors present the material in this text. This supplement will include the following:

- Sample Test Questions and Answers
- Critical Thinking Discussion Tips
- Answers for Chapter Study Questions and Classroom Activities
- Power Point Presentations
- 40 Electronic Images (transparencies will also be available)

The guiding principle throughout the writing of this text has been that nutrition is and increasingly will be one of the core disciplines for health care as we continue in the 21st century. Not everyone takes medications, not everyone undergoes surgery or other extraordinary procedures, but everyone needs good nutrition. It is the single most important factor in the care of the well and the ill client. Medical nutrition therapy saves health care dollars while improving the quality of lives. As previously stated, the aim has been to make this body of information more accessible and useful to the people who need it most, the health care providers. I would be very interested in your views concerning how well the objectives of this textbook have been met and how future editions might be improved. Please write in care of W.B. Saunders Company with your suggestions.

Nancy J. Peckenpaugh, MSEd, RD, CDN, CDE

Acknowledgments

The long history of this textbook began with Alberta Shackelton, who authored the first four editions. Charlotte Poleman served as a co-author for the fourth through the eighth editions. These two remarkable women continue to serve as an inspiration in the writing of this current edition. Special recognition goes to Charlotte who first brought me on as her co-author for the sixth edition. The diligence and insight of the editorial staff of the W.B. Saunders Company and its parent company, Elsevier Science, have further allowed growth of this textbook as a solid core in the training of future health care professionals. In particular, the expertise and support of Yvonne Alexopoulos, Editor, Danielle Frazier, Associate Developmental Editor, and Jamie Lyn Thornton, Project Manager, in the revision process was greatly appreciated. The suggestions and feedback of the many reviewers of the early drafts of the revision work served to make this a stronger textbook. A final tribute goes to family and friends who provided support in innumerable ways.

Nancy J. Peckenpaugh, MSEd, RD, CDN, CDE

Reviewers

Mary Babcock, MS, RD
Medical Nutrition Therapist
Wilkes-Barre Veterans Administration
  Medical Center
Wilkes-Barre, Pennsylvania
Adjunct Professor
Wilkes University
Wilkes-Barre, Pennsylvania

Bonita E. Broyles, RN, BSN, EdD
Instructor
Department of Associate Degree
  Nursing
Piedmont Community College
Roxboro, North Carolina

Margaret M. Gingrich, BSN, MSN
Associate Professor
Department of Nursing
Harrisburg Area Community College
Harrisburg, Pennsylvania

Betty Kenyon, RD, LMNT
Consultant Dietitian
Panhandle Community Services
Gering, Nebraska

Anne O'Donnell, MS, MPH, RD
Instructor
Diet Tech Program Coordinator
Department of Consumer and Family
  Studies
Santa Rosa Junior College
Santa Rosa, California

Sue G. Thacker
Professor
Department of Nursing
Wytheville Community College
Wytheville, Virginia

Contents

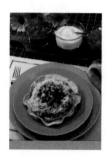

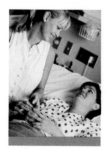

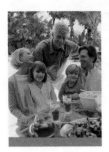

NUTRITION ESSENTIALS

and Diet Therapy

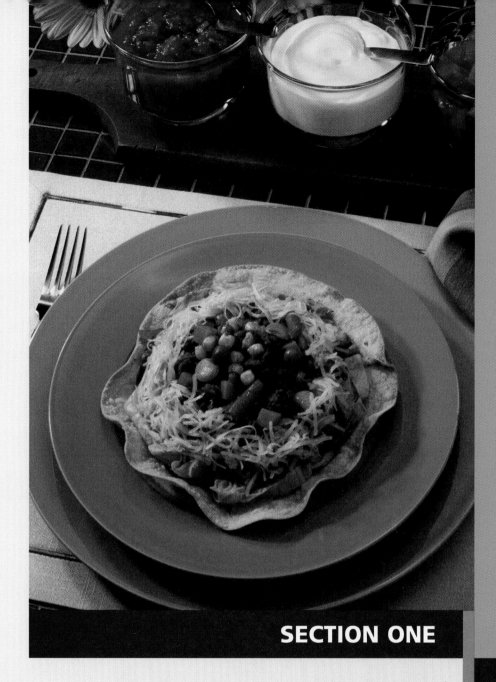

The Art and Science of Nutrition in Health and Disease

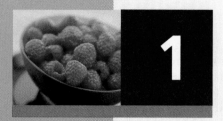

1

Guides for Good Food Choices in a Family Meal Environment

OBJECTIVES

After completing this chapter, you should be able to:

- Define terms used in the study of nutrition.
- Identify biopsychosocial influences on nutritional intake and health.
- Evaluate a daily diet for moderation, variety, and balance.
- Explain the significance of nutrition labeling.
- Recognize and differentiate between the various food guides available.
- Describe the role of vegetarianism on health.
- Describe the affect of snacking on health.
- Describe how to include fast foods in a healthy diet.
- Describe the affect of alcohol on health.
- Identify your personal strengths and weaknesses in nutrition knowledge
  and application.

TERMS TO IDENTIFY

Biopsychosocial	Grazing	Medical nutrition therapy
Chronic disease	Kilocalorie (kcalorie or kcal)	Nutrient density
Cleft palate	Learned food aversions	Vegan
Daily values (DVs)	Medical genealogy	Vegetarian

INTRODUCTION

We are a nation of immigrants and, as such, our genetically based health problems can be traced back to the roots of our many heritages, whether our families originate from Northern Europe, Southern Europe, Africa, or other parts of the world. Even Native Americans are believed to have originally migrated from Asia. Although there may not be a direct familial link, persons with common ancestry share a common gene pool and, hence, may resemble one another (biochemically and physically) more than they resemble people from other groups. Diabetes, high blood pressure, obesity, and atherosclerosis appear in families for genetic reasons. This is referred to as **medical genealogy**.

We all have different family **biopsychosocial** factors (differences in genetics and in psychologic and social factors). The application of the science of nutrition becomes an art form when the various biopsychosocial factors are taken into consideration. Effective health care professionals respect the differences in individuals and plan health care messages accordingly.

Around the world it has been shown that a change to a more Westernized diet and lifestyle with increased kilocalories (kcals), fat, sugar, and reduced fiber and activity level results in obesity and increased rates of diabetes. Obesity often has a genetic component, but the environment allows this tendency to be realized. The same can be said for diabetes. This tendency has been found among persons whose ancestors came from areas near the equator, including persons of African, Spanish, Asian, Pacific Island, and Native American heritage. Alaskan natives and aboriginal Australians are two groups who, in this century, have gone from issues of starvation to rampant growth of obesity and diabetes.

As we learn more about medical genealogy, our ability to provide precise and accurate information about nutrition will be increased for various population groups whose nutritional needs differ from the population at large. For example, the simple public health message that encourages a low-fat and high-carbohydrate diet can be detrimental for people with the insulin resistance syndrome (see Chapter 6).

A return to or maintenance of plant-based diets is being promoted around the world. Traditional ethnic cooking is often based around legumes that have been a mainstay of cooking for centuries. Other traditional food habits—such as eating dandelion greens, having baked beans every Saturday, or taking a spoonful of cod liver oil—are seldom found today in the United States. The change in our food supply and the nutrients we consume continues to affect world health. Hawaii, for example, with one of the highest rates of obesity worldwide since the diet changed to one high in fat and sugar, has been advocating a return to traditional Hawaiian foods.

The definition of healthy eating has changed over the years. In the 1940s, there were seven recommended food groups and butter was one of them. In the 1950s, the time the baby-boom generation was being born, the Basic Four Food Groups classification (meat, grains, dairy, and vegetables and fruits) was developed by the U.S. Department of Agriculture (USDA) to replace the older concept of seven food groups. In 1990, the USDA replaced the Basic Four with the Food Guide Pyramid (see inside front cover). The Food Guide Pyramid met with an uproar from the meat and dairy industries because less consumption of meat and milk was being advocated by their position in the smaller portion of the pyramid. The dried bean and lentil industry was not pleased either because legumes were placed in the upper portion of the pyramid rather than at the base with other plant foods. Nutritionists also agree that legumes are a healthy substitute for meat and should be recommended for more use, not less. Nevertheless, the Food Guide Pyramid generally represents a healthy eating plan for the majority of persons. Individual changes to this plan may be warranted with guidance from a registered dietitian.

WHAT ARE THE BASIC TERMS TO UNDERSTAND IN THE STUDY OF NUTRITION?

1. *Nutrition* is the sum of the processes by which the body uses food for energy, maintenance, and growth. *Good nutritional status* implies appropriate intake of the macronutrients—carbohydrates, proteins, and fats, and the various vitamins and minerals—often referred to as micronutrients as they are needed in small quantities. If there is good digestion, absorption, and cellular metabolism of these nutrients in the diet, a person can generally achieve good nutritional status.
2. *Malnutrition* or *poor nutritional status* is a state in which a prolonged lack of one or more nutrients retards physical development or causes the appearance of specific clinical conditions (anemia, goiter, rickets, etc.). Excess nutrient intake creates another form of malnutrition when it leads to conditions such as obesity, heart disease, hypertension, and hypercholesterolemia.
3. *Optimal nutrition* means that a person is receiving and using the essential nutrients to maintain health and well-being at the highest possible level.
4. A *nutrient* is a chemical substance that is present in food and needed by the body. Proteins, carbohydrates, fats, vitamins, minerals, and water are included in the more than 50 known nutrients needed by the body.
5. A **kilocalorie** (or kcal) is a unit of measure used to express the fuel value of carbohydrates, fats, and proteins. The large calorie (or kcal) used in nutrition represents the amount of heat necessary to raise the temperature of 1 kg of water 1° C. One pound of body fat equates to 3500 kcal. Carbohydrates, proteins, fats, and alcohol are the only sources of kcals.
6. *Health* is currently recognized as being more than the absence of disease. High-level health and wellness is present when an individual is actively engaged in moving toward the fulfillment of his or her potential.
7. *Public health* is the field of medicine that is concerned with safeguarding and improving the health of the community as a whole. Public health nurses may work out of public health departments or private health organizations. Other public health programs have been developed for various population groups such as women who are pregnant or the elderly (see Chapter 15).
8. *Holistic health* is a system of preventive medicine that takes into account the whole individual. It promotes personal responsibility for well-being and acknowledges the total influences—biologic, psychologic, and social—that affect health, including nutrition, exercise, and emotional well-being.

9. **Medical nutrition therapy** (referred to in the past as diet therapy) is the treatment of disease through nutritional therapy by registered dietitians. Registered dietitians are uniquely qualified to provide medical nutrition therapy because of their extensive training in food composition and preparation, nutrition and biochemistry, anatomy and physiology, as well as life-cycle concerns and disease states.

WHAT ARE BIOPSYCHOSOCIAL CONCERNS IN HEALTH CARE?

Biopsychosocial concerns address the interplay between external environmental and internal forces. For example, the diagnosis of diabetes is primarily a biochemical or internal problem, but for the person hearing this diagnosis it involves psychologic issues of acceptance versus denial and anger and social concerns of healthy living in an environment that may be stressful and that may provide little opportunity for low–saturated-fat, low-sugar food choices (external problems or social forces). The biochemical problem of either very high or very low blood sugars can also affect the ability to think (cognitive functioning) and the emotions. The incidence of depression, for example, increases with poor blood sugar control. The nurse or other health care professional who is aware of the interplay between external and internal forces will be a much more effective team member in the health care system.

WHAT IS MEANT BY MODERATION, VARIETY, AND BALANCE?

Moderation means avoidance of too much or too little of any food or nutrient. This implies that any food can be worked into a healthy way of eating. There are no good foods or bad foods. Foods that are higher in fat and sugar should be eaten in smaller amounts or less frequently than foods that are nutrient dense. Variety refers to eating a number of different foods within each of the food groups of the Food Guide Pyramid—not just the same two or three types of vegetables, for example. Balance refers to the amount of macronutrients and micronutrients in the diet in relation to individual needs. Selecting a variety of low-processed foods from each of the three lower levels of the Food Guide Pyramid will allow for a balanced diet (see inside front cover). The lowest level promotes intake of grain; the second level promotes vegetables and fruits. Thus the base of the Food Guide Pyramid promotes a plant-based diet as the foundation of a healthy diet. Intake of fat and sugar is portrayed in the upper, small tip of the Food Guide Pyramid, indicating that fats and sugars should constitute a small portion of the diet. In other words, small amounts of fat and sugar are generally acceptable in the diet.

HOW DO FOOD AND DIETARY PATTERNS DEVELOP?

Sound nutrition begins in infancy through the influence of food culture. Persons of various cultural communities consume differing types and amounts of foods. (See Table 1-1 for common and regional food habits.) The family affects the growing child's meal environment and exposure to food.

In the ideal scenario, the infant is exposed to a variety of foods and is fed in a manner that promotes positive meal association. The infant then is more likely to become a child who learns to like a variety of foods that are of high quality and dense in nutrients. When a child has been allowed to eat on the basis of his or her own hunger and satiety cues in a positive meal environment, eating takes place according to growth needs; thus an appropriate quantity of food intake is maintained (see Chapter 13 for more detailed information on child development and nutritional needs).

Many factors can change this ideal scenario. Children may have food allergies or food intolerances and these foods become associated with physical discomfort. Learned food aversions fall into this classification. For example, a food that is eaten before the onset of an illness that is unrelated to the food (such as a viral illness) becomes mistakenly associated with the illness. If this food is avoided in the future, the phenomenon is appropriately termed a **learned food aversion**.

Many barriers to adequate nutrient intake are external in nature and they may stem from a variety of causes:

- *Economic* (inadequate money to purchase food)
- *Physical* (lack of food storage facilities or physical impairment such as loose-fitting dentures or no teeth, or **cleft palate**—a birth defect in which there is an opening in the roof of the mouth, lips, or both)
- *Cultural* (lack of exposure to a variety of food because of limited parental offerings or overemphasis on meat or high-fat and high-sugar foods)
- *Ecologic* (droughts, floods)
- *Emotional* (television advertisements depicting nonnutritious foods as appealing)
- *Religious* (adherence to restrictive food codes)
- *Political* (food boycotts, forced starvation for military purposes)

How Can the Health Care Professional Facilitate Positive Meal Environments?

The health care professional can help promote harmonious family mealtimes, which will allow the innate satiety cues to function more effectively and also promote the association of eating with positive feelings, by making the following recommendations to family members:

- Focus on positive conversations during mealtimes; avoid points of potential conflict and friction.
- Use soft music, candles, or both to facilitate a quiet, relaxed atmosphere.
- Eat as a family as much as possible rather than eating on the run.
- Encourage children to eat with the family, but do not force them to eat; encourage the *one-taste rule* and emphasize that taste is learned.
- Serve food that looks appealing by using a combination of colors, textures, and sizes (e.g., orange carrot "coins," white chicken, crisp lettuce wedges, warm biscuits, and cold milk).

TABLE 1-1

ETHNIC AND REGIONAL FOOD PATTERNS ACCORDING TO THE BASIC FOOD GROUPS OF THE FOOD GUIDE PYRAMID

ETHNIC GROUP	BREAD AND CEREAL	EGGS, MEAT, FISH, POULTRY	DAIRY PRODUCTS	FRUITS AND VEGETABLES	SEASONINGS AND FATS
Italian	*Northern Italy*: Crusty white bread Cornmeal and rice *Southern Italy*: Pasta	Beef, chicken, eggs, fish, anchovies	Milk in coffee, cheese	Broccoli, zucchini, other squash, eggplant, artichokes, string beans, legumes,* tomatoes, peppers, asparagus, fresh fruit	Olives and olive oil, balsamic vinegar, salt, pepper, garlic, capers, basil
Puerto Rican	Rice, beans, noodles, spaghetti, oatmeal, cornmeal	Dry salted cod fish, meat, salt pork, sausage, chicken, beef	Hot milk in coffee	Starchy root vegetables, green bananas, plantains, legumes,* tomatoes, green pepper, onion, pineapple, papaya, citrus fruits	Lard, herbs, oil, vinegar
Near Eastern	Bulgur (wheat)	Lamb, mutton, chicken, fish, eggs	Fermented milk, sour cream, yogurt, cheese	Nuts, grape leaves	Sheep's butter, olive oil
Greek	Plain wheat bread, phyllo dough	Lamb, pork, poultry, eggs, organ meats	Yogurt, cheese, butter	Onions, tomatoes, legumes,* fresh fruit	Olive oil, parsley, lemon, vinegar

*Legumes are also counted as a meat substitute.

- Watch portion sizes; smaller portions are useful for small appetites and for weight control.
- Provide rest and calming activities just before and after meals.

fact FALLACY

Fallacy: Children who do not "clean their plates" should not have dessert.

Fact: This commonly practiced principle may work in the short term to coerce children to eat their meals, but the long-term implications outweigh any benefits. This approach implicitly conveys to children that desserts have more value than other foods because dessert is being used as a reward. Parents should be reminded that desserts can be nutritious, such as fresh fruit, a colorful fruit salad, or a piece of pumpkin pie or carrot cake. The "clean the plate" philosophy can also contribute to overeating and excess weight gain. Children (and many adults) need to learn to stop eating when they are comfortably full.

TABLE 1-1

ETHNIC AND REGIONAL FOOD PATTERNS ACCORDING TO THE BASIC FOOD GROUPS OF THE FOOD GUIDE PYRAMID—cont'd

ETHNIC GROUP	BREAD AND CEREAL	EGGS, MEAT, FISH, POULTRY	DAIRY PRODUCTS	FRUITS AND VEGETABLES	SEASONINGS AND FATS
Mexican	Lime-treated corn tortillas	Little meat (ground beef or pork), poultry, fish	Cheese, evaporated milk as beverage for infants	Pinto beans,* tomatoes, potatoes, onions, lettuce, black beans	Chili pepper, salt, garlic
Chinese	Rice, wheat, millet, corn, noodles	Little meat and no beef; fish (including raw fish); eggs of hen, duck, and pigeon; tofu and soybeans	Water buffalo milk occasionally, soybean milk, cheese	Soybeans,* soybean sprouts, bamboo sprouts, soy curd cooked in lime water, radish leaves, legumes,* vegetables, fruits	Sesame seeds, ginger, almonds, soy sauce, peanut oil
African American or Southern United States	Hot breads, pastries, cakes, cereals, white rice	Chicken, salt pork, ham, bacon, sausage	Milk and milk products (often lactose-free for African heritage)	Kale, mustard, turnip, collard greens; hominy; grits; sweet potatoes; watermelon; black-eyed peas	Molasses
Jewish	Noodles, crusty white seed rolls, rye bread, pumpernickel bread	Kosher meat (from forequarters and organs from beef, lamb, veal); fish (except shellfish)	Milk and milk products Milk not eaten at same meal as meat	Vegetables—usually cooked with meat; fruits	

*Legumes are also counted as a meat substitute.

What Are Some Cultural and Societal Influences on Nutritional Intake?

Changing Food Habits in the United States

Because more women are working outside of the home, increasing numbers of men are now shopping for and preparing food (Figure 1-1). Changing demographics also have an effect on the nutritional status of the United States as a whole, which in turn affects food choices. The increasing number of elderly and minority persons affects the rate of chronic health concerns. Households composed of single persons are growing, with an increased demand for more ready-to-use foods, which are often high in fat and salt.

Americans now eat far more sugar than our ancestors did. In the mid-1990s, Americans aged 2 years and older consumed the equivalent of 20 tsp to over ¾ c of sugar per day. Adolescents had the highest intakes (averaging 20% of total energy from added sweeteners). The largest source of added sweeteners was regular soft drinks (Guthrie and Morton, 2000). Unfortunately, our society tends to overvalue many foods with empty kcals. Schools often reward academic

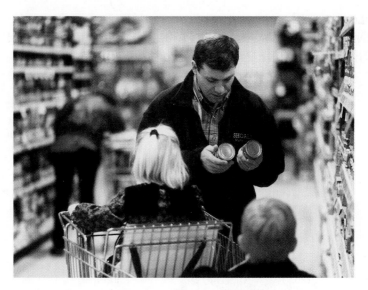

FIGURE 1-1 Men are becoming more involved in food shopping and meal preparation, which has increased their concern with the nutritional value of foods.

achievement with candy, divorced parents may give their children extra treats in an attempt to lessen their guilt, and television advertisements tell us, "Go ahead, you deserve it!" Because of this reward system and because people like the taste of sweets, many Americans overconsume low-nutrient foods that are high in fat and sugar.

Effect of Regional, Ethnic, Cultural, and Religious Dietary Habits in Studying Nutrition and Meal Planning

In many countries and cultures it is still common to find daily use of legumes (dried beans and peas), greens, and fish. Lentils are one of the oldest foods known, having been eaten for at least 8000 years. From Northern Africa, through the Mediterranean, to Syria, people commonly sit down to half a plate of spinach, not a small dollop as Americans typically eat, if they eat it at all. In England, people to this day love baked beans on toast. Sardines, salmon, herring, mackerel, anchovies, cod, and cod liver oil were basic foods to many of our ancestors, although they no longer are commonly consumed in the United States. Religious holiday dietary practices have long been observed, such as 24-hour fasting for the Jewish holiday Yom Kippur, abstaining from meat on Fridays among Catholics (which has developed into the Friday Fish Fry), or giving up chocolate for Lent.

The population of the United States includes many ethnic groups. They come from all parts of the world and have varied eating habits. Immigrants from Yugoslavia at the turn of the century did not know how to eat a banana. Currently, many young Americans have never had any of a variety of vegetables, such as Swiss chard, lentils, or even basic vegetables such as brussel sprouts and broccoli. Persons from the South are more likely than others to eat okra, collard greens, kale, pinto beans, and black-eyed peas. Those who were born before World War II (before the process of hydrogenation was introduced) remember stirring their peanut butter. Some ethnic foods, such as Italian and Mexican, have become popular with broad groups of Americans. Unfortunately, these foods often become Americanized, with excess amounts of cheese and meat added. Chinese meals in China are low in fat, but Chinese restaurants in the United States increasingly serve food high in fat, with large portions not typical in China. One Chinese buffet restaurant in the United States was recently observed to serve chocolate cake and green gelatin.

Foods familiar in other countries may be rare and expensive in the United States and, consequently, may be omitted from the diet after immigration. If an ethnic group gives up some of its own food habits and adopts those of the new country, the poorest of the new country's nutritional habits are frequently chosen, such as a preference for excessive sweets and fats. For example, Korean Americans report an increase in the consumption of beef, dairy products, coffee, soda, and bread, as well as a decrease in the intake of fish and rice and other grains, compared with diets in Korea. As a group, Korean Americans generally meet the recommended dietary guidelines for most nutrients, except for dietary fiber and calcium (Kim et al., 2000). It is important to acknowledge this desire to try new foods, but consumers should ideally focus on maintaining the low–saturated-fat, low-sugar, low-salt, and high-fiber foundation of the diet according to the Dietary Guidelines for all Americans. Table 1-1 shows how the five food groups of the Food Guide Pyramid are incorporated into different types of eating patterns. A typical day's diet for any ethnic, regional, or religious group may be evaluated nutritionally by checking it against an acceptable meal plan such as the Food Guide Pyramid.

What Are Some Positive Ethnic Eating Habits That Follow the Dietary Guidelines for Americans?

Chinese. Traditional Chinese meals include tofu or other soybean products at least daily, if not with all three meals. Rice, vegetables, and fish are principal parts of the diet. Dessert often consists of legumes that have minimal amounts of sugar added. Fat and sugar intake is expected to rise as American food products increasingly become available in the Chinese market.

French. The French are known for their pastries and cheese. However, their portions tend to be much more limited than those of Americans and they eat plenty of vegetables. Wine provides phytochemicals that are believed to reduce the risk of heart disease. It is difficult to find soda pop or a junk food aisle in grocery stores in France.

Japanese. The Japanese typically eat fish and vegetables for breakfast. The traditional diet centers around rice and vegetables, but also includes noodles, seaweed, and soybean products. A food that is considered a bar snack in Japan is lightly steamed soybeans in the pods, which are then pulled through the teeth, allowing the beans but not the pods to be consumed. Raw fish is a favorite in Japan.

Mediterranean Region. The traditional Mediterranean diet is based around beans and greens. Vegetables and grains are key elements of the Mediterranean diet. Beans and nuts are regularly consumed and both are good sources of protein. The consumption of lean red meat historically was limited to a few times per month and fish about once a week. Sweets are eaten in small amounts on special occasions only. Olives and olive oil are used liberally, but they are low in saturated fat and cholesterol free, yet high in monounsaturated fats. The amount of cheese used historically has been moderate.

HOW DOES NUTRITION LABELING AID THE CONSUMER?

Mandatory nutrition labeling went into effect in 1994 with the goal of helping consumers adhere to the Dietary Guidelines for Americans (see the following section). The change is aimed at reducing the prevalence and complications of chronic illnesses, such as heart disease, hypertension, and diabetes (see Chapters 8 and 9). Nutrition labeling is a valuable tool for learning to apply nutrition information in a practical way. A health-conscious shopper uses the percentages shown on the label to determine how well each serving of the food fulfills recommended nutritional requirements. For example, if one serving of a food has 25% of a particular nutrient listed, it means that each serving is good for one fourth of a person's recommended daily intake for that nutrient.

Ingredients are still listed in order of content in a product. If sugar is listed as the first ingredient, the amount of sugar in the product is greater than the amount of any of the other ingredients. It is also easy now to quantify exactly how much is included in a serving of food. For example, 1 tsp of sugar equates to 4 g on the food label; therefore a can of soda pop containing 40 g of sugar is equivalent to 10 tsp of sugar. Consumers need to learn how to interpret food labels (Figure 1-2).

To help the consumer calculate the kcals in a given food, the food label on larger food packages also lists the conversion factor to change grams into kcals—that is, fat 9, carbohydrate 4, protein 4 (refer also to Chapter 2). Thus 1 tsp of sugar contains 16 kcals (4 g carbohydrate multiplied by 4).

If consumers use the food labels when making food purchases, they will be promoting their health through the inclusion of adequate nutrient intake (proteins, carbohydrates, vitamins, and minerals) while reducing their risk of chronic illness through a reduction of fat, salt, and sugar and an increase in fiber. Food labels used in conjunction with the Food Guide Pyramid can be a highly effective and ultimately simple means to promote health.

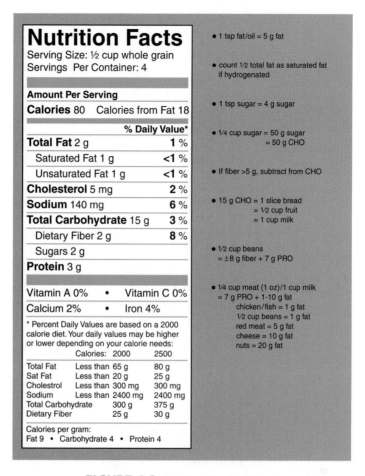

FIGURE 1-2 Reading the food label.

The health claims that can be made on food labels under the labeling law are as follows:

1. Fiber: Foods high in fiber may reduce the risk of cancer and heart disease.
2. Fat: A low-fat diet may reduce the risk of cancer and heart disease.
3. Sodium: A low-sodium diet may help prevent high blood pressure.
4. Calcium: Foods high in calcium may help prevent osteoporosis.
5. Folate leads to decreased neural tube defects.
6. Sugar alcohols reduce dental caries.
7. Soy protein reduces cardiovascular disease.

Foods exempt from nutrition labeling include those sold in restaurants, cafeterias, and airplanes, unless a health claim is made. Coffee, tea, spices, and foods produced by small businesses or packaged in small containers are not required to carry a nutrition label.

What Are Daily Values?

Daily values (DVs) is a term developed for the new food labels. These DVs can be found on the new food labels for vitamins A and C and the minerals calcium and iron (see Figure 1-2).

Daily values also include the recommended amounts of fat, saturated fat, total carbohydrate, and dietary fiber based on preset kcal levels of 2000 and 2500 on food labels, as follows:

- Fat is based on 30% of kcals.
- Saturated fat is based on 10% of kcals.
- Carbohydrate is based on 60% of kcals.
- Fiber is based on 11.5 g of fiber per 1000 kcal.

The reference quantity for sodium intake on the new food labels is 2400 mg/day. This amount will meet required sodium needs in all healthy Americans without providing excess, although up to 3000 mg of sodium per day for most individuals is also reasonable. Medical conditions may necessitate a smaller or larger intake of sodium. Cholesterol is another DV not based on kcal intake (300 mg).

WHAT ARE THE DIETARY GUIDELINES FOR AMERICANS?

In 1980, the Public Health Service of the Department of Health and Human Services, together with the USDA, published the first edition of *Dietary Guidelines for Americans*. This report, revised every 5 years, includes recommendations that address the relationship between diet and **chronic diseases**. The most recent version of the *Dietary Guidelines for Americans* includes 10 specific goals within a broader ABC format: *A*im for fitness, *B*uild a healthy base, and *C*hoose sensibly (Figure 1-3). Table 1-2 shows the frequency of foods consumed that allow the Dietary Guidelines to be followed.

HOW DOES THE FOOD GUIDE PYRAMID RELATE TO THE RECOMMENDED DIETARY ALLOWANCES AND THE DIETARY GUIDELINES?

The USDA's Food Guide Pyramid, which was released in the 1990s, portrays the Dietary Guidelines for Americans by emphasizing optimal amounts of foods (see inside front cover). Nutritional adequacy can be met by including the minimum number of recommended food servings in the Food Guide Pyramid if low-processed foods are chosen wisely. Choosing a wide assortment of foods from the two lower levels of the pyramid (foods that are high in carbohydrate and fiber and low in fat), moderate amounts of foods from the third level (the protein foods, which generally contribute fat as well), and minimal amounts from the upper tip of the pyramid (added fats and sugars) is advised. Selecting foods in this manner

Nutrition and Your Health:
DIETARY GUIDELINES FOR AMERICANS

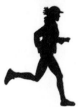

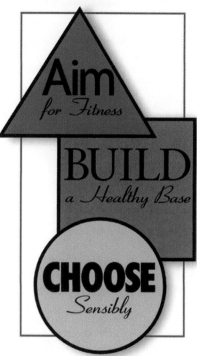

Aim *for Fitness*

BUILD *a Healthy Base*

CHOOSE *Sensibly*

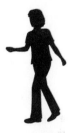

AIM FOR FITNESS...

▲ Aim for a healthy weight.

▲ Be physically active each day.

BUILD A HEALTHY BASE...

■ Let the Pyramid guide your food choices.

■ Choose a variety of grains daily, especially whole grains.

■ Choose a variety of fruits and vegetables daily.

■ Keep food safe to eat.

CHOOSE SENSIBLY...

● Choose a diet that is low in saturated fat and cholesterol and moderate in total fat.

● Choose beverages and foods to moderate your intake of sugars.

● Choose and prepare foods with less salt.

● If you drink alcoholic beverages, do so in moderation.

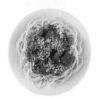

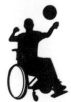

...for good health

FIGURE 1-3 Dietary Guidelines for Americans for good health.

TABLE 1-2
FREQUENCY OF USE OF FOODS FOR IMPLEMENTING DIETARY GUIDELINES

FOOD GROUPS	CHOOSE MORE OFTEN	CHOOSE LESS OFTEN	MAJOR CONTRIBUTIONS
Fats	Corn, cottonseed, olive, sesame, soybean, safflower, sunflower, peanut, canola oils Mayonnaise or salad dressing (made from above oils) Avocado Olives	Butter, lard Margarine made from hydrogenated or saturated fats Coconut or palm oil Hydrogenated vegetable shortening Bacon Meat fat/drippings, gravy, sauces	Vitamin A, calories, essential fatty acids
Soups	Lightly salted soups with fat skimmed Cream-style soups (with low-fat milk)	Commercially prepared soups and mixes	Fluid, calories (may contain a variety of vitamins, minerals, and protein, depending upon type)
Sweets and desserts	Desserts that have been sweetened lightly and/or contain only moderate fat, such as puddings made from skim milk, angel food cake, fruit-based desserts	Desserts high in sugar and/or fats, candy, pastries, cakes, pies, whole-milk puddings, cookies	Calories (fats, carbohydrates)
Beverages	Water Unsweetened soft drinks Decaffeinated drinks	Sweetened beverages Caffeine-containing beverages Alcoholic beverages	Fluid, calories (unless sugar-free)
Milk and milk products	Low-fat or skim milk Low-fat cheeses Low-fat yogurt	Whole milk Whole-milk cheeses Whole-milk yogurt Ice cream	Calories, calcium, protein, phosphorus, vitamins A and D, riboflavin
Vegetables, including starchy vegetables	Fresh, frozen, or canned; potatoes—baked or boiled Include one dark green or deep orange vegetable daily	Deep-fat fried vegetables, chips Pickled vegetables Highly salted vegetables or juices	Calories, vitamins A and C, dietary fiber, potassium, zinc, cobalt, folic acid
Fruits	Unsweetened fruits or juices Include one citrus fruit/juice or one tomato/juice daily	Sweetened fruits or juices Coconut Avocado	Calories, dietary fiber, vitamins A and C
Breads, starches, and cereals	Whole-grain breads or cereals Muffins, bagels, tortillas Enriched pasta, rice, grits, or noodles	Snack chips or crackers Sweetened cereals Pancakes, doughnuts, biscuits	Calories, B-complex vitamins, magnesium, copper, iron, dietary fiber
Meats or substitutes	Lean meats, fish, shellfish, poultry without skin Low-fat cheeses (such as cottage cheese and part-skim mozarella) Peanut butter Soybeans, tofu Dry beans and peas	Fried or fatty meats/fish Fried poultry or poultry with skin High-fat cheeses (such as cheddar and processed cheeses) Eggs Nuts	Calories, protein, iron, zinc, copper, B-complex vitamins
Miscellaneous	Herbs, spices, flavorings	Salt and salt/spice combinations	Sodium

can allow adherence to the *Dietary Guidelines for Americans* while meeting nutrient needs. Table 1-3 shows the evaluation of an adequate diet for an adult.

Other countries have similar guides that vary with cultural food habits and the availability of foods. Canada's new food guide is represented as a rainbow and is also shown on the page facing the inside front cover. The *Guide to Good Eating* by the National Dairy Council (Figure 1-4) uses the five food groups and can be used in conjunction with the Food Guide Pyramid. This guide is useful for low-literacy persons as it uses pictorial representation of food portions.

Similar guides have been developed around the world, including the Mediterranean and Asian pyramids, which emphasize legumes and oils as basic parts of a healthy diet, with the Greek Columns food guide specifically recommending legumes 6 days a week.

How Do the Food Pyramid Groups Supply Needed Nutrients?

As shown in Figures 2-1 and 4-3, all of the needed nutrients can be found in the lower three levels of the Food Guide Pyramid. Complete analytic data regarding food supply and human needs are available for key nutrients (see Appendix 5 for food composition tables).

Foods within the five food groups can also be identified by their macronutrient and vitamin and mineral content. For example, animal products in the milk and meat groups (third level of the pyramid) have more protein and fat than foods found in the fruit, vegetable, bread, and grain groups. Foods in the second level (vegetables and fruits) provide the main source of vitamins A, C, and folic acid, whereas the foods in the base of the pyramid are the main source of carbohydrate and the B vitamins. The following chapters in this section will go into more detail on the body's need for these nutrients.

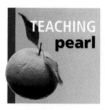

TEACHING pearl   A useful analogy to use with children is to explain that some foods (those high in fat and sugar—shown in the tip of the Food Guide Pyramid to indicate that they should be consumed in a small amount) help us grow outward, whereas plant foods (in the lower part of the Food Guide Pyramid) help us grow upward. Using your hands to describe these changes graphically is very effective in aiding children's understanding.

WHAT IS THE FOOD EXCHANGE SYSTEM AND HOW DOES IT COMPARE WITH THE FOOD GUIDE PYRAMID?

The Exchange System for Meal Planning, developed by the American Dietetic Association and the American Diabetes Association, is a food guide aimed at managing diabetes and weight (see Chapters 7 and 9 for more information and Appendix 9 for the complete Dietary Exchange System). The Dietary Exchange System groups foods according to the amounts of the macronutrients (carbohydrates, proteins, and fats) that they contain. The Food Guide Pyramid puts less emphasis on amounts of carbohydrates and fats in foods.

TABLE 1-3
EVALUATION OF THE FOUNDATION OF AN ADEQUATE DIET FOR AN ADULT

| | AVERAGE SERVING | | | | | |
	HOUSEHOLD MEASURE	WEIGHT (g)	KCALS	PROTEIN (g)	FAT (g)	CARBOHYDRATE (g)
DAIRY						
Milk (whole or equivalent)	1 pt	488	300	16	16	22
MEAT GROUP						
Eggs	1	50	80	6	6	1
Meat, poultry, fish[1]	3 oz (cooked)	85	322	19	26	0
VEGETABLE AND FRUIT GROUP						
Vegetables: Deep green or orange[2]	1 salad or cooked	50 raw or cooked	23	0.9	trace	5
Other cooked[3]	½ c	85	52	2.5	trace	13
Potato, peeled and boiled	1 medium	122	90	3	trace	20
Fruits: Citrus[4]	1 serving	125	50	0.3	trace	13.5
Other (fresh and canned)[5]	1 serving	135	99	0.4	trace	25
BREAD AND CEREAL GROUP						
Cereal (whole-grain and enriched)[6]	½ c cooked	25 (dry)	80	2.2	1	16
Bread (whole grain and enriched)	3 slices 1 whole wheat 2 white	78	170	7	3	40
TOTALS[7]			1266	57.3	52	180.5
RECOMMENDED DAILY DIETARY ALLOWANCES*						
Man (age 25-50 years: wt. 174 lb; ht. 70 in.)			2900	63		
Woman (age 25-50 years: wt. 138 lb: ht. 64 in.)			2200	50		

Data from Nutritive Value of Foods, Home and Garden Bulletin No. 72, U.S. Department of Agriculture.
*From National Academy of Sciences, National Research Council: Recommended Dietary Allowances, ed 10, Washington, DC, National Academy of Sciences, National Academy Press, 1989.
[1]Evaluation based on figures for cooked (lean and fat) beef, lamb, and veal.
[2]Evaluation based on lettuce, cooked carrots, green beans, winter squash, and broccoli.
[3]Evaluation based on average for cooked peas and beets.
[4]Evaluation based on Florida oranges and white and pink grapefruit—whole and juice.

	MINERALS				VITAMINS	
CALCIUM (mg)	IRON (mg)	A (RE)	ASCORBIC ACID (mg)	THIAMIN (mg)	RIBOFLAVIN (mg)	NIACIN (mg)
582	0.2	152	4	0.18	0.8	0.4
28	1	78	0	0.04	0.15	trace
9	2	trace	—	0.09	0.19	4.6
20	0.5	2644	9	0.03	0.06	0.3
19	1.1	54	4.8	0.04	0.26	0.4
8	0.7	trace	22	0.12	0.05	1.6
23	0.4	28	50	0.07	0.03	0.31
8	0.6	23	6	0.03	0.04	0.36
6	0.65	379	4.5	0.20	0.18	1.5
90	2	trace	trace	0.29	0.15	2.4
793	9.61	3358[8]	100.3	1.09[9]	1.9	11.9[10,11]
800	10	1000	60	1.5	1.7	19
800	15	800	60	1.1	1.3	15

[5]Evaluation based on canned peaches, applesauce, raw pears, apples, and bananas.
[6]Evaluation based on oatmeal and corn flakes.
[7]With the addition of more of the same foods, or other foods, to meet calorie requirement, the totals will be increased.
[8]With the use of liver, this figure will be markedly increased.
[9]With the use of pork, legumes, and liver, this figure will be markedly increased.
[10]The average diet in the United States, which contains a generous amount of protein, provides enough tryptophan to increase the niacin value by about one third.
[11]These figures are expressed as niacin equivalents, which include dietary sources of the preformed vitamin and the precursor, tryptophan.

The Exchange System for Meal Planning counts cheese in the meat group based on the similar protein content, but in recognition of the higher fat content. Cheese is not included in the milk group in the Dietary Exchange System because, unlike milk, it does not contain carbohydrates. The Food Guide Pyramid counts equivalent amounts of milk and cheese based on calcium content.

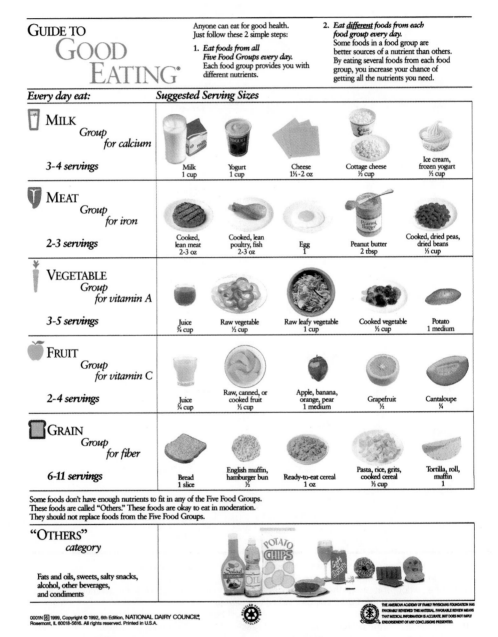

FIGURE 1-4 Guide to good eating from the National Dairy Council.

The Exchange System for Meal Planning counts legumes in the starch and bread group based on the comparable carbohydrate content ($\frac{1}{2}$ c of legumes contains about 15 g of available carbohydrates). Because of the high protein content of legumes (about 5 g per $\frac{1}{2}$ c serving), the Food Guide Pyramid includes legumes in the meat group.

Carbohydrate content of the fruit group is not considered in the Food Guide Pyramid. The pyramid counts one whole banana as a serving, whereas the Dietary Exchange System counts only one half of a banana as a serving. The Dietary Exchange System calculates 15 g of carbohydrates for one serving of fruit.

The Dietary Exchange System counts a fat serving as 5 g of fat, which is equivalent to 1 tsp of added fat. Foods that are naturally high in fat such as avocados, nuts, and bacon are found in the fat group of the Dietary Exchange System. The Food Guide Pyramid does not specifically state portion sizes for fats and includes nuts in the meat group and avocados in the fruit group.

WHAT IS THE EFFECT OF VEGETARIANISM ON HEALTH?

People who follow a **vegetarian** diet that is planned around legumes, whole grains, a variety of fruits and vegetables, and low-fat milk products can improve their health through the reduction of cholesterol levels. Good planning is needed to ensure a healthy vegetarian diet. Just because a person avoids meat does not mean he or she is following a healthy diet.

Vegetarians may have lower intakes of protein, saturated fat, cholesterol, niacin, and vitamins B_{12} and D, and higher fiber and magnesium intakes (Barr and Broughton, 2000). It is vital to ensure adequate vitamin B_{12} to prevent permanent neurologic damage. A higher intake of vitamin B_{12} is needed by the vegetarian because of a low intake of methionine, which is found in meat. Both vitamin B_{12} and folate are needed in the diet to prevent build-up of homocysteine, which is associated with heart disease (see Chapters 4 and 8 for more information). Adequate vitamin B_{12} is easy to obtain if milk, milk products, and eggs are included in a vegetarian diet.

Who Follows Vegetarian Diets?

Two religious groups that forgo consumption of meat and other animal products are Seventh-Day Adventists and Muslims. Many persons of the Jewish faith adopt a vegetarian eating plan to help them follow a kosher diet. Others follow vegetarian diets for health, political, cultural, or economic reasons, or a combination of these.

How Do Vegetarian Diets Differ?

There are three main classifications of vegetarian diets:

1. *Lacto-ovo vegetarian.* Plant foods (whole grains, legumes, fruits, and vegetables) are supplemented with dairy products and eggs. This is probably the most common type of vegetarian diet. *Lacto* comes from the word *lactose*

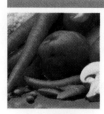

**BOX 1-1
NUTRITIOUS
SAMPLE
MENU FOR A
VEGAN DIET**

BREAKFAST

Oatmeal with soy milk

Whole wheat toast with peanut butter

Orange juice

Half a grapefruit

Herbal tea

LUNCH

Minestrone soup

Apple slices

Pecans and raisins

Whole wheat bread

Glass of soy milk

SUPPER

Tofu stir-fry with snow peas and carrot wedges

Fresh spinach salad with croutons and dressing

Couscous

Cantaloupe wedges

Herbal iced tea

SNACK

Almonds

Whole-wheat crackers

Glass of soy milk

(milk sugar) and *ovo* comes from *ovum* (egg). Lacto-ovo vegetarians may also eat fish and chicken.

2. *Lacto-vegetarian.* Dairy products are included, but eggs are not.

3. *Total vegetarian* (**vegan**). Animal food sources (including eggs and dairy products) are completely excluded. For this reason, the diet may be low or inadequate in iodine, vitamin B_{12}, iron, calcium, zinc, riboflavin, and vitamin D. Good meal planning can allow for a healthy vegan diet that includes legumes, nuts, whole grains, and soy products for complementary proteins over the course of the day. Vegans should also include vitamin B_{12}-fortified foods.

How Should an Individual Plan a Vegetarian Diet?

Because meat provides protein, a variety of B vitamins, and minerals, alternative foods high in these nutrients need to be included in the vegetarian diet for health (Table 1-4). The minimum amount of meat in the Food Guide Pyramid is 4 oz daily or the equivalent amount in meat substitutes. Meat is replaced with an increased intake of legumes (dried beans and peas), nuts, meat analogues such as soybean burgers, eggs, and milk products. One-half c of legumes is equivalent to 1 oz of meat. One egg, $\frac{1}{4}$ c nuts, 2 tbsp of peanut butter, or 1 c of milk contains a similar amount of protein as 1 oz of meat. The minimum number of servings (2 c of milk and 4 oz of meat equivalent) will easily meet, and actually exceed, protein needs. Soy milk may replace cow's milk as a high source of protein and calcium. Vitamin D fortified soy milk is advised for optimal calcium absorption.

Vegans need to emphasize legumes, nuts, and whole grains to meet the dietary need for complete protein (Box 1-1). These foods are also high in B vita-

■ TABLE 1-4
■ FOOD SOURCES FOR IMPORTANT NUTRIENTS IN THE VEGETARIAN DIET

NUTRIENT	SOURCES
Calcium*	Milk and milk products, particularly cheese and yogurt; fortified soy milk; dark green leafy vegetables such as parsley, kale, mustard, dandelion, and collard greens
Iron	Legumes, dark green leafy and other vegetables, whole-grain or enriched cereals or breads, some nuts, and dried fruits (many factors may affect absorption of this nutrient)
Riboflavin (Vitamin B$_2$)	Milk, legumes, whole grains, and certain vegetables
Vitamin B$_{12}$	Milk and eggs, fortified soybean milk, and fortified soy products, Marmite™
Zinc	Nuts, beans, wheat germ, and cheese
Protein	Eggs, milk, nuts and seeds, legumes, especially soybeans and tofu

*See Table 1-5.

■ TABLE 1-5
■ SOURCES OF CALCIUM IN THE VEGETARIAN DIET

FOOD SOURCE	AVERAGE CALCIUM (mg)
4 oz tofu*	110
½ c almonds*	175
½ c peanuts*	50
1 c greens (except spinach)*	200
1 c dried apricots*	100
1 c dates*	130
1 tbsp blackstrap molasses*	135
½ c oysters	110
3 oz salmon	165
3 oz sardines	370

*Appropriate for vegan diet.

mins and minerals. Calcium and vitamin D are particular nutritional challenges for vegans because they avoid milk products. Soy remains the best alternative for calcium for a vegan, but other food alternatives are available (see the list of vegetarian calcium sources in Table 1-5). If adequate calcium and vitamin D intake is not possible, supplementation may be required. Foods fortified with vitamin B$_{12}$ should be included. Brewer's yeast is a natural source of vitamin B$_{12}$, but should not be relied on for adequate intake by vegans. A spread used to put on crackers in England, Marmite™, is a yeast product that contains vitamin B$_{12}$. Marmite™ may be found in larger U.S. grocery stores carrying British foods. Vegans may be best served by taking a vitamin B$_{12}$ supplement.

Because of their restrictive food code, it is of the utmost importance that vegetarians primarily consume nutrient-dense foods. The use of whole grains is critical to provide all of the needed essential amino acids for complementary protein. Empty kcal foods (foods high in kcals, but low in nutrients) should be avoided, unless kcal needs are high and all essential nutrients are being consumed in the diet.

By combining different foods in vegetarian diets, complete proteins can be formed from the available amino acids over a 24-hour period. Emphasis should be on the inclusion of legumes and whole grains at a minimum, and if possible, the inclusion of eggs, dairy, and nuts can help ensure adequate protein.

HOW DOES SNACKING AFFECT NUTRITION?

Many people find it more convenient to eat when they can and snacking has become part of our culture. The term **grazing** is sometimes applied to the frequent all-day eating in which many people engage. The daily morning coffee break, which often includes donuts, is a popular custom for people working in various organizations. Persons of British heritage usually partake of tea in the late afternoon with some sort of sweet cake or cookie.

When an individual eats generally does not matter for the healthy population. Rather, it is more important to consider *what* is eaten and *how much*, remembering the principles of moderation, balance, and variety. Three meals daily may be satisfactory for some people, but others find that the best way to receive adequate and appropriate amounts of kcals and nutrients is to eat more often. Snacking can be beneficial for children and older adults alike, especially if appetites are small in relation to physical needs. As a general rule, snacks with low **nutrient density** should not replace nutrient-dense foods.

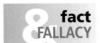

Fallacy: A late-night snack or meal causes weight gain.

Fact: The time when food is eaten has little effect on weight. What is more important is the total kcal and fat content of meals and snacks. Saving all the day's kcals for one late-night meal may be a problem. Rather, the kcals should be spread out over the day, with inclusion of at least three meals throughout the day. This can help promote a higher metabolic rate (see Chapters 3 and 7).

How Should Snacks Be Chosen?

There is no single perfect snack, but some snacks are more nutritious than others and careful selection is necessary to avoid potential problems. Snacks should be planned according to the needs of each member of the family. An individual who nibbles food during food preparation or cleanup may find it easy to put on unwanted pounds and hard to succeed in a weight reduction program. Conversely, planned snacking can be an effective means for meeting the energy and nutrient needs of a growing or very active child or adolescent and may be an effective weight management strategy.

Snacks should be chosen from the five food groups. Foods such as sticky sweets, which have been found to increase susceptibility to tooth decay, should be avoided. A piece of fresh fruit or a handful of low-fat, whole-grain crackers can be an appropriate snack. Rinsing the mouth with water is important after any kind of carbohydrate-based snack to help prevent dental decay (see Chapter 13).

HOW DO FAST FOODS AFFECT NUTRITION?

People of various cultures eat at fast-food restaurants (Figure 1-5). As long as an individual remembers the goals of balance, variety, and moderation, fast-food meals can safely be included in the diet (Box 1-2). Obesity can result from excess fat and sugar intake.

What Is the Definition of Fast Foods?

Fast foods simply mean that they are quickly obtained. Unfortunately, fast foods are often referred to as *junk food.* Junk foods usually are thought of as being low in nutrient density, especially for the amount of kcals present, such as in high-sugar or high-fat foods. Although these types of foods can be found in any restaurant, healthy meal choices can be found on fast-food menus. The Food Guide Pyramid concept can easily be applied to fast food. To illustrate: a small cheeseburger on a bun with lettuce, tomato, and onion, plus juice, represents the five food groups; a taco is composed of a shell made from grain, with ground beef, shredded cheese, shredded lettuce, and tomato; pizza has a crust made from grain, plus tomato sauce, cheese, and various vegetable and meat toppings; a typical fried chicken dinner with mashed potato, coleslaw, a roll, and a glass of milk

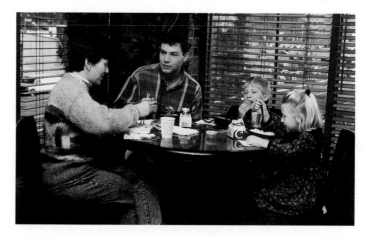

FIGURE 1-5 Restaurant eating is often a family socialization experience in the United States.

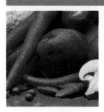

**BOX 1-2
NUTRITIOUS
MENU
INCLUDING
FAST FOOD**

BREAKFAST (AT HOME)
Toasted English muffin with natural
    peanut butter

Banana slices dipped in wheat germ*
Glass of 1% or skim milk

LUNCH (CAFETERIA)
Chili con carne
Mixed salad greens with Italian
    dressing

Piece of cornbread
Glass of 1% or skim milk or 8 oz yogurt

AFTERNOON SNACK
Bunch of grapes (brought from home)

SUPPER (FAST-FOOD RESTAURANT)
Small cheeseburger
Small orange juice
Coleslaw

Soft ice cream or frozen yogurt for
    dessert

SNACK (AT HOME)
Herb-seasoned low-fat popcorn

Small glass apple cider

*Wheat germ has a nutty flavor and crunchy texture and is found in the cereal section of the grocery store. One tablespoon contains about 10% of the recommended dietary allowance for vitamin B_1, folic acid, vitamin E, zinc, and phosphorus. It is also high in magnesium.

also represents at least four of the five food groups. To help include fast foods in a manner consistent with the Food Guide Pyramid, the following tips may help:

- Focus on smaller portions of meat and cheese dishes.
- Remove the skin from cooked chicken.
- Look for bean-based dishes and salads or other vegetables or fruits.
- Use lemon instead of salad dressing or butter.
- Choose a small or low-sugar beverage.

Fast foods can meet nutrient density criteria and the Dietary Guidelines if chosen wisely. Serving sizes are important. See Appendix 4 for a nutritional analysis of selected fast foods.

HOW DOES ALCOHOL AFFECT NUTRITIONAL STATUS?

Excessive alcohol consumption affects health through two general, broad modes. One is the altered food intake resulting from factors such as decreased or increased appetite, replacement of the kcals in food for those in alcohol (a concern for weight control or loss of appetite for food associated with heavy intake of alcohol), or the use of available food money for alcohol. The other major influence is impaired absorption, reduced storage, altered metabolic needs, and impaired use of nutrients (see Chapter 3). Thiamin deficiency is often a result of excess alcohol and too little food (see Chapter 4). The same holds true for other minerals, such as magnesium. A moderate amount of alcohol is acceptable and potentially desirable as long as there is little risk of alcohol abuse.

WHAT IS THE ROLE OF THE NURSE OR OTHER HEALTH CARE PROFESSIONAL IN THE FAMILY MEAL ENVIRONMENT?

Family eating behaviors fall in a spectrum from ideal to poor. The ideal diet consists of a balance of high-quality, nutritionally dense foods in appropriate quantities and variety to support normal growth and repair while inhibiting the development of chronic disease. Most families have a combination of ideal and poor food habits. All health care professionals can reinforce the positive food habits by giving ideas about how to incorporate well-liked nutritious foods into daily lifestyle.

The nurse or other health professional should be aware of nutritional inadequacies or excesses as represented in the Food Guide Pyramid. For persons who require a higher kcal intake, the addition of more foods from the base of the Food Guide Pyramid (whole grains and fruits) would be the wisest choice, although added sugars and liquid unsaturated fats may also be appropriate as a kcal source. Many patients will require dietary modification for various conditions, such as cardiovascular disease, which may require a lower sodium intake. Foods needed for long-term health, however, should still fall within the parameters of the Food Guide Pyramid. In the case of limiting sodium intake, it would be appropriate for a nurse to advise reading labels for sodium content. Emphasis should be placed on the food groups needed for health, but with specific guidelines provided, such as noting that fresh and frozen vegetables are low in sodium whereas canned vegetables are high in sodium. Problems with patient adherence to the goals of nutrition or multiple therapeutic diets beyond normal nutrition should be documented and the patient should be referred to a registered dietitian.

The nurse plays a vital role in assessing and identifying patient and family needs while facilitating solutions using a counseling approach. Meal planning can be relatively simple when few or no negative forces are influencing a family. The more likely scenario, however, is a combination of internal and external barriers to good nutrition, which can best be overcome through a total health care team approach. Many community services are available that can complement the skills of the health care team.

A nurse's contacts with patients in any situation provide unlimited teaching opportunities to promote better nutrition. The nurse's own dietary habits, attitudes, and state of nutrition are reflected in his or her interest and approach in helping patients understand the importance of a basic normal or modified diet. Success will more likely occur if the nurse starts with good attitudes about the importance of nutrition. By having a good basic knowledge of nutrition and by keeping informed, the nurse can do much to combat the misinformation forced on the public by slanted advertising, food faddists, quacks, and untrained self-termed "health specialists," among others.

What Is Your Nutrition IQ as You Begin the Study of Nutrition?

Some of the following statements are true and some are false. Read each question and then write your answer in the blank before you consult the list of correct answers on page 29. Relevant chapter numbers are provided for further information.

_____ 1. A daily diet for weight reduction should have adequate amounts of protein, carbohydrates, fat, minerals, and vitamins, but should furnish less than the daily requirements for kcals (Chapter 7).

_____ 2. Margarine and butter contain the same number of calories (Chapter 2).

_____ 3. Food allergies and food intolerances are the same thing (Chapter 5).

_____ 4. A well person who eats the right kinds and amounts of foods every day generally does not need to take vitamin pills to meet the Recommended Dietary Allowance (Chapter 4).

_____ 5. Skipping meals is a good way to lose weight safely (Chapter 7).

_____ 6. Children should not have dessert unless they clean their plates (Fact & Fallacy, Chapter 1, page 8).

_____ 7. Calcium supplements are the best way to increase calcium intake if the individual does not like milk (Chapter 4).

_____ 8. The risk of heart disease can be reduced by following a diet low in saturated fat, cholesterol, and sodium (Chapter 8).

_____ 9. White bread is the same as wheat bread (Chapter 2).

_____ 10. Olives, olive oil, avocados, and most nuts are low in saturated fat and moderate amounts are fine for a low-cholesterol diet (Chapter 2).

_____ 11. People with diverticulosis should eat dried beans and peas because they are high in fiber, depending on individual tolerance (Chapter 3).

_____ 12. An obese woman should lose weight if she becomes pregnant (Chapter 12).

_____ 13. Children should be forced to eat vegetables for their own good (Chapter 13).

_____ 14. Baby teeth are not important and therefore good dental care and oral hygiene should wait until children are old enough to brush their own teeth (Chapter 13).

_____ 15. It is possible for elderly people to develop muscle mass (Chapter 14).

_____ 16. Not all food additives are harmful (Chapter 15).

_____ 17. If a survivor of breast cancer gains weight, it is always because of consumption of too many kcals (Chapter 11).

_____ 18. Natural sweets such as honey may be eaten freely by people with diabetes (Chapter 9).

_____ 19. Drinking water at mealtimes may aid digestion if the water is not used to wash down food (Chapter 3).

_____ 20. A teenager needs more milk every day than does a preschooler (Chapter 13).

What Is Your Nutrition IQ as You Begin the Study of Nutrition?—cont'd

Correct Answers to the Nutrition IQ

1. T	8. T	15. T	Number correct answers _____
2. T	9. T	16. T	Number incorrect answers _____
3. F	10. T	17. F	How good do you think your
4. T	11. T	18. F	Nutrition Score is? _____
5. F	12. F	19. T	
6. F	13. F	20. T	
7. F	14. F		

CHAPTER STUDY QUESTIONS AND CLASSROOM ACTIVITIES

1. Explain what is meant by the following statement: "Good meal planning is both a science and an art."
2. How would you advise a patient to overcome food dislikes or avoidances?
3. Analyze food advertisements in magazines. To whom are the ads appealing? How?
4. Become familiar with the ethnic, religious, or regional diet assigned to you by the instructor and summarize information about it to present to the class. Be prepared to discuss this ethnic diet in terms of the five food groups of the Food Guide Pyramid and Dietary Guidelines for Americans. What are the good points? How could the diet be improved? Use the following chart to record important information about each diet presented in class.

Ethnic Dietary Habits

Regional or ethnic diet (list foods):

Characteristics and main dish:

Good nutritional features:

Desirable nutritional improvements:

5. Students might tell about the food customs and dietary habits of their country or countries of heritage and possibly demonstrate the ethnic dishes popular in their personal family meals. Markets of a city, ethnic food sections of large grocery stores, and ethnic restaurants afford good opportunities for learning about foods used by families with different ethnic backgrounds. The class might prepare a traditional Italian/Mediterranean meal or determine if any traditional Italian foods (such as bean-based dishes) can be found on local menus.

6. Bring some sample nutrition labels to class to discuss how you would use the percentage values on the label in planning a day's menu for yourself.

7. Referring to a food label, determine how much protein is needed to meet the 2000-kcal guidelines of 65 g of fat and 300 g of carbohydrate.

8. Plan a day's menu using the maximum recommended number of servings in the Food Guide Pyramid for a total intake of about 2000 kcal.

9. Assess the following menu for the questions below:

Breakfast	**Lunch**	**Dinner**
Banana	Hot dog on roll	Cheeseburger
Corn flakes	Mustard and relish	French fries
Whole milk	Chocolate chip cookies	Coleslaw
Sugar	Coke	Milkshake
Toast, butter, and jelly		

10. Judge the meals according to the Food Guide Pyramid.

11. What suggestions would you make to this menu to have it meet the Dietary Guidelines for Americans?

Case Study

CRITICAL THINKING

A.J. was sitting in health class, learning about the Food Guide Pyramid. He thought it odd that beans were placed in the meat group, as he knew his dad ate beans, such as ceci beans (otherwise called chickpeas or garbanzo beans), instead of bread because of the carbohydrates. He had also just studied photosynthesis in science class that morning and knew that plant foods contain carbohydrates. Why, then, were beans in the protein group of the Food Pyramid? Although A.J. did not know the answer, he did not want to ask the teacher and look stupid in front of that cute girl with the longest hair he had ever seen.

Critical Thinking Applications

1. Describe how family and culture influence food choices.

2. Describe why legumes (beans) might replace either meat or bread and identify the food guides that explain the difference.

3. Describe how health professionals can assist in the public's gaining knowledge of nutrition.

"My Food and Nutrition Experience Diary"

To help make you food and nutrition minded as you study nutrition, (1) jot down in the space provided any food and nutrition comments, questions, or experiences you encounter in discussions with individuals out of a classroom setting and later as you give nutritional care to patients (checking menus, setting up or observing and serving trays, feeding patients, and so on); and (2) assemble in a notebook (preferable), folder, or file box any available food and nutrition booklets, clippings, or other printed materials.

Date   Food and Nutrition Experience   Comments

REFERENCES

Barr SI, Broughton TM: Relative weight, weight loss efforts and nutrient intakes among health-conscious vegetarian, past vegetarian and nonvegetarian women ages 18 to 50. J Am Coll Nutr. November-December 2000; 19(6):781-788.

Guthrie JF, Morton JF: Food sources of added sweeteners in the diets of Americans. J Am Diet Assoc. January 2000; 100(1):43-51, quiz 49-50.

Kim KK, Yu ES, Chen EH, Cross N, Kim J, Brintnall RA: Nutritional status of Korean Americans: implications for cancer risk. Oncol Nurs Forum. November-December 2000; 27(10):1573-1583.

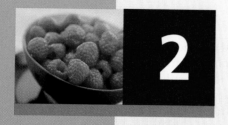

2

Carbohydrate, Protein, and Fat: The Energy Macronutrients of Balanced Meals

OBJECTIVES

After completing this chapter, you should be able to:

- Describe the macronutrient content of various foods and meal items.
- Describe the function and general recommendations for carbohydrate, protein, and fat in health prevention and disease management.
- Describe the role of the nurse or other health care professional in promoting an appropriate carbohydrate, protein, and fat intake in a meal context.

TERMS TO IDENTIFY

Arachidonic acid
Biologic value
Cholesterol
Complete protein
Dietary fiber
Diglycerides
Disaccharides
Dyslipidemia
Empty calories
Essential amino acids
Essential fatty acids
Glycemic index
Glycerol

Gout
Hydrogenated
Hyperinsulinemia
Incomplete protein
Ketosis
Kwashiorkor
Linoleic acid
Linolenic acid
Macronutrients
Marasmus
Monoglycerides
Monosaccharides
Monounsaturated fat

Nitrogen balance
Omega-3 fatty acid
Phospholipids
Polysaccharides
Postprandial
Prostaglandins
Protein-energy malnutrition
Starch
Sterols
Sugar
Sugar alcohols
Trans fatty acid
Triglycerides

INTRODUCTION

The energy (measured in *kilocalories* [kcals]) in the food we eat comes from *carbohydrate, protein,* and *fat,* otherwise called **macronutrients** (Figure 2-1). Balanced meals contain all three macronutrients or ideally at least one serving from each of the three lower levels of the Food Guide Pyramid (see the inside front cover and Chapter 1). The macronutrients provide the fuel for body functioning (although of the three, proteins serve this function the least efficiently). All three macronutrients contain the elements carbon, hydrogen, and oxygen. Protein differ from carbohydrate and fat in that protein also contain nitrogen. Carbohydrate and protein provide 4 kcal/g, and fat provides 9 kcal/g, as noted on many food labels (see Figure 1-2). *Alcohol* provides 7 kcal/g. Although alcohol is produced from a source of carbohydrate, the body uses it differently once the carbohydrate is fermented into alcohol.

WHERE ARE THE THREE MACRONUTRIENTS FOUND?

Carbohydrate is made through the process of *photosynthesis* (in which the sun's energy allows plant leaves to take in carbon dioxide [CO_2] from the air and water

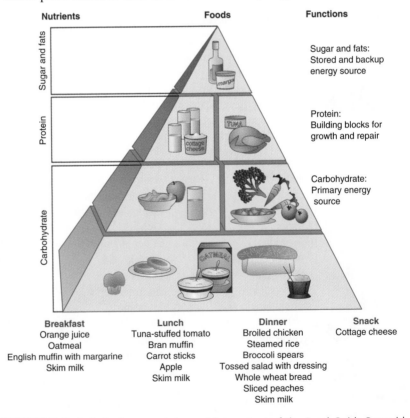

FIGURE 2-1 Carbohydrate, protein, and fat content of the Food Guide Pyramid.

[H$_2$O] through the roots). Carbon (*carbo-*) and water (*-hydrate*) are formed into carbohydrate and the plant gives off oxygen as a result. Hence, carbohydrate is mainly found in foods of plant origin. Although we do not think of sugar as growing out of the ground, it does come from a plant. Even honey comes ultimately from plant matter, produced from the nectar of flowers by bees. The only non-plant source of carbohydrate is milk, which makes sense if you consider that baby animals need a source of carbohydrate before they are able to eat solid foods.

The carbohydrate found in table sugar is, however, very concentrated (½ c of sugar contains 95 g—without any other nutritional value—whereas ½ c of most plant foods contain only 15 g or less and are concentrated in the micronutrients vitamins and minerals). Sugar is an example of an **empty calorie** food, supplying carbohydrate calories, but no other nutrients.

Protein is produced in the body from *amino acids*. The greatest source of amino acids and protein is muscle, thus all forms of meat (red, white, and fish) are high in protein. Legumes (beans) and nuts are plant material and thus contain carbohydrate (as do all plant-based foods), but legumes also have the ability to draw nitrogen from the air, making them high in protein. Therefore legumes and nuts are included in the meat group of the Food Guide Pyramid (see Chapter 1). Other rich sources of protein are eggs, milk, and cheese.

Whole grains and vegetables supply small amounts of protein, but can add up to a significant quantity, depending on the amount consumed. Grains and vegetables do not contain complete protein, as do meat, milk, and eggs. Fruits are very low in protein. This is why most fresh fruits have fewer kcals than bread, even though they have the same amount of carbohydrate on a per-volume basis.

Fat is found in many foods containing protein and is added through cooking or flavoring foods. The amount of fat found in grains, vegetables, and most fruits is insignificant. Fats extracted from vegetable sources (such as corn, safflowers, soybeans, and olives) are usually found in liquid form and generally are not harmful to health unless they are **hydrogenated** (turned into solid fats). Fats that are solid (found mostly in animal products such as butter and red meat) need to be limited to help prevent or manage a variety of health conditions.

CARBOHYDRATE: FUNCTIONS AND RECOMMENDATIONS FOR APPROPRIATE INTAKE

What Are the Functions of Carbohydrate?

Carbohydrate is readily converted to energy. The carbon chains found in it serve as the source of energy burned by humans and are similar to the carbon found in coal. In fact, the human body is made up of millions of microscopic body cells that act as small furnaces to burn our food energy. Thus the primary function of carbohydrate is to meet the body's specific needs for energy (Table 2-1). One gram of carbohydrate yields 4 kcal. Carbohydrate has the following functions as well:

1. *Sparing* the burning of protein for energy (proteins have more important functions, such as building and repairing body structures).

2. In *aiding* in the more efficient and complete oxidation (burning) of fats for energy.
3. As sugar, *producing* energy quickly.
4. As starch, *providing* an economical and abundant source of energy after being changed to glucose. Sugar and starch are both digested quickly in less than an hour.

TABLE 2-1
TYPES AND SOURCES OF CARBOHYDRATE

TYPE	DESCRIPTION	SOURCES
MONOSACCHARIDES (SIMPLE SUGARS)		
Glucose (blood sugar)	The end product of most carbohydrate digestion. One form in which carbohydrates are absorbed, resulting from its being the only fuel the central nervous system can use.	Found in fruits, certain roots, corn, and honey. Also found in blood as the product of starch digestion.
Fructose (fruit sugar)	Gives honey its characteristic flavor. Combined with glucose in table sugar.	Found in fruit, honey, and vegetables.
Galactose	A byproduct of lactose digestion.	Naturally found only in mammalian milk.
DISACCHARIDES (DOUBLE SUGARS)		
Sucrose (table sugar)	Composed of glucose and fructose. Commonly known as table sugar, which is made from sugar cane.	Found in sugar cane, sugar beets, molasses, maple sugar, maple syrup, many fruits and vegetables, and added to foods as table sugar.
Lactose (milk sugar)	Produced only by mammals. It is less soluble and less sweet than cane sugar and is digested more slowly. Composed of glucose and galactose.	Found in milk and unfermented milk products.
Maltose (malt sugar)	Formed when starch is changed to sugar during digestion. Composed of two glucose molecules.	Found in malt and malt products; not free in nature.
POLYSACCHARIDES (STARCH, COMPLEX CARBOHYDRATES)		
Complex carbohydrate (starch)	The reserve store of carbohydrates in plants; changed to glucose during digestion (through intermediate steps of dextrin and maltose).	Found in grains and grain products, seeds, roots, potatoes, green bananas, and other plants.
Dextrin	Formed from starch breakdown.	Cooked starch (toast).
Dietary fiber	Indigestible; provides bulk and stimulation for the intestines and helps prevent or manage many chronic illnesses.	Insoluble found in skins and seeds of fruits, vegetables, and grains. Soluble found in large amounts in legumes, greens, citrus fruits, oatmeal, and barley.
Glycogen	The reserve store of carbohydrates in animals; changed to glucose as needed.	Stored small amounts in the liver and muscles.

5. As lactose, *having* a certain laxative action (remains in the intestines longer and encourages desirable bacterial growth) and aids in the absorption of calcium.
6. As dietary fiber (insoluble and indigestible), *aiding* in the normal functioning of the intestines by adding bulk. Soluble forms, in significant amounts, lower serum cholesterol levels (see Chapter 8) and lessen the **postprandial** (after-meal) rise in blood glucose (see Chapter 9). One study found that thick oat flakes had a significantly lower effect on glucose levels than did bread (Granfeldt et al., 2000). Soluble fiber, in particular, slows down the time of digestion, which helps promote *satiety* (the feeling of fullness or satisfaction after eating) and allows for more stable blood sugar levels. Increased intake of water is needed if fiber intake increases.

Because it slows digestion, soluble fiber is said to have a low glycemic index. The **glycemic index** relates to the expected rise in blood sugar from different foods and macronutrients. Carbohydrate have a higher glycemic index than do foods with protein and fat. Carbohydrate foods high in soluble fiber have a lower glycemic index than do liquid forms such as fruit juice.

What Are the Three Basic Forms of Carbohydrate?

1. **Sugars**, or simple carbohydrates, are single or double molecules made up of carbon, hydrogen, and oxygen ($C_6H_{12}O_6$) and may also be referred to as **monosaccharides** (single units) and **disaccharides** (double units or double sugars). Disaccharides are found in food and must break apart into monosaccharides before they can be absorbed into the bloodstream.
2. **Starch**, often still called a complex carbohydrate, consists of several units of sugar linked together in a long chain—also referred to as a **polysaccharide** (multiple unit). Based on the results of a long-term diabetes study (see Chapter 9), it is now known that starch is digested as rapidly as sugar.
3. **Dietary fiber** is the most complex form of carbohydrate. Although it is a polysaccharide like starch, the complexity of the polysaccharide chain in fiber makes digestion by humans nearly impossible. An analogy for such a fiber chain is that of a twisted gold chain necklace. Just as it is difficult to unravel such a chain, the human digestive system cannot unravel a polysaccharide chain. A cow's digestive system can unravel such a chain because they have the equivalent of four stomachs. This is why cows can derive nutritional value from grass, but humans cannot.

Because fiber passes through the human intestinal tract virtually undigested, it does not raise blood glucose levels (see Chapter 9). The two types of fiber are defined according to their solubility in water. Insoluble fiber (in celery and apple skins, for example) tends to be crunchy, whereas soluble fiber (in oatmeal, baked beans, applesauce, or the white of the apple) tends to be gummy. Insoluble fibers include cellulose and hemicellulose, primarily found in the skin and seeds of plant-based foods. Soluble fibers include gums, lignins, and pectins.

■ **BOX 2-1**
■ **FOOD SOURCES OF VARIOUS FIBER COMPONENTS**

CELLULOSE
Whole-wheat flour
Bran
Cabbage family
Peas and beans
Apples
Root vegetables

HEMICELLULOSE
Bran
Cereals
Whole grains

GUMS
Oatmeal
Dried beans
Brown rice
Barley
Pectin
Apples
Citrus fruits
Strawberries

LIGNIN
Mature vegetables
Wheat

Plant foods contain both soluble and insoluble fibers. Some foods are higher in one than in the other. See Box 2-1 for a general listing of fiber content of various plant foods.

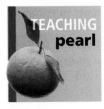

TEACHING pearl

To describe the difference between soluble and insoluble fiber, say to the patient, "If you put the peel of an apple in a glass of water, it will sit there day after day. That is insoluble fiber, or roughage. But if you put the white part of the apple into water, it will dissolve into little particles. This is soluble fiber, known as pectin, which is used to thicken fruit juice into jam. Soluble fiber dissolves in the digestive tract and helps to thicken and slow the movement of food through the intestinal tract, which is particularly helpful in controlling blood sugar levels and cholesterol. Legumes have at least twice as much soluble fiber as fruit, but they have the same amount of total carbohydrates."

What Are the Recommendations for Carbohydrate Intake?

Most authorities advise that a person should derive 50% to 60% of their kcals from carbohydrate. For those with insulin resistance, there is some evidence that lowering the carbohydrate level to 40% may be warranted. One study found that with this reduced carbohydrate intake and an emphasis on complex forms (high fiber), two conditions associated with insulin resistance, **gout** (high levels of uric acid) and **dyslipidemia** (high triglycerides with low high-density lipoprotein [HDL] cholesterol), were improved (Dessein et al., 2000). Chapter 6 goes into detail on insulin resistance.

The lowest recommended amount of carbohydrate intake is 40% of total kcals or a minimum of 100 g to prevent **ketosis** (rapid breakdown of body fat leading to a lowered pH, or increased acidity level of the blood). Guidelines found on food labels promote 60% or 300 g for a 2000-kcal diet. The recommendation for carbohydrate in the Food Guide Pyramid, not including added sugars, is about 150 to 300 g (using the range of minimum to maximum recommended number of servings for each food group; see the inside front cover and Chapter 1).

Sugar is now considered appropriate as part of total carbohydrate intake as long as the minimum micronutrient needs are being met (consumption of the minimum number of food servings in the Food Guide Pyramid) and weight and level of health allow for added sugar. Infants, however, should not consume honey because of the possible presence of botulism spores. For example, some persons benefit by limiting carbohydrate intake to 200 g/day. This equates to the minimum Food Guide Pyramid servings (150 g) plus the addition of ¼ c of sugar (50 g, which is approximately the equivalent of one can of soda pop or 10 tsp of sugar). Foods that are high in sugar but low in fiber, protein, and fat are digested rapidly—especially if in liquid form, such as soda pop or fruit juice. This can be a problem for people with *reactive hypoglycemia* (a condition in which the body overreacts to excess carbohydrate by producing too much insulin, also called *hyperinsulinemia*). This can cause symptoms such as weakness and shakiness (see Chapter 9) and can contribute to high levels of triglycerides (see Chapters 6 and 8).

The recommended amount of fiber (20 to 35 g) can be met by including in the daily diet the recommended number of food servings of the Food Guide Pyramid (with 2 g of fiber on average for each serving of whole grain, vegetable, and fruit. Legumes provide up to 10 g of fiber per ½-c serving). The fiber in grains is found in the germ and the bran layer, where most of the overall nutritional value in whole grains is found (Figure 2-2). With any increase in fiber intake, an increase in water intake is needed to prevent fecal impaction.

What Is Carbohydrate Counting?

Carbohydrate counting is the newest tool in diabetes self-management. By focusing on the chief factor of elevated blood glucose—carbohydrate—meal choices become simpler and persons with diabetes can be more effective in managing blood glucose (see Chapter 9).

What Quantities of Food Are Needed to Meet the Carbohydrate Recommendations?

To help translate carbohydrate grams into real food recommendations, either the Dietary Exchange System or the Food Guide Pyramid may be used (see Chapter 1). The carbohydrate content of plant foods can be determined by assessing three factors: water content, level of sweetness, and density (see Box 9-3). Generally speaking, there are approximately 15 g of carbohydrate for every ½ c of grain or fruit or every whole cup of milk or plain yogurt. Most vegetables provide 5 g of carbohydrates per ½ c when cooked or per whole cup when raw (Figure 2-3).

Dry plant material, such as potatoes and bread products, contains on average 15 g of carbohydrates per ½ c. Sweet potatoes (yams) are dry like white potatoes, so they also contain at least 15 g per ½ c. The fact that they are also sweet doubles

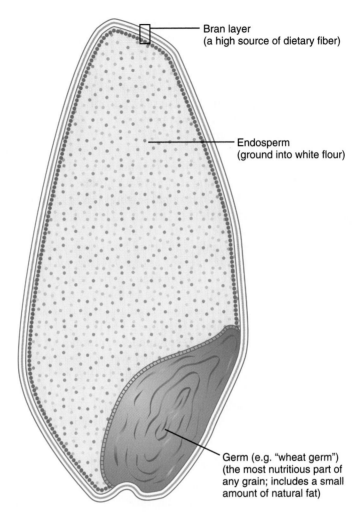

Bran layer
(a high source of dietary fiber)

Endosperm
(ground into white flour)

Germ (e.g. "wheat germ")
(the most nutritious part of
any grain; includes a small
amount of natural fat)

FIGURE 2-2 Anatomy of a grain. Whole grains include all three portions of the grain.

the carbohydrate value to 30 g per ½ c. Grains that have a lot of air allow a larger volume for the same amount of carbohydrates (for example, 3 c of popcorn or 1 c of puffed cereals). A slice of bread provides a good size analogy for estimating carbohydrate values—for example, a piece of pizza that is the size of a slice of bread contains one serving of starch (about 15 g of carbohydrate).

Most fruits are not dry like grains, but they are sweet. There is generally 15 g of carbohydrate for every ½-c serving of fruit, which is why fruit has a caloric content closer to that of bread than to that of most vegetables. Fruits that are very high in water content (such as watermelon or cantaloupe) contain 15 g of carbohydrate

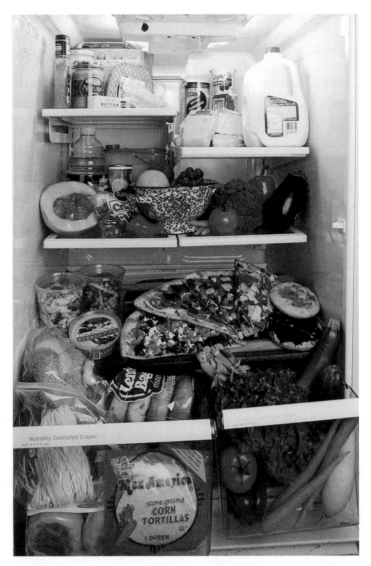

FIGURE 2-3 Vegetables low in carbohydrates are those that are high in water content and relatively low in sweetness as shown in the lower drawer of the refrigerator. Grains are found in a variety of forms, such as those in the lower bread drawer (tortillas [corn tortillas may serve as a grain substitute because of their carbohydrate content], bagels, English muffins, pasta, and bread; grain is also found in pizza crust, on the lower shelf). Mixed dishes like pizza and the five-bean salad, as shown on the lower shelf, provide carbohydrate, protein, and some fat. Fruits and vegetables, as shown on the middle shelf, are generally fat-free. On the top shelves, dairy foods, meat, peanut butter, and eggs are all protein-rich foods that contain variable amounts of fat. (Eggs should be stored either in a leakproof container—as shown in the plastic container—or on the bottom shelf to prevent cross-contamination with salmonella in case they crack.) Solid fats, such as butter, contain mostly saturated fat, whereas mayonnaise and liquid salad dressing contain mostly unsaturated fat.

per cup, whereas only ¼ c of dry fruit or ⅛ c of dry sweet fruit (e.g., raisins) contains the same amount (see Box 9-3).

Because vegetables grow out of the ground, they are also a source of carbohydrate as a result of photosynthesis. However, most vegetables are high in water content and low in sugar and thus have the lowest carbohydrate content (see Table 9-3). High-carbohydrate vegetables are the dry potato, legumes, sweet corn, and sweet peas. This is why they are often referred to as *starchy vegetables* (remember, they have the same 15 g of carbohydrates for a ½-c serving as starches have). Examples of low-carbohydrate vegetables are those that sound odd when the word *sweet* is used with them. It sounds odd to say sweet spinach, sweet broccoli, or sweet cabbage, all of which are low in carbohydrate (5 g per ½-c cooked serving). Carrots, which are sweet, contain only 10 g of carbohydrate, because the high water content displaces some of the carbohydrate.

It is now recognized that fiber may be subtracted from the total carbohydrate values listed on food labels because the human body cannot digest it. The carbohydrate found in many nuts and seeds consist mainly of fiber; therefore they do not provide significant amounts of carbohydrate that can be counted in terms of kcals or that can have an effect on blood glucose (see Chapter 9). A minimal amount of fiber is digested through bacterial fermentation in the colon, which allows for some contribution of kcals from fiber, but is generally considered insignificant.

Ordinary table sugar, molasses, maple syrup, corn syrup, and honey are concentrated sources of carbohydrate, but provide mainly empty calories, meaning they contain carbohydrate, but few vitamins or minerals. Blackstrap molasses is the one exception, in that it is relatively high in some nutrients such as iron, calcium, and potassium and it also contributes some B vitamins. Sugar can be noted on food labels as sugar, syrup, or any word that ends in *-ose* (except cellulose, which is a type of fiber). Fruit sugar is called *fructose,* milk sugar is *lactose,* and table sugar is *sucrose.* Honey is a combination of fructose and glucose (glucose is also known as *blood sugar*). One teaspoon of sugar contains 4 g of carbohydrates (and therefore 16 kcal). In carbohydrate counting, sugar may be included as part of the known need or tolerance for carbohydrates (determined by self-monitoring of blood glucose; see Chapter 9).

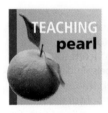

TEACHING pearl

To clarify carbohydrate content during patient education you could say, "You can almost feel the water content of green beans when you eat them and you would never call them 'sweet.' You also wouldn't say 'sweet asparagus' or 'sweet celery.' These are all examples of low-carbohydrate (and thus low-calorie) vegetables because they are high in water content and not sweet." Or you might say, "The number of prunes in one fruit exchange can be determined by the number of plums that fit into ½ c (about three small plums), which means three prunes equals one fruit exchange or 15 g of carbohydrates."

No significant animal sources of carbohydrate exist except for lactose found in milk. Cheese does not contain carbohydrate because the liquid whey is drained off during production and what lactose remains is converted into lactic acid during fermentation. This is why the Food Exchange System counts cheese as equivalent to meat; there is equal protein to meat, but no carbohydrate as in milk. Yogurt contains simple carbohydrate, but minimal lactose, because the double sugar is converted into simple sugar by the bacterial culture used to make the yogurt. About 15 g of carbohydrate are contained in 1 c of milk or yogurt. (Actually, most milk has 12 g of carbohydrate and plain yogurt has 17 g, but it is easier for the consumer to remember 15 g).

Sugar substitutes come in two main forms: nutritive (providing a source of carbohydrate) and nonnutritive (containing insignificant amounts of carbohydrate). **Sugar alcohols** are nutritive and are easy to recognize by their names, which all end in -*ol* and sound like *alcohol*. The main sugar alcohols are sorbitol, mannitol, and xylitol. Sugar alcohols do not contribute to dental decay, but otherwise have little advantage over sugar. One problem with sugar alcohols is that they can induce diarrhea with as little as 8 g, as noted on food labels. Saccharin, aspartame, and acesulfame-K are all nonnutritive sweeteners that are useful for the management of diabetes.

What Problems Are Associated with Excess Carbohydrate Intake?

Obesity is the primary concern whenever a person consumes an excess of kcals. This is true for any of the macronutrients, but usually carbohydrate and fat are the chief kcal sources leading to obesity.

Persons who graze on carbohydrate foods throughout the day are more prone to dental caries. Good oral hygiene can help compensate for a person who chooses to eat in this manner (see Chapter 13). Both sugars and starches are *cariogenic* (promoting dental cavities).

A high-serum **triglyceride** (a form of fat in the blood) level will improve if one avoids an excessive carbohydrate intake. Avoiding excess sugar intake is important for persons who are being treated for *hypertriglyceridemia,* in part because sugar is a concentrated form of carbohydrate.

Some individuals with diabetes need a moderate or low carbohydrate intake to maintain normal blood glucose levels. Persons with diabetes can monitor their blood glucose levels to determine the ideal amount of carbohydrate for their individual needs (see Chapter 9).

Although it is still in research stage, there is growing evidence that persons with insulin resistance and the consequent **hyperinsulinemia** (excess insulin in the blood) associated with a high-carbohydrate diet will benefit from a moderate intake of carbohydrate (about 50% of kcals, or 250 g of carbohydrates for a 2000-kcal diet). Because carbohydrate is the primary cause of the rise in postprandial blood glucose levels, carbohydrate induces insulin production. A decrease of carbohydrate intake will lower the need for insulin. For persons with insulin resistance, lowering carbohydrate intake may help to reduce the risk of heart disease (see Chapter 8).

Fallacy: Only fats are fattening.

Fact: Starches and sugars (complex and simple carbohydrates) are comparable to protein in energy value, as both contribute 4 kcal/g. In excess, both can cause excess caloric intake and lead to weight gain. Fat, which provides 9 kcal/g, is the most concentrated source of food energy, supplying at least 1000 kcal for each ½ c. High-sugar foods, however, are also high in kcals because they are a concentrated carbohydrate source (½ c sugar equates to almost 100 g) and thus provide 400 kcal for a ½-c serving of, for example, a small handful of jellybeans. You might want to place a ½-c measuring cup in the palm of your hand to better estimate this portion size.

How Does Alcohol Differ from Carbohydrates?

Alcohol is an additional fuel source for the human body because it is a source of kcals. It provides 7 kcal/g. The caloric content of alcohol is close to that of fat, which provides 9 kcal/g. Alcohol is derived from a carbohydrate source, such as barley for beer and grapes for wine. However, once the carbohydrate is fermented into alcohol, it is no longer used in the same fashion. This is why it is found in the fat exchange group of the Food Exchange System (see Chapter 1).

PROTEIN: FUNCTIONS AND RECOMMENDATIONS FOR APPROPRIATE INTAKE

What Are the Functions of Protein?

The nitrogen found in protein is what sets it apart from the other macronutrients. Nitrogen gives protein its unique function of building and repairing all of the various body tissues, allows for the production of hormones and digestive enzymes, and is needed for a strong immune system. Although this is protein's primary role, it can also be broken down and stripped of its nitrogen to be used as an energy source. Unless adequate carbohydrates and fats are provided, some of the protein ingested will be used for energy needs rather than for building and repairing body tissues. Protein has numerous functions:

1. *Repairing* or *replacing* worn-out tissues
2. *Supplying* material for growth and tissue building
3. *Providing* some energy (4 kcal/g), but not as well equipped for this purpose as are carbohydrate and fat
4. *Constructing* and properly *maintaining* important body compounds (enzymes, hormones, hemoglobin, antibodies, other blood proteins, and glandular secretions)

What Are the Types of Protein?

The term **biologic value** describes how well a particular protein food approximates the amount and combination of **essential amino acids** in the body. Essential amino acids cannot be produced by the body and hence need to be included in the diet. A **complete protein** is said to contain all of the nine essential amino acids, whereas an **incomplete protein** has some of the essential amino acids but is lacking others.

Generally speaking, animal sources of protein such as meat, fish, poultry, and dairy products (see Figure 2-3) contain complete proteins of high biologic value. Incomplete yet good sources of protein foods that are lacking one or more of the essential amino acids include whole grains, legumes, nuts, and seeds. Combining incomplete protein foods over the course of the day can give the body all of the essential amino acids needed for adequate protein levels. Therefore vegetarians can receive adequate protein without eating meat if they make wise food choices (see Chapter 1).

What Are Amino Acids?

Protein, necessary for building and repairing body tissue in humans and for the formation of enzymes, is made up of 22 amino acids. They are often called the building blocks of protein. They can be found in varying amounts and combinations in the food we eat and the human body can synthesize most of them. However, the following amino acids are essential, which means they cannot be synthesized and must therefore be obtained from the diet:

Valine	Phenylalanine	Isoleucine
Lysine	Threonine	Leucine
Methionine	Tryptophan	Histidine (required for children)

There are 13 nonessential amino acids; that is, those that can be synthesized by the body in adequate amounts:

Alanine	Cystine	Hydroxyproline
Arginine	Glutamic acid	Proline
Asparagine	Glutamine	Serine
Aspartic acid	Glycine	Tyrosine
Cysteine		

Fallacy: Phenylalanine, as found in the sugar substitute Aspartame, is a poison.

Fact: Phenylalanine is an essential amino acid needed in the formation of protein. Some persons are born with a metabolic defect in which excess phenylalanine can cause mental retardation (see Chapter 13). A routine test is performed at birth to determine infants with this metabolic disorder, called *phenylketonuria* (PKU). Such persons need to avoid excess phenylalanine throughout life. Cautions about Aspartame (brandname Equal™), which contains phenylalanine, are provided to help protect persons with PKU. Persons without PKU are not harmed by increased consumption of this essential amino acid.

What Are the Recommendations for Protein Intake?

The protein allowance is based on the amount necessary to maintain nitrogen balance. Generally, 45 to 60 g of protein will meet the health needs of most adults. **Nitrogen balance** refers to a condition in which the nitrogen consumed in the form of protein is equal to the nitrogen lost daily in the urine and other body secretions. At this point, intake is considered to be meeting the body's needs. The requirement is then increased to account for the *mixed protein diet* (protein from a variety of foods). The allowance is 0.8 g of protein for each kilogram of body weight (weight in kilograms is calculated by dividing weight in pounds by 2.2). This translates into 63 g of protein for a man weighing 79 kg and 50 g for a woman weighing 63 kg.

For infants, the allowances are based on the amount of protein provided by the quantity of milk required to ensure a satisfactory rate of growth. This is estimated to be 2.24 g/kg per day during the first month of life and falls gradually to about 1.5 g/kg per day by the sixth month. The protein requirement during growth is greater than that in adulthood because the formation of new tissue requires more nitrogen. The allowances for children and adolescents are calculated from information on growth rates and body composition. The allowances decrease gradually from 1.5 g/kg per day between 6 months and 1 year to 0.8 g/kg per day by the eighteenth year.

During pregnancy, at least 60 g of protein daily is recommended. Some authorities advocate as much as 100 g in the pregnant woman's daily diet. The dietary protein allowance for a lactating woman is about the same as that for a pregnant woman.

The protein requirement is increased for any condition in which body proteins are broken down, such as hemorrhages, burns, poor protein nutrition, previous surgery, wounds, and long convalescence. Protein deficiency over a long period results in muscle loss, reduced resistance to disease, skin and blood changes, slow wound healing, and a condition known as *nutritional edema*.

What Quantities of Food Are Needed to Meet the Protein Recommendations?

The minimum number of food servings in the Food Guide Pyramid provides 60 g of protein, more than enough for most people. Every serving of grains provides 2 to 3 g of protein, vegetables provide 2 g, milk 8 g, and 1 oz (¼ c) of meat or cheese provides 7 g (1 egg, ½ c of beans, or ¼ c of nuts equates to 1 oz of meat).

What Problems Are Associated with Inadequate Protein Intake?

The term **kwashiorkor** refers to a condition in which the individual may have an adequate caloric intake, but lacks adequate dietary protein. However, protein deficiency is frequently associated with a deficiency in calories as well. When the diet is low in calories, protein is used as a source of energy, leaving little of this nutrient to build and repair tissues and maintain immune function. Such a condition is termed **protein-energy malnutrition** (also called **marasmus**) and is prevalent in most developing countries (see Chapter 15). This condition occurs often during physiologic stress (see Chapter 5) and is also seen in hospitalized patients.

What Problems Are Associated with Excess Protein Intake?

Excess protein is generally a problem for persons with renal insufficiency (see Chapter 10) and end-stage liver disease (see Chapter 3). Excess nitrogen from protein foods that must be excreted through the kidneys can place a burden on these organs. Excess protein may also limit the body's ability to use calcium. Also, because most protein foods contain fat (see Figure 2-3), excess protein intake can lead to an excess fat intake, which promotes obesity, cardiovascular disease, and cancer.

Protein intake should be about 10% to 15%, up to a maximum of 20%, of the total daily caloric intake. (See the later section on calculating grams of protein into percentages of total kcals.) The protein content of the recommended servings in the Food Guide Pyramid ranges from a minimum of 60 g to a maximum of 115 g (see the inside front cover and Chapter 1).

FAT AND CHOLESTEROL: FUNCTION AND RECOMMENDATIONS FOR APPROPRIATE INTAKE

What Are the Functions of Dietary Fats?

The primary function of fat is to serve as a concentrated source of heat and energy. About one third to one half of the kcals in the current average American diet comes from fat. Body cells, with the exception of the cells of the nervous system and erythrocytes, can use fatty acids directly as a source of energy. In addition, fats perform the following functions:

1. *Furnishing* essential fatty acids (Table 2-2)
2. *Sparing* burning of protein for energy
3. *Adding* flavor and palatability to the diet
4. *Giving* satiety value to the diet (fat slows the digestive process and retards the development of hunger)
5. *Promoting* absorption of fat-soluble vitamins
6. *Providing* a structural component of cell membranes, digestive secretions, and hormones
7. *Insulating* and controlling body temperature in the form of body fat
8. *Protecting* body organs

Animal fats and fortified margarines not only contain some of the fat-soluble vitamins (A, D, E, and K), but also aid in their absorption. They also play a role in the absorption of fatty acids. Excess fat stored in the body as adipose tissue insulates and protects organs and nerves. Fats also lubricate the intestinal tract. Fat-like substances that have important roles in the body include **phospholipids** (fat plus the mineral phosphorus) and **sterols** (*ergosterol* in plants and **cholesterol** in animal fat).

TABLE 2-2
FATTY ACIDS AND THEIR COMMON FOOD SOURCES

FATTY ACIDS	COMMON FOOD SOURCES
SATURATED	
Lauric	Coconut, palm kernel oil
Myristic	Coconut
Palmitic	Palm oil, beef
Stearic	Cocoa butter, beef
MONOUNSATURATED FATTY ACID	
Oleic	Olive oil, grapeseed (canola) oil, beef
POLYUNSATURATED FATTY ACIDS	
Linoleic	Corn oil, cottonseed oil, safflower oil, sunflower oil
Linolenic acid	Green leafy vegetables, soybean oil, soybean products (tofu), canola oil
Eicosapentaenoic acid	Mackerel, sardines, lake trout
Docosahexaenoic acid	Salmon, tuna, bluefish, halibut

Monounsaturated fats are becoming increasingly favored over both saturated and polyunsaturated fats, because monounsaturated fats help prevent the lowering of HDL, or "good," cholesterol and are not associated with cancer, as are high intakes of polyunsaturated fats (see Chapter 11). Table 2-2 and Figure 2-4 show how food fats break down in saturated, monounsaturated, and polyunsaturated fat percentages—note that you can visually determine this based on degree of solidity versus liquidity at cold temperatures (see Figure 2-3).

What Are the Functions of Essential Fatty Acids?

Essential fatty acids are necessary for the nutritional well-being of all animals and must be supplied in the diet. The principal essential fatty acid for humans is called **linoleic acid** and is found in vegetable oils. Two others, **arachidonic acid** and **linolenic acid**, are essential, but the body can usually produce them if adequate linoleic acid is consumed.

These essential fatty acids have multiple purposes, including maintenance of the functioning and integrity of cellular and subcellular membranes, cholesterol metabolism regulation, and acting as the precursor of a group of hormone-like compounds (**prostaglandins**).

What Are the Functions of Cholesterol?

Cholesterol has an essential role in the structure of adrenal and sex hormones and in increasing the body's production of vitamin D through the exposure of

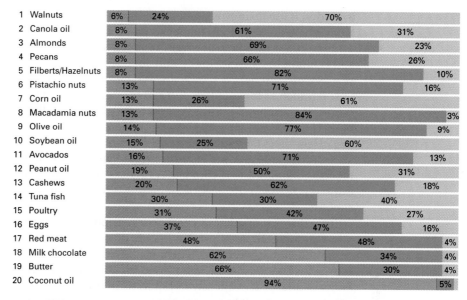

FIGURE 2-4 Degree of saturation in common foods (in percentages). Percentages are based on the total amount of saturated, monosaturated, and polyunsaturated fats. *Purple,* saturated fat; *green,* monounsaturated fat; *orange,* polyunsaturated fat. Reference for fat content modified from Jean AT, Pennington, Bowes, and Church: Food values of portions commonly used, ed 17, Philadelphia, JB Lippincott, 1997.

ultraviolet light to the skin. It is made and stored in the liver and also occurs in the form of a lipoprotein in the blood. In susceptible individuals, excess cholesterol intake contributes to fatty deposits in blood vessels and arteries, which in turn contributes to cardiovascular disease. There is, however, growing evidence that cholesterol in food is not as harmful to health as was once thought (see Chapter 8).

What Is the Difference Between Fat and Cholesterol?

Fat is similar to carbohydrate in that it is composed of carbon, hydrogen, and oxygen. However, it differs from carbohydrate in that it contains a greater concentration of carbon, which leads to higher energy values (at least 9 kcal/g versus 4 kcal/g for carbohydrate). Saturated fat contains more hydrogen than does unsaturated fat. Fat is listed on food labels as total fat and is then broken down into the saturated, monounsaturated, and polyunsaturated forms (often the unsaturated fats are added together on the food label). If saturated fatty acids predominate, the fat is called saturated; if unsaturated fatty acids predominate, the fat is called unsaturated or, more specifically, either polyunsaturated or mono-unsaturated. Oleic acid, which is found in nuts, seeds, olives, canola oil, and avocados, is the main type of monounsaturated fat (olives and avocados also contain carbohydrate, but are higher in fat content).

Polyunsaturated fat is generally referred to as linoleic and linolenic fatty acids and is found in corn, safflower, and sunflower oils (see Table 2-2). Saturated fat (e.g., stearic and butyric fatty acids) is typically found in products containing animal fat, such as milk, butter, and red meat. It is important to note that mineral oil is not considered a food fat because it cannot be digested and used by the body. If used as a laxative, it should never be taken near mealtime because it can negatively affect fat-soluble vitamin absorption.

Lipids include all types of fats and fat-related compounds. Cholesterol is a fat-related compound that contains zero kcals. It is found only in animal fats because it is made in the liver of animals. Fat from plant sources does not contain cholesterol.

Fats that are of a liquid consistency at room temperature are usually called oils. Oils are composed predominantly of the unsaturated fatty acids; the solid fats are the saturated forms. The most unsaturated form of fat is called **omega-3 fatty acid**. Fish from cold-water areas are high in this kind of unsaturated fat. Polyunsaturated fats will stay in liquid form if placed in the refrigerator, monounsaturated fats will become viscous, and saturated fats will become so hard that you have to cut them.

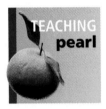

TEACHING pearl

The fat in cold-water fish is mainly of the most unsaturated form, called omega-3 fatty acids, which does not solidify in the cold arctic waters. Imagine what would happen to these fish if their body fat consisted of saturated fat—they would solidify and sink. Thus fish from cold arctic waters have to be high in omega-3 fatty acids to survive.

The difference in degree of saturation relates to the amount of hydrogen in the fat molecule. Hydrogen atoms can be added to unsaturated liquid oils to make them more solid. By adding hydrogen, the oil becomes a spread, or margarine. These are called hydrogenated fats. This form of fat contains **trans fatty acid**, which may contribute to a higher risk of cardiovascular disease. Solid stick margarines have the most hydrogen added, with tub margarines having less, and liquid margarines having the least. All liquid oils in moderation are heart healthy and can lower a person's cholesterol level as long as no weight gain occurs.

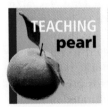

TEACHING pearl

A tip for explaining hydrogenation to patients is to say, "Hydrogen is found in water. When clothes are hanging on the clothesline and soaking wet, we could say they are saturated with water, just as fat containing a great deal of hydrogen is saturated. The more hydrogen in a fat, the more saturated it is."

Both fats and oils are composed principally of triglycerides and various fatty acids in various proportions. These differences contribute to flavor and other properties of food and have health implications. Triglycerides consist of a base of glycerol with three fatty acids and are the main type of fat circulating in the bloodstream. **Diglycerides** have two fatty acids, whereas **monoglycerides** have one.

Fats are insoluble in water. **Glycerol** is a small, water-soluble carbohydrate. The addition of glycerol to fats in the body assists in the transport through the water-based bloodstream, but contributes insignificant amounts of carbohydrate.

Fallacy: It is better to use butter because we now know margarine also contributes to heart disease.

Fact: Although margarine does contain trans fatty acids, which promote cardiovascular disease, butter is no better. Butter contains both saturated fat and cholesterol, increasing the risk of heart disease. Liquid margarines contain insignificant amounts of hydrogen when compared with the harder margarines and therefore contain less trans fatty acids. We might adopt the practice of Italian cuisine, in which bread is dipped in olive oil rather than butter or margarine, thereby avoiding saturated and hydrogenated fats. Traditional Italian restaurants and many restaurants in California offer olive oil on the table for use with bread.

What Are the Recommendations for Intake of Fats and Cholesterol?

There are no specific requirements for fat other than the body's need for the essential fatty acids, which is usually met through a diet that contains appropriate food fats. A minimum of 20 g of fat can meet the body's need for essential fatty acids if the appropriate fats are consumed. The Committee on Diet and Health of the Food and Nutrition Board has recently recommended that individual intake not exceed 10% of kcals for either polyunsaturated or saturated fats. The balance of fat should come from monounsaturated fats, with many advocates recommending that these fats should account for up to 20% of kcals. Most authorities recommend a maximum of 30% of total caloric intake from fat, with equal distribution of polyunsaturated, monounsaturated, and saturated fats. Some individuals may benefit from a higher fat intake—up to 35%—as long as monounsaturated or omega-3 fatty acids predominate (see Chapters 6 and 8). The Step One Diet of the National Cholesterol Education Program (NCEP) recommends less than 10% saturated fat and less than 300 mg of cholesterol per day, whereas the Step Two diet recommends lowering intake of saturated fat to 6% to 7% of total kcals (see Chapter 8) and cholesterol to less than 200 mg per day. A diet low in both saturated fatty acids and trans fatty acids should be promoted.

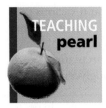

In patient education, you might explain that peanuts are cholesterol free because they grow in the ground. You can add to this by saying that cholesterol is found only in animal fats. Most nuts can be safely eaten when a higher intake of monounsaturated fat is acceptable, such as in the treatment of hyperlipidemia when HDL cholesterol levels are low (see Chapter 8). Nuts that contain mainly monounsaturated fats are grown in the temperate climate zones (tropical nuts such as brazil nuts and cashews contain relatively high amounts of saturated fat), whereas the nut of the coldest climate zones (the walnut) contains mainly polyunsaturated fat (see Figure 2-4).

What Quantities of Food Are Needed to Meet the Fat Recommendations?

The fat content of the recommended servings in the Food Guide Pyramid ranges from a low of about 20 g (if the minimum number of food servings is consumed using skim milk, lean meat, and unprocessed grain products) to 80 g if whole milk and high-fat meats are used. It is not unusual for Americans to consume 100 to 150 g of fat per day.

There are 5 g of fat in each teaspoon of added fat or oils and on average 5 g for every ounce of red meat (but only 1 to 2 g for white meat, fish, and legumes; see Figure 4-1). Steak contains 8 g of fat per ounce (which is why it is so tender and juicy), whereas stew beef has only 3 g per ounce (which is why you have to cook it in liquid for a long time to tenderize the meat). Thus a person eating a pound of white-meat chicken (without the skin) will consume only 16 g of fat (with about 5 g of saturated fat—about 30% of the total fat—see Figure 2-4), whereas someone eating the same amount of steak will consume 128 g of fat— literally ½ c of lard (and 64 g of saturated fat—3 days' worth—or about 50% of the total fat). A food containing 3 g or less of fat per serving is considered a low-fat food. This includes grains that do not have significant amounts of fat added, such as sliced bread used to make sandwiches, pasta, vegetables, most cereals, and most fruits (except coconuts, avocados, and olives). Also low in fat is 1% milk because it contains less than 3 g of fat per cup.

What Are the Recommendations for Fat Substitutes?

Simplesse consists of very small particles of protein, generally of milk origin. These microparticles of protein provide a creamy consistency similar to fat. Simplesse is all natural and fat free, although it is not free of kcals because it contains protein. Simplesse will increasingly be found in food products because of its acceptability. It is generally safe to use, even in large quantities, except for persons with an allergy to milk, because Simplesse contains milk protein (see Chapter 5).

Olestra is another fat substitute that still has some unresolved problems because it is not digestible. The consequence is that excess intake can cause unpleasant gastrointestinal problems such as diarrhea and many experts feel it may contribute to inadequate absorption of food nutrients such as fat-soluble vitamins. Moderate intake of products containing olestra appears appropriate. For this reason, it has received approval by the FDA and is now being used in food products such as potato chips.

HOW ARE PERCENTAGES OF THE MACRONUTRIENTS IN THE DIET CALCULATED?

The percentage of kcals from protein in relationship to the total dietary intake is calculated by first multiplying the number of grams of protein in the diet by 4 (to find the number of kcals) and then dividing that number by the total caloric intake from all foods consumed in one day. For example, a 2000-kcal diet containing both animal and vegetable sources of protein in the form of 3 c of milk (24 g protein), 6 slices of bread (18 g protein), 3 vegetables (6 g protein), and 4 oz of meat (28 g protein) for a total of 76 g of protein would be calculated as follows:

$$76 \times 4 = 304 \text{ kcal}$$
$$304 \div 2000 \text{ kcal} = 0.15 = 15\% \text{ protein}$$

The same calculation can be used to find carbohydrate percentage (excluding fiber content because fiber is not digestible and therefore provides no kcals). For calculating the fat percentage, the number of fat grams should be multiplied by 9 because fats yield 9 kcal/g.

WHAT IS THE ROLE OF THE NURSE OR OTHER HEALTH CARE PROFESSIONAL IN EDUCATING THE PUBLIC ABOUT CARBOHYDRATE, PROTEIN, AND FAT INTAKE?

The goal of a nurse or other health care professional should be to educate patients about the positive role of carbohydrate, protein, and fat in their diets and to promote proper consumption of different sorts of foods, as based on the Food Guide Pyramid. The health care professional should use good interviewing skills in determining a patient's current dietary habits and the reasons such practices are being followed (for example, adherence to physician advice, which may have been given years ago; dental problems; or health beliefs). Some patients may be receptive to dietary change when given a reason, whereas others may resist strongly. The nurse should never argue or give the impression of arguing, but rather should indicate respect for a patient's food choices and health beliefs while introducing new ideas about healthy diets.

Promoting consumption of complex carbohydrate and dietary fiber food sources (with adequate fluids) and providing information on current thinking related to fiber constitutes an appropriate role for the health care professional. The minimum number of food servings portrayed at the base of the Food Guide Pyramid provide adequate carbohydrate and fiber. Sugar, although a carbohydrate, should be promoted as the Food Guide Pyramid portrays: as the tip of the diet, not something to fill up on.

The health care professional can help reeducate the public about how much protein in the daily diet the body really needs. The amount of protein we consume can generally be safely decreased, but an assessment of a patient's usual dietary intake should be made before automatically recommending a reduced amount. In the past, the emphasis in meal planning was to have meat as the main part of the meal with side dishes such as starchy foods and vegetables. It is now recommended that we view meat as the side dish and emphasize vegetables and grains.

Many individuals are now aware that controlling the fat content of their diet plays a key role in the prevention and management of chronic diseases such as obesity, cardiovascular disease, and cancer. However, the health care professionals can help the public recognize that not all fats are bad and that too much of a reduction in fat intake can have adverse health implications. Beyond this awareness, individuals need to learn what foods are low in saturated fat and cholesterol; these foods should be promoted in a way that makes them practical and appealing to consume. Alternatives to meat, such as legumes, can be promoted simply by indicating verbally that they can be a delicious part of a meal (as bean burritos or baked beans, for example).

Finally, the health care professional should recognize when referral to a qualified nutritionist or registered dietitian is appropriate for highly motivated individuals or those at risk for obesity, cardiovascular disease, diabetes, cancer, or those who have not had success on a low-fat diet.

CHAPTER STUDY QUESTIONS AND CLASSROOM ACTIVITIES

1. What are the three different kinds of carbohydrate?
2. What is the difference between soluble and insoluble fiber? Provide examples of foods with the two types of fiber.
3. Write a healthy day's menu that provides 20 to 30 g of fiber.
4. How does protein differ from carbohydrate and fat?
5. What is the difference between a complete and an incomplete protein?
6. What are some of the nutritional problems associated with excess and insufficient protein intakes?
7. Describe the texture of saturated versus unsaturated fats.
8. *Class activity.* Students are to bring in a sample of crackers and their respective food labels. In class, students will estimate how many crackers would take up the same amount of space as a slice of bread. Compare this estimate with the food label (how many crackers does it take to equal 15 g of carbohydrates?). Then compare fat content and texture of the various crackers (hard or crumbly) for one serving of starch.
9. If a food label states that one bagel contains 60 g of carbohydrate, how many servings of grain would it contain?

CRITICAL THINKING

Case Study

Anna and her friends were having a discussion while eating lunch. Was it better to eat a submarine sandwich without mayonnaise or a quarter pounder with cheese, no bun? Anna was saying that there was a better alternative to either type of meal. The traditional Mediterranean style of eating she grew up with had been a major factor in getting her dad's diabetes under control. She knew that her own battle with weight needed a balance between carbohydrate and fat and that she benefited from fiber, which neither the sub or the burger provided. She added up the carbohydrate in a 12-inch sub—120 g, or over one third of the day's recommended amount—which her father's dietitian had taught the family. The burger with cheese was not much better, having no carbohydrate but at least 15 g saturated fat, with the daily guideline being less than 20 g. She saw some nods of acceptance of her suggestion that beans and greens and moderate amounts of monounsaturated fat such as those found in olive oil and nuts were the best compromise for short- and long-term health goals and needs. They all eagerly dipped their bread into the olive oil that was on the table at the restaurant.

Critical Thinking Applications

1. Describe what type of restaurant might serve olive oil for dipping bread.
2. Discuss family experience of students regarding low-fat versus low-carbohydrate diets.
3. Discuss experience of students regarding satiety value of low-fat, low-fiber meals such as pasta versus high-fat, high-fiber meals such as bean burritos and guacamole.

REFERENCES

Dessein PH, Shipton EA, Stanwix AE, Joffe BI, Ramokgadi J: Beneficial effects of weight loss associated with moderate calorie/carbohydrate restriction, and increased proportional intake of protein and unsaturated fat on serum urate and lipoprotein levels in gout: a pilot study. Ann Rheum Dis. July 2000; 59(7):539.

Granfeldt Y, Eliasson AC, Bjorck I: An examination of the possibility of lowering the glycemic index of oat and barley flakes by minimal processing. J Nutr. September 2000; 130(9):2207.

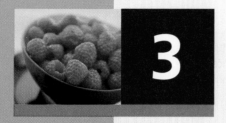

3 Digestion, Absorption, and Metabolism in Health and Disease

OBJECTIVES

After completing this chapter, you should be able to:

- Describe the mechanical and chemical processes of digestion, absorption, and metabolism of foods.
- Describe the digestion and metabolism of carbohydrates, proteins, and fats.
- Summarize the role of the mouth, stomach, and intestines in the digestive process in health and disease states.
- Describe the role of enzymes and the endocrine system on digestion, absorption, and cell metabolism.
- Describe the metabolism and effect of alcohol on digestion, absorption, and metabolism of food nutrients.
- Describe the role of the nurse or other health care professional in aiding the digestive and metabolic processes.

TERMS TO IDENTIFY

Absorption	Cholecystitis	Diverticulosis
Achalasia	Cholelithiasis	Duodenum
Albumin	Chyme	Dyspepsia
Amino acids	Cirrhosis	Dysphagia
Anabolism	Cleft palate	Encopresis
Ascites	Constipation	Endocrine system
Aspiration pneumonia	Crohn's disease	Enzyme
Basal metabolism	Counterregulatory	Esophageal reflux
Bile	hormones	Esophageal varices
Capillaries	Cystic fibrosis	Fatty acids
Catabolism	Diarrhea	Gastritis
Celiac sprue	Digestion	Gliadin
Cholecystikinin	Diverticulitis	Gluconeogenesis

Continued

INTRODUCTION

Good nutrition goes beyond obtaining and consuming appropriate amounts of carbohydrate, protein, and fat. Without adequate digestion, absorption in the intestinal tract, and metabolism at the cell level, the energy macronutrients cannot be used for their intended biologic functions. Vitamins and minerals found in food also require absorption through the gastrointestinal (GI) tract and are necessary for optimal use of the energy macronutrients. The specifics on vitamins and minerals essential for good health is reviewed in the following chapter.

The GI tract is much more than a long tube with a few attachments (the liver, the gallbladder, and the pancreas) that allows food to pass through. It is a major endocrine gland, producing a wide variety of hormones and digestive enzymes that control how food is digested, absorbed, and metabolized. The process of digestion and cellular metabolism can affect nutritional status and health as much as food choices can. Health care professionals need to be aware of the effect of digestion and metabolism on the use of food nutrients.

WHAT IS MEANT BY THE DIGESTION, ABSORPTION, AND METABOLISM OF FOODS?

Digestion is the change of food from a complex to a simpler form and from an insoluble to a soluble state in the digestive tract. These changes facilitate absorption through the intestinal walls into circulation for eventual use by the body cells (Figure 3-1). The processes of digestion occur simultaneously:

1. *Physical (mechanical)*: During the physical, or mechanical, process, food is broken into small particles in the mouth, then mixed with digestive juices by a churning action in the stomach, and then propelled through the digestive tract in rhythmic movements known as **peristalsis**.

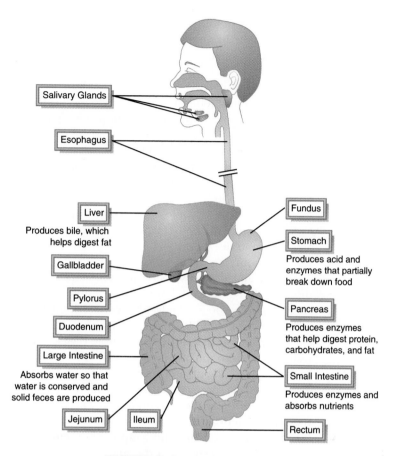

Salivary Glands

Esophagus

Liver
Produces bile, which
helps digest fat

Gallbladder

Pylorus

Duodenum

Large Intestine
Absorbs water so that
water is conserved and
solid feces are produced

Jejunum   Ileum

Fundus

Stomach
Produces acid and
enzymes that partially
break down food

Pancreas
Produces enzymes
that help digest protein,
carbohydrates, and fat

Small Intestine
Produces enzymes and
absorbs nutrients

Rectum

FIGURE 3-1 The digestive system.

2. *Chemical:* During the chemical process, enzymes in digestive juices change food nutrients into simple soluble forms that can be absorbed: carbohydrate to simple sugars, fat to fatty acids and glycerol, and protein to amino acids. This chemical breakdown, called **hydrolysis**, involves adding water to molecules. Water, simple sugars, salts, vitamins, and minerals require no digestion.

Each digestive **enzyme** (chemicals produced by the body to break food down in preparation for absorption in the intestinal tract) has a specific action and optimal conditions under which it acts. The name of each group of enzymes ends in *ase*: amylases act on starch, lipases act on fat, and proteases act on protein. Other enzymes include lactase (to digest lactose) and sucrase (to digest sucrose). If there is inadequate digestion of the macronutrients, absorption in the intestinal tract cannot take place. Abdominal cramping and diarrhea can result from inadequate digestion, especially with carbohydrates and fats.

Other chemical substances assist in the physical and chemical processes, such as hydrochloric acid and mucin in the gastric secretion. **Bile**, which promotes the digestion of fat, is excreted from the liver into the gallbladder where it is stored and then released into the small intestine after intake of a meal containing fat. Certain **hormones** (chemicals produced by the body) influence the body's use of nutrients found in food.

Digestibility of food refers to the rapidity and ease of digestion and to its completeness. Liquid foods and thoroughly masticated solid foods are more rapidly digested than are foods left in large pieces. The well-masticated food begins to leave the stomach 15 to 30 minutes after ingestion. Forms of liquid sugar such as fruit juice leave an empty stomach almost immediately.

Foods that stay in the stomach longer have a higher **satiety** (satisfaction from eating) value. Small meals move out of the stomach faster than do larger ones. Solid foods stay in the stomach longer than liquids. The amount and type of food eaten at one time also affect the rapidity of digestion.

Of the three macronutrients, carbohydrates are digested and leave the stomach most rapidly (about 1 hour), proteins are digested and leave less rapidly (about 2 hours), and fats require the longest time for digestion (about 4 hours). Thus a balanced meal stays in the stomach longer than a meal of only carbohydrate foods. Foods containing a large amount of soluble fiber are digested more slowly than are low-fiber foods. A meal high in both fat and fiber takes the longest to digest and leave the stomach.

Absorption is the passage of soluble digested food materials through the intestinal walls into the blood, either directly or through osmosis by way of the lymphatic system. The greater part of absorption takes place in the small intestine. Tiny fingerlike projections called **villi**, which contain small **capillaries** (tiny blood vessels), line the intestinal wall. The villi are in constant motion and trap the tiny nutrients, which are then taken in by the adjacent cells and transported through the circulatory and lymphatic system to every body cell. Microvilli are even smaller projections on the surface of the villi (Figure 3-2).

Simple sugars, amino acids, a few fatty acids, minerals, and water-soluble vitamins reach the general circulation through the capillaries. Water is absorbed from the large intestine. Absorbed materials are carried by the blood to the liver and from there to various organs and tissues to be used as needed. The body is able to digest and absorb about 90% to 98% of an average mixed diet.

Metabolism is a general term covering all physical and chemical changes that food nutrients undergo after their absorption from the GI tract and use at the cell level. Simple sugars, amino acids, fatty acids, and glycerol are all used by the body cells either for energy needs or for building of new tissue.

If the metabolic change is of a constructive nature, resulting in the building up of new substances, it is called **anabolism**; if it is of a destructive or oxidative nature, resulting in the release of energy, it is called **catabolism**. Energy metabolism refers to the oxidation of the macronutrients (carbohydrate, protein, and fat) within the body resulting in the release of heat and energy. **Metabolic rate** refers to the rate in which food energy is burned, with a high metabolic rate requiring a high amount of calories and low metabolic rate requiring few calories to sustain life.

All metabolism happens at the cell level with the human body cells acting like small furnaces to burn food energy (catabolism) and allow for anabolism. It is at

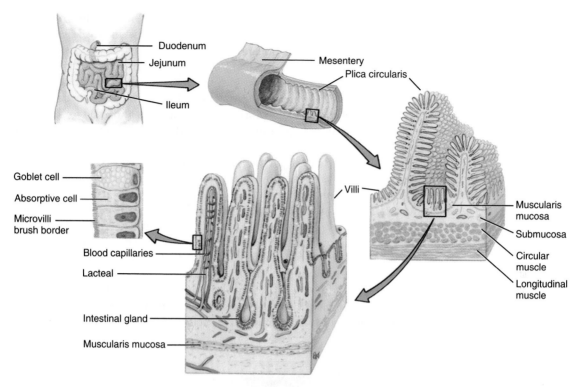

FIGURE 3-2 Wall of the small intestine. (From Applegate EJ: The Anatomy and Physiology Learning System, ed 2, Philadelphia, 2000, WB Saunders, Figure 16-9, p. 339.)

the cell level that very complex biochemical reactions take place. Food nutrients must enter the body cells in order for the body to metabolize or use these nutrients. Thus good digestion and absorption of food nutrients is essential for proper metabolism at the cellular level.

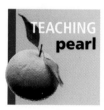

TEACHING pearl   If you "fan a fire" you know it will burn better. This is somewhat like our own increased intake of air or oxygen from aerobic exercise—our metabolic rate increases because we are "fanning the fire" in the body cells.

What Is Basal Metabolism?

The body needs energy for the internal, involuntary activities of organs and tissues and oxidation within the tissues. Energy is also needed for circulation, respiration, digestion, elimination, and maintenance of muscle tone, heartbeat, and so on. All internal activities continue 24 hours a day, both while a person is asleep and awake. The amount of energy required to sustain these processes alone is known as the **basal metabolism**.

The basal metabolic rate is influenced by body composition, body size, and age. The more muscle tissue a person has, the more calories are needed. The basal metabolic rate varies from person to person, but on the average it amounts to approximately 1200 to 1400 kilocalories daily for women and 1600 to 1800 kcal daily for men. Total energy requirements and weight management are discussed in Chapter 7.

A simple and relatively accurate method of estimating daily basal metabolism is to multiply weight in kilograms by 0.9 for women and 1.0 for men and then by 24 (the number of hours in a day). This estimate is generally accurate enough, except during times of physiologic stress (see Chapter 5). In large institutions, metabolic carts are used to measure a person's oxygen intake and carbon dioxide output. This technique can precisely measure the basal metabolic kilocalorie needs. Various measurements of oxygen intake and carbon dioxide output have been used over the years to determine basal metabolic rate (Figure 3-3).

The process of digestion and absorption requires energy. Total food intake alters metabolism. Increased eating raises metabolism and vice versa. This is referred to as the **specific dynamic action**. This action raises the total energy needs

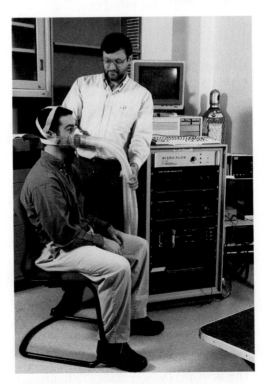

FIGURE 3-3 Measuring metabolic rate.

about 10% for a person who eats a mixed diet. With hunger, low blood sugar can result. This is associated with a reduced metabolic rate and reduced levels of the hormone **cholecystikinin** that curbs hunger (Szekely, 2000).

HOW ARE THE MACRONUTRIENTS DIGESTED AND ABSORBED?

Carbohydrates

Carbohydrates (except for fiber) are easily digested and the degree of absorption is high. Digestion of starch starts in the mouth with ptyalin and is completed in the small intestine. **Glucose** (blood sugar), which is normally formed from carbohydrates eaten in food, is absorbed into the bloodstream through the walls of the small intestine and is metabolized as shown in Figure 3-4.

Simple sugars such as glucose and fructose are ready for absorption in the digestive tract without digestion. Double sugars such as sucrose must be changed to simple sugars for absorption, which is a quick process when there is adequate enzyme production. Double sugars are digested and absorbed in the small intestine (Figure 3-5).

Complex carbohydrates such as starch require two digestive steps to be changed to simple sugar (glucose) for absorption in the intestinal tract. Cooking starch facilitates digestion because it breaks down the cell walls, which makes the action of the digestive enzymes easier.

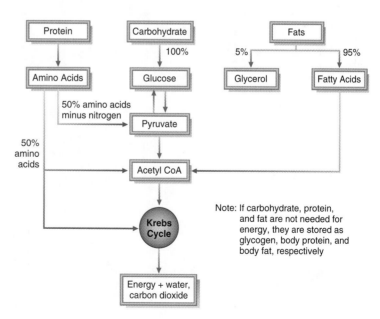

FIGURE 3-4 Metabolic pathways.

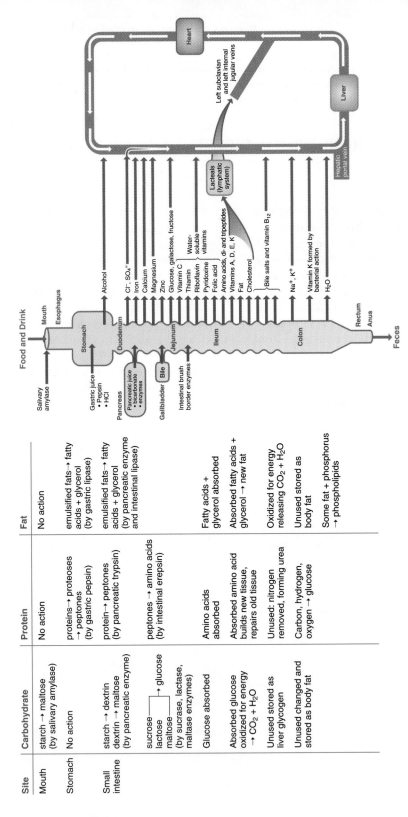

FIGURE 3-5 Digestive process of carbohydrate, protein, and fat. (Key: Cl⁻ = chloride; CO_2 = carbon dioxide; HCl = hydrochloric acid; H_2O = water; K⁺ = potassium; Na⁺ = sodium; SO_4 = sulfate.) (Modified from Mahan LK: Krause's food, nutrition, and diet therapy, ed 10, Philadelphia, WB Saunders, 2000, Figure 1-8, p. 16.)

Dietary fiber is essentially indigestible and passes through the intestinal tract virtually unchanged. Bacteria naturally found in the GI tract do allow for minimal digestion of fiber. Because most unprocessed plant foods contain fiber, the process of digestion is slower for them than for sugar and low-fiber plant food products such as white bread.

The carbon part of carbohydrate is used as energy in animal cells, similar to the burning of carbon in coal and wood in actual furnaces. The black substance formed in burnt toast is carbon.

Protein

The protein in the daily diet must be broken down by digestion into the component parts, the **amino acids** and small peptides. Once protein is digested, it can be absorbed into the bloodstream from the small intestine. Digestion of protein is started in the stomach by enzymes in the gastric juice and is continued and completed in the small intestine by enzymes from the pancreatic and intestinal juices (see Figure 3-5).

Fat

Fats, because they are insoluble in water, require special treatment in the GI tract before absorption can take place. No digestion of fat takes place in the mouth and only finely emulsified fats (such as those found in butter, cream, and egg yolk) can start to be digested in the stomach. For the most part, fats must be emulsified by bile (produced in the liver and stored in the gallbladder for use in fat digestion) and bile salts before they are digested in the small intestine by enzymes from the pancreatic juice. Fats are changed to **glycerol** and **fatty acids** during digestion (see Figure 3-4).

Fatty foods are generally digested without difficulty, but they require a longer time for digestion than do carbohydrates. Softer fats are more completely digested and absorbed than are harder fats. Fried foods are not necessarily indigestible, but are more slowly digested. The presence of carbohydrates in the diet is necessary for the complete **oxidation** of fats (the chemical step in releasing energy from fat) in the tissues; otherwise, ketone bodies accumulate and ketosis results.

How Are Macronutrients Converted to Energy?

When the body cells need energy, a series of complex metabolic reactions occur called the **Krebs cycle** (see Figure 3-4, which shows the central pathways of energy metabolism). Oxygen is necessary for the release of energy by the cells in the body. The process of combining oxygen with a molecule is called oxidation. A person needs hemoglobin to supply oxygen to the cells, and a low level of hemoglobin means oxygen is not available for energy production, which results in a tired feeling. An increased intake of air into the body, such as that achieved with aerobic exercise, tends to raise the body's rate of metabolism through the process of oxidation (see Chapter 7).

WHAT ROLE IS PLAYED BY EACH PART OF THE DIGESTIVE TRACT?

The Mouth

The teeth provide the first mechanical function of chewing, with the cutting action of the anterior teeth (incisors) and the grinding action of the posterior teeth (molars). Chewing aids the digestion of food for a simple reason; that is, the digestive enzymes act only on the surface of food particles and thorough chewing increases the amount of food surface area available to these enzymes.

Another mechanical function is performed by saliva, which moistens food and prepares it for swallowing. A chemical function of the mouth is changing cooked starch to dextrin and then to maltose by the salivary enzyme ptyalin (amylase).

Physical disorders can begin where digestion starts—in the mouth, or oral cavity. One type of birth defect with the oral cavity is **cleft palate** (an opening or hole in the roof of the mouth sometimes extending to the lip). Babies born with cleft palate have difficulty creating a suction seal around their mother's nipple or a bottle nipple, which leads to inadequate ingestion of breast milk or formula. Severe cases may require surgical correction. Babies with less severe forms of cleft palate, however, may benefit from special bottle nipples that do not require suction or from a slightly larger hole in the bottle nipple. Mothers who are motivated to continue nursing until the problem is resolved should be encouraged to do so with supplemental bottle feedings as needed (see Chapter 12 for more ideas).

Missing teeth or severe dental caries can adversely affect food choices. Persons with dental problems may have a low fiber intake because of difficulty in chewing. Without adequate nutritional knowledge, omitting food groups may not seem important to a person with dental problems. Alternatives should be discussed, such as eating applesauce in place of fresh apples, or eating cooked or soft vegetables in place of raw or hard-to-chew vegetables. Prevention of dental caries is addressed in Chapter 13.

Swallowing problems, referred to as **dysphagia**, are often related to stroke, head injury, cerebral palsy, and other conditions (Figure 3-6). Inability to swallow correctly may result in aspiration of food into the lungs. **Aspiration pneumonia** is a frequent complication of dysphagia. Dysphagia requires a review of the swallowing process to determine the best means of feeding. A speech pathologist is trained to help assess swallowing problems. An x-ray examination called **videofluoroscopy** is used in conjunction with a barium swallow to objectively diagnose dysphagia. Liquids are usually the most difficult food to swallow for persons with dysphagia. Liquids thickened with a commercial product such as THICK-IT™ or with baby rice cereal or other thickener may be easier for a patient with dysphagia to swallow. Feeding positions can also help (see Chapter 5). Table 3-1 lists food consistency considerations.

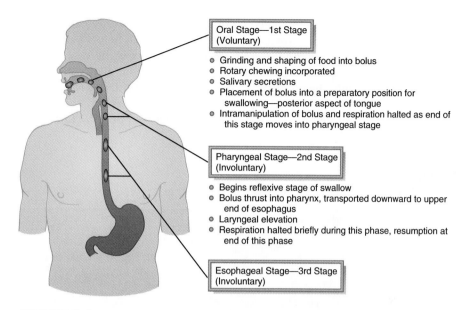

Oral Stage—1st Stage
(Voluntary)

- Grinding and shaping of food into bolus
- Rotary chewing incorporated
- Salivary secretions
- Placement of bolus into a preparatory position for
  swallowing—posterior aspect of tongue
- Intramanipulation of bolus and respiration halted as end of
  this stage moves into pharyngeal stage

Pharyngeal Stage—2nd Stage
(Involuntary)

- Begins reflexive stage of swallow
- Bolus thrust into pharynx, transported downward to upper
  end of esophagus
- Laryngeal elevation
- Respiration halted briefly during this phase, resumption at
  end of this phase

Esophageal Stage—3rd Stage
(Involuntary)

FIGURE 3-6 The stages of swallowing as they relate to appropriate food pathways.

Fallacy: Washing food down with water is a good habit.

Fact: Food must be chewed thoroughly so that it can be mixed with saliva, which aids digestion. However, a glass of water at mealtime is beneficial to the digestive process, as long as it does not take the place of mastication.

Esophagus

In general, swallowing can be divided into the following three stages: (1) the voluntary stage, which initiates the swallowing process, or *mechanical function*; (2) the pharyngeal stage, which is involuntary and involves the passage of food through the pharynx to the esophagus; and (3) the esophageal stage, which involves passage of food through the esophagus to the stomach through peristaltic wave contractions.

The esophagus transfers food from the oral cavity to the stomach. This process is complicated and can go awry with neurologic or neuromuscular disorders. Respiration is generally only minimally stopped during the act of swallowing. Poorly chewed food, however, increases the risk of obstruction of the airway, especially for persons with an impaired swallowing reflex, in whom oxygen deprivation can occur as breathing and swallowing cannot be done simultaneously.

In **achalasia,** the lower part of the esophagus fails to relax and swallowing difficulty occurs. The individual senses fullness in the sternal region and may vomit; then there is danger that the contents of the esophagus may be aspirated into the respiratory passages. Weight loss may become a problem that requires nutritional intervention. Dilation of the esophagus or surgical intervention can improve the condition. Including semisolid foods can help a person manage this condition.

The condition of **esophageal reflux** is the opposite of achalasia. The lower esophageal sphincter is incompetent and allows stomach matter to regurgitate into the esophagus. Gastroesophageal reflux disease (GERD) is considered common in the elderly and may present various symptoms, such as heartburn and regurgitation. The sphincter pressure may become low from a variety of causes in-

TABLE 3-1
FOOD CONSISTENCY CONSIDERATIONS

TYPE OF DIET	EXAMPLE	POTENTIAL EFFECT ON ORAL FUNCTION
Thin foods and liquids	Soup broth, juice	More difficult to control within mouth, especially with limited tongue control (i.e., quickly runs to all areas of mouth); often promotes excessive food loss
Thick foods	Pudding, yogurt, applesauce	Improved control within oral cavity because of reduced flow and increased sensory input (i.e., weight and texture)
Pastelike or sticky foods	Peanut butter, thick cheese sauce	May be more difficult to move in oral cavity with limited tongue movement; may stick to the roof of the mouth, especially with a high, narrow palate
Slippery foods	Pasta, Jell-O	Often difficult to control and either triggers reflexive swallow too quickly or runs out of oral cavity before the swallow
Smooth textures	Pudding, pureed foods	Relatively easy to swallow; promotes minimal tongue and jaw movement, especially over time
Coarse textures	Creamed corn, ground foods, Sloppy Joe filling	Increases sensory input to stimulate more jaw and tongue movement; coarseness of food should be carefully graded
Varied textures	Soups with noodles or chunks of vegetables	Difficult to manage in oral cavity, especially with limited tongue movement or decreased oral sensitivity (i.e., liquid is swallowed and solid pieces remain in the mouth)
Scattering textures	Grated carrots, rice, coleslaw, corn bread	Very difficult to manage with limited tongue movement and decreased oral sensitivity
Crisp solids	Carrot sticks, celery sticks	Requires sophisticated biting and chewing to grind pieces into consistency that is safe to swallow
Milk-based substances	Milk, ice cream	Appear to coat mucous membranes in oral-pharyngeal cavities to interfere with swallowing
Broth	Meat broth, chicken broth	Appears to cut mucus in oral-pharyngeal cavity and facilitate swallowing
Dry foods	Bread, cake, cookie	May be difficult to chew or swallow with insufficient saliva
Whole, soft foods	Slice of bread	Requires the ability to bite off appropriately sized pieces

Courtesy of the Occupational Therapy Department of the J.N. Adam Developmental Center, Perrysburg, NY.

cluding a high-fat diet and central obesity with resulting regurgitation. Medications and hormonal variations can also play a role. Treatment may include weight loss to decrease abdominal pressure on the stomach. Additional treatment includes small, frequent meals to avoid stomach distention and avoidance of chocolate and fats, which reduce sphincter competence. Avoidance of caffeine and alcohol may help reduce stomach acidity. Drinking liquids between meals and remaining upright after eating also help.

The Stomach

The presence of food in the stomach stimulates functioning of the digestive tract. Food is kept in motion by the muscular walls of the stomach, which bring it into contact with the gastric juice secreted by stomach cells. The fundus of the stomach acts as a temporary storage place for food.

Various gastric juice enzymes work in the stomach to digest the different macronutrients. Complex proteins are partially digested by pepsin (protease); milk protein is coagulated by renin and then is partially digested by pepsin. Emulsified fats are digested to fatty acids and glycerol by lipase. Hydrochloric acid aids these digestive enzymes and increases the solubility of calcium and iron. Mucus protects the lining of the stomach from the hydrochloric acid. Once solid food is reduced to a semiliquid state (**chyme**), it is passed from the stomach to the small intestine.

Functional disorders of the stomach (reflex disorders) involve a change in body functions without detectable changes in structural tissue. One example is **dyspepsia** (indigestion). Alterations in hydrochloric acid content of gastric juice is another functional disorder.

A **hiatal hernia** is a protrusion of a part of the stomach through the esophageal hiatus (opening) of the diaphragm (Figure 3-7). Persons with this disorder sometimes complain of heartburn because of the reflux of gastric contents into the esophagus. Medical treatment includes ingestion of antacids to neutralize or inhibit gastric secretions and possibly surgery. Small, frequent meals are recommended to reduce symptoms, although dietary modifications cannot eliminate the cause. No food is advised for approximately 3 hours before bedtime and the person should remain in the upright position after eating. For the obese person, weight loss is indicated to help relieve pressure on the diaphragm. Any source of pressure on the abdomen, such as bandages or clothes that fit too tightly, should be eliminated.

Gastritis (acute or chronic) is an inflammation of the lining of the stomach that results in abdominal pain, nausea, and vomiting. It may be caused by food poisoning, overeating, excessive intake of alcohol, or bacterial and viral infections. A chronic condition may be related to other disease states. It often precedes the development of ulcers or cancer. Acute gastritis, which usually heals within a few days, is often treated first with antibiotics and neutralization of the stomach contents. The stomach is allowed to rest for a while and then the patient drinks clear fluids for the first day or two.

A **peptic ulcer** is an eroded lesion in the lining (mucosa) of the stomach (gastric ulcer) or duodenum (duodenal ulcer). Excess use of nonsteroidal antiin-

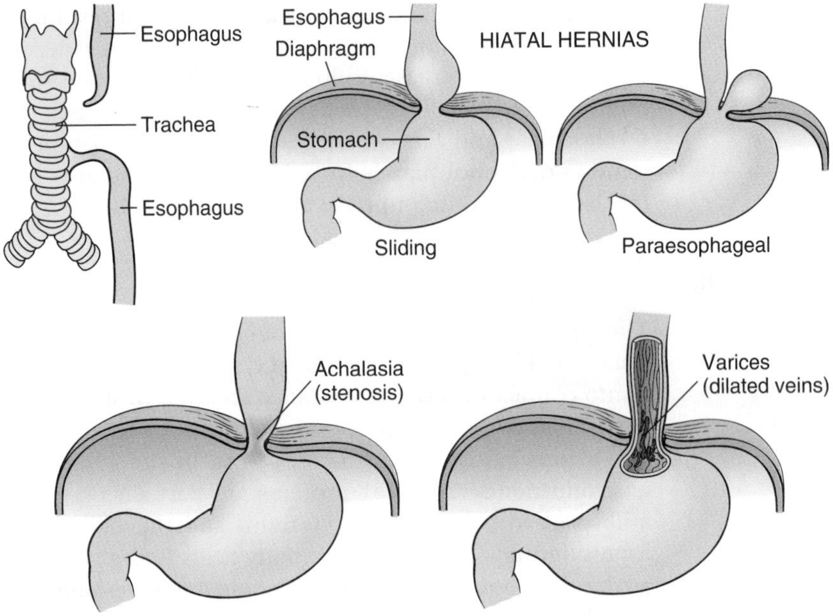

FIGURE 3-7   Sketch of hiatal hernia. (From Damjanov I: Pathology for the health-related professions, ed 2, Philadelphia, WB Saunders, 2000.)

▌TABLE 3-2
▌DIETARY TREATMENT OF PEPTIC ULCERS

GUIDELINE	RATIONALE
Eat three regular meals or six small meals	Inhibits stomach distention
Avoid caffeine-containing beverages, decaffeinated coffee	Decreases gastric secretions
Avoid alcohol	Reduces damage to stomach lining
Avoid black pepper, chili powder, cloves, nutmeg, curry powder, mustard seed	Reduces irritation to stomach lining
Avoid aspirin	Reduces irritation of stomach lining
Avoid cigarette smoking	Promotes healing of ulcer
Eat in a relaxed atmosphere	Reduces stress

flammatory drugs (NSAIDs) can contribute to the erosion of the mucosal lining. In recent years, the *Helicobacter pylori* infection has been increasingly recognized as being involved in the development of peptic ulcers. Symptoms include burning or gnawing pain in the pit of the stomach. While an ulcer is bleeding, no food is allowed; instead, the patient may be given intravenous feedings of dextrose and amino acids. As the condition improves, the patient usually progresses from a full liquid diet to a regular diet with the omission of irritants based on individual tolerances. Common intolerances include caffeine, alcohol, and spicy foods, but some individuals have no adversity with these substances (Table 3-2).

The Small Intestine

The small intestine is 20 ft long and is made up of the **duodenum** (the upper section), the **jejunum** (the middle section), and the **ileum** (the lower section). The food mass from a meal remains in the intestine for 3 to 8 hours, although liquids and pure carbohydrate foods pass more quickly. The gallbladder, pancreas, and liver are all connected with the small intestine.

Chyme mixes with the digestive juices of the small intestine and with pancreatic juices. Bicarbonate ions neutralize the chyme. Bile is excreted into the duodenum; it prepares unemulsified fats for digestion. Pancreatic enzymes finish starch and fat digestion and partially digest protein. The intestinal enzymes complete protein and carbohydrate digestion. Digested food moves with peristaltic waves through the small intestine where absorption of food nutrients occurs. The pancreas also produces hormones such as insulin that allows use of glucose as an energy source at the cell level after absorption occurs. Unused food, waste materials, and water move to the large intestine.

Lactose intolerance, the inability to digest milk sugar (lactose), is caused by a low amount of the enzyme lactase, which is necessary for converting lactose into glucose and galactose in the GI tract. Symptoms include bloating, flatulence, cramping, and diarrhea. Different populations show variations in degrees of lactase deficiency, usually occurring after 5 years of age. Lactase deficiency is more common among persons of African, Asian, Mediterranean, Hispanic, and Native American heritage than among persons of Northern European heritage.

Lactase deficiency can occur with anyone who has GI distress such as from the intestinal flu. Severe cases of lactase deficiency require avoidance of all foods containing lactose (see Box 3-1 for a sample menu). Many grocery stores now carry 100% lactose-free milk. The milk will taste sweeter than regular milk because the lactose is broken down into simple sugars. There will be no long-term health problem if lactose is accidentally ingested, however, because the condition is an intolerance, not an allergy.

The patient with lactose intolerance should be encouraged to try small amounts of milk products such as low-fat cheese or yogurt. These are often tolerated in mild forms of lactose intolerance. Repeated, small amounts of milk can increase the natural production of lactase by some individuals.

Celiac sprue, also called **nontropical sprue**, is a malabsorptive disorder and is characterized by destruction of intestinal villi from a protein known as **gliadin**, found in foods containing gluten. In this disorder the villi of the intestinal tract are damaged, resulting in impaired absorption of digested food. Symptoms include diarrhea, steatorrhea, and weight loss. **Gluten** is the protein portion of wheat, oats, rye, and barley.

The exact cause of celiac disease is unknown, but it occurs more frequently among persons of British heritage than among other groups. There is some evidence that stressful events precede the onset of this disease. Measurement of antigliadin antibody is useful in diagnosis, but an intestinal biopsy is required for final diagnosis. The patient is prescribed a gluten-free diet, in which all products containing gluten or gliadin are eliminated. This includes all foods containing the grains wheat, oat, rye, and barley or flavorings that are wheat based. Oat

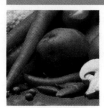

**BOX 3-1
SAMPLE
MENU FOR
A LACTOSE-
FREE DIET**

BREAKFAST

½ c orange juice
½ c farina
1 egg, soft cooked
2 slices Vienna bread toasted

2 tsp milk-free margarine
1 tbsp jelly
2 tsp sugar
Coffee or tea

LUNCH

2 oz sliced chicken
½ c rice
½ c green beans
½ sliced tomato on lettuce
2 tsp mayonnaise
1 slice Vienna bread

2 tsp milk-free margarine
½ c canned peaches
1 slice angel food cake
1 tsp sugar
Coffee or tea

MIDAFTERNOON SNACK

1 c apple juice

SUPPER

3 oz roast beef
½ c cubed white potatoes
¼ c beef broth gravy
½ c peas and carrots
¾ c tossed lettuce salad
1 tbsp oil and vinegar

1 slice Vienna bread
2 tsp milk-free margarine
Small banana
1 tsp sugar
Coffee or tea

EVENING SNACK

Popcorn

products of U.S. origin are often contaminated with wheat. Even dried fruit may be a problem if the fruit comes in contact with a flour-dusted conveyor in food packaging companies. Box 3-2 provides a sample gluten-free diet.

Lactose intolerance often accompanies celiac sprue because of the inflammatory condition of the intestinal tract with untreated celiac sprue. The patient's condition improves dramatically on a gluten-free diet. Once healing of the villi has occurred, lactose is usually tolerated again, but may need to be introduced slowly. Dietary counseling must include a discussion of foods allowed, reading labels for even small amounts of gluten in various foods, and using alternative flours (e.g., rice, corn, and potato) in recipes. Other substitutes include tapioca and soybean and arrowroot flours. The gluten-free diet is very tedious and referral to celiac organizations is highly recommended (see Appendix 1).

Crohn's disease (regional enteritis) is another inflammatory bowel disease, the cause of which is unknown. However, it is becoming more common, especially in young adults, and is felt to be an autoimmune disease in which the body

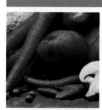

**BOX 3-2
SAMPLE
MENU FOR
A GLUTEN-
RESTRICTED
DIET**

BREAKFAST

½ c grapefruit juice
½ c corn grits
1 egg, soft cooked
Rice cake
1 tsp butter or margarine

1 tbsp grape jelly
1 c 1% milk (or lactose-reduced milk as
    needed)
2 tsp sugar
Coffee or tea

LUNCH

2 oz sliced turkey
1 c rice
½ c green beans
½ sliced tomato on lettuce
1 tsp butter or margarine
Fresh apple

Puffed rice bar
1 c 1% milk (or lactose-reduced milk as
    needed)
Rice muffin
Coffee or tea

SUPPER

3 oz roast beef
1 c cubed white potato
½ c cooked broccoli
¾ c tossed lettuce salad
1 tbsp oil and lemon juice

Rice muffin
2 tsp butter or margarine
1 c 1% milk (or lactose-reduced milk as
    needed)
Coffee or tea

attacks itself. Crohn's disease can affect any part of the intestinal tract, but inflammation usually occurs in the terminal ileum. Diarrhea, abdominal cramps, fever, and weakness are common symptoms. Malnutrition is likely caused by inadequate dietary intake, decreased absorption of nutrients, and excessive losses from the GI tract.

The goal of dietary treatment of Crohn's disease is to maintain good nutritional status, promote healing, and reduce inflammation. A well-balanced, high-calorie, high-protein diet is suggested. However, an elemental diet, which requires no digestion, may be used in the treatment of Crohn's disease. The theory behind elemental diets is that inflammation of Crohn's disease may arise from an immunologic response to dietary protein antigens. A vitamin and mineral supplement that meets the recommended dietary allowance (RDA) is beneficial because of the malabsorption that occurs with Crohn's disease. The prescribed diet is low in residue, especially during the acute stages. The patient should be taught the importance of documenting foods eaten in relation to symptoms.

The Large Intestine

The large intestine consists of the cecum, the colon, the rectum, and the anal canal. Water is drawn out of the contents of the large intestine and absorbed and solid feces are formed. Waste, including indigestible residue, undigested food

BOX 3-3
LOW-RESIDUE DIET AS MODIFIED WITH FOOD GROUPS FROM THE FOOD GUIDE PYRAMID

GRAINS
Emphasize refined grain products such as white bread, white rice, pasta, and cereals that are not whole grain.

VEGETABLES/FRUITS
Emphasize those without skins or seeds such as canned fruits and fruit juice.

MILK
Drink or use 2 c or more as tolerated per day.

MEAT
Emphasize tender meats; avoid fried meats or those with gristle. Avoid legumes and nuts.

particles, meat fibers, and decomposition products, is eliminated. Because no enzymes are produced in the large intestine, no digestion takes place there.

Diarrhea is the passage of frequent stools of liquid consistency. Persons experiencing severe diarrhea are told to abstain from consuming any food for up to 48 hours. This will give the intestinal tract a chance to rest. Intravenous solutions of dextrose may be required for severe cases of diarrhea to help replace fluids. Clear liquid may be given after this time. Once diarrhea has diminished, the patient can progress to a diet that is restricted in residue (insoluble fiber) and high in protein, calories, nutrients, and fluids. Box 3-3 shows how residue can be restricted using the food groups of the Food Guide Pyramid. These restrictions are gradually replaced by a regular normal diet as soon as the person is able to tolerate it.

Antibiotic treatment can cause diarrhea because it kills helpful and harmful bacteria. The intestinal tract normally contains certain types of bacteria that help digest food matter. A person in this situation will benefit from consuming yogurt with live bacterial culture (***Lactobacillus* culture**).

Constipation is a condition in which the waste matter in the large intestines or bowels is difficult to pass or the emptying time of the feces is so delayed that discomfort or uncomfortable symptoms result. A high-fiber diet (Box 3-4) and increased water intake are used in the treatment of constipation. Two liters of water daily, or the equivalent, is needed by most adults. Fiber provides bulk and water promotes softer stools which both help in elimination of fecal material. A variety of high-fiber foods from a variety of sources is recommended, with 20 to 35 grams (g) of fiber recommended for adults and "age plus five" grams of fiber advised for children. An increase of fluid intake is of further importance in controlling constipation. If fiber intake is increased, it is imperative that fluid intake

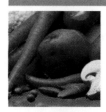

**BOX 3-4
SAMPLE
MENU FOR A
HIGH-FIBER
DIET**

BREAKFAST

Raisins	1 tbsp jam
½ c bran cereal	1 c 1% milk
1 slice toast, 100% whole wheat	1 tsp sugar
1 tsp butter or margarine	Coffee or tea

LUNCH

Tuna sandwich on 2 slices toast, 100% whole wheat	Tomato slices
¾ c lettuce salad	½ c canned peaches
½ c green beans	Oatmeal cookie

MIDAFTERNOON SNACK

Fresh orange

SUPPER

½ c split pea soup	1 slice bread, 100% whole wheat
2 oz roast beef	1 tsp butter or margarine
1 baked potato with skin	Fig bar
½ c cooked carrots	1 c 1% milk
1 c tossed salad	Coffee or tea
1 tbsp French dressing	

EVENING SNACK

½ c bran cereal	½ c 1% milk
1 tsp sugar	

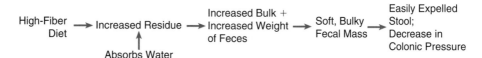

FIGURE 3-8 How a high-fiber diet helps correct and prevent constipation.

also increase. Figure 3-8 shows how fiber helps in the correction or prevention of constipation.

Prolonged constipation is called **obstipation**. Symptoms include nausea, heartburn, headache, general malaise, or distress in the rectum or intestine as a result of the nerves reacting when the rectum is distended by the contained matter.

Atonic constipation is characterized by the loss of rectal sensibility and weak peristaltic waves. It commonly occurs in elderly or obese persons, pregnant women, persons who abuse or overuse laxatives, and postoperative patients. Factors contributing to its occurrence include a low-fiber diet, irregular meals, inadequate fluid intake, lack of exercise, lack of time allowed for evacuation of stool, and prolonged use of chemical laxatives.

Spastic constipation (also known as **irritable bowel syndrome**, spastic colitis, and mucous colitis) is characterized by irregular contractions of the bowel, resulting in either diarrhea or constipation. A high soluble fiber intake with frequent meals can be helpful.

Encopresis is a condition of chronic constipation that afflicts children. Encopresis is characterized by a fecal impaction consisting of a semi-fitting "plug" of feces that allows more liquid fecal material to seep around and soil the child's pants. Parents may not understand this physiology and may wonder if their child is misbehaving. A high-fiber diet with use of laxatives after a complete bowel clean out may be helpful. Mineral oil, if used, should be infrequent because of associated malabsorption of food nutrients.

For the management of irritable bowel syndrome the emphasis is on soluble fiber. Soluble fiber absorbs water and has a gummy texture, which allows for more stable GI transit time. Other forms of constipation will benefit with either type of fiber (soluble or insoluble). Figure 3-8 shows how this is accomplished.

Steatorrhea is diarrhea characterized by excess fat in stools and results from a malabsorption syndrome caused by disease of the intestinal mucosa or pancreatic enzyme deficiency. Steatorrhea usually indicates a more serious underlying organic disease. It may be seen in pancreatitis or following gastric or intestinal resection. It is often associated with diseases of the liver or gallbladder or with malabsorptive diseases such a nontropical sprue (celiac disease—see earlier section) or regional enteritis. It sometimes occurs after GI radiation. All of these disorders may involve problems with fat digestion or absorption. It is generally diagnosed from a fecal fat test, which may require 3 to 4 days of fecal material collection. A simple test of fat malabsorption is if the person's stools float in the toilet because fat floats on water.

In diet planning for steatorrhea the emphasis is on low-fat foods. The treatment of steatorrhea may also involve the use of **medium-chain triglycerides (MCTs)**, which are fats that contain 8 to 10 carbon atoms (as opposed to the 12 to 18 carbon atoms found in long-chain triglycerides [LCTs]). The MCTs are used in the treatment of steatorrhea because they are more easily digested, absorbed, and transported than are LCTs. This can be accomplished with the use of commercially available products. The two principal forms of MCT are Portagen, which is a powdered formula that can be mixed and served as a supplement to meals, and MCT oil, which can replace vegetable oil in recipes.

Diverticulosis is a condition involving the formation of outpockets of small sacs (diverticula) protruding from the wall of the large intestines. They are found mainly in the sigmoid colon. Low-fiber diets favor the development of diverticulosis because intraluminal pressure is exerted against the colon wall instead of longitudinally, resulting in pouches (Figure 3-9). These outpockets do not disappear. Thus a person with diverticulosis will always have diverticulosis, but can experience **diverticulitis** (the inflammation stage) in cycles.

The high-fiber diet is used for prevention and management of diverticulosis. The effect of fiber and liquids is expected to reduce the incidence and symptoms

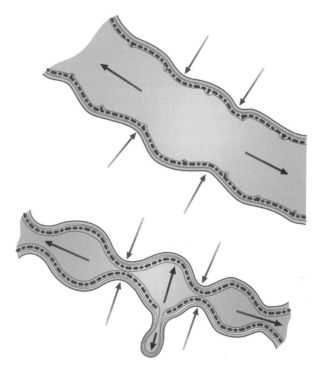

FIGURE 3-9 Mechanism by which low-fiber, low-bulk diets might generate diverticula. Where colon contents are bulky *(top)*, muscular contractions exert pressure longitudinally. If lumen is smaller *(bottom)*, contractions can produce occlusion and exert pressure against colon wall, which may produce a diverticular "blow-out."

of diverticular disease by reducing pressure inside the intestinal tract. Until recently, the diet restricted intake of seeds, skins, and nuts. If these foods are consumed, thorough chewing should be advised.

Diverticulitis requires temporary management with a low-fiber diet to avoid inflammation of diverticula. Symptoms include abdominal pain, usually in the lower left quadrant, and occasionally fever. Diverticulitis is a temporary condition of inflammation.

Ulcerative colitis is a chronic disease characterized by inflammation and ulceration of the mucosa of the large intestine. The cause of this disease is unknown. The inclusion of fatty fish such as albacore tuna and salmon are known to reduce the inflammation process and may be of benefit in treating ulcerative colitis. Emphasis on soluble fiber, versus insoluble fiber can be of further help. For management of severe cases of ulcerative colitis a tube feeding of an elemental diet or total parenteral nutrition (TPN) may be necessary (see Chapter 5). Symptoms of ulcerative colitis include rectal bleeding, diarrhea, fever, anorexia, dehydration, and weight loss.

What Are Common Digestive Issues And Suggestions?

Poor Appetite

1. Encourage good oral hygiene before and after meals.
2. Promote a pleasant meal setting. Play soft music. Use candles if possible. Make meals visually attractive with a variety of food colors and textures.
3. Note times when appetite is the best—often mornings—and provide larger portions or more nutritious foods at these times.
4. Try well-seasoned foods. Sometimes salt or fat restrictions are discontinued to promote adequate intake.
5. Provide calorie-dense foods such as ice cream, milkshakes, or liquid supplements.
6. Evaluate reasons for poor appetite such as depression; use medications as needed.

Dry or Sore Mouth

1. Avoid foods that are irritating such as hard, salty, or hot-spiced foods.
2. Provide soft, moist foods for ease in chewing. Moisten dry foods, such as dry toast, in beverages or add gravy or cream sauces to foods.
3. Include cold foods such as ice cream, sherbet, and iced beverages.
4. Encourage good oral hygiene. Dry mouth can lead to dental decay.

Diarrhea

1. Rule out causes such as fat malabsorption; ask if the person's stools "float." If so, pancreatic enzymes with meals can help with fat digestion and absorption.
2. Rule out excess sugar alcohol intake (a form of sugar substitute such as sorbitol and mannitol).
3. Rule out GI illness. If this is the cause, an initial clear liquid diet may be necessary for 24 hours or longer to provide bowel rest. See Chapter 5. Low-residue, lactose-free liquid supplements may be tolerated and needed for extended bowel rest.
4. If intestinal irritation exists, initially restrict irritants such as caffeine, alcohol, spicy foods, skins and seeds of fruits and vegetables, bran and whole grains, and nuts.
5. Increase soluble fiber such as bananas, oatmeal, and small legumes such as lentils.
6. Avoid lactose (milk sugar).
7. Include plain, lemon, or vanilla yogurt with active bacterial cultures if diarrhea is induced from antibiotics.

Excess Gas Production (Flatulence and/or Belching)

1. Ensure no swallowing of air by chewing with the mouth closed.
2. Reduce fiber intake until symptoms abate; resume in small amounts to build up digestibility for decreased gas production by intestinal bacteria.
3. Try a low-lactose diet.
4. Avoid carbonated drinks.

Constipation

1. Assess fiber and fluid intake and physical activity; advise as needed to increase fiber, fluid, and exercise.

The Liver

The liver is involved with the metabolism and storage of the macronutrients carbohydrate, protein, and fat, as well as vitamins and minerals after the process of digestion and absorption is completed.

The liver stores glucose in the form of glycogen that can then be released back into the bloodstream as glucose. The liver can also make glucose from protein in the process called **gluconeogenesis**. The end products of protein digestion, amino acids, are formed back into complete protein by the liver. The liver can manufacture the nonessential amino acids (see Chapter 2). The liver produces lipids such as cholesterol and triglycerides and bile salts, essential for fat digestion.

The liver detoxifies harmful substances such as changing ammonia, created from protein metabolism, into urea that can then be cleared into the urine by the kidneys. Life cannot exist without the functions of the liver.

Hepatitis is inflammation and injury to liver cells caused by infections, drugs, or toxins. Symptoms include anorexia, fatigue, nausea, vomiting, fever, diarrhea, and weight loss. The symptoms during the early stage of hepatitis make it difficult for the patient to consume adequate nutrients. Tube feedings (see Chapter 5) may be required until the patient can tolerate the oral intake of food. Once oral intake is resumed, a diet high in calories, protein, vitamins, and minerals with moderate fat is planned for the patient. Several small meals are usually better tolerated than are three large ones.

Cirrhosis is a chronic liver disease in which normal liver tissue is replaced by inactive fibrous tissue. Because liver tissue is not able to function normally, there may be **jaundice** (a buildup of bile in the body causing yellowing of the skin and eyes), a prolonged bleeding time, fatty infiltration of liver tissue, lower serum albumin levels, and other complications (depending on the severity of tissue function impairment). Symptoms sometimes include nausea, vomiting, anorexia, **ascites** (accumulation of fluid in the abdomen), and **esophageal varices** (enlargement of the veins in the esophagus because of poor portal vein blood circulation).

Because carbohydrate metabolism is often affected by this condition, the diet for cirrhosis should be adequate in energy and nutrients to prevent further deterioration of the liver. As much as 300 to 400 g of carbohydrates may be necessary, as well as 45 to 50 kcal per kilogram of body weight to spare protein. The fat intake may need to be lowered because of malabsorption of fats. Table 3-3 shows daily food allowances for a 50 g, low-fat diet.

When liver function becomes severely impaired, ammonia levels become abnormally high and toxic to brain tissue. Protein may be restricted to 35 to 50 g per day (see Box 3-5 for a sample menu). The amount of protein is gradually increased in increments of 10 to 15 g as liver function improves. Supplements of branched-chain amino acids may be used.

TABLE 3-3
DAILY FOOD ALLOWANCES FOR 50 G FAT DIET

FOOD	AMOUNT	APPROXIMATE FAT CONTENT (g)
Skim milk	2 c or more	0
Lean meat, fish, poultry	6 oz or 6 equivalents	18
Whole egg or egg yolks	3 per week	3
Vegetables	3 servings or more, at least 1 or more dark leafy green or orange	0
Fruits	3 or more servings, at least 1 citrus	0
Breads, cereals	As desired	0
Fat	5-6 tsp fat or oil daily	25-30
Desserts and sweets	As desired from permitted list	0
	Total fat	46-51

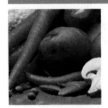

**BOX 3-5
SAMPLE
MENU FOR A
35-g PROTEIN
MEAL**

BREAKFAST
½ c fruit or juice
½ c cereal with ½ c milk, sugar

1 slice toast with margarine and jelly
Coffee or tea

LUNCH
1 small potato with margarine
½ c vegetable
Tossed salad with Italian dressing

1 slice bread with margarine
½ c fruit
½ c milk

SUPPER
1 oz meat or 1 egg
1 small potato
½ c vegetable
Fruit salad

1 slice bread with margarine
½ c fruit
½ c milk
Coffee or tea

*On a 20-g protein meal pattern, 1 oz of meat and 1 c of milk would be omitted. Extra margarine, concentrated sweets, low-protein bread and pasta, and possibly carbohydrate supplements help to provide adequate kilocalories in the diet.

Vitamin and mineral supplementation is often necessary. Sodium and fluids are restricted if edema and ascites develop. It is not unusual for the sodium to be limited to 500 to 1500 mg per day. Fluids are restricted to 100 to 1500 mL per day, depending on the severity of the condition. Foods high in roughage (whole grains and vegetables and fruits with skin and seeds) may need to be restricted with esophageal varices to prevent rupture of these tiny blood vessels.

A state of unconsciousness may result because of a build-up of blood toxins. This is known as **hepatic coma**. Contributing factors include GI bleeding, excessive dietary protein, severe infection, and surgical procedures. Symptoms include confusion, irritability, delirium, and flapping tremors of the hands and feet.

Methionine, an essential amino acid has to be metabolically activated into S-adenosylmethionine (SAMe), which is impaired by liver disease. Thus SAMe rather than methionine is the compound that must be supplemented in the presence of significant liver disease (Lieber, 2000).

WHAT ARE DISEASES OF THE GALLBLADDER?

The release of bile for fat digestion can cause severe pain if there are gallstones or inflammation. **Cholelithiasis** is the formation of gallstones. Sometimes the gallstones block the bile duct and interfere with the flow of bile. Symptoms include pain in the right upper quadrant as the gallbladder contracts and jaundice if the bile duct is obstructed. **Cholecystitis** is an inflammation of the gallbladder. It can be caused by a bacterial infection or stones in the gallbladder. Symptoms include acute pain in the upper-right quadrant, nausea, belching, vomiting, fever, and jaundice if the bile duct is blocked.

During an acute attack of cholecystitis or cholelithiasis, food may be withheld for up to 24 hours. Food is introduced gradually, starting with a clear liquid diet. As food tolerance improves, patients progress to a minimum-fat diet that contains 50 g of fat or less (see Table 3-3).

Excess fat intake will cause the gallbladder to contract, which can be very painful if gallstones are present. Therefore foods high in fat may not be tolerated, including foods such as sausages, bacon, and peanut butter. Other food intolerances, such as with onions, may exist in certain individuals. If stone removal by surgery or by ultrasonic or chemical dissolution is necessary, the patient should follow a low-fat diet until the procedure is performed.

After stone removal, the patient should follow a low-fat diet for several weeks until fat digestion is normalized. Thereafter, a normal diet is usually well tolerated and should be encouraged, although a 50-g fat diet is appropriate for long-term use.

WHAT ARE DISEASES OF THE PANCREAS?

The pancreas produces digestive enzymes for metabolism of proteins, carbohydrates, and fats; bicarbonate ions to neutralize chyme; and hormones such as insulin (see Chapter 9).

Cystic fibrosis (also called cystic fibrosis of the pancreas) consists of an insufficiency or abnormality of some essential hormone or enzyme. Excessive thick mucus is produced by the exocrine glands and interferes with breathing and digestion.

Fats are poorly digested and absorbed and a common symptom is frequent fatty, bulky, and odorous feces. Recurrent respiratory infections and excessive loss of sodium and chloride from the sweat glands are common. Pancreatic insufficiency may develop. The MCTs are more easily absorbed and therefore are the best source of fat in the diet for cystic fibrosis. Pancreatic enzyme tablets given at mealtimes, however, allow for more normal intake of dietary fats and can therefore promote growth of children with cystic fibrosis.

The fat-soluble vitamins (A, D, E, and K) and a high-protein, high-kilocalorie diet are the cornerstones of diet therapy for this condition. Children who have cystic fibrosis often have a good appetite, which allows for adequate intake of kilocalories and protein.

Pancreatitis is inflammation of the pancreas. It is caused by digestion of pancreatic tissue by its own pancreatic digestive enzymes. The reason for this is not fully understood. Chronic alcoholism and triglyceride levels over 1000 mg/dL are often associated with pancreatitis. Symptoms include abdominal pain, fever, malaise, nausea, and vomiting. Treatment is aimed at resting the pancreas. A low-fat diet is often implemented during acute pancreatitis. Pancreatic insufficiency may develop; it is treated by the administration of pancreatic enzyme at each meal.

Diabetes mellitus is related to inadequate amounts or use of insulin produced by the islets of Langerhans found in the pancreas (see Chapter 9). Because this is a complex disease, Chapter 9 has been devoted to a full discussion of its management.

WHAT ARE HEREDITARY DISEASES OF THE BLOOD?

Sickle cell disease is a serious hereditary, chronic condition that is found mainly in African Americans, but sometimes in persons of Mediterranean, Middle Eastern, and Asian Indian ancestry. It is now believed, historically, persons with the sickle cell trait had a survival advantage to ward off malaria.

In persons with this disease, the red blood cells (erythrocytes) are rigid and crescent, or sickle, shaped and have difficulty passing through the small arterioles and capillaries. The cells clump together and obstruct blood vessels, causing pain. The major symptoms are anemia, periodic joint and extremity pain (sometimes with edema), and severe bouts of abdominal pain with vomiting and distention. The patient is prone to infection. In one study 15% of those with sickle cell disease had low folate (a B vitamin; see Chapter 4) levels in the red blood cells, despite daily folate supplementation, which may increase the risk for vascular damage and stroke (Kennedy et al., 2001).

Thalassemia is a hereditary condition in which red blood cells are small and contain less hemoglobin than is normal. The relationship of vitamin E to thalassemia is being studied, especially because this vitamin has an antioxidant effect on cells and may improve red blood cell survival.

WHAT IS THE ROLE OF CELLULAR METABOLISM?

Metabolism is the rate in which food calories are used as energy in the body cells. A slow metabolic rate can result in obesity and a high metabolic rate can result in undesirable weight loss. Metabolism goes beyond use of kilocalories, however. Numerous, complex biochemical changes occur within the cells in both anabolic and catabolic processes.

WHAT IS THE ROLE OF THE ENDOCRINE SYSTEM IN METABOLISM?

The **endocrine system** is a major control system of the body. More than a dozen hormones that the body produces regulate metabolism and the use of nutrients. Insulin is the only hormone that lowers glucose levels. The hormones that raise glucose levels are referred to as **counterregulatory hormones**, as they work counter to insulin. Some hormones that have significance to nutrition and diet are as follows:

Insulin. This hormone is produced in the pancreas and allows carbohydrates to be metabolized for energy by facilitating the entry of blood sugar (glucose) into the cells where the Krebs cycle takes place. Insulin also affects the metabolism of fat. Insulin stimulates protein synthesis and decreases protein degradation. Insulin deficiency decreases the body's ability to metabolize carbohydrates and fats and it contributes to weight loss.

Glucagon. This is the primary hormone produced when the body perceives the blood glucose level is dropping too far. Glucagon is one of several hormones that promotes the breakdown of **glycogen** (stored sugar) in the liver to raise blood glucose levels. Insulin and glucagon are the primary hormones involved in maintaining **homeostasis** (the regulation of body functions or processes) of blood glucose levels.

Epinephrine (also referred to as adrenalin). This hormone is produced mainly by the adrenal glands and helps release stored sugar in the liver in response to low blood sugar or stress. Energy metabolism is increased in response to epinephrine because of the resultant increased heart rate and oxygen intake. Excess epinephrine may raise the blood glucose too high if there is insufficient insulin for the metabolism of carbohydrates (see Chapter 9).

Cortisol. This hormone is also produced by the adrenal gland. It is often produced in increased amounts during the early morning hours. As a result, blood sugar levels tend to run higher first thing in the morning (this is referred to as the dawn phenomenon; see Chapter 9). An increased production of insulin may occur in the early morning hours to compensate for the dawn phenomenon, especially if large amounts of simple sugar are consumed. Steroid medications are similar to the cortisol hormone because they tend to increase the appetite and their use is related to weight gain (see Chapter 7). They also raise blood glucose levels.

Growth hormone. This hormone is produced by the pituitary gland. It raises the rate of metabolism and is associated with protein anabolism, which produces a positive nitrogen balance. It is also referred to as diabetogenic because it works against insulin in muscle tissue. Adolescents have an increased need for insulin because of increased levels of growth hormone. This hormone contributes to the dawn phenomenon as well.

Estrogen. This hormone is produced mainly in the ovaries and helps retain bone calcium, which results in a decreased risk of osteoporosis (see Chapters 13 and 14). Estrogen tends to cause blood glucose levels to rise because of its inhibiting effect on insulin. Premenstrual syndrome (PMS; see Chapter 12) may be caused in part by lowered levels of estrogen after ovulation. Without estrogen, insulin is able to lower the blood sugar level more effectively. Lowered blood sugar levels can result in the irritability, hunger, and headaches that often are associated with PMS.

Thyroxine. This is one of the hormones produced in the thyroid that raises the rate of metabolism. A high level of thyroxine increases the metabolic rate in part because it increases oxygen consumption. The thyroid hormones also help regulate lipid (fat) metabolism. Low levels of thyroxine may be reflected in raised levels of blood cholesterol (see Chapter 8). Iodine binds to thyroxine, so measuring the amount of protein-bound iodine found in a blood sample is one technique for measuring the basal metabolic rate. The more iodine found bound to thyroxine, the more active the thyroid gland, therefore the greater the metabolic rate.

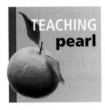

TEACHING pearl

Blood glucose and glycogen stores can be equated to the fuel in a motorcycle. There is no gas gauge on the tank of a motorcycle. If the motorcycle accidentally runs out of fuel, the rider can flip a switch to a small reserve tank of fuel. If blood glucose levels fall, the body will "flip a switch" to allow access to a reserve source of glucose. The switch involves the production of glucagon, adrenalin, and other hormones. The back-up fuel is the glycogen stored in the liver, which is then released as glucose into the blood stream.

HOW DOES ALCOHOL AFFECT DIGESTION, ABSORPTION, AND METABOLISM?

Alcohol is toxic to the body when consumed in excess and thus impairs the entire process of digestion, absorption, and metabolism. This can affect nutritional status by interfering with normal use of food nutrients. Poor food choices with lower nutrient intakes also occur as smoking and drinking increase (Ma et al., 2000). Chronic alcohol abuse is an important risk factor for oral cancer that can impair intake of food (Bode and Bode, 2000).

In the small intestine, alcohol abuse interferes with the absorption of glucose, amino acids, lipids, water, sodium, and vitamins (especially thiamin and folic acid). Alcohol damages the villi in the intestinal system leading to poor absorption of nutrients. This inhibition of absorption of nutrients may contribute to nutritional deficiencies frequently observed in alcoholics. **Wernicke-Korsakoff syndrome** (also called Wernicke's encephalopathy) is a condition caused by alcoholism and compounded by a deficiency of vitamin B_1 (thiamin).

Alcohol is widely known to harm the liver, which affects how protein is metabolized. Because protein is a vital component of all body cells, including digestive enzymes and hormones, alcohol toxicity directly impairs all normal body processes. A low-serum **albumin** (a form of protein found in the blood and a measure of protein status) will be found when there is inadequate protein intake for the body's needs or if the liver is too damaged to metabolize protein.

A less well-known problem with alcohol is its propensity to damage the pancreas. This damage can develop into secondary diabetes if the pancreas loses its ability to produce insulin (see Chapter 9).

In moderation, alcohol is generally not harmful and may be beneficial. Persons who are not on diabetes medication may benefit with moderate amounts of alcohol because of its positive effects on insulin resistance, high-density lipoprotein (HDL) cholesterol (also known as the "good" cholesterol), and reduced tendency to form blood clots. Because alcohol intake decreases glucagon production, persons who take diabetes medication should consult their physician for guidance on alcohol use (Rasmussen et al., 2001). Moderate intake for men is two drinks or less per day, and for women, is one drink or less.

How Is Alcohol Metabolized?

Two principal enzymes are known to be involved in the metabolism of alcohol: alcohol dehydrogenase (ADH) and aldehyde dehydrogenase (ALDH). The ADH is responsible for the metabolism of ethanol to acetaldehyde. The ALDH catalyzes the conversion of acetaldehyde to acetate. The presence of an inactive form of ALDH2 is thought to be responsible for an increase in acetaldehyde levels in the body. Acetaldehyde is considered responsible for the facial flushing reactions often observed among Asians who have consumed alcohol. This may deter further consumption because of the unpleasant sensation. Asians who possess the ALDH2*2 genotype are considered to have some protection against alcoholism (Segal, 1999).

What Are Risk Factors for Development of Alcoholism?

Research into the genetics of alcoholism is a relatively recent scientific endeavor. A low level of response to alcohol is genetically influenced and is a characteristic of children of alcoholics. This appears to predict alcoholism 10 and 15 years later (Schuckit et al., 2001). Thus persons who may tout their ability to "hold their liquor" may, in fact, be predisposed to alcoholism.

Primary depression and secondary alcoholism has been associated within families (Kasperowicz-Dabrowiecka and Rybakowski, 2001). A study involved with depressed patients found that their brains used an energy source other than glucose (Lambert et al., 2000). The decreased ability to use glucose, by the brain, in persons suffering depression may predispose them to alcohol abuse. Alcohol may serve as an alternative energy or calorie source for such persons. Unipolar mood disorders are frequently secondary to alcoholism (Preisig et al., 2001).

It is for the concern of alcoholism that recommendations cannot be made to the public to start drinking moderate amounts of alcohol unless it is known the person does not have alcoholic tendencies. As a better understanding of alcoholism develops, public health advice may change in the future. For now, individuals who already consume alcohol should be encouraged to drink moderate amounts for the best health outcomes.

WHAT IS THE ROLE OF THE NURSE OR OTHER HEALTH PROFESSIONAL IN PROMOTING POSITIVE NUTRITIONAL INTAKE AND METABOLISM?

The nurse or other health care professional in an institutional setting can indirectly promote the digestive process by providing a relaxed and unhurried atmosphere where patients can feel at ease to thoroughly chew their food. Direct intervention might include emphasizing the importance of thorough chewing.

The health care professional should be aware of possible issues of digestion in patients, such as swallowing problems and intestinal or gastric surgery, and should be alert to signs of malabsorption such as chronic diarrhea and unexplained weight loss. Patients with these types of problems should be referred to a registered dietitian once the attending physician makes a diagnosis. Digestive or intestinal problems, such as chronic constipation, may also be improved with medical nutrition therapy.

The nurse and other health care professional can have a positive role in the prevention of alcoholism by assessing family risk and helping persons suffering from alcoholism through involvement of the total health care team. (See Chapter 5 for more information on coordination of the health care team.) The planning and implementation of nutritional care must always be individualized.

CHAPTER STUDY QUESTIONS AND CLASSROOM ACTIVITIES

1. What is the purpose of digestion?
2. What is absorption? In what part of the body does it take place?
3. In what form are all carbohydrates absorbed? All fats? All proteins?
4. Name the enzymes involved in the digestion of maltose and sucrose.
5. Why would a low-fiber and then a high-fiber diet be helpful for someone with diverticulitis?
6. Why is a low-fat diet used to treat gallbladder disease?
7. Discuss class experiences of alcohol use and abuse on campus.

Practical Application

Trace the digestion of a meal composed of a ham sandwich on whole wheat bread, a glass of low-fat milk, and a fresh apple. Describe the mechanical and chemical processes that occur and name the enzymes involved.

Case Study

CRITICAL
THINKING

Joey sat in class at UCLA. His stomach felt so uncomfortable. He was getting to the point that he didn't dare eat. He would get terrible stomach cramping and diarrhea on some days. He couldn't figure out what was going on. He hoped that it was just stress related and would go away after he and his new bride moved back to his old hometown. He chuckled as he thought about how the old townies were going to massacre her name with a real twang, nasal-sounding "A." Andrea, pronounced "Ondrea," was in for a culture shock after growing up in California. He hoped they could find some good Mexican restaurants, or maybe he would just have to cook for them at home. He was looking forward to getting Grandma Brown's baked beans again and told his family he would be sure to keep them in steady supply because the rest of the family were going to continue living out here because his dad's job paid well. Although, after the events of September 11th, his family was talking about moving back to be closer to the rest of the family.

Critical Thinking Applications

1. Describe what the symptoms of cramping and diarrhea might indicate.
2. How might soluble fiber from legumes assist with the management of diarrhea?
3. Discuss the effect of regional food variability—what foods can you find in one part of the country and not in others or from urban to rural food access and how can this affect health?
4. Discuss food options in common restaurants for someone with digestive issues such as lactose intolerance or poor-fitting dentures.
5. Discuss how families' and friends' food preferences and habits may affect nutritional status.
6. Have students describe changes in their eating habits since attending college.

REFERENCES

Bode JC, Bode C: Alcohol, the gastrointestinal tract and pancreas, Ther Umsch. April 2000; 57(4):212.

Kasperowicz-Dabrowiecka A, Rybakowski JK: Beyond the Winokur concept of depression spectrum disease: which types of alcoholism are related to primary affective illness?, J Affect Disord. March 2001; 63(1-3):133-138.

Kennedy TS, Fung EB, Kawchak DA, Zemel BS, Ohene-Frempong K, Stallings VA: Red blood cell folate and serum vitamin B_{12} status in children with sickle cell disease, Am J Pediatr Hematol Oncol. March 2001; 23(3):165-169.

Lambert G, Johansson M, Agren H, Friberg P: Reduced brain norepinephrine and dopamine release in treatment-refractory depressive illness: evidence in support of the catecholamine hypothesis of mood disorders, Arch Gen Psychiatry. August 2000; 57(8):787.

Lieber CS: ALCOHOL: its metabolism and interaction with nutrients, Annu Rev Nutr. 2000; 20:395.

Ma J, Betts NM, Hampl JS: Clustering of lifestyle behaviors: the relationship between cigarette smoking, alcohol consumption, and dietary intake, Am J Health Promot. November-December 2000; 15(2):107.

Preisig M, Fenton BT, Stevens DE, Merikangas KR: Familial relationship between mood disorders and alcoholism, Compr Psychiatry. March-April 2001; 42(2):87.

Rasmussen BM, Orskov L, Schmitz O, Hermansen K: Alcohol and glucose counterregulation during acute insulin-induced hypoglycemia in type 2 diabetic subjects, Metabolism. April 2001; 50(4):451.

Schuckit MA, Edenberg HJ, Kalmijn J, Flury L, Smith TL, Reich T, Bierut L, Goate A, and Foroud TA: Genome-wide search for genes that relate to a low level of response to alcohol. Alcohol Clin Exp Res. March 2001; 25(3):323.

Segal B: ADH and ALDH polymorphisms among Alaska Natives entering treatment for alcoholism, Alaska Med. January-March 1999; 41(1):9-12

Szekely M. The vagus nerve in thermoregulation and energy metabolism. Auton Neurosci. December 20, 2000; 85(1-3):26.

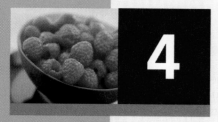

4

Food as the Source of Vitamins, Minerals, Phytochemicals, and Water

OBJECTIVES

After completing this chapter, you should be able to:

- Describe the main difference between the fat-soluble and water-soluble vitamins.
- Recognize at least one known function of each of the vitamins and minerals.
- List foods high in the various vitamins and minerals.
- Describe the function and common sources of electrolytes.
- Describe the importance of water and explain how to include an appropriate amount in the diet.
- Describe how the nurse or other health care professional can most appropriately promote the intake of vitamins, minerals, phytochemicals, electrolytes, and water.

TERMS TO IDENTIFY

Acid-base balance
Adequate Intake (AI)
Anemia
Antioxidants
Beriberi
Cardiomyopathy
Carotene
Cheilosis

Cretinism
Dietary Reference Intakes (DRI)
Deoxyribonucleic acid (DNA)
Electrolyte
Elemental
Enrichment

Estimated Average Requirement (EAR)
Fat-soluble vitamins
Fortification
Goiter
Heme iron
Hemoglobin
Hyperosmotic diarrhea

Continued

INTRODUCTION

As we become more knowledgeable about our vitamin and mineral needs, it is helpful to keep the history of that knowledge in perspective. Initially, food was recognized as the important element in health. One of the first major discoveries about the role of vitamins was that the use of lemons and limes offered protection against the dreaded scurvy that plagued ocean voyagers. Before this revelation, sailors often developed this severe vitamin C deficiency, which resulted in internal bleeding and death. The effect of toxic vitamin levels was noted when Arctic explorers died from ingesting polar bear liver, which has a high level of vitamin A.

It was not until the twentieth century that vitamins were chemically identified. This author had the rare opportunity of talking personally to a retired scientist who recalled being one of the first people asked to chemically isolate vitamin C during the 1920s. He and his colleagues laughed at the foolishness of this idea at the time. We may no longer laugh about the importance of vitamins, but we cannot expect that all has been learned in one lifetime about the complexity of the body's need for vitamins.

Minerals, the seeming equivalent of vitamins in the consumer's eye, are inorganic substances that have some similarities to vitamins, but also have many differences. The most notable difference is that minerals are **elemental**, which means that they do not break down. This characteristic of minerals prevents their destruction by heat and air—destruction to which vitamins are susceptible. All minerals are elements found in the chemical periodic table. In the saying "Ashes to ashes, dust to dust," the ashes are the minerals found in the body.

Vitamins and minerals become available to body cells from foods we eat after the processes of digestion and absorption. Vitamins and minerals are integral to the function of metabolic enzymes at the cellular level for basic life processes.

Food is the ideal medium for intake of vitamins and minerals. Food such as whole grains, dark green leafy and orange vegetables, orange fruits, and legumes are very concentrated sources of vitamins and minerals. A variety of foods best allows inclusion of all known nutrients for health. Plant-based foods are also a source of **phytochemicals** (substances in foods that are beneficial to health, but are not vitamins or minerals). It is believed there are many phytochemicals yet to be identified in food. Low-processed foods in balanced meals with an emphasis on variety will likely meet all known needs for the many nutrients needed for health.

Persons electing to take additional amounts of vitamins and minerals through supplements need to do so with caution. The Dietary Supplement Health and Education Act of 1995 (DSHEA—pronounced D-Shay) distinguished dietary supplements from drugs or food additives and allowed for a less restrictive regulatory environment for supplements (Radimer et al., 2000). Furthermore, it is potentially very easy to take toxic doses from supplements, which is virtually impossible from food. An excess of one vitamin or mineral can compete with another; for example, zinc competes with copper, and vitamin E can inhibit the activity of vitamin K.

Vitamin and mineral supplements, which are usually unnecessary, should be within 100% to 200% of the recommended amounts (see the table inside the back cover). Exceptions to these guidelines should be made only with a warranted medical condition and the advice of a physician or registered dietitian. Many health conditions associated with the need for vitamins and minerals are better resolved through food because the human body is extremely complex and the nutrient composition of food best matches this need. Health care professionals are in a unique position to positively influence a patient's nutrient intake. This chapter is aimed at increasing appreciation for the micronutrients in food that our bodies require.

WHAT ARE THE DIETARY REFERENCE INTAKES?

The U.S. Recommended Dietary Allowances (RDAs) and Canadian Recommended Nutrient Intake (RNIs) are being replaced by **Dietary Reference Intakes (DRIs)**, the term used collectively to describe four measures of recommended dietary intake. The new DRIs will be used by both the United States and Canada. Nutrient intake amounting to less than the lower end of the range of the RDAs may lead to nutrient deficiency. Intake amounting to more than the upper limit may give rise to toxic effects, especially with trace minerals (Figure 4-1). The DRIs should not be confused with requirements for a specific individual because requirements vary considerably. Problems such as premature birth, inherited metabolic disorders, infections, chronic diseases, and the use of medications may require special dietary modifications. The specific reference values that comprise the DRIs are as follows:

Estimated Average Requirement (EAR): the amount of a nutrient estimated to meet half of the healthy individuals' needs based on life stage and gender.
Recommended Dietary Allowance (RDA): the average daily dietary intake level that meets the nutrient requirement of more than 97% of the healthy population in a particular life stage and gender group.

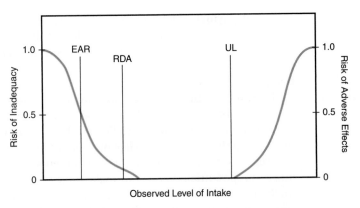

FIGURE 4-1 Dietary reference intakes. This figure shows that the Estimated Average Requirement (EAR) is the intake at which the risk of inadequacy to an individual is 50%. The Recommended Dietary Allowance (RDA) is the intake at which the risk of inadequacy is very small (2% to 3%). The Adequate Intake (AI) does not bear a consistent relationship to the EAR or the RDA because it is set without being able to estimate the average requirement. It is assumed the AI is above the RDA if it could be calculated. At intakes between the RDA and Tolerable Upper Intake Level (UL), the risks of inadequacy and of excess are both close to 0. At intakes above the UL the risk of adverse effects increases.

Adequate Intake (AI): a recommended intake of vitamins and minerals based on observations of nutrient intake by a group of healthy persons that is assumed to be adequate (when an RDA cannot be determined).

Tolerable Upper Intake Level (UL): the highest level of daily nutrient intake that is likely to pose no risk of adverse health effects in almost all individuals in the general population.

HOW ARE VITAMINS AND MINERALS BEST INCLUDED IN THE DIET?

Reliance on food sources for vitamins and minerals (Table 4-1 through 4-4) offers little risk of ingesting toxic amounts and provides a good balance of vitamins and minerals. The Food Guide Pyramid (see Chapter 1) is a strategy to plan healthy meals. The base of the Food Guide Pyramid provides the B vitamins (especially thiamin and niacin) with whole grains, which also provide a wide variety of minerals such as chromium and zinc. The second level of the Food Pyramid, composed of vegetables and fruits, supplies a variety of vitamins, such as vitamin C, and minerals, such as potassium. The dark green leafy vegetables are especially high in potassium, magnesium, and vitamins A (in the carotene form) and C, as well as the B vitamin, folate. Deep orange fruits and vegetables such as sweet potatoes, carrots, and cantaloupe are very high in carotene. Citrus fruits are very high in vitamin C. The third level of the Food Pyramid shows the high-calcium milk group, which also provides the primary source of vitamin B_2. The addition of legumes, meat, or other protein-rich foods further round out the nutritional needs, providing B vitamins and many minerals, such as iron.

Text continued on p. 101

TABLE 4-1
FAT-SOLUBLE VITAMINS

FUNCTIONS	GOOD SOURCES	SYMPTOMS OF DEFICIENCY	SYMPTOMS OF TOXICITY
VITAMIN A (NOMENCLATURE: PREFORMED—RETINOL, RETINAL, RETINOIC ACID; PRECURSOR—CAROTENE)			

Maintenance of epithelial cells and mucous membranes
Constituent of visual purple, important for night vision
Necessary for normal growth, development, and reproduction
Necessary for adequate immune response
	Preformed vitamin A: liver
	Carotene (dark green leafy):
	  Spinach
	  Broccoli
	  Kale
	  Swiss chard
	  Turnip greens
	  Collard greens
	Carotene (deep orange):
	  Carrots
	  Sweet potatoes
	  Orange winter squash
	  Pumpkin
	  Tomatoes
	  Apricots
	  Watermelon
	  Cantaloupe
		Nyctalopia (night blindness)
		Keratinized skin (rough, dry skin)
		Dry mucous membranes
		Xerophthalmia (an eye disease)
			Appetite loss
			Hair loss
			Dry skin
			Bone and joint pain
			Enlarged liver and spleen
			Fetal malformations
			Headache
			Weakness
			Vomiting
			Irritability
			Hydrocephalus (children)
			Brittle nails
			Gingivitis
			Cheilosis
			Ascites

VITAMIN E (NOMENCLATURE: TOCOPHEROL)			
Prevents oxidative destruction of vitamin A in the intestine Protects red blood cells from rupture (hemolysis) Helps maintain normal cell membranes by reducing the oxidation of polyunsaturated fatty acids	Wheat germ Vegetable oils Nuts Whole grains	Breakdown of red blood cells	Decreased thyroid hormone level Modest increases in triglycerides
VITAMIN K (NOMENCLATURE: MENADIONE [VITAMIN K_3], PHYLLOQUINONE [VITAMIN K_1])			
Necessary for formation of prothrombin and other factors necessary for blood clotting	Dark green leafy vegetables Cauliflower Soybean oil Green tea Synthesis of intestinal bacteria	Hemorrhage	No toxicity known
VITAMIN D (NOMENCLATURE: ERGOCALCIFEROL [VITAMIN D_2], CHOLECALCIFEROL [VITAMIN D_3]; PRECURSORS—ERGOSTEROL [PLANTS], 7-DEHYDROCHOLESTEROL [IN SKIN])			
Aids in absorption of calcium and phosphorus Regulates blood levels of calcium Promotes bone and teeth mineralization	Fortified milk Fish liver (e.g., cod liver oil) or whole fish with livers such as small sardines or anchovies	Rickets (children) Osteomalacia (adults)	Calcification of soft tissues Hypercalcemia Renal stones Appetite and weight loss Nausea and fatigue Growth failure in children

From the National Research Council: Diet and health, Washington, DC, National Academy Press, 1989; Davis J, Sherer K: Applied nutrition and diet therapy for nurses, ed 2, Philadelphia, WB Saunders, 1994; and Mahan KL, Escott-Stump S: Krause's food, nutrition, and diet therapy, ed 10, Philadelphia, WB Saunders, 2000.

TABLE 4-2
WATER-SOLUBLE VITAMINS

FUNCTIONS	GOOD SOURCES	SYMPTOMS OF DEFICIENCY	SYMPTOMS OF TOXICITY
VITAMIN B$_1$ (NOMENCLATURE: THIAMIN)			
Plays a role in carbohydrate metabolism Helps the nervous system, heart, muscles, and tissue to function properly Promotes a good appetite and good functioning of the digestive tract	Whole grains Wheat germ Enriched white flour products Organ meats Pork Legumes Brewer's yeast	Polyneuritis Beriberi Fatigue Depression Poor appetite Poor functioning of intestinal tract Nervous instability Edema Spastic muscle contractions Wernicke's encephalopathy Korsakoff's psychosis	No toxicity known
VITAMIN B$_2$ (NOMENCLATURE: RIBOFLAVIN [FORMERLY VITAMIN G])			
Essential for certain enzyme systems that aid in the metabolism of carbohydrates, proteins, and fats	Milk and milk products Eggs Green leafy vegetables Organ meats (liver, kidney, heart) Dry yeast Peanuts Peanut butter Whole grains	Tongue inflammation Scaling and burning skin Sensitive eyes Angular stomatitis and cheilosis Cataracts	No toxicity known in humans
VITAMIN B$_3$ (NOMENCLATURE: NIACIN, NICOTINIC ACID)			
Part of two important enzymes that regulate energy metabolism Promotes good physical and mental health and helps maintain the health of the skin, tongue, and digestive system	Meats and organ meats Whole-grain flour products Enriched white flour products Legumes Brewer's yeast	Pellagra (rare) with skin and mouth manifestations Gastrointestinal disturbances Photosensitive dermatitis Depressive psychosis	Flushing caused by vasodilation Nausea and vomiting Abnormal glucose metabolism Abnormal plasma uric acid levels Abnormal liver function tests Gastric ulceration Anaphylaxis (swelling, pain, fever, or asthmatic symptoms caused by physical sensitivity) Circulatory collapse

From the National Research Council: Diet and health, Washington, DC, National Academy Press, 1989; Davis J, Sherer K: Applied nutrition and diet therapy for nurses, ed 2, Philadelphia, WB Saunders, 1994; and Mahan KL, Escott-Stump S: Krause's food, nutrition, and diet therapy, ed 10, Philadelphia, WB Saunders, 2000.

TABLE 4-2
WATER-SOLUBLE VITAMINS—cont'd

FUNCTIONS	GOOD SOURCES	SYMPTOMS OF DEFICIENCY	SYMPTOMS OF TOXICITY
VITAMIN B$_6$ (NOMENCLATURE: PYRIDOXINE, PYRIDOXAL, PYRIDOXAMINE)			
Important in metabolism of proteins and amino acids, carbohydrates, and fats Essential for proper growth and maintenance of body functions	Liver and red meats Whole grains Potatoes Green vegetables Corn	Not fully established, but believed to lead to convulsions, peripheral neuropathy, secondary pellagra, possible depression, oral lesions	Sensory nerve damage Numbness of extremities Ataxia Bone pain Muscle weakness
VITAMIN B$_{12}$ (NOMENCLATURE: COBALAMIN)			
Aids in hemoglobin synthesis Essential for normal functioning of all cells, especially nervous system, bone marrow, and gastrointestinal tract Important in energy metabolism, especially folic acid metabolism	Foods of animal origin Meats Organ meats Dry milk and milk products Whole egg and egg yolk Not found in significant amounts in plant sources	Pernicious (megaloblastic) anemia Subacute combined degeneration of the spinal cord Various psychiatric disorders May cause anorexia	No toxicity known
FOLACIN (NOMENCLATURE: FOLIC ACID)			
Functions in the formation of red blood cells and in normal functioning of gastrointestinal tract Aids in metabolism of protein	Glandular meats Yeast Dark green leafy vegetables Legumes Whole grains	Impaired cell division Alterations of protein synthesis with possible neural tube defect Various psychiatric disorders Megaloblastic anemia Supplements mask the symptoms of pernicious anemia, but not the neurologic manifestations	No toxicity known
CHOLINE			
A constituent of several compounds necessary for certain aspects of nerve function and lipid metabolism	Synthesized from methionine (an amino acid)	Occurs only when protein intake (methylamine) is low	No toxicity known in humans

Continued

■ **TABLE 4-2**
■ **WATER-SOLUBLE VITAMINS—cont'd**

FUNCTIONS	GOOD SOURCES	SYMPTOMS OF DEFICIENCY	SYMPTOMS OF TOXICITY
		PANTOTHENIC ACID	
Essential part of complex enzymes involved in fatty acid metabolism	Animal products Liver Eggs Whole grains Legumes White potatoes Sweet potatoes	Nutritional melalgia (burning foot syndrome) Headache Fatigue Poor muscle coordination Nausea Cramps	Possible diarrhea
		BIOTIN (NOMENCLATURE: ONCE KNOWN AS VITAMIN H)	
Essential for activity of many enzyme systems Plays a central role in fatty acid synthesis and in the metabolism of carbohydrates and protein	Liver Meats Milk Soy flour Brewer's yeast Egg yolk (raw egg white destroys biotin) Bacteria in the intestinal tract also produce biotin	Rare, but includes certain types of anemia, depression, insomnia, muscle pain, dermatitis	No toxicity known in humans
		VITAMIN C (NOMENCLATURE: ASCORBIC ACID, DEHYDROASCORBIC ACID)	
Helps protect the body against infections and in wound healing and recovery from operations Is important for tooth dentin, bones, cartilage, connective tissue, and blood vessels	Citrus fruits Tomatoes Strawberries Cantaloupe Currants Green leafy vegetables Green peppers Broccoli Cabbage Potatoes	Anemia Swollen and bleeding gums Loose teeth Ruptures of small blood vessels (bruises) Scurvy (rebound scurvy can occur when large doses, or megadoses, are suddenly stopped)	Urinary stones Diarrhea Hypoglycemia Interferes with tests for fecal and urinary occult blood Will provide a false positive test for glucosuria

TABLE 4-3
MAJOR MINERALS (MACRONUTRIENTS)

FUNCTIONS	SOURCES	DEFICIENCY SYMPTOMS	TOXICITY SYMPTOMS
MINERAL AND ELEMENTAL SYMBOL: CALCIUM (Ca^{2+})			
Helps muscles to contract and relax, thereby helping to regulate heartbeat Plays a role in the normal functioning of the nervous system Aids in blood coagulation and the functioning of some enzymes Helps build strong bones and teeth May help prevent hypertension	Primarily found in milk and milk products; also found in dark green leafy vegetables, tofu and other soy products, sardines, salmon with bones, and hard water	Poor bone growth and tooth development, leading to stunted growth and increased risk of dental caries, rickets (bowing of legs) in children, osteomalacia (soft bones) and osteoporosis (brittle bones) in adults, poor blood clotting, and possible hypertension	Kidney stones in predisposed individuals
MINERAL AND ELEMENTAL SYMBOL: CHLORIDE (Cl^-)			
Involved in the maintenance of fluid and acid-base balance Provides an acid medium, in the form of hydrochloric acid, for activation of gastric enzymes	Major source is table salt (sodium chloride); also found in fish and vegetables	Disturbances in acid-base balance, with possible growth retardation, psychomotor defects, and memory loss	No toxicity known
MINERAL AND ELEMENTAL SYMBOL: MAGNESIUM (Mg^{2+})			
Helps build strong bones and teeth Activates many enzymes Participates in protein synthesis and lipid metabolism Helps regulate heartbeat	Dark green leafy vegetables, nuts and legumes, whole grains and wheat bran, bananas and apricots, seafoods, coffee, tea, cocoa, and hard water	Rare, but in disease states may lead to central nervous system problems (confusion, apathy, hallucinations, poor memory) and neuromuscular problems (muscle weakness, cramps, tremor, cardiac arrhythmia)	Increased calcium excretion

From the National Research Council: Diet and health, Washington, DC, National Academy Press, 1989; Davis J, Sherer K: Applied nutrition and diet therapy for nurses, ed 2, Philadelphia, WB Saunders, 1994; and Mahan KL, Escott-Stump S: Krause's food, nutrition, and diet therapy, ed 10, Philadelphia, WB Saunders, 2000.

Continued

TABLE 4-3
MAJOR MINERALS (MACRONUTRIENTS)—cont'd

FUNCTIONS	SOURCES	DEFICIENCY SYMPTOMS	TOXICITY SYMPTOMS
MINERAL AND ELEMENTAL SYMBOL: PHOSPHORUS (P)			
Helps build strong bones and teeth Present in the nuclei of all cells Helps in the oxidation of fats and carbohydrates (energy metabolism) Aids in maintaining the body's acid-base balance	Milk and milk products, eggs, meats, legumes, whole grains, soft drinks (used to make the fizz)	Rare, but with malabsorption can cause anorexia, weakness, stiff joints, and fragile bones	Hypocalcemic tetany (muscle spasms)
MINERAL AND ELEMENTAL SYMBOL: POTASSIUM (K⁺)			
Plays a key role in fluid and acid-base balance Transmits nerve impulses and helps control muscle contractions and promotes regular heartbeat Needed for enzyme reactions	Apricots, bananas, oranges, grapefruit, raisins, broccoli, carrots, greens, potatoes, meats, milk and milk products, peanut butter, legumes, molasses, coffee, tea, and cocoa	May cause impaired growth, hypertension, bone fragility, central nervous system changes, renal hypertrophy, diminished heart rate, and death	Hyperkalemia (excess potassium in the blood) with cardiac function disturbances
MINERAL AND ELEMENTAL SYMBOL: SODIUM (Na⁺)			
Plays a key role in the maintenance of acid-base balance Transmits nerve impulses and helps control muscle contractions	Salt (sodium chloride) is the major dietary source; minor sources occur naturally in foods such as milk and milk products and several vegetables	Hyponatremia (too little sodium in the blood)	May cause hypertension, which can lead to cardiovascular diseases and renal (kidney) disease; in the form of salt tablets, can cause gastric irritation
MINERAL AND ELEMENTAL SYMBOL: SULFUR (S)			
Part of three amino acids and the B vitamins thiamin and biotin Plays a role in oxidation reduction reactions Regulates cell membrane permeability	Protein-rich foods (meat, eggs, milk)	None documented in humans	Unlikely to cause significant symptoms

TABLE 4-4
TRACE MINERALS (MICRONUTRIENTS)

FUNCTIONS	SOURCES	DEFICIENCY SYMPTOMS	TOXICITY SYMPTOMS
MINERAL AND ELEMENTAL SYMBOL: CHROMIUM (Cr^{3+})			
Activates several enzymes Enhances the removal of glucose from the blood	Liver and other meats, whole grains, cheese, legumes, and brewer's yeast	Weight loss, abnormalities of the central nervous system, and possible aggravation of diabetes mellitus	Liver damage and lung cancer caused by industrial exposure
MINERAL AND ELEMENTAL SYMBOL: COBALT (Co^{2+})			
An essential component of vitamin B$_{12}$ Activates enzymes	Figs, cabbage, beet greens, spinach, lettuce, watercress	Pernicious anemia	Polycythemia (excess number of red corpuscles in blood) Hyperplasia of bone marrow Increased blood volume
MINERAL AND ELEMENTAL SYMBOL: COPPER (Cu^{2+})			
Aids in the production and survival of red blood cells Part of many enzymes involved in respiration Plays a role in normal lipid metabolism	Shellfish—especially oysters—liver, nuts, seeds, raisins, whole grains, chocolate, and legumes	Anemia, central nervous system problems, abnormal electrocardiograms, bone fragility, impaired immune response; may be a factor in failure to thrive in premature infants	In Wilson's disease, copper accumulation causes neuron and liver cell damage
MINERAL AND ELEMENTAL SYMBOL: FLUORINE (F^-)			
Helps the formation of solid bones and teeth, thereby reducing incidence of dental caries (see Chapter 13) and may help prevent osteoporosis	Fluoridated water (and foods cooked in fluoridated water), fish, tea, gelatin	Increased susceptibility to dental caries	Fluorosis and mottling of teeth

From the National Research Council: Diet and health, Washington, DC, National Academy Press, 1989; Davis J, Sherer K: Applied nutrition and diet therapy for nurses, ed 2, Philadelphia, WB Saunders, 1994; and Mahan KL, Escott-Stump S: Krause's food, nutrition, and diet therapy, ed 10, Philadelphia, WB Saunders, 2000.

Continued

TABLE 4-4
TRACE MINERALS (MICRONUTRIENTS)—cont'd

FUNCTIONS	SOURCES	DEFICIENCY SYMPTOMS	TOXICITY SYMPTOMS
MINERAL AND ELEMENTAL SYMBOL: IODINE (I^-)			
Helps regulate energy metabolism as a part of thyroid hormones Essential for normal cell functioning, helping to keep skin, hair, and nails healthy	Primarily from iodized salt, also found in saltwater fish, seaweed products, vegetables grown in iodine-rich soils	Goiter, cretinism in infants born to iodine-deficient mothers, with accompanying mental retardation and diffuse central nervous system abnormalities	Little toxic effect in individuals with normal thyroid gland functioning Goiter may also occur in toxic states
MINERAL AND ELEMENTAL SYMBOL: IRON (Fe^{3+})			
Essential to the formation of hemoglobin, which is important for tissue respiration and ultimately growth and development and proteins in the body	Heme sources: organ meats, especially liver; red meats; and other meats Nonheme sources: iron-fortified cereals, dark green leafy vegetables, legumes, whole grains, blackstrap molasses, dried fruit, and foods cooked in iron pans	Iron-deficiency anemia and possible alterations that impair behavior	Idiopathic hemochromatosis, which can lead to cirrhosis, diabetes mellitus, and cardiomyopathy Part of several enzymes
MINERAL AND ELEMENTAL SYMBOL: MANGANESE (Mn^{2+})			
Need for normal bone structure, reproduction, normal functioning of cells, and the central nervous system A component of some enzymes	Nuts, whole grains, vegetables and fruits, coffee, tea, cocoa, and egg yolks	None observed in humans	Parkinson's-like symptoms have been noted in miners
MINERAL AND ELEMENTAL SYMBOL: MOLYBDENUM (Mo)			
A component of three enzymes Important for normal cell functioning	Organ meats, legumes, whole grains, dark green vegetables	Vomiting, tachypnea (fast breathing), tachycardia, coma, hypermethioninemia in premature infants (methionine is an amino acid)	No toxicity known

TABLE 4-4

TRACE MINERALS (MICRONUTRIENTS)—cont'd

FUNCTIONS	SOURCES	DEFICIENCY SYMPTOMS	TOXICITY SYMPTOMS
MINERAL AND ELEMENTAL SYMBOL: SELENIUM (Se)			
Part of an enzyme system Acts as an antioxidant with vitamin E to protect the cells from oxygen	Protein-rich foods (meat, eggs, milk, nuts), whole grains, and garlic	Keshan's disease (a human cardiomyopathy) and Kashin-Beck disease (an endemic human osteoarthropathy)	Physical defects of the fingernails and toe-nails and hair loss Nausea Abdominal pain Diarrhea Peripheral neuropathy Fatigue Irritability
MINERAL AND ELEMENTAL SYMBOL: ZINC (Zn^{2+})			
Plays a role in protein synthesis Essential for normal growth and sexual development, wound healing, immune function, cell division and differentiation, and smell acuity	Whole grains, wheat germ, crabmeat, oysters, liver and other meats, brewer's yeast	Depressed immune func-tion, poor growth, dwarfism, impaired skeletal growth and delayed sexual matura-tion, acrodermatitis	Severe anemia, nausea, vomiting, abdominal cramps, diarrhea, fever, hypocupremia (low blood serum copper), malaise, fatigue Impaired immunity also found in toxic states Renal damage

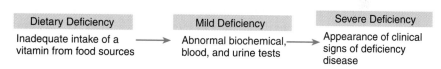

FIGURE 4-2 The progression of the development of vitamin deficiencies.

WHAT IS THE ROLE OF VITAMINS IN NUTRITION?

The body requires vitamins only in minute amounts, but proper growth and de-velopment and optimal health are impossible without them. Some vitamins may be synthesized by the body, but for the most part they must be supplied in the daily diet of normal healthy persons. Early attention was paid to the clear-cut manifestations of diseases caused by vitamin deficiencies (Figure 4-2).

Vitamins, although organic in nature, do not provide energy (kilocalories). But they do help in the metabolism of the kilocalorie-containing macronutrients:

carbohydrate, protein, and fat. In this role, vitamins are thought to act as catalysts.

Vitamins are classified as *body regulators* because of the following functions:

1. *Regulating* the synthesis of many body tissues (bones, skin, glands, nerves, brain, and blood).
2. *Participating* in the cell metabolism of proteins, carbohydrates, and fats.
3. *Preventing* nutritional deficiency diseases and allow for optimal health at all ages.
4. *Serving* as **antioxidants** to reduce damage at the cell level from the process of oxidation.

What Is the Difference Between Fat-Soluble and Water-Soluble Vitamins?

Generally, vitamins are classified into two groups: **fat-soluble** (vitamins A, D, E, and K) and **water-soluble** (B-complex vitamins and vitamin C). The fat-soluble vitamins are stored in body fat and can reach toxic levels, whereas water-soluble vitamins are not stored in any significant amounts in the body, which means that they need to be included in the diet on a daily basis. Deficiencies of fat-soluble vitamins in healthy individuals are less likely to occur than deficiencies of water-soluble vitamins.

The absorption of fat-soluble vitamins is enhanced by dietary fat (Table 4-5). Individuals who are afflicted with malabsorption of fat or who consume an extremely small amount of fat are at higher risk for development of fat-soluble vitamin deficiencies. Fat-soluble vitamins are generally more stable than water-soluble vitamins and are less prone to destruction by heat, air, and light.

What Are the Fat-Soluble Vitamins?

Vitamin A

Vitamin A can be obtained in two forms. The **precursor** form is **carotene**, which is found in abundance in dark green leafy vegetables and deep orange vegetables and fruits. The color of carotene is orange, which is why those foods high in carotene are of similar color and why the skin can turn orange when these foods are eaten in abundance. This is innocuous and fades away once carotene foods are decreased in the diet. Carotene is later converted into vitamin A in the liver and is often simply referred to as vitamin A.

Preformed vitamin A, also called *retinol,* is found in animal products such as liver, milkfat, butter, and egg yolks and is able to produce toxicity in large amounts (see Table 4-1 and Figure 4-3 for other specific food sources).

Deficiency of vitamin A has long been known to increase the risk of infection and is associated with night blindness, as well as total blindness in many countries (see Chapter 15). It is now known that a good intake of vitamin A helps with bone growth, a healthy immune system, improved vision, and reproduction. Inadequate vitamin A nutrition during early pregnancy may account for some congenital abnormalities with the heart, central nervous system, and other structures including the circulatory, urogenital, and respiratory systems; the development of skeleton and limbs may possibly be impaired as well (Zile, 2001).

TABLE 4-5
SOME NUTRIENT INTERACTIONS WITH VITAMINS AND MINERALS

NUTRIENT	INHIBITING NUTRIENT	ENHANCING NUTRIENT
VITAMINS		
Vitamin A (carotene)	Excess vitamin E, deficiency of protein, iron, and zinc	Dietary fat
Vitamin D		Dietary fat
Vitamin E		Dietary fat
Vitamin K	Excess vitamin E	Dietary fat
Vitamin B$_1$	Tannins (as found in coffee)	
Vitamin B$_2$	Excess vitamin B$_1$	
Vitamin B$_3$	Deficiency of vitamin B$_6$	
Vitamin B$_6$	Excess choline and leucine	Deficiency of vitamin C
Vitamin B$_{12}$	Excess vitamin C, deficiency of vitamin B$_6$	
Folacin	Thiamin hastens decomposition in supplements	
Biotin	Pantothenic deficiency	
Choline	Excess inositol	
Vitamin C	Deficiency of vitamin B$_6$	
MINERALS		
Calcium	Excess sodium, protein, phosphorus, oxalates	Vitamin D, lactose, and
Phosphorus	Excess iron	certain amino acids
Magnesium	Excess sodium, calcium, vitamin D, phosphate, protein, and alcohol	
Iron	Excess manganese	Vitamin C, copper, cobalt
Zinc	Excess iron, copper, tin, folic acid, tannins, and possibly calcium	Possible fluoride role
Copper	Excess zinc, molybdenum, and vitamin C	Possible fluoride role Estrogen increases copper serum levels
Molybdenum	Excess sulfur	

How is Vitamin A measured? **Retinol equivalents (REs)** and **international units (IUs)** are two different methods of describing the amount of vitamin A in foods. The use of IUs indicates that both preformed vitamin A and carotenoids are measured; this is still a common method used in food composition tables and diet planning. Because the biologic activities of carotenoids and vitamin A are different, however, REs began to be used. Simply put, numbers used in the IU system are about five times those expressed in the RE system.

Vitamin D

Vitamin D has many physiologic roles beyond those related to bones, including regulating blood pressure and acting as a tumor suppressant. The recommended amount of vitamin D has recently increased for adults over age 50 (Fuller and Casparian, 2001). Vitamin D deficiency leads to secondary hyperparathyroidism, increased bone turnover, bone loss, and, when severe, to osteomalacia.

Vitamin D has been known to prevent **rickets** (bowing of the legs caused by increasing weight on the soft bones of growing children who do not receive

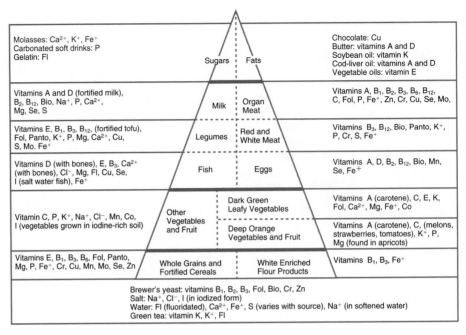

FIGURE 4-3 Vitamin and mineral content of the Food Guide Pyramid (listed in the following order: fat-soluble vitamins, water-soluble vitamins, major minerals, and trace minerals). (Key: *Bio*, biotin; Ca^{2+}, calcium; Cl^-, chloride; *Co*, cobalt; *Cr*, chromium; *Cu*, copper; Fe^+, iron; *Fl*, fluorine; *Fol*, folate; *I*, iodine; K^+, potassium; *Mg*, magnesium; *Mn*, manganese; *Mo*, molybdenum; Na^+, sodium; *P*, phosphorus; *Panto*, pantothenic acid; *S*, sulfur; *Se*, selenium; *Zn*, zinc.)

enough vitamin D) since the early part of this century although rickets in children had been recognized for centuries before (Figure 4-4). After vitamin D was chemically isolated in 1935, it was eventually added to milk, which ultimately replaced cod liver oil as a means to prevent rickets (1 tsp of cod liver oil provides about 100% of the RDA for vitamin D and vitamin A). Milk is an appropriate food to fortify with vitamin D because this vitamin greatly enhances the absorption of calcium, of which milk is the best source.

Sunlight also contributes to vitamin D levels by starting the conversion of a cholesterol-related vitamin D precursor in the skin to an active form. This conversion varies according to the length and intensity of sun exposure and the color of the skin. Institutionalized elderly persons are at high risk for vitamin D deficiency because of negligible exposure to the sun and may therefore benefit from supplementation. Patients with renal (kidney) disease may also require supplementation because of impairment of the final steps of vitamin D synthesis, which occur in the kidneys (see Chapter 10). With aging, the ability of the body to produce vitamin D from sunlight exposure becomes impaired.

Vitamin D analogues are useful in topical therapy of psoriasis (Durakovic et al., 2001). Vitamin D has immunoregulatory properties that may explain the association with accelerated bone loss in persons with rheumatoid arthritis

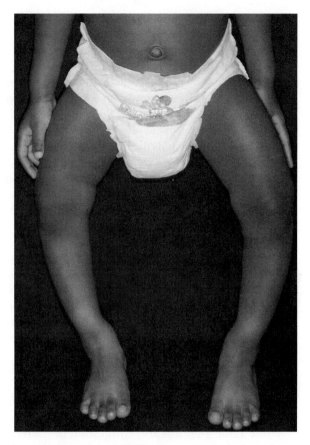

FIGURE 4-4 Nutritional vitamin D deficiency rickets in young child. (From Shah BR, Laude TA: Atlas of pediatric clinical diagnosis, ed 1, Philadelphia, WB Saunders, 2000.)

(Garcia-Lozano et al., 2001). Vitamin D deficiency resulting from malabsorption may be a factor in the biology of low bone mineral density (BMD) in patients with cystic fibrosis (Lark et al., 2001).

Vitamin D deficiency is considered a public health problem. Risk of vitamin D deficiency increases in those who follow vegan diets or in others who do not consume vitamin D-fortified milk. This is especially a risk during the winter months or in other conditions where skin is not adequately exposed to sunlight, such as with veiled Arab women. Evidence suggests that the daily oral intake of vitamin D in sunlight-deprived individuals should exceed 600 IU; most probably it should be 1000 IU per day (Glerup et al., 2000).

Vitamin E
Vitamin E was initially recognized as essential for reproduction in rats. Vitamin E acts as an antioxidant and appears to have a role in preventing cell damage from oxidation. Although known toxic effects from excess ingestion of vitamin E are limited primarily to premature infants, persons receiving anticoagulant

medications such as coumadin may have complications associated with mega-doses of vitamin E because it inhibits the clotting action of vitamin K. At this time, there is not enough medical justification for the use of large doses of vitamin E, particularly as it is widely distributed in common foods. A mere ¼ cup of almonds provides 100% of the RDA for vitamin E.

Vitamin E deficiency is now associated with neurologic problems including spinocerebellar, retinal, and peripheral nerve deficits, particularly in conjunction with protein-energy malnutrition (Kalra et al., 2001). A form of neurodegenerative ataxia with vitamin E deficiency related to a mutation in a transfer protein gene was reported. Therefore measurement of serum vitamin E concentration should be included as part of the investigations in children with progressive ataxia, even in the absence of fat malabsorption. Early treatment with vitamin E may protect such children against further neurologic damage (Alex et al., 2000).

Vitamin K

Vitamin K was first recognized as an antihemorrhagic factor. Because vitamin K is essential for the formation of **prothrombin** (a clotting factor), defective blood coagulation is the main symptom of vitamin K deficiency. Vitamin K is also involved in other physiologic processes, including vascular function and bone metabolism. Vitamin K—with vitamin D and calcium—was found to be useful in increasing the bone density of the lumbar spine in postmenopausal women with osteoporosis (Iwamoto et al., 2000).

Because the vitamin K requirement of bones and vessel walls is higher than that of the liver (where the clotting factors are produced), it has been suggested that RDA values for vitamin K be redefined (Vermeer and Schurgers, 2000). This vitamin is not only found in dietary sources such as dark green leafy vegetables (see Table 4-1), it is also synthesized by bacteria in the jejunum and ileum. Vitamin K deficiency is most likely to occur in individuals receiving antibiotics over an extended period who are not able to absorb fat and who have a low intake of foods containing vitamin K. Infants are also at risk because of low levels of the vitamin K-synthesizing bacteria in the intestinal tract. Vitamin K injections are recommended for newborn infants and infant formulas are now routinely supplemented with this vitamin. Persons receiving antibiotic therapy should be considered for vitamin K supplementation. Persons who take coumadin to reduce the risk of blood clot formation need a consistent intake of vitamin K to maintain stable prothrombin rates.

Water-Soluble Vitamins

The **vitamin B complex** refers to all water-soluble vitamins except ascorbic acid (vitamin C). Vitamin B_1 was the first of this group to be discovered and was found to prevent **beriberi** (a condition involving inflammation of the nerves). With further study, vitamin B proved to be not a single substance, but a combination of substances, each one of which was given a letter or a descriptive term, or later a chemical designation as its chemical nature became known.

Several factors in the vitamin B complex are recognized today. These include thiamin (vitamin B_1), riboflavin (B_2), niacin (B_3), pyridoxine and related substances (collectively known as vitamin B_6), cobalamin (B_{12}), and folacin (see the DRI table on the inside back cover). Important functions in the body have been assigned to biotin, choline, and pantothenic acid, but no definite daily allowances have been established, although estimated safe and AIs are now given.

A lack of B-complex vitamins is one of the most widespread forms of malnutrition. Because of the similar distribution of these vitamins in foods, a deficiency of several is observed more often than is a deficiency of a single one. The interrelationship of many of these vitamins in life processes means that signs of dietary deficiency are often similar when the diet lacks any one of several factors (Figure 4-5). Many physiologic and pathologic stresses influence the need for the B vitamins, but generally an adequate diet including whole grains will meet these needs. The

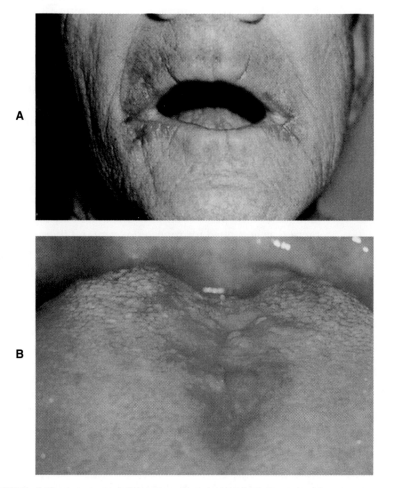

FIGURE 4-5 Vitamin B deficiencies. **A**, Angular cheilosis caused by vitamin B complex deficiency. **B**, Depapillation of the tongue from the same cause. (**A** from Callen JP, Greer KE, Hood AF, Paller AS, and Swinyer LJ: Color atlas of dermatology, Philadelphia, WB Saunders, 1993; **B** from Murphy GF, Herzberg AJ: Atlas of dermatopathology, Philadelphia, WB Saunders, 1996.)

germ portion of grain kernels is especially rich in nutrients such as the B vitamins. Wheat germ can be found in the cereal section of grocery stores and has a nutty flavor and crunchy texture that can be added to a wide variety of foods.

Thiamin (Vitamin B$_1$)

The requirement for thiamin is small, but important, and is based on the caloric requirements. Thiamin is needed in increased amounts during pregnancy and breastfeeding, but these levels are easy to achieve through an increased food intake. Deficiency of this vitamin does occur when unenriched processed white flour and white rice or sugar is consumed as a main staple of the diet. Deficiency characteristics include beriberi (muscle wasting from nerve damage or edema), mental confusion, anorexia, and enlarged heart. Alcoholics can also develop Wernicke-Korsakoff syndrome (see Chapter 3). Although Wernicke's encephalopathy is most commonly associated with alcoholism, other causes have also been implicated: excessive vomiting, drastic weight-reducing diet, renal colic in a postpartum woman, colonic surgery, and chronic hemodialysis (Merkin-Zaborsky et al., 2001). **Neuropathy** is associated with deficiency of thiamin. Neuropathy includes problems of the peripheral nervous system and is commonly found in persons with diabetes unrelated to thiamin deficiency.

The classic signs of thiamin deficiency only occur in states of extreme depletion and are unreliable indicators for early treatment of alcoholic patients at risk. Thiamin deficiency sufficient to cause irreversible brain damage has been noted. Decreased intake of foods containing thiamin, malabsorption, reduced storage, and impaired utilization further reduce the chances of recovery. Even large oral doses of thiamin may be inadequate for rapid replacement of depleted brain thiamin levels. To provide an effective treatment for Wernicke's encephalopathy there may be a need for repeated parenteral therapy with adequate doses of thiamin (Thomson, 2000).

The only known toxicity is from intravenously administered thiamin. However, the potential for toxicity exists in extremely large doses readily available in supplement form, especially with long-term, chronic use of very high amounts.

Riboflavin (Vitamin B$_2$)

The requirement for riboflavin is also related to caloric requirements. Riboflavin is involved in many enzyme reactions that allow for energy use at the cellular level. It is important for healthy eyes, skin, lips, and tongue. Deficiency symptoms are associated with skin changes such as **cheilosis** (see Figure 4-5) and vulval and scrotal skin changes and general dermatitis. Without an adequate consumption of milk and milk products, riboflavin intake is likely to be impaired. The metabolism of riboflavin is dependent on a variety of minerals such as vanadium (Swavey and Gould, 2000). There are no known toxic levels of this vitamin.

Niacin (Nicotinic Acid or Vitamin B$_3$)

Niacin requirements are related to caloric intake and are essential for energy metabolism at the cellular level. Niacin needs are met in part by the conversion of the amino acid tryptophan, found in milk and eggs.

The niacin deficiency disease **pellagra** is a syndrome of various skin, digestive, and mental disturbances. Pellagra is caused by a deficiency of nicotinamide or of its precursor tryptophan. Pellagra leads to the triad of dermatitis, diarrhea, and dementia, eventually followed by death. Because of the diversity of pellagra's signs and symptoms, diagnosis is difficult. The combination of homelessness, alcohol abuse, and failure to eat regularly is associated with the development of pellagra (Kertesz, 2001).

Pyridoxine, Pyridoxal, and Pyridoxamine and Related Substances (Vitamin B$_6$)

Vitamin B$_6$ is necessary for normal cell membrane function and stability. Vitamin B$_6$ functions primarily in the cellular metabolism of protein and amino acids. It is also important in energy metabolism. Vitamin B$_6$ may be of importance in regeneration of red blood cells and the normal functioning of the nervous system. This vitamin also lowers levels of homocysteine, a risk factor for cardiovascular disease (see Chapter 8). In addition, vitamin B$_6$ helps to convert tryptophan to niacin.

A deficient status of this vitamin adversely alters the function and structure of endothelial cells of the vascular lining (Chang, 2000). Widespread structural defect of collagen in connective tissue has been noted with vitamin B$_6$ deficiency and excess cortisol levels (Masse et al., 2000). Excess pyridoxine can be related to neuropathy. Women who take 500 to 5000 mg of vitamin B$_6$ per day to treat premenstrual syndrome (PMS, see Chapter 12) have shown peripheral neuropathy within a few years. The use of vitamin B$_6$ at doses less than 100 mg per day appears safe for adults.

Three interrelated substances—pyridoxine (from plants), pyridoxal, and pyridoxamine (from animal products)—are collectively known as vitamin B$_6$. The need for vitamin B$_6$ increases with high-protein diets, pregnancy, certain tuberculosis therapies, certain medications, and some contraceptives.

Fallacy: Women experiencing premenstrual syndrome (PMS) should be advised to take a vitamin B$_6$ supplement.

Fact: There is no scientific evidence to support this hypothesis. Women who are insistent on this approach would be better off increasing their vitamin B$_6$ intake through the use of whole grains, wheat germ, or legumes. A balanced diet, evenly spaced throughout the day to help maintain blood glucose levels, may also be helpful to minimize symptoms of PMS. Supplement use should not exceed 100 mg per day, which is the upper limit (UL) for this vitamin.

Cobalamin (Vitamin B$_{12}$)

Cobalt, a mineral, is an essential part of vitamin B$_{12}$. **Pernicious anemia** (a form of anemia that can lead to permanent neurologic impairment and death) is caused by a lack of **intrinsic factor**, a glycoprotein secreted in the stomach that attaches to vitamin B_{12} to aid its absorption. Decreased amounts of intrinsic factor are common among elderly persons (see Chapter 14). Vitamin B_{12} is found bound to protein in foods of animal origin. There is relatively little in vegetables, which is why strict vegetarians (also known as *vegans*) may need a vitamin B_{12} supplement. Intestinal malabsorption can also cause a deficiency, because the ileum is the main site of vitamin B_{12} absorption. Latin American and black patients have food cobalamin malabsorption more often than do white and Asian American patients (Carmel et al., 2001).

Mild hyperhomocysteinemia (associated with cardiovascular disease—see Chapter 8) can be a consequence of vitamin B_{12} deficiency, as found with vegans (see Chapter 1). In conditions of low methionine intake (methionine is an amino acid found in animal protein sources and, in low amounts, in plant proteins), a pathway of homocysteine metabolism prevails that is vitamin B_{12}- and folate-dependent. Thus the combination of low methionine and low vitamin B_{12} levels in a vegan diet contributes to hyperhomocysteinemia (Krajcovicova-Kudlackova et al., 2000). Ability to absorb vitamin B_{12} decreases with age.

Psychotic symptoms have also been associated with deficiency of vitamin B_{12}. A treatment of vitamin B_{12} in combination with folic acid was found to correct the psychosis. This emphasizes the need to measure this vitamin in geriatric patients, especially when they have a severe infection and organic mental symptoms (Buchman et al., 1999).

Folate

The active form of folate is folic acid, which is formed from folate by vitamin C. Many forms of this water-soluble vitamin exist. Folate aids in the metabolism of protein and **deoxyribonucleic acid (DNA)**, a basic structure of genes found in all cells. Studies with human cells clearly show that folate deficiency causes fragile chromosomes and chromosomal breaks (Fenech, 2001).

Folate helps prevent **spina bifida**, a condition that starts during the first month of pregnancy when the spinal cord is not fully enclosed. It is recommended that all women of childbearing age consume 0.4 mg folic acid daily. Grain products that are fortified with B vitamins now must also be fortified with folic acid.

Alcoholic patients going through withdrawal with low levels of folate and high blood alcohol concentrations were found to be at increased risk for withdrawal seizures. Those most at risk for seizures were best identified by a high homocysteine level upon admission (Bleich et al., 2000). In normal, healthy adults, supplemental folate can be considered nontoxic. Those on antiepileptic medications should consult their physicians. Other concerns related to supplemental folate include potential problems identifying a B_{12} deficiency resulting in neurologic damage, reduced zinc absorption, and interactions with drugs designed to inhibit folate metabolism.

Folate got its name from the word *foliage,* because all dark green leafy vegetables are high in folate. Ideally, raw, fresh, dark green leafy vegetables such as spinach or broccoli should be consumed because folate may be lost in cooking. Legumes and wheat germ are also high sources of folate.

Choline

Choline is a constituent of several compounds that are necessary for certain aspects of nerve function and lipid metabolism. No RDA has been established, but AI and UL values can be found in the DRI table inside the back cover. An enzyme containing choline was found to help prevent the degeneration of nerves in the genetic condition called *Huntington's disease*—of which Woody Guthrie died (Kosinski et al., 1999). Fatty liver has been found to be induced by consumption of a choline-deficient diet and is associated with a lower level of antioxidants. Starvation combined with choline deficiency appears to allow increased oxidative injury to the fatty liver (Grattagliano et al., 2000). Mixed diets are estimated to provide adults with 400 to 900 mg of choline daily and such diets are evidently adequate. In addition, the body can synthesize choline from methionine.

Pantothenic Acid

Pantothenic acid is an essential constituent of complex enzymes involved in fatty acid metabolism and synthesis of certain products. It is widely distributed in food and occurs abundantly in animal sources, whole-grain cereals, and legumes. The AI levels can be found in the DRI table inside the back cover. Dietary deficiencies are unlikely, but marginal ones may exist in generally malnourished individuals, as well as deficiency of other B-complex vitamins. The usual dietary intake is between 5 and 20 mg daily.

Biotin

Biotin is a sulfur-containing vitamin that is essential for the activity of many enzyme systems. It is widely distributed in nature and is bound to protein in foods and tissues. It plays a central role in synthesis of fatty acids and participates in several metabolic reactions at the cellular level. The AI levels may be found in the DRI table inside the back cover.

The uptake and transport of biotin in the small intestine is shared with pantothenic acid. Both biotin and pantothenic acid are synthesized by colonic microflora of the large intestine (Said, 1999). Biotin deficiency may be aggravated by pantothenic acid deficiency (Ramakrishna, 1999).

Biotin deficiency has been shown to be induced by excess intake of raw egg white or by long-term parenteral nutrition (see Chapter 5). Insufficient biotin intake results in symptoms such as loss of appetite, nausea and vomiting, hair loss, dermatitis, and an increase in cholesterol. There is no known toxicity.

Vitamin C (Ascorbic Acid)

Vitamin C, also called ascorbic acid, is a water-soluble derivative of glucose and performs a variety of functions. It is an essential cofactor for a range of enzymes involved in diverse metabolic pathways. Vitamin C aids in the formation and maintenance of the intracellular cement substance of body tissues, thus is important for tooth dentin, bones, cartilage, connective tissue, and blood vessels. Through its role of promoting skin integrity, it is thought to help protect the body against infections. Vitamin C helps heal wounds, which is critical for a patient recovering from a surgical operation. Consumption of foods rich in vitamin C (fruits and vegetables) is associated with decreased risk of cardiovascular disease, many types of cancer, and possibly neurodegenerative disease. Whether this effect is because of the vitamin C content of these foods or other substances found in these foods is uncertain. To date, there is no strong evidence that vitamin C supplements decrease the oxidative damage to DNA (Halliwell, 2001).

Higher levels may be necessary during conditions of stress, with certain medications, or in persons who smoke. However, these increased needs can easily be met with an extra serving of a food high in vitamin C. Citrus fruits, melons, dark green leafy vegetables, potatoes, and green pepper are all high in vitamin C. Foods containing vitamin C also contain other vitamins and minerals needed for health.

Inadequate vitamin C intake may eventually lead to swollen and bleeding gums, loose teeth, and ruptures of small blood vessels (Figure 4-6), which are early forerunners of *scorbutus,* also known as scurvy. Vitamin C is generally not toxic. However, some individuals are at risk of toxicity. About one eighth of men with African, Asian, Sephardic Jewish, or Mediterranean heritage are born with glucose-6-phosphate dehydrogenase deficiency. In these individuals, megadoses of vitamin C will instantly affect red blood cells and can lead to death within hours. In addition, megadoses of vitamin C can precipitate an acute sickle cell crisis in those with **sickle cell disease** (a disease in which red blood cells take on a sickle shape). Also, because megadoses of vitamin C cause **hyperosmotic diarrhea** (in which excess substances attract water in the intestinal tract through the process of osmosis, resulting in watery stools), persons with preexisting diarrhea—such as those with AIDS—can go into hypovolemic shock.

A safe dose of vitamin C is less than 1000 mg daily, 500 mg being already nearly ten times the recommended daily amount. Very high amounts of vitamin C increase oxalate and urate excretion, which can promote the development of renal stones (see Chapter 10). **Rebound scurvy** may occur if the body has be-

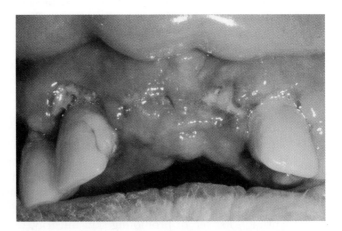

FIGURE 4-6 Scorbutic gingivitis. (From Neville BW, Damm DD, Allen CM, Bouquot JE: Oral and maxillofacial pathology, ed 2, Philadelphia, WB Saunders, 2002.)

come accustomed to high doses of vitamin C that result in high blood plasma levels and the dose is then discontinued. Instead, health professionals recommend that people in this category gradually decrease from high doses. Much more research is needed on the safety of high doses of vitamin C and other vitamins. A more prudent approach at the present time is to obtain vitamin C, as well as other vitamins and minerals, from food sources to help avoid toxicity problems.

Fallacy: People who have colds should take megadoses of vitamin C (1 g per day).

Fact: Although cold symptoms may lessen to a minor degree, the risks of large doses of vitamin C can outweigh any possible benefits. A 1 g dose is more than ten times the RDA for vitamin C, which is less than 100 mg per day. This quantity can result in rebound scurvy when the dosage is stopped. Also, a vitamin C supplement that is in chewable pill form promotes dental decay because the acidity of vitamin C is very destructive to dental enamel.

WHAT IS THE ROLE OF MINERALS IN NUTRITION?

Minerals function as building material in the following:

Bony tissue: Calcium, magnesium, and phosphorus in bones and teeth; fluoride in teeth
Soft body tissue (muscles, nerves, and glands): All salts, especially phosphorus, potassium, sulfur, and chloride
Hair, nails, and skin: Sulfur
Blood: All salts, as well as iron for hemoglobin and copper for red blood cells
Glandular secretions: Chloride in gastric juice, sodium in intestinal juice, iodine in thyroxine, manganese in endocrine secretions, and zinc in enzymes

Minerals also function as regulators of the following:

Fluid pressure: All salts, especially sodium and potassium
Muscle contraction and relaxation: Calcium, magnesium, potassium, sodium, phosphorus, and chloride
Nerve responses: All salts, with a balance between calcium and sodium
Blood clotting: Calcium
Oxidation in tissues and blood: Iron and iodine
The acid-base balance: A balance between acidic compounds—chloride, sulfur, and phosphorus—and basic compounds—calcium, sodium, potassium, and magnesium
Coenzymes: zinc, magnesium, potassium, calcium, and chloride

How Are Minerals Classified?

Minerals are usually classified into two groups: *major minerals* and *trace minerals*. The major minerals are those present in the human body in amounts greater than 5 g. The trace minerals are found in the human body in amounts less than 5 g. See Tables 4-3 and 4-4 for lists of the major and trace minerals, their functions and sources, and symptoms of deficiency and toxicity. The known DRIs for minerals can be found inside the back cover. Other trace minerals are now thought to be essential, but no DRI has been set for amounts needed for health. These minerals include aluminum, arsenic, boron, bromine, cadmium, germanium (used in semiconductors, which muscle and nerve cells essentially are), lead, lithium, nickel, rubidium, silicon, tin, and vanadium. Because minerals are meant to be found in the body only in small amounts, chronic excess ingestion has potential for toxicity. An adequate diet allows for a safe intake of these trace minerals, especially if whole grains, legumes, and leafy green vegetables are consumed regularly.

Major Minerals

Calcium

Stored in the form of calcium phosphate, calcium is the major mineral constituent of the body—99% of which is found in bones and teeth (giving rigidity), with the remainder found in the blood, other body fluids, and soft tissues. In conjunction with the other minerals, calcium facilitates passage of materials into and out of cells. Vitamin D is required for proper absorption and use of dietary calcium. Inadequate calcium in the diet leads to poor bone growth and tooth development, stunted body growth, rickets in children (see Figure 4-4), osteomalacia and osteoporosis in adults, thin and fragile bones, and poor blood clotting. However, variability in calcium balance is more a consequence of absorption than of actual calcium intake. It has long been believed that excess dietary phosphorus and protein inhibit calcium absorption. However, more recent work disputes this assumption (Heaney, 2000).

Calcium is effective in reducing blood pressure in various types of hypertension, including that which is induced by pregnancy. Inadequate vitamin D and calcium intake could play a contributory role in the pathogenesis and progression of hypertension and cardiovascular disease in elderly women (Pfeifer et al., 2001). Low levels of calcium in the blood can lead to **tetany**, a condition of muscle twitches, cramps, and convulsions. The condition is not likely caused by inadequate calcium intake but rather by **hypoparathyroidism** (reduced function of the parathyroid gland), some bone diseases, certain kidney diseases, or low serum protein. High levels of calcium can be caused by hyperparathyroidism or excess vitamin D from excessive milk or supplement intake.

Milk, the best source for calcium, is also a major contributor of protein, vitamin D, riboflavin, potassium, and magnesium. For this reason, milk intake is a major contributor to health. Calcium supplements cannot replace the nutritive value of milk. One concern with reliance on calcium supplements versus milk is the purity of the supplement. An analysis of 136 brands of supplements that were purchased in 1996 found that two thirds of them failed to meet the 1999 California criteria for acceptable lead levels. Antacids and infant formulas had the lowest lead concentrations (Scelfo and Flegal, 2000).

Calcium absorption is enhanced by stomach acid released in digestion (see Chapter 3).

Individuals who cannot tolerate milk can use alternatives such as low-lactose milk and fortified soy milk. For persons who are weight-conscious or trying to control their fat intake, low-fat or skim milk can be used. Figure 4-3 shows where calcium foods are found in the Food Guide Pyramid. Although dark green leafy vegetables are high in calcium, the calcium in chard, beet greens, spinach, and rhubarb generally is not available to the body because an insoluble salt forms with the oxalic acid found in these foods.

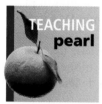

TEACHING pearl

An interesting experiment (and a useful teaching technique) is to soak a chicken bone in vinegar, which leaches the calcium from the bone. This activity clearly demonstrates how calcium lends rigidity to the bone, because without it the bone becomes extremely soft and pliable.

fact FALLACY

Fallacy: Butter and eggs are high in calcium because they are dairy products.

Fact: Butter comes from milkfat and does not contain a significant amount of calcium. Eggs do not have any significant amount of calcium.

Magnesium

Magnesium affects many cellular functions, including transport of potassium and calcium ions, and modulates nerve signal transduction, energy metabolism, and cell proliferation. In addition to the other minerals, magnesium is vital for the metabolism of adenosine triphosphate (ATP) and thus plays a role in metabolic processes at the cellular level and in muscle contractions. The major food sources of magnesium are those containing chlorophyll, such as the dark green leafy vegetables (magnesium is a part of the green chlorophyll molecule).

Magnesium deficiency is relatively common among the general population. Its intake has decreased over the years, especially in the western world. Magnesium supplementation or intravenous infusion may be beneficial in various diseased states. There is special interest in the role of magnesium status in alcoholism, eclampsia, hypertension, atherosclerosis, cardiac diseases, diabetes, and asthma (Saris et al., 2000). Magnesium deficiency is associated with oxidative damage (Kharb and Singh, 2000).

Magnesium deficiency can occur as a result of frequent urination, as found in uncontrolled diabetes and with the use of diuretics. Low levels of magnesium in the blood can also be caused by alcoholism, malabsorption, hyperthyroidism, use of steroids, and massive blood transfusions.

High levels of magnesium can be caused by renal failure, heavy use of laxatives and antacids containing magnesium, dialysis, total parenteral nutrition (TPN, see Chapter 5), and inadequate amounts of the hormone aldosterone. Reduced renal function in general among the elderly population increases the risk for toxicity symptoms as a result of excessive retention of magnesium. Antacids, laxatives, or other drugs containing magnesium should be used cautiously in such individuals.

Food sources high in magnesium include dark green leafy vegetables, legumes, whole grains, and fish (see Table 4-3).

Phosphorus

Phosphorus helps enzymes act in energy metabolism. Among minerals, the amount of phosphorus in the body is second only to the amount of calcium. The largest amount of phosphorus is found with calcium in the bones; the remainder is in soft tissues and fluids. A wide variation in the ratio of calcium to phosphorus is tolerated in the adult diet that includes adequate vitamin D. A ratio of 1.5:1 is recommended in early infancy to prevent tetany caused by **hypocalcemia** (low blood levels of calcium). Newer evidence, however, has shown that a high phosphorus intake does not significantly alter bone-related hormones (Grimm et al., 2001). Phosphorus is widely available in most foods. Thus deficiency is not a problem in the United States.

Potassium

Potassium is an *electrolyte* (a substance that conducts electric flow through the body, discussed later in this chapter). Potassium is necessary for intracellular enzyme reactions and the synthesis of proteins.

Serum potassium fluctuations can be fatal because potassium affects the heartbeat. This is one reason that taking potassium supplements—such as those found in salt substitutes (e.g., potassium chloride)—should be based on a physician's recommendation. It is imperative that individuals who are taking potassium-depleting diuretics receive additional potassium, preferably through food and again on the advice of a physician. Persons taking hypertensive medications called ACE inhibitors retain potassium and thus need to avoid use of salt substitutes containing it. These ACE inhibitors often end in the suffix *-il*, such as enalapril and captopril.

There is no DRI for potassium; however, the recommended intake is about 1500 to 6000 mg, which is easily met by a variety of food sources.

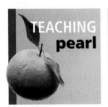

TEACHING pearl

Based on kilocalories and carbohydrate content, leafy green vegetables contain far more potassium than the usually recommended bananas and orange juice for a person taking a potassium-depleting diuretic. One average banana contains 120 kcal and 30 g of carbohydrate. For the same amount of potassium, ½ c spinach or broccoli provides only 25 kcal and 5 g carbohydrate.

Sodium

Sodium is an electrolyte, and as such is vital to health. It is naturally found in low levels in food, although rather significant levels are found in some foods such as milk and certain vegetables. The major dietary sources are table salt (sodium chloride) and foods with added salt, such as processed meats, convenience foods, and canned vegetables and soups (canned fruit is low in sodium). One teaspoon of salt contains about 2400 mg of sodium.

The recommended Daily Value for sodium, as found on food labels, is 2400 mg (see Figure 1-2). An intake up to 4000 mg is generally safe for healthy adults.

Reducing salt intake has been recommended for calcium-stone–forming patients with hypercalciuria and osteopenia (Martini et al., 2000). Increased sodium intake can increase loss of calcium into the urine. See Chapter 8 for a more detailed discussion of sodium as it relates to heart disease.

Trace Minerals

Fluoride
This mineral helps in the formation of solid bones and teeth. It also helps reduce the incidence of dental caries (see Chapter 13). There is some evidence that it aids calcium in bone formation. The Food and Nutrition Board recommends fluoridation of public water supplies if natural fluoride levels are low. The American Dental Association recommends fluoride supplements until about age 13 or until the adult teeth are fully formed. Like other trace minerals, fluoride is toxic when consumed in excessive amounts. The DRIs have now been established, as listed in the DRI table inside the back cover.

Iron
More than one half of the 4 to 5 g of iron in the body is in hemoglobin found in the bloodstream. **Hemoglobin** facilitates tissue respiration by carrying oxygen from the lungs to the tissue cells and by carrying the carbon dioxide formed in oxidation away from cells. Copper, protein, vitamin B_{12}, B_6, and folate are necessary for hemoglobin synthesis. Tests for levels of hemoglobin indicate whether iron deficiency **anemia** (a condition of reduced oxygen delivery to the body cells) is present.

Iron comes in two forms: heme and nonheme. **Heme iron**—found in high quantities in red meat and organ meats such as liver, kidney, and heart—is absorbed extremely well by the body. In contrast, *nonheme iron*—found in plant foods such as blackstrap molasses, whole grains, iron-fortified cereals, and legumes—is poorly absorbed unless vitamin C foods or meat are consumed at the same meal. For example, orange juice or coleslaw, each with a high vitamin C content, would enhance the iron absorption from a peanut butter sandwich or other nonheme iron source. The use of iron cooking pans is also known to increase the iron content of food greatly; the amount of that increase is related to the length of cooking time and acidity of the food.

During periods of rapid growth—such as with infants older than 6 months, children through the preschool years, adolescents, and pregnancy—the need for iron increases. Loss of blood (e.g., in menstruating women) increases the need for iron.

Excess iron inhibits absorption of zinc (see Table 4-5). True toxicity from food sources has been documented only from long-term ingestion of home-brewed alcohol made in iron stills. However, toxic overdoses from iron supplements do occur in the United States. Genetically some persons are at risk for **iron overload** (idiopathic hemochromatosis) and has recently been recognized as a common disorder. From 1979 to 1997, the rate of hemochromatosis-associated hospitalizations was 2.3 per 100,000 persons in the United States (Brown et al., 2001). Iron overload is highly prevalent among males of northern European descent, but has also been found among Hispanics and African Americans. The liver is a principal target for iron toxicity because it is chiefly responsible for taking up and storing excessive amounts of iron. Heavy iron overload, as occurs in primary (hereditary) or secondary forms of hemochromatosis, may cause cirrhosis, liver failure, and hepatocellular carcinoma (Bonkovsky and Lambrecht, 2000). Problems related to hemochromatosis can be averted by early detection if those affected avoid excess iron intake with regular blood donation. To assess if a person has iron overload, health professionals are recommended to measure the transferrin index, which is the serum iron level divided by measured transferrin. Values greater than 1.0 are associated with this disorder.

Iodine

Iodine is found in thyroid hormones involved in general metabolism. An antioxidant function of iodide has been recognized in the stomach, breast, and thyroid gland. A correlation was found between a decrease in the stomach cancer rate in Italy and eating iodine-rich fish (Venturi et al., 2000). Iodized salt and saltwater fish are the most common sources of iodine. Inadequate iodine intake leads to **goiter**, a disease of the thyroid gland (Figure 4-7). A form of mental retardation, **cretinism** was once a relatively common phenomenon in infants born to mothers who had iodine deficiency during pregnancy. With the advent of fortification, iodine was added to salt and goiter and cretinism have virtually disappeared in the United States. The present intake of iodine in the United States is

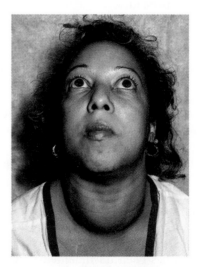

FIGURE 4-7 Goiter. (From Swartz MH: Textbook of physical diagnosis, ed 3, Philadelphia, WB Saunders, 1997.)

considered adequate, although use of iodized salt is still important, especially in noncoastal regions where fish intake is limited.

Selenium

Selenium has a close metabolic relationship with the antioxidant vitamin E, but other functions are likely to exist. Selenium is important in providing protection against oxidative damage. Selenium is one of the essential nutrients that may have beneficial effects on health at dietary intakes higher than the established RDAs in the United States (Neve, 2000). The selenium requirement for adults appears to be related to body weight. The RDA for selenium was first set in 1989 and DRI values may be found in the table inside the back cover.

Selenium toxicity and deficiency have been noted mainly as a result of soil selenium content. Selenium deficiency was first noted in China, where it was associated with **cardiomyopathy** (a form of heart disease). Hair loss and toxic defects in fingernails and toenails have been found in regions where there is a high content of selenium in the soil.

Zinc

Zinc is a component of more than 50 enzymes. It promotes cell division and differentiation, mainly because of its role in protein synthesis. The retina contains particularly high amounts of zinc, suggesting a pivotal role in this tissue. There is also suggestive evidence that zinc deficiency in humans may result in abnormal dark adaptation and age-related macular degeneration; however, excess zinc acts as a toxin (Ugarte and Osborne, 2001). Zinc is required for normal taste perception and sexual development. Zinc deficiency induces a decrease of myelinated nerve fibers (Gong and Amemiya, 2001).

Although zinc is stored primarily in bone, it is poorly mobilized, and therefore regular dietary intake is crucial. Zinc is found in high amounts in the germ portion of grains, in nuts, and animal protein foods (see Table 4-4).

Individuals with malabsorption, such as those with chronic diarrhea, chronic pancreatitis, *celiac sprue* (a condition involving the intestinal tract that is caused by an allergy-like reaction to gluten found in certain grains; see Chapter 3), *Crohn's disease* (an inflammatory disease of the intestinal tract; see Chapter 3), and short bowel syndrome, are at particular risk for zinc deficiency. Zinc absorption is also impaired by excessive intake of iron, copper, tin, folic acid, and possibly calcium. Persons who have polyuria from uncontrolled diabetes (see Chapter 9) or who take diuretics may be predisposed to loss of zinc in the urine.

Other Trace Minerals

The following minerals do not have established DRIs at present, but are essential to the body. Including a variety of low-processed foods will likely meet health needs of these trace minerals.

Chloride

Chloride is found in extracellular fluids. It is an electrolyte and is found in gastric juice. Deficiency is generally found only in association with sodium depletion occurring with excessive fluid loss such as in diarrhea, vomiting, or excessive sweating. The only excess known to occur results from water-deficiency dehydration.

Chromium

Chromium activates several enzymes. It is an essential nutrient required for carbohydrate and lipid metabolism. Chromium supplementation in humans has been reported to improve glucose metabolism, improve serum lipids, and reduce body fat; however, this has not been borne out in research (Amato et al., 2000).

Good sources of chromium include brewer's yeast, liver, whole grains, meat, and cheese. Most of the chromium is removed from grains during the processing of white flour products and is not returned during the enrichment process.

Chromium exists in different forms. There are low rates of cancer with chromium(0) and chromium(III). Chromium(VI), on the other hand, has been known for more than a century to be associated with induction of cancer in humans, but massive exposure is required (De Flora, 2000). The most serious health effect associated with chromium(VI) is lung cancer, which has been associated with some occupational exposure scenarios, whereas chromium(III) is an essential nutrient with a broad safety range and low toxicity (Rowbotham et al., 2000).

Cobalt

Cobalt is an essential component of vitamin B_{12}, which is found in animal protein foods such as meat, fish, eggs, and milk. Inadequate intake of cobalt may result in pernicious anemia with a vitamin B_{12} deficiency. No other deficiency symptoms or toxicities are known.

Copper

Copper aids in the absorption of iron from the intestinal tract and in the production and survival of red blood cells and is also an essential part of many enzymes. It is an essential trace element in the maintenance of the cardiovascular system and there is also evidence that it helps prevent heart disease. Copper-deficient diets can elicit structural and functional changes that are comparable to those observed in coronary heart disease (Hamilton et al., 2000).

Manganese

Manganese is essential for normal bone structure, reproduction, and functioning of the central nervous system. It is a component of some enzymes. In general, there is low risk of toxicity, but workers exposed to manganese dust or fumes have been known to develop central nervous system problems.

Molybdenum

Molybdenum is a component of an enzyme (xanthine oxidase). The role of this essential mineral in humans is not well understood, but deficiency may be implicated in certain neurologic dysfunctions by its essential presence in various enzymes. There is insufficient knowledge about the demands of molybdenum in infancy. Because of substantial retention observed at higher intakes, upper limits should be set for preterm infant formulas (Sievers et al., 2001). The foods known to be high in this mineral include legumes, milk, and whole grains.

Sulfur

Sulfur is a component of skin, hair, nails, cartilage, and some organ tissue. It is a component of all body proteins. Protein-rich foods are the primary source of sulfur. Little is known about the effect on human health of a deficiency or toxicity.

Nickel, Tin, Vanadium, and Silicon

Findings produced in experimental animal feeding suggest that these elements are essential, but the implications for human nutrition are not well known. Vanadium may affect the activity of various intracellular enzyme systems and alter their physiologic functions. There have been accounts of vanadium, in the form of vanadyl sulfate, having insulin-like properties or promoting insulin signaling in cells and therefore helping in blood glucose management (see Chapter 9). However, in animals, vanadyl sulfate was found to be ineffective in controlling glucose levels except when given together with insulin (Shafrir et al., 2001). The potential for vanadium toxicity precludes recommendations for high doses of this supplement for diabetes management in humans.

What Are Electrolytes?

An **electrolyte** is a compound that, when dissolved in water, separates into charged particles (ions) capable of conducting an electric current. Within the body, electrolytes play an essential role in maintaining fluid and **acid-base balance** (a state of equilibrium in the body between acidity and alkalinity of body fluids [Figure 4-8]). Diet, however, is considered to play only a small role in maintaining an appropriate acid-base balance.

The chief electrolytic ions are sodium, potassium, calcium, magnesium, chloride, and phosphate. All body fluids contain electrolytes. The chief extracellular (outside the cell) electrolytes are sodium and chloride, whereas potassium, magnesium, and phosphate are found in large intracellular (inside the cell) amounts.

Changes in the electrolyte composition of body fluids create electric charges and these in turn are responsible for electrochemical reactions such as transmission of nerve impulses, contraction of muscles, and glandular cell secretions. Shifts in the electrolyte balance that cause either an excess or a deficiency of electrolytes may occur as the result of various disease conditions. Alterations in

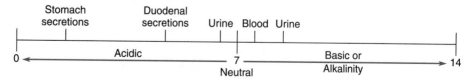

FIGURE 4-8 The pH of various body fluids.

electrolyte balance can cause death. Thus careful monitoring of the blood levels of electrolytes is necessary, especially during times of illness.

Correction of malnutrition, as with the initiation of nutrition support, can cause shifts in electrolyte balance. The refeeding syndrome (see Chapter 5 for details) is related to electrolyte shifts from extracellular to intracellular. Extracellular serum phosphorus levels, for example, can become low as phosphorus moves back into the cell.

Are There Any Harmful Minerals?

All minerals are harmful in excess. Arsenic is probably the best known of the harmful minerals; it is, however, probably important for health in very trace amounts. In addition, excess mercury and lead need to be avoided. For this reason, some fish products need to be used sparingly because of their mercury content; bone meal supplements, which tend to be high in lead, should be avoided. Other potential lead contaminant sources are wine decanters with lead crystal (storage of wine in decanters is discouraged); ceramic dishes with a lead glaze; food left in opened cans that have lead solder; household water pipes that are either made from lead (such as those found in older homes) or have lead in the solder (running the tap water for 1 to 2 minutes before use each morning is advised); lead paint (now illegal in the United States, but still found in older homes); lead-based fuel, including its fumes; and dirt and dust contaminated with lead residue. Younger children are particularly susceptible to lead poisoning, in part because of an increased risk of exposure from playing in dirt contaminated with lead (one reason that washing hands before eating is so important) and from eating peeling lead paint, which has a sweet taste. As previously noted, minerals in excess are generally harmful.

HOW CAN VITAMINS AND MINERALS BE PRESERVED IN FOOD PREPARATION?

The following food-handling practices will enhance vitamin and mineral retention:

1. Store vegetables properly to avoid wilting and drying out, which cause loss of vitamins A and C.
2. Cook vegetables whole as often as possible. Cutting and peeling release oxidative enzymes and increase surfaces from which water-soluble vitamins and minerals leach out.
3. Use cooking water and canned food juices to conserve soluble nutrients, or preferably, steam fresh or frozen vegetables to lessen the leaching of water-soluble vitamins and minerals.
4. Avoid use of baking soda in cooking vegetables, as it is destructive to thiamin and ascorbic acid. Avoid long cooking for the same reason. Cooling meat drippings before use allows one to easily remove solidified fats without sacrificing thiamin and niacin.

5. Store fats covered—and preferably refrigerated—to prevent them from becoming rancid, which destroys vitamin A.
6. Keep milk in glass containers away from light, which is destructive to riboflavin, or put in opaque containers. Waxed cardboard containers for milk prevent destruction of riboflavin by light.
7. Keep fruit juices covered and cold to prevent oxygen from destroying vitamin C.
8. While cooking foods containing vitamin C, avoid stirring because oxygen destroys it.
9. Cook vegetables quickly in a covered container just until fork-tender. Store leftovers covered.
10. Cook vegetables in the microwave or in a steamer.

WHAT IS FOOD FORTIFICATION?

The question sometimes posed in the war among cereal brands—"How many bowls of your cereal does it take to equal one of ours?"—is an example of food fortification. This differs from **enrichment**, a method to replace known nutrients lost in processing such as B vitamins and iron in white-flour products. In contrast, **fortification** means "to make stronger; to fortify" and involves either adding nutrients in higher amounts than naturally occur or adding nutrients that are generally not present, such as adding calcium to orange juice. Food fortification does play an important role in the promotion of the health of our society. With the advent of fortification, many deficiency diseases such as goiter have been overcome in the United States, although goiter itself is still found in some other areas of the world. Iron-fortified cereal and infant formula help prevent iron deficiency anemia. Processed grain products are now fortified with folic acid in an attempt to reduce the birth defect spina bifida.

The food industry generally has a profit motive rather than society's health as its basis for food fortification. Advertisements that promote fortified food as the best alternative can mislead the public. To use the preceding example, calcium-fortified orange juice is not a replacement for milk because milk offers many other nutrients. Also, because we know that overconsumption of vitamins and minerals can be harmful, if not toxic, indiscriminate use of and reliance on fortified foods is not a healthful practice, particularly if those foods are used as a replacement for a balanced, varied diet.

HOW ARE VITAMIN AND OTHER DIETARY SUPPLEMENTS REGULATED?

Under the Nutrition and Labeling Education Act (NLEA), dietary supplements are eligible for health claims authorized by the Food and Drug Administration (FDA). In 1995, when DSHEA was passed, it expanded and clarified the definition of dietary supplements. However, because of DSHEA, there are only voluntary regulations on labeling requirements—what is listed in the ingredients does not legally have to be found inside the container. Supplement manufacturers do not need FDA approval to market their products. The FDA must prove that a supplement is not safe after it is on the market before it can intervene and restrict sales. Since DSHEA there has been an explosion of products on the market. This is reflected in the overall increased use of nutrient and botanic dietary supplements. Common supplements used are for heart disease (vitamin E, folic acid, and garlic), cancer (selenium, vitamin E, and garlic), and certain birth defects (folic acid). Other supplements are used for short-term benefits such as sleep management (valerian, melatonin) and enhanced physical performance (pyruvate, creatine) (Hathcock, 2001).

HOW CAN HERBAL PRODUCTS BE USED IN ACHIEVING HEALTH?

In the Western world, medicinal herbs are becoming increasingly popular. Their role in the achievement and maintenance of health is still controversial. There is little scientific research outlining the specific active compounds found in herbs as they relate to health. For example, most of the health claims found on the World Wide Web for one herb in particular were based on folklore or indirect scientific evidence and could not be validated by scientific research (Veronin and Ramirez, 2000).

A great deal of variation in known compounds found in herbs occurs because of different growing conditions such as amount of sun, level of soil acidity, and amount of rain. Thus an herb originally grown in China can have different actions if grown in another part of the world. Furthermore, as a result of DSHEA (see earlier section), herbs are regarded in this country as dietary supplements, which means consumers can purchase any and as much as they want. This is in contrast to China and other countries, where herbs are regulated (Lee, 2000). One scientist, working on developing consistency in labeling to ensure what is listed on the label actually reflects the contents of the container, called the degree of correspondence between label statements and actual content a "crap shoot." As noted previously, it is advisable for consumers who choose to take herbs to ensure quality and purity with the United States Pharmacopeia (USP) guidelines or to verify the product has been chemically assayed by calling the herbal company or looking for this statement on the label.

Much of the public is unaware of the strong biologic compounds found in herbs. Some can have a positive role, such as that found in the long history of treating rheumatism with salicylates that first originated from extracts of herbs and plants such as willow bark or leaves (Vane, 2000). Many herbs such as Chinese red yeast rice can reduce oxidation of LDL cholesterol (see Chapter 8). However, large-scale clinical trials have been advised to assess the public health potential of this herbal supplement (Heber, 2001). Eight different herbs, including saw palmetto, have shown a strong estrogenic activity, which can serve as an another tool in the management of prostate cancer patients (De la Taille et al., 2000). A significant number of patients scheduled for an elective surgical procedure were found to be self-administering supplements, some of which having the potential to cause serious drug interactions and instability during surgery. It is advised that patients self-administering these medications be identified before surgery (Kaye et al., 2000). Many herbs and dietary supplements can inhibit platelet function and may predispose surgical patients to excessive bleeding (Norred and Finlayson, 2000).

WHAT IS THE NUTRITIONAL FUNCTION OF WATER?

Water is the principal constituent of the body. One half to three quarters of body weight is water. Most water is intracellular; the remainder is found in blood, lymph, various secretions and excretions, and around cells. The water requirement for adults is 1 mL/kcal and for infants is 1.5 mL/kcal. Fluid balance is essential—intake must equal output. Fluid requirements are closely related to salt requirements; intake of increased amounts of water is needed under conditions of extreme heat or excessive sweating. Water is absorbed in the small intestine and colon with digested food. Because water is not stored, daily intake is necessary. Water requirements are increased for infants receiving high-protein formulas; comatose patients; those with fever, polyuria, or diarrhea; or those on high-protein diets. Water is normally lost through urine, in expired air, in feces, and through the skin. Water serves a number of functions in the body:

- *Helping* every organ to function properly.
- *Aiding* digestion, absorption, circulation, and excretion.
- *Serving* as a solvent for body constituents and as a medium for all chemical changes in the body.
- *Carrying* nutrients to and waste products from cells as part of the blood.
- *Participating* in the regulation of body temperature.
- *Contributing* to the lubrication of the moving parts of the body.

Water can be found in varying quantities (anywhere from 10% to 98%) in foods; it is formed in the body's metabolic processes and is an end product of oxidation. The average diet with milk (87% water) contains about 1000 mL of water daily. With the addition of 1 quart (4 c) of water, the recommended 2000 mL of water can be met. Beverages containing caffeine or alcohol should not generally be counted as fluid because these substances promote diuresis and do not contribute to the body's need for fluid as much as water does.

WHAT IS THE ROLE OF THE NURSE OR OTHER HEALTH CARE PROFESSIONAL IN EDUCATING THE PUBLIC ON VITAMINS AND MINERALS?

The nurse or other health care professional needs to be aware of how positive nutritional messages about food can be conveyed in informal settings, such as while a patient is eating a meal. Emphasis should be on positive messages such as, "That cantaloupe looks really good. Did you know that half a cantaloupe has all the vitamin A and vitamin C that you need for the day?" or "No milk? Can I get you something else in the dairy group—pudding, yogurt, cheese?" These types of messages reinforce good nutritional practices.

It is a disservice to consumers to speak of minerals as if they alone can cure some of humanity's ills. Claims such as "Calcium prevents osteoporosis," "Selenium prevents cancer," or "Zinc promotes sexual performance," have an element of truth, but are simplistic messages at best. Rather, a better approach would be to take facts, put them in their proper perspective, and apply them to the relevant food sources. For example, a nurse might say, "Milk and milk products help prevent osteoporosis," "Fruits and vegetables are known to reduce cancer risk," or "Wheat germ and legumes help promote sexual maturation." This approach promotes good nutrition without placing undue emphasis on one mineral over another. This is particularly important in our pill-popping society, in which mineral interactions or excess intake can lead to toxicity or imbalances.

The health care professional should also assess supplement usage. Are excessive amounts being taken, particularly of the fat-soluble vitamins? For persons concerned with their vitamin needs, a quick comparison of their diet to the foods in the Food Guide Pyramid can decrease fears of vitamin deficiency. People need to be reminded that nature supplies us with our needed vitamins, minerals, and other nutrients through food; the vitamin pill industry is a profit-oriented one that does not have the experience of Mother Nature. It may be helpful to point out that an excess of one vitamin or mineral (in supplement form) can have a negative effect on the body's use of other vitamins or minerals. Also, it cannot be stressed enough that if a person chooses to take a supplement, it should not exceed 100% to 200% of the RDA unless advised by a physician. Referral to a medical doctor or a registered dietitian is appropriate for high-risk individuals (those with an impaired ability to excrete excess vitamins, such as persons with renal disease, elderly individuals, pregnant women, or younger children).

**CHAPTER
STUDY
QUESTIONS
AND
CLASSROOM
ACTIVITIES**

1. Bring vitamin bottles to class to identify the RDI percentage of various vitamins and minerals. Do amounts vary from one brand to another? Why might this be? Do any labels show megadoses (greater than 10 times the RDI)?
2. Why do minerals not break down when cooked, as some vitamins do?
3. Why must some foods containing vitamins be eaten daily? Which vitamins can be stored by the body? Which ones cannot be stored?
4. What is meant by the vitamin B complex? What foods need to be included in the diet to ensure an adequate amount of the B-complex vitamins?
5. List the foods in the Food Guide Pyramid that will help meet your vitamin and mineral requirements, as well as the correct numbers of servings.
6. Calculate the calcium content of your diet. How could you meet the RDA for calcium without relying on supplements?
7. Name several procedures in food care, preparation, and cooking that will help retain water-soluble vitamins and minerals.

8. Role-play in class, portraying each of three characteristics detrimental to nutrition (lack of knowledge, food dislikes, or inadequate food habits), singly or in combination, to practice strategies to encourage an AI of foods high in vitamin A.

9. On the table of DRIs printed on the inside back cover of this text, underline in red pencil the figures that indicate the requirements for calories and each of the nutrients for a person of your age. You will be referring to these figures throughout the course.

Case Study

CRITICAL THINKING

Sean opened the magazine and was reading about pills that would increase energy levels. He read through the article, "You can no longer get enough vitamins and minerals in foods grown today. This specially patented supplement containing antioxidants and other energy-boosting vitamins and minerals will make you feel your youth once again. Order now toll-free ..." I must admit, he thought to himself, I sure do need some energy. Maybe I'll ask my son's father-in-law to ask his dietitian what she thinks about my taking a nutritional supplement to boost my energy. I have some golf tournaments coming up and I want to be in good form.

Critical Thinking Applications

1. How might you respond to a person interested in taking a vitamin and mineral supplement for increased energy levels?
2. Survey 10 students on campus about their beliefs on the use of supplements for increased energy; report findings in class.
3. Discuss how health messages may pass from one person to the next.

How Have Your Food Habits and Nutritional Attitudes Changed As You Have Studied About Nutrients and Foods Necessary for Good Nutrition?

Now is a good time for you to check your food habits.

1. Keep a record of your food intake (at meals and between meals) for 1 week.
2. Score your diet for each day, using the accompanying Food Selection Score Card, and determine your average score for the week. Repeat this activity later in the semester and compare the scores to see if you have improved your eating habits.
3. Analyze and comment on your last food selection score in the space provided.

Food Groups	Perfect Score	My Score	Comments
Milk group			
Meat group			
Vegetable group			
Fruit group			
Bread and cereal group			
Water			

- What thought did you give to the principles of meal planning as you selected the necessary foods for your various meals?
- What improvements have you made in your food selection habits thus far?
- What further improvements would you like to make?

Note to Instructor: Each student should keep and score a week's food intake at least once more (preferably twice) before the end of the course.

4. Why are good food habits important? How are they formed? How can they be improved?
5. What are five good food habits for *you* to acquire and follow daily?

Food Selection Score Card

Score your diet for each day and determine your average score for the week. If your final score is between 85 and 100, your food selection standard has been good. A score of 75 to 85 indicates a fair standard. A score lower than 75 indicates a low standard.

Maximum Score for Each Food Group	Credits	Columns for Daily Check
20	**Milk Group:** Milk (including foods prepared with low-fat milk, part-skim cheese, and yogurt) Adults: 1 glass, 10; 1½ glasses, 15; 2 glasses, 20 Children: 1 glass, 5; 1½ glasses, 10; 2 glasses, 15; 4 glasses, 20*	

*Count ½ c milk in creamy soups, puddings, cream pies.

How Have Your Food Habits and Nutritional Attitudes Changed As You Have Studied About Nutrients and Foods Necessary for Good Nutrition?—cont'd

Maximum Score for Each Food Group	Credits	Columns for Daily Check
25	**Meat Group:** Eggs, meat, cheese, fish, poultry, dry peas, dry beans, and nuts 1 serving of any one of above, 10 1 serving of any two of above, 20	
35	**Vegetable and Fruit Group:** Vegetables: 1 serving, 5; 2 servings, 10; 3 servings, 15 Potatoes may be included as one of the preceding servings If dark green or orange vegetable is included, extra credit, 5 Fruits: 1 serving, 5; 2 servings, 10 If citrus fruit, raw vegetable, or canned tomatoes are included, extra credit, 5[†]	
15	**Bread and Cereal Group:** Bread—dark whole grain, enriched or restored Cereals—dark whole grain, enriched or restored 2 servings of either, 10; 4 servings of either, 15	
5	**Water** (total liquid including milk, decaffeinated coffee and tea, or other beverage): Adults: 6 glasses, 2½; 8 glasses, 5 Children: 4 glasses, 2; 6 glasses, 5	
100	**Final Score**	

[†]Count ½ serving vegetables in soups or fruit in salad.
Deductions from final score: Each meal omitted, 10; excessive consumption of soft drinks, 10.

REFERENCES Alex G, Oliver MR, Collins KJ: Ataxia with isolated vitamin E deficiency: a clinical, biochemical and genetic diagnosis. J Paediatr Child Health. October 2000; 36(5):515-516.

Amato P, Morales AJ, Yen SS: Effects of chromium picolinate supplementation on insulin sensitivity, serum lipids, and body composition in healthy, nonobese older men and women. J Gerontol A Biol Sci Med Sci. May 2000; 55(5):M260-M263.

Bleich S, Degner D, Bandelow B, von Ahsen N, Ruther E, Kornhuber J: Plasma homocysteine is a predictor of alcohol withdrawal seizures. Neuroreport. August 21, 2000; 11(12):2749-2752.

Bonkovsky HL, Lambrecht RW: Iron-induced liver injury. Clin Liver Dis. May 2000; 4(2):409-429.

Brown AS, Gwinn M, Cogswell ME, Khoury MJ: Hemochromatosis-associated morbidity in the United States: an analysis of the National Hospital Discharge Survey, 1979-1997. Genet Med. March-April 2001; 3(2):109-111.

Buchman N, Mendelsson E, Lerner V, Kotler M: Delirium associated with vitamin B_{12} deficiency after pneumonia. Clin Neuropharmacol. November-December 1999; 22(6):356-358.

Carmel R, Aurangzeb I, Qian D: Associations of food-cobalamin malabsorption with ethnic origin, age, *Helicobacter pylori* infection, and serum markers of gastritis. Am J Gastroenterol. January 2001; 96(1):63-70.

Chang SJ: Vitamin B_6 antagonists alter the function and ultrastructure of mice endothelial cells. J Nutr Sci Vitaminol (Tokyo). August 2000; 46(4):149-153.

De Flora S: Threshold mechanisms and site specificity in chromium(VI) carcinogenesis. Carcinogenesis. April 2000; 21(4):533-541.

De la Taille A, Hayek OR, Burchardt M, Burchardt T, Katz AE: Role of herbal compounds (PC-SPES) in hormone-refractory prostate cancer: two case reports. J Altern Complement Med. October 2000; 6(5):449-451.

Durakovic C, Malabanan A, Holick MF: Rationale for use and clinical responsiveness of hexafluoro-1,25-dihydroxyvitamin D_3 for the treatment of plaque psoriasis: a pilot study. Br J Dermatol. March 2001; 144(3):500.

Fenech M: The role of folic acid and Vitamin B_{12} in genomic stability of human cells. Mutat Res. April 18, 2001; 475(1-2):57-67.

Fuller KE, Casparian JM: Vitamin D: balancing cutaneous and systemic considerations. South Med J. January 2001; 94(1):58.

Garcia-Lozano JR, Gonzalez-Escribano MF, Valenzuela A, Garcia A, Nunez-Roldan A: Association of vitamin D receptor genotypes with early-onset rheumatoid arthritis. Eur J Immunogenet. February 2001; 28(1):89-93.

Glerup H, Mikkelsen K, Poulsen L, Hass E, Overbeck S, Thomsen J, Charles P, Eriksen EF: Commonly recommended daily intake of vitamin D is not sufficient if sunlight exposure is limited. J Intern Med. February 2000; 247(2):260-268.

Gong H, Amemiya T: Optic nerve changes in zinc-deficient rats. Exp Eye Res. April 2001; 72(4):363-369.

Grattagliano I, Vendemiale G, Caraceni P, Domenicali M, Nardo B, Cavallari A, Trevisani F, Bernardi M, Altomare E: Starvation impairs antioxidant defense in fatty livers of rats fed a choline-deficient diet. J Nutr. September 2000; 130(9):2131-2136.

Grimm M, Muller A, Hein G, Funfstuck R, Jahreis G: High phosphorus intake only slightly affects serum minerals, urinary pyridinium crosslinks, and renal function in young women. Eur J Clin Nutr. March 2001; 55(3):153-161.

Halliwell B: Vitamin C and genomic stability. Mutat Res. April 18, 2001; 475(1-2):29.

Hamilton IM, Gilmore WS, Strain JJ: Marginal copper deficiency and atherosclerosis. Biol Trace Elem Res. Winter 2000; 78(1-3):179-189.

Hathcock J: Dietary supplements: how they are used and regulated. J Nutr. March 2001; 131(3s):1114S-1117S.

Heaney RP: Dietary protein and phosphorus do not affect calcium absorption. Am J Clin Nutr. September 2000; 72(3):758-761.

Heber D: Herbs and atherosclerosis. Curr Atheroscler Rep. January 2001; 3(1):93-96.

Iwamoto J, Takeda T, Ichimura S: Effect of combined administration of vitamin D_3 and vitamin K_2 on bone mineral density of the lumbar spine in postmenopausal women with osteoporosis. J Orthop Sci. 2000; 5(6):546-551.

Kalra V, Grover JK, Ahuja GK, Rathi S, Gulati S, Kalra N: Vitamin E administration and reversal of neurological deficits in protein-energy malnutrition. J Trop Pediatr. February 2001; 47(1):39-45.

Kaye AD, Clarke RC, Sabar R, Vig S, Dhawan KP, Hofbauer R, Kaye AM: Herbal medicines: current trends in anesthesiology practice—a hospital survey. J Clin Anesth. September 2000; 12(6):468-471.

Kertesz SG: Pellagra in two homeless men. Mayo Clin Proc. March 2001; 76(3):315-318.

Kharb S, Singh V: Magnesium deficiency potentiates free radical production associated with myocardial infarction. J Assoc Physicians India. May 2000; 48(5):484-485.

Kosinski CM, Cha JH, Young AB, Mangiarini L, Bates G, Schiefer J, Schwarz M: Intranuclear inclusions in subtypes of striatal neurons in Huntington's disease transgenic mice. Neuroreport. December 16, 1999; 10(18):3891-3896.

Krajcovicova-Kudlackova M, Blazicek P, Babinska K, Kopcova J, Klvanova J, Bederova A, Magalova T: Traditional and alternative nutrition—levels of homocysteine and lipid parameters in adults. Scand J Clin Lab Invest. December 2000; 60(8):657-664.

Lark RK, Lester GE, Ontjes DA, Blackwood AD, Hollis BW, Hensler MM, Aris RM: Diminished and erratic absorption of ergocalciferol in adult cystic fibrosis patients. Am J Clin Nutr. March 2001; 73(3):602-606.

Lee KH: Research and future trends in the pharmaceutical development of medicinal herbs from Chinese medicine. Public Health Nutr. December 2000; 3(4A):515-522.

Lips P, Duong T, Oleksik A, Black D, Cummings S, Cox D, Nickelsen T: A global study of vitamin D status and parathyroid function in postmenopausal women with osteoporosis: baseline data from the multiple outcomes of raloxifene evaluation clinical trial. J Clin Endocrinol Metab. March 2001; 86(3):1212-1221.

Martini LA, Cuppari L, Colugnati FA, Sigulem DM, Szejnfeld VL, Schor N, Heilberg IP: High sodium chloride intake is associated with low bone density in calcium-stone-forming patients. Clin Nephrol. August 2000; 54(2):85-93.

Masse PG, Delvin EE, Hauschka PV, Donovan SM, Grynpas MD, Mahuren JD, Watkins BA, Howell DS: Perturbations in factors that modulate osteoblast functions in vitamin B_6 deficiency. Can J Physiol Pharmacol. November 2000; 78(11):904-911.

Merkin-Zaborsky H, Ifergane G, Frisher S, Valdman S, Herishanu Y, Wirguin I: Thiamine-responsive acute neurological disorders in nonalcoholic patients. Eur Neurol. 2001; 45(1):34-37.

Neve J: New approaches to assess selenium status and requirement. Nutr Rev. December 2000; 58(12):363-369.

Norred CL, Finlayson CA: Hemorrhage after the preoperative use of complementary and alternative medicines. AANA J. June 2000; 68(3):217-220.

Pfeifer M, Begerow B, Minne HW, Nachtigall D, Hansen C: Effects of a short-term vitamin D_3 and calcium supplementation on blood pressure and parathyroid hormone levels in elderly women. J Clin Endocrinol Metab. April 2001; 86(4):1633-1637.

Radimer KL, Subar AF, Thompson FE: Nonvitamin, nonmineral dietary supplements: issues and findings from NHANES III. J Am Diet Assoc. April 2000; 100(4):409.

Ramakrishna T: Vitamins and brain development. Physiol Res. 1999; 48(3):175-187.

Rowbotham AL, Levy LS, Shuker LK: Chromium in the environment: an evaluation of exposure of the UK general population and possible adverse health effects. J Toxicol Environ Health B Crit Rev. July-September 2000; 3(3):145-178.

Said HM: Cellular uptake of biotin: mechanisms and regulation. J Nutr. February 1999; 129(2S Suppl):490S-493S.

Saris NE, Mervaala E, Karppanen H, Khawaja JA, Lewenstam A: Magnesium. An update on physiological, clinical and analytical aspects. Clin Chim Acta. April 2000; 294(1-2):1-26.

Scelfo GM, Flegal AR: Lead in calcium supplements. Environ Health Perspect. April 2000; 108(4):309-319.

Shafrir E, Spielman S, Nachliel I, Khamaisi M, Bar-On H, Ziv E: Treatment of diabetes with vanadium salts: general overview and amelioration of nutritionally induced diabetes in the *Psammomys obesus* gerbil. Diabetes Metab Res Rev. January-February 2001; 17(1):55-66.

Sievers E, Oldigs HD, Dorner K, Kollmann M, Schaub J: Molybdenum balance studies in premature male infants. Eur J Pediatr. February 2001; 160(2):109-113.

Swavey S, Gould ES: Electron transfer. 140. Reactions of riboflavin with metal center reductants. Inorg Chem. January 24, 2000; 39(2):352-356.

Thomson AD: Mechanisms of vitamin deficiency in chronic alcohol misusers and the development of the Wernicke-Korsakoff syndrome. Alcohol Alcohol Suppl. May-June 2000; 35 Suppl 1:2-7.

Ugarte M, Osborne NN: Zinc in the retina. Prog Neurobiol. June 2001; 64(3):219-249.

Vane JR: The fight against rheumatism: from willow bark to COX-1 sparing drugs. J Physiol Pharmacol. December 2000; 51(4 Pt 1):573-586.

Venturi S, Donati FM, Venturi A, Venturi M, Grossi L, Guidi A: Role of iodine in evolution and carcinogenesis of thyroid, breast, and stomach. Adv Clin Path. January 2000; 4(1):11.

Vermeer C, Schurgers LJ: A comprehensive review of vitamin K and vitamin K antagonists. Hematol Oncol Clin North Am. April 2000; 14(2):339-353.

Veronin MA, Ramirez G: The validity of health claims on the World Wide Web: a systematic survey of the herbal remedy Opuntia. Am J Health Promot. September-October 2000; 15(1):21-28.

Zile MH: Function of vitamin A in vertebrate embryonic development. J Nutr. March 2001; 131(3):705.

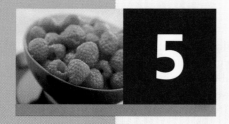

5 The Nutrition Care Process in the Health Setting

OBJECTIVES

After completing this chapter, you should be able to do the following:

- Describe what total health care means and how best to use this approach.
- Describe the steps of the nursing process as it relates to nutrition care.
- Describe good interviewing skills.
- Identify patient risk factors for poor nutritional status.
- Describe differences and management of food intolerances versus allergies.
- Describe appropriate nutrition interventions for families.
- Describe different types, methods, and uses of nutritional support.
- Describe the differences in acute-care versus long-term care settings.

TERMS TO IDENTIFY

Active listening
Activities of daily living (ADL)
Acquired immunodeficiency syndrome (AIDS)
Affective
AIDS-related complex (ARC)
Albumin
American Heart Association (AHA)
Anaphylactic shock
Anthropometry
Aspiration
Change agent
Cholesterol
Cognitive
Dementia
Diuretics
Elemental
Elimination diets

Enteral nutrition
Expanded Food and Nutrition Education Program (EFNEP)
Food allergens and antigens
Food allergy
Food intolerances
Gastrostomy
Human immunodeficiency virus (HIV)
Hyperalimentation
"I" versus "You" statements
Immunoglobulin E (IgE) antibody
Jejunostomy
Megaloblastic anemia
Metabolic
Nasogastric tube
Nonverbal communication
Nursing process

Nutrition care process
Nutrition Program for the Elderly
Nutritional support
Percutaneous endoscopic gastrostomy (PEG) tube
Peripheral parenteral nutrition (PPN)
Phlebitis
Physiologic stress
Psychomotor
Refeeding syndrome
Sepsis
Therapeutic nutrition
Thrush
Total parenteral nutrition (TPN)
Tube feeding
Women, Infants, and Children (WIC) Supplemental Food Program

133

INTRODUCTION

Imagine yourself, as a health care professional, meeting a new patient or consumer. What do you say? Where do you begin? What questions should you ask? How do you help the person to be open about expressing health and nutrition needs and concerns? Do you present yourself as very professional and aloof, informal and witty, or perhaps a combination? What are you trying to achieve through contact with the patient? These are just some of the questions that face a new nurse or practicing health care professional.

Good nutritional status is vital to promote health and well-being. Poor nutritional status must be improved during treatment of illness or injury for optimal recovery. Food provides the basic nutrients needed for health and well-being. Nutrients in food also help prevent and treat a variety of illnesses. Specific guidelines on medical nutrition therapy should be provided by a registered dietitian (RD) who will look at the total nutritional needs in relation to therapeutic needs.

HOW IS NUTRITION AN ASPECT OF TOTAL HEALTH CARE?

The total needs and care of the patient as a person and community member, rather than in terms of diagnosis, continue to be emphasized in health care education. Nutrition is considered an integral part of patient care, with the physical, social, psychiatric, and economic aspects. The patient (the term *patient* will be used throughout this book to mean client, consumer, and so on) requires adequate nutritional intake to maintain an already good nutritional state or to improve a poor one. For many patients, food is the single most important factor used to restore good health.

Patient-centered educational activities are the accepted approach in choosing learning experiences by the health professional. As a result, the patient has a better understanding of medical nutrition therapy in illness and recovery and in everyday living. Nutrition education strategies, as noted in the sections titled "Teaching Pearl" provided throughout this textbook, can later be applied in patient education settings.

Improvement in food selection patterns for bettering one's health frequently means changing established habits. This is a slow, step-by-step, almost never-ending process necessitating a real desire to change, a deep conviction that change is important, and the willingness to substitute desirable food habits for undesirable ones. Health care professionals dealing with nutritional improvement, although primarily concerned with the **metabolic** (biochemical) role of food in health, must also have some understanding of the circumstances under which dietary habits are acquired and the various meanings that food may have for different individuals. This is especially true in dealing with patients who suffer from a disorder or disease that requires drastic, long-term changes in dietary habits.

A registered dietitian (RD) is of special importance when there are complex factors or medical conditions that interfere with nutritional status. Other professionals may need to be consulted as well, such as the family physician (for medically related factors), the occupational therapist (OT) or speech pathologist (for physical factors such as cleft palate), and the social worker or mental health worker (for negative family dynamics and finances). To make the best use of these professional resources, the nurse or other health care professional should first identify the patient's nutritional needs by describing the factors that are negatively influencing the family's ability to feed itself adequately. This role particularly suits the nurse or other health care professional who has regular, frequent contact with patients.

What Is the Health Care Team?

The health care team comprises all the health care professionals that work with a given patient or patients and their families toward the common goal of patient health. This includes the medical part of the team (physician, nurse, dietitian, physical therapist [PT], and pharmacist), the social professionals (social worker, psychologist, and OT), and other community resource personnel who play a role in facilitating good health. Because each type of health care professional has a unique perspective on needs assessment and health care planning, a team approach is most effective in eliciting positive changes in a person's well-being.

The patient should also be considered part of the health care team; in fact the patient may arguably be the most important member. This is especially true in managing chronic illness, when the patient must make day-to-day management decisions regarding lifestyle changes. Lifestyle changes, no matter how small, can have either a positive or a negative effect on health. It is critical that patients feel they have choices in their health care intervention and they should be considered integral to the health care team in the planning and implementation stage. The patient needs to be encouraged to contribute fully to the assessment phase and be actively involved in the planning stage. This will increase patient cooperation and health outcomes by facilitating compliance through identifying realistic health care changes.

The Physician

Generally, the person with the most broad-based knowledge related to patient health care is the medical doctor (MD), otherwise referred to as the physician. The physician knows the patient's medical history and has a general understanding of the relationship between disease states and other health concerns. Often, however, it is in the best interest of the patient for the physician to refer patients to other complementary health services, such as an RD for medical nutrition therapy. Doctors may not have the office time or the skills that another health professional might provide. The physician needs to be kept abreast of the health services the patient receives. This may be in the form of written documentation in a hospitalized patient's chart, through standardized written correspondence from a community agency or other health care provider, or through telephone contact when there is an urgent need to discuss patient needs between the physician and the health care provider. Final health care decisions often are in the realm of the physician, who should be kept informed of concerns of the health care team and their recommendations for individual patient care.

The Nurse

The nurse generally has the most contact with individual patients and their families. The nurse can provide other members of the health care team with good insight into patient needs because of this in-depth patient contact. Ongoing assessment and monitoring of patient eating habits and health status are important roles of the nurse.

The Social Worker

The social worker is the health care professional who has expertise in the area of community resources including financial, counseling, technical support, and educational services. The social worker often can help patients identify and express barriers—whether perceived or actual—they may be facing to meet the goal of achieving health and wellness. Many times the patient is not ready to hear health care advice because of the need to resolve and come to terms with a chronic or acute illness.

The Physical Therapist

Assisting in promoting mobility and physical movement to control pain is part of the role of the PT. A PT may be involved with helping a person enhance the physical capabilities that have been impaired by illness or trauma. The PT may suggest exercise that is appropriate for the individual to promote weight loss or increase muscle strength.

The Occupational Therapist

The OT emphasizes the remaining strengths of the individual and identifies adaptive devices that would enhance independent functioning, such as large-handled spoons and reaching devices. The OT works to increase the amount or types of **activities of daily living** (**ADL**) a patient is involved with, such as personal hygiene and eating. This is of particular importance after a person has suffered a stroke or other physical injury that impairs or prevents independent living.

The Speech Pathologist

The professional to consult when assessing the seemingly simple act of swallowing is the speech pathologist. Swallowing, a series of interrelated steps, can be seriously impaired by stroke or other neurologic damage (see Chapter 3). Aspiration of food (inhaling food into the lungs) is of serious consequence and can lead to partial or full airway obstruction or to pneumonia. A speech pathologist can help determine the degree of risk for aspiration and make appropriate care plans that other health care professionals can use in developing their plans. For example, the PT may be enlisted to help the patient position correctly for good swallowing, the OT may promote the use of eating utensils designed for special feeding needs, and the dietitian may need to plan certain food consistencies to facilitate effective swallowing.

The Pharmacist

The registered pharmacist is responsible for preparing the nutritional solutions that the physician orders. These solutions are administered through veins or enteral routes (see Nutrition Support later in this chapter). The dietitian often makes recommendations in consultation with the physician on the solution used to provide appropriate amounts of nutrients for the specific patient's needs. Because of the pharmacist's specialized knowledge about drugs and their actions, she or he is able to serve as a resource person concerning drug and nutrient interactions.

The Registered Dietitian

The RD is the health care professional best qualified to interpret the science of how food is used by the body in health and disease states and to evaluate how changes in the diet can improve a patient's health status. The RD is trained to work with culturally diverse populations in adapting customary foods to meet ongoing health concerns for effective medical nutrition therapy.

The Nutritionist

A nutritionist is an educator, as well as a counselor, who usually works in a public health setting and who typically has at least a bachelor's degree in nutrition. The legal credential certified or licensed nutritionist is used in some states to help indicate qualified nutritionists. All RDs are nutritionists.

THE NUTRITION CARE PLANNING PROCESS

The **nutrition care process** of assessment, planning, intervention, and evaluation is the same as the **nursing process** with the omission of diagnosis. It is both a science and an art. By following the steps of the nursing process you will be a more effective health care professional. With practice and experience it will become easier, but your own unique style can either help or hinder the process of patient nutrition health care. Being very observant of **nonverbal communication** (facial expressions or other body language) and verbal communication from the patients you work with can guide you to becoming an effective change agent in patient compliance. A positive **change agent** is one who is directly and indirectly involved in promoting improved health of patients and consumers. Nurses and other health care professionals need to become culturally competent and work with the patient to plan appropriate goals that are based on the individual patient's values, beliefs, and practices. Generally, each step of the nursing process or nutrition care process should be followed in order. There is also a degree of integration between each step of the process and the process is usually repeated several times during the course of patient intervention. This chapter emphasizes the importance of developing patient rapport by using good communication skills in the process of assessment, planning, intervention, and evaluation.

A summary of the nutrition assessment process is shown in Table 5-1. Figure 5-1 shows a sample nutrition assessment and planning form that may be used to document the nutrition assessment and care plan.

Assessing the Patients' Needs

Identification of previous or current health concerns is important. This is best done with a variety of tools including reading of patient medical charts, discussion with other health care team members, and interviewing the patient. One simple assessment is determining if the patient is overweight or underweight or has had a change in weight that may be indicative of a problem. Lab values—such as those for hemoglobin (to determine iron status), **albumin** (to determine protein status), **cholesterol** and other blood fats such as triglycerides, blood glucose (BG), and other lab values—can help determine health needs that should be addressed in the later intervention phase. Physical signs of poor nutritional status may also be evident (Table 5-2). These physical findings relate to the *bio* part of biopsychosocial concerns.

For effective intervention, assessment should also include the psychosocial issues that may be contributing to physical health concerns and may need to be addressed before realistic changes can take place in patient health care. For example, social events or poor self-esteem may be causing negative food choices. This part of the assessment phase requires excellent communication skills to promote patient disclosure of potentially sensitive and personal lifestyle issues (see following section on interviewing and communication). Developing rapport and trust is critical to effective nutrition assessment and intervention. The more thorough the assessment phase, the more likely that appropriate and well-focused intervention strategies can be identified and implemented. A "hit-or-miss" interven-

▌TABLE 5-1
▌SUMMARY OF THE NUTRITIONAL ASSESSMENT PROCESS

AREA OF SCREENING	METHOD	INFORMATION GATHERED
Diet history	Patient family interview	Food preferences and intolerances; taste, appetite, and recent weight changes; desired weight and usual weight; estimation of typical kilocalorie and nutrient intake
Clinical	Physical examination	Indicators of malnutrition: appearance of hair, skin, oral cavity, fingernails, presence of edema
	Radiography Anthropometry	Skeletal condition size, weight, and height
Biochemical	Laboratory tests of blood and urine	Composition of blood to compare with normal ranges for hemoglobin, albumin, transferrin, total plasma protein, and so on; nitrogen content in 24-hour urinary output
	Skin tests	Immunity to certain diseases, response to antigens; possible identification of vitamin and mineral deficiencies

tion plan is not only potentially a waste of time, energy, and money, but can even be harmful to the patient.

Acquired immunodeficiency syndrome (AIDS) or **AIDS-related complex (ARC)** is an example of a chronic illness that involves biopsychosocial concerns and requires a total health care team approach. These conditions occur as the

Nutritional Assessment and Care Plan

Name: _____   Date: _____
D.O.B.: _____   Age: _____   Diagnoses: _____

Subjective Data

Food habits: _____
_____

Fluid intake: _____
Activity level: _____

Objective Data

Diet order: _____   Meal pattern: _____
Consistency: _____   Breakfast   Lunch   Supper
Medications: _____   _____
Supplements: _____   _____
                                             Male/Female: _____
Bowel/bladder functions: _____   Weight HX: _____

Laboratory values: _____   Weight: _____   Height: _____
_____   Physical indicators:_____
_____   _____
_____   _____
Meal observations: _____   _____
_____

Medical factors affecting nutritional status: _____
_____
_____

Physical limitations: _____
_____
_____

Problem	Goal	Intervention

Recommendations: _____
_____

Signature: _____

FIGURE 5-1 Sample nutrition assessment and care plan.

TABLE 5-2
PHYSICAL SIGNS INDICATIVE OR SUGGESTIVE OF MALNUTRITION

	NORMAL APPEARANCE	SIGNS ASSOCIATED WITH MALNUTRITION	POSSIBLE DISORDER OR NUTRIENT DEFICIENCY	POSSIBLE NONNUTRITIONAL PROBLEM
Hair	Shiny; firm; not easily plucked	Lack of natural shine; dull and dry Thin and sparse Dyspigmented Flag sign Easily plucked (no pain)	Kwashiorkor and, less commonly, marasmus	Excessive bleaching of hair Alopecia
Face	Skin color uniform; smooth, healthy appearance; not swollen	Nasolabial seborrhea (scaling of skin around nostrils) Swollen face (moon face) Paleness	Riboflavin Kwashiorkor	Acne vulgaris
Eyes	Bright, clear, shiny; no sores at corners of eyelids; membranes a healthy pink and moist; no prominent blood vessels or mound of tissue or sclera	Pale conjunctiva Bitot's spots Conjunctival xerosis (dryness) Corneal xerosis (dullness) Keratomalacia (softening of cornea) Redness and fissuring of eyelid corners Corneal arcus (white ring around eye) Xanthelasma (small yellowish lumps around eyes)	Anemia (e.g., iron) Vitamin A Riboflavin, pyridoxine Hyperlipidemia	Bloodshot eyes from exposure to weather, lack of sleep, smoke, or alcohol
Lips	Smooth, not chapped or swollen	Angular cheilosis (white or pink lesions at corners of mouth)	Riboflavin	Excessive salivation from improper fitting dentures

From Mahan LK, Escott-Stump S: Krause's food, nutrition and diet therapy, ed 10, Philadelphia, WB Saunders, 2000, p. 375.

immune system is destroyed from **human immunodeficiency virus (HIV)** virus. Although nutrition support (see later section) will be needed to extend life expectancy, there are many issues that will need to be identified and interventions that will need to be planned.

Body Weight. This measurement is often expressed as relative weight, desirable weight, or as a percentage of usual weight. Any assessment of body weight can be misleading if the patient is retaining fluid or is dehydrated. Significant weight

TABLE 5-2

PHYSICAL SIGNS INDICATIVE OR SUGGESTIVE OF MALNUTRITION—cont'd

	NORMAL APPEARANCE	SIGNS ASSOCIATED WITH MALNUTRITION	POSSIBLE DISORDER OR NUTRIENT DEFICIENCY	POSSIBLE NONNUTRITIONAL PROBLEM
Tongue	Deep red in appearance; not swollen or smooth	Magenta tongue (purplish)	Riboflavin	Leukoplakia
			Folic acid	
		Filiform papillae atrophy or hypertrophy—red tongue	Niacin	
Teeth	No cavities; no pain; bright	Mottled enamel	Fluorosis	Malocclusion
		Caries (cavities)	Excessive sugar	Periodontal disease
		Missing teeth		Health habits
Gums	Healthy; red; do not bleed; not swollen	Spongy, bleeding	Vitamin C	Periodontal disease
		Receding gums		
Glands	Face not swollen	Thyroid enlargement (front of neck swollen)	Iodine	Allergic or inflammatory enlargement of thyroid
		Parotid enlargement (cheeks become swollen)	Starvation Bulimia	
Nervous system	Psychological stability; normal reflexes	Psychomotor changes	Kwashiorkor	
		Mental confusion		
		Sensory loss		
		Motor weakness		
		Loss of position sense		
		Loss of vibration		
		Loss of ankle and knee jerks	Thiamin	
		Burning and tingling of hands and feet (paresthesia)		
		Dementia	Niacin, vitamin B_{12}	

loss that is reflective of malnutrition is an unplanned weight loss of 5% or more in 30 days or 10% or more in 6 months. Weight loss is best expressed in terms of percentage of weight change:

$$\text{Amount of weight loss} \div \text{usual weight} \times 100$$

Anthropometry. The science that deals with body measurements, such as size, weight, and proportions, is called anthropometry. It is especially useful in screening

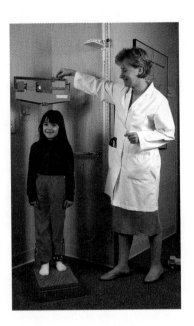

FIGURE 5-2 Monitoring patient weight. (From Jarvis C: Physical examination and health assessment, ed 3, Philadelphia, WB Saunders, 2000.)

hospitalized patients who may have varying degrees of protein-energy malnutrition (kwashiorkor and marasmus are two forms, see Chapter 2). This condition is most likely to develop when the patient is under the stress of an acute illness or major surgery, at which time the desire or ability to eat is impaired.

It is especially important to regularly monitor weights and heights of children (Figure 5-2) and any undesirable changes should be noted with the child's family. Assessment of stature can be difficult, for example, with persons with developmental disabilities such as cerebral palsy and contractures of the muscles (see Figure 5-3 and Chapter 13). Such physical contractures prevent usual height measurements and, instead, require segmental measures taken from joint to joint with a flexible measuring tape. Growth charts are based on percentiles, which are taken from measures of normal growth or "norms." To elaborate, a child with Down syndrome (Figure 5-3) will have a shorter stature than other children, but may still have normal growth as compared with other children with Down syndrome. Growth charts are available for Down syndrome, though other genetic disorders have not yet had growth charts developed. Thus the science of anthropometry is, in part, an art. The RDs are best qualified to assess nutritional intake and individual needs when they are outside of normal values. The other members of the health care team, however, are vital in helping to identify issues with developmental disorders or other conditions that involve difficulty with food behaviors, chewing, or swallowing abilities.

Ongoing growth assessments, such as those in school settings, can help identify inappropriate athletic weight goals or risk of childhood eating disorders as reflected in rapid weight loss or weight cycling up and down. In long-term care settings, such as nursing homes, weight monitoring should be done on a weekly

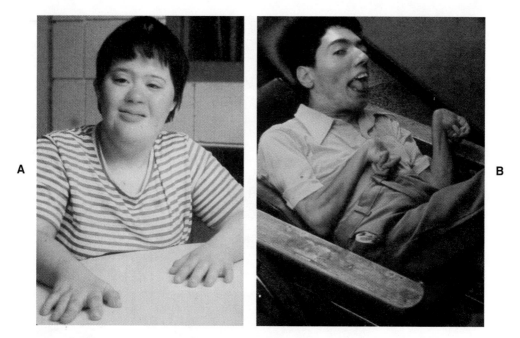

FIGURE 5-3 A, Client with Down syndrome. **B**, Client with cerebral palsy. (Personal Touch Slides, courtesy of Ross Products Division, Abbott Laboratories.)

or monthly basis. High-risk hospitalized patients can benefit from daily weight monitoring, which can give health professionals the information they need to aggressively treat fluid problems. Patients in hospitals or long-term care settings may be weighed using a Hoyt lift or bed scale (Figure 5-4).

The dietitian is one professional trained in anthropometry. Measurements are taken of elbow breadth, skin-fold thickness, and midupper-arm circumference to help determine the extent of the body's fat and protein stores in relation to body frame size and height. A discussion of various anthropometric measurements follows.

Triceps Skin Fold.   This is an index of the body's fat or energy stores. A low skin-fold thickness measurement may indicate malnutrition. Figure 5-5 shows how the measurement is taken. This technique is used for both men and women. The most common site for measuring skin-fold thickness is the posterior side of the upper arm at the midpoint. Accuracy and consistency of measurement are paramount.

Mid-Arm Circumference.   Taking a measurement of the mid-arm circumference of the upper arm indicates the level of the body's protein stores, which are found mainly in the muscles. The nondominant arm is flexed at a 90-degree angle and the circumference is measured with a nonstretchable measuring tape after the midpoint of the upper arm is determined (see Figure 5-5).

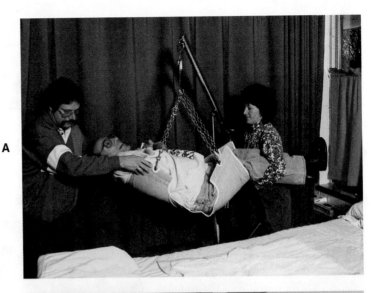

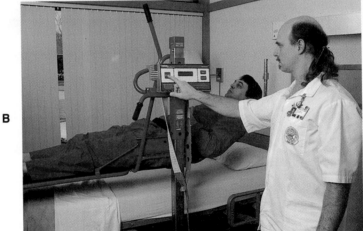

FIGURE 5-4 **A**, Weighing a nonambulatory person in a Hoyt lift. **B**, Using a bed scale to assess body weight. (From Lindeman C, McAthie M: Fundamentals of contemporary nursing practice, Philadelphia, WB Saunders, 1999.)

Elbow Breadth. This measurement determines body frame size. It is a reliable measurement that changes little with age and is not affected by body fat stores. The elbow breadth measurement is helpful in determining desirable weight ranges because body frame size reflects factors that influence weight, such as bone thickness, muscularity, and length of trunk in relation to total height. Calipers are applied to either side of the two prominent bones of the elbow while the forearm is bent upward at a 90-degree angle. The fingers are straight and the

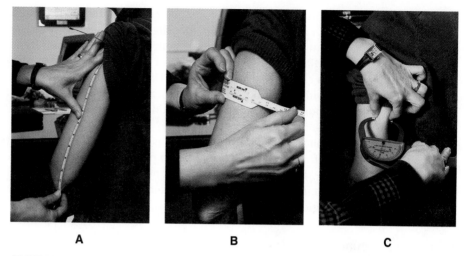

A   **B**   **C**

FIGURE 5-5 **A** and **B**, Measuring midarm circumference. **C**, Triceps skin-fold thickness.

inside of the wrist is turned toward the body. Most persons have a medium frame size. With experience, it is easy to visually determine when a person has a small or large frame size. See Appendix 11 for frame size measurements.

Accurate body composition measurements can be more difficult to obtain for obese people than for thin people because of the compression factor involving the use of the calipers. However, anthropometric measurements are very useful because they can help justify the use of special nutritional support when a patient is shown to be at risk for development of protein-energy malnutrition.

Biochemical and Clinical Data. Several lab tests of the blood, urine, and skin are used in assessing nutritional status. Protein-energy malnutrition in its various forms can be detected by monitoring the blood serum levels of albumin, transferrin, and lymphocytes. These elements are all associated with body protein status. A person's level of immunity is discovered with skin antigen tests.

A nitrogen balance study can also be helpful in determining nutritional status. A negative nitrogen balance signifies that the body is using some of its protein reserves for energy. Nitrogen balance is determined from the urinary urea nitrogen content of a 24-hour urine collection. Clinical dietitians can calculate nitrogen balance with this information and determine patient protein needs to promote healing or preserve lean muscle mass. Certain vitamin and mineral deficiencies may also be detected with lab tests when the tests are evaluated in conjunction with physical findings and dietary assessment of usual intake.

Diet History. This assessment is typically done by an RD, but other health professionals can assist. For example, if a person likes milk and reports an intake of

2 to 3 cups per day, this can be corroborated with clinical outcomes such as growth in children or bone density in older adults. A variety of ways exist to assess nutritional intake from 24-hour food recalls to food frequency checklists and food diaries. No one approach will provide complete information because food habits change for most persons. Thus diet histories should be used in conjunction with physical parameters of health. The RDs are trained to take a multitude of factors into account when making nutritional assessments.

Minimum Data Set Forms. Used in long-term care settings (see later section), these forms were designed to help promote a total health care team approach to ensure long-term care residents' health. These forms help to organize critical health information useful in resident care meetings and to reassess intervention strategies in achieving health goals.

What Are Planning Strategies?

The planning stage of the nursing process brings together all the findings of the assessment phase, starting with identifying priority health concerns, long-term health goals, and short-term objectives. Identifying small, achievable, and measurable objectives aimed at long-term goals and specified health outcomes is important for facilitating behavioral change by patients. When the health care professional is clear on the goals and the rationale for change, appropriate objectives and means of intervention can be determined.

Objectives are the steps needed to achieve long-term health goals. They should include measurable action verbs combined in a statement of intent or expected health outcome. For example, the action verbs *identify, state,* and *demonstrate* can all be used in patient objectives. The expected time frame for achievement of the objectives is sometimes also included. Objectives for the patients might read as follows:

- Identify foods high in salt using food labels.
- Substitute low-salt foods for high-salt foods.
- Determine foods high in sugar versus foods high in fiber.
- Correlate after-meal blood glucose values to meal intake.
- Describe low-fat food alternatives.

These objectives might be evaluated or measured through follow-up counseling sessions, through observation, or from improved lab values. Although objectives are aimed at short-term, measurable activities or outcomes, goals should be more broadly based, such as "Patient will achieve a triglyceride level less than 150 mg/dL." Writing out the planning process is important because it increases the effectiveness of the intervention and communicates the care plan to other members of the health care team (see Figure 5-1).

The short-term objectives may need to be prioritized, starting with the most important change. A patient is more likely to implement easy changes than more complex changes or too many changes at once. As objectives are met in the intervention and evaluation phases, the patient should receive positive reinforcement for these changes and should, then, be encouraged to meet the others as needed.

The evaluation plan is also determined before the intervention phase. Evaluation ultimately means changes in lab values or other clinical health outcomes. Because funding is limited, the health care field now demands effective patient intervention and documented positive health outcomes.

The intervention phase can begin once the planned health outcomes are written or at least thought out or expressed verbally with the patient. A review with the patient of goals, objectives, and means of evaluation as based on the assessment phase can help promote compliance.

What Are Intervention Strategies?

Intervention approaches often begin with simple, brief, reinforcing messages. One question might be "Have you tried the new low-fat snacks of hot pretzels or herb-seasoned popcorn?" A more general question might also be asked, such as "Have you ever tried to lower your fat or sugar intake?" Suggestions can then be built on the patient's earlier attempts or changes in eating habits.

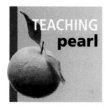

TEACHING **pearl** | Quality of life versus quantity of life might be addressed by asking an assessment question such as "How do you feel about eating less cheese and butter to bring down your cholesterol level?" You might add the statement, "Eating less fat will also help you lose weight and bring down your triglyceride level. Are you willing to try low-fat cheese and to use less butter?"

Patient retention of information is enhanced by combining different modes of information given. It is known that people remember best what they have heard, seen, and practiced. Therefore verbal reinforcement of written educational material is more effective than simply giving patients a brochure. Reviewing food labels and having patients describe the amount of sodium, sugar, or fat in the food product is another exercise that can be very effective in patient compliance.

Asking patients what has been successful in the past in their attempts to improve their health is also useful. This allows reinforcement of the positive attempts or changes made in the past.

Through identifying individual or group goals and objectives, messages can be kept to a few key points. Prioritizing messages and offering sequential information needed to elicit patient health and eating changes are important. Simple concepts can later be built upon with more complex concepts. For example, decision-making skills regarding meal planning are advanced concepts and need to be stressed after there is a general understanding of the rationale for change.

Messages given should offer positive reinforcement for behavior change. Scare tactics can cause inappropriate behaviors for health improvement, such as denial or tuning out the message. Follow-up reinforcement or referral to other appropriate services can assist patients to continue developing more positive health habits (Table 5-3).

TABLE 5-3
COMMON FAMILY NUTRITION PROBLEMS AND POSSIBLE SOLUTIONS

PROBLEM	REFERRALS TO OR SOURCES OF SOLUTIONS
Inadequate economic resources for purchasing food	The Food Stamp Program The **Women, Infants, and Children (WIC) Supplemental Food Program**—a program for lower-income families that includes food coupons and nutrition education Food pantries and soup kitchens The **Expanded Food and Nutrition Education Program (EFNEP)**—a program of the Cooperative Extension Service that can be referred to for budgeting assistance Use food models to determine if excess intake in one food group (such as meat) can be reduced to allow for increase in other foods
Physical constraints to obtaining food	**Nutrition Program for the Elderly** for meal delivery for homebound older adults Local grocery stores with delivery service Public Health Nursing for professional home-based assessment
Inadequate cooking equipment or storage facilities	EFNEP for recipes and meal ideas
Food dislikes	A qualified nutritionist (or RD) for food alternatives Explain that tastes are learned; suggest the one-taste approach to facilitate acceptance
Inadequate time to prepare food	Suggest use of nutritious, but convenient, food ideas Vitamin A ideas: carrot sticks, apricots, cantaloupe, watermelon Protein ideas: cheese (low-fat or moderate amounts of natural cheese), peanut butter, eggs, or egg whites
Too much sodium in diet	The local **American Heart Association (AHA)**, an organization promoting heart health, for recipe ideas An RD for individualized meal plans and behavioral change strategies Suggest use of frozen or fresh vegetables, Swiss cheese instead of high-sodium processed cheese; spices and herbs or jelly to enhance the natural flavor of food Explain that our taste for salt is both learned and unlearned Explain that salt substitutes should be used only on the advice of an MD because of potential harm from the potassium content
Too much sugar in diet	Encourage gradual sugar reduction while tastes change: use of one half or three fourths of usual amount in baking or at the table; suggest use of fresh fruit or fruit canned in light syrup Explain that spices such as cinnamon or nutmeg can enhance the natural flavor without added sugar Encourage the use of ice water, flavored waters, iced tea, or diet soda as a replacement for soft drinks
Too much cholesterol, fat, and saturated fat	The American Heart Association for recipe ideas Suggest a gradual change from 4% (whole milk) to 2% (reduced-fat) to 1% (low-fat) or skim milk (fat-free) while tastes change Suggest use of less butter, margarine, mayonnaise, and oil Explain that although cholesterol is found only in animal foods, saturated fats should be mainly avoided; food products with ingredient labels that say *liquid oil* are better than those that say *hydrogenated* oil (see Chapters 3 and 8 for more details)
Negative effects of commercials on food-buying practices	Explain that advertisements are meant to sell products; they generally are not concerned with healthy dietary habits Explain to children that many foods they see advertised help them to grow outward, not upward (a representation with your hands can be helpful to children)

What Are Evaluation Strategies?

The final step of evaluation should be considered during the planning and intervention phases. The effectiveness of the plan in terms of the patient's progress must then be documented and evaluated. This is based on information and skills gained by the patient and by the outcomes of lab blood tests or other measures. Examples might be achieving a 10% weight loss, a fasting blood sugar level under 110 mg/dL, or a blood cholesterol level of less than 200 mg/dL. The evaluation process can help the health care professional determine if further intervention is needed.

Many forms of evaluation may be performed. Measuring health outcomes, one important form of evaluation, might be done with ongoing, informal evaluation through observation (such as at mealtimes or in other social settings) or through informal conversation (for example, a discussion of food likes and dislikes). More formal evaluation may involve monitoring lab values.

Monitoring the growth in children and weight changes in adults is a simple, but effective, means of measuring nutritional status. Evaluation may also focus on knowledge gained through verbal or written questions. Before-and-after tests can evaluate the outcome of a planned intervention, but should be used with caution, as many adults do not like to be quizzed.

The nutrition care plan (see Figure 5-1) should always be incorporated into the total patient care plan. This plan should be formulated by the health care team as soon as possible to establish patient-centered goals to be met. In summary, the nutrition care planning process includes making a nutrition assessment, identifying nutritional needs, planning how to meet nutritional needs using goals and objectives, carrying out the plan of care, and evaluating nutritional care.

INTERVIEWING AND COMMUNICATION SKILLS

How Are Good Communication Skills Important in Health Care?

Both the assessment phase and the intervention phase require using good communication skills with patients. The planning stage also requires good written and verbal communication skills in working with other health care professionals in the coordination of patient care. Nonverbal communication is also involved. Using an authoritative manner is not as effective as using an empathetic approach with active listening techniques. Active listening techniques use open-ended questions, such as, "Can you tell me more about ..."

To promote patient discussion of personal health concerns, the following strategies are helpful (Figure 5-6):

- Use a warm, friendly, positive approach.
- Sit in comfortable proximity, neither too close nor too far away.
- Use good eye contact, with eyes intent, but not staring.
- Face the patient and lean forward.

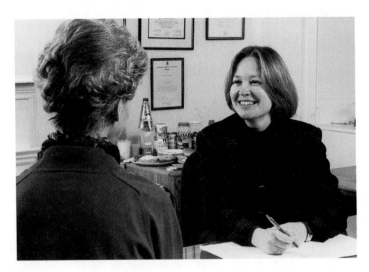

FIGURE 5-6 Effective nutrition care starts with good patient communication and rapport development.

- Have arms unfolded and resting in a relaxed manner.
- Carefully listen to what the patient is saying, using affirming responses to encourage the patient to clarify comments made.
- Allow pauses in the conversation; take as long a pause as needed to consider how to best make replies—it shows that you are interested in giving correct and appropriate replies.

Terminology used in the intervention stage can further promote or hinder patient openness. Using overly technical medical jargon can discourage the patient's understanding and willingness to ask questions. As much as possible, the health care professional should use terms and expressions that are understood and used by the patient in everyday settings. Observing the nonverbal communication signals that the patient exhibits can assist the health care professional in determining and fine-tuning messages given based on patient needs. A patient who initially is very talkative, but who becomes very quiet or begins to look at the clock is sending a powerful message. The health care professional needs to observe the patient's verbal and nonverbal communication and respond accordingly.

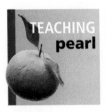

TEACHING pearl

Using simple analogies can diffuse any growing tension and help redirect the message based on the patient's needs. In describing the complex medical condition diabetes, for example, you might say, "There are little doors into the body's cells that allow insulin and sugar to get in. The insulin is sometimes referred to as the key that allows glucose through the doors of the cell. These doors are called receptor sites if you do much reading on diabetes." (See Chapter 9.)

What Are Some Interviewing Tips?

In the process of nutritional assessment, the following three realms should not be overlooked in patient care: (1) **cognitive** (knowledge), (2) **affective** (attitudes), and (3) **psychomotor** or behavioral (behaviors). Does the family have adequate knowledge about good nutritional practices? Does the family value good nutrition? What constraints does the family have in gaining access to and consuming a balanced diet? What is the patient's family meal environment in general? Can the patient shop and cook? Is the patient's ability to chew, swallow, and digest food appropriate?

A variety of interviewing and assessment methods can be used to identify these three areas (cognitive, affective, and psychomotor), such as diet history and questions based on active listening techniques (see the next section). It is important to be aware that patients sometimes combine misconceptions with accurate information. Asking patients to provide an example of a learned concept—for example, to interpret a food label—is useful in evaluating their understanding and ability to apply learned nutrition concepts.

What Is Active Listening?

Active listening is a manner of questioning and responding to a person that promotes full disclosure of opinions, feelings, emotions, and beliefs. This form of assessment can take time, but the information gathered allows for planning the most effective intervention methods. A few key questions can result in a wealth of information. Active listening is nonjudgmental and uses open-ended questions that elicit feelings and thoughts rather than yes or no responses. The following are examples of effective active listening questions:

Good Interviewing Questions
How do you feel about _____?
Can you tell me what you know about _____?
How is _____ a problem for your family?
Can you tell me more about _____?

How Can "I" Versus "You" Statements Help in the Nursing Process?

"I" versus "You" statements complement active listening techniques. "You" statements can sound judgmental and authoritarian, which can cause the patient or client to react defensively. Rephrasing "you" statements to "I" statements will promote patient interaction and communication.

An example of a "you" statement changed to an "I" statement is as follows: "You have a problem with fat intake" changed to "I am concerned about what appears to be a high-fat diet." Using the word *concerned* indicates empathy for the patient, especially when coupled with the use of *I*. Follow this comment with an active listening questioning such as "How do you feel about your diet?" for a very effective communication strategy.

An "I" statement is your opinion, which makes the statement less threatening and final. Your position as an authority figure can prevent many patients from questioning statements that sound official, even if they feel that your statements are in error. A defensive reaction by the patient will essentially end your effectiveness in bringing about health changes. If patients feel that their opinions are being listened to, through the use of active listening techniques, they also will be more likely to listen to your opinions.

Does Choice Help in Patient Compliance?

Chronic illness often is best controlled or managed through ongoing support services. Developing goals and small achievable objectives is important. It is also important for the patient or client to have a feeling of choice in making health care decisions. A verbal commitment (action) from a patient can further increase the likelihood that the patient will believe in and adopt the agreed upon health change.

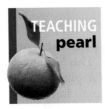

TEACHING pearl   Choice is important for people of all ages. Even 2-year-olds are more likely to eat vegetables if given a structured choice such as "Which do you want to eat tonight, carrots or broccoli?" This same principle can be applied to an adult situation, such as saying, "One salty food can be worked into your low-salt meal plan. Which would you prefer?" Or the choice might be between having the saturated fat of cheese one day and that of red meat the next to keep the total amount of saturated fat down.

What Is the Importance of Honesty and Respect in Patient Care and Education?

It is okay to admit lack of knowledge when questioned by a patient. There is a lot to know regarding how food and nutrition affect health. It is much better to admit you do not know an answer than to give inaccurate information. This can forever damage your credibility as a patient educator. Instead, you might say, "That's an interesting question. Perhaps we can find the answer in this brochure."

The most important aspect of patient communication is respect. Without respect, all attempts at effective communication will be lost. For example, if you have to leave the room, tell the patient. Do not assume the patient knows you will return. If the patient makes a comment unrelated to his or her health care needs, respond anyway. Showing respect for a patient's feelings and thoughts will greatly enhance the nutrition care process.

fact FALLACY   **Fallacy:** Doctors are always the best source for nutrition information.

Fact: Most doctors receive little nutrition information in medical school, especially in the area of nutrition education. Physicians, other health care professionals, and even patients and their families should use the unique services of an RD when the health need arises, even if only to make a phone call and ask a question.

WHAT IS THE ROLE OF THERAPEUTIC NUTRITION?

Therapeutic nutrition is the use of food and nutrition in the treatment of various diseases and disorders. Also referred to as medical nutrition therapy or a **therapeutic diet**, it involves the modification or adaptation of the normal or basic diet according to the needs of the individual.

Medical nutrition therapy may be necessary for one or more of the following reasons:

1. To maintain or improve nutritional status
2. To improve clinical or subclinical nutritional deficiencies
3. To maintain, decrease, or increase body weight
4. To rest certain organs of the body
5. To eliminate particular food constituents to which the individual may be allergic or intolerant
6. To adjust the composition of the normal diet to meet the ability of the body to absorb, metabolize, and excrete certain nutrients and other substances

Tables 5-4 and 5-5 list information about the basic hospital diets, uses of hospital diets, and foods allowed and omitted. Some differences exist from hospital to hospital in the foods allowed in each category, as well as in the number of kinds of diets. When a patient is admitted to the hospital, the physician will select the type of diet, often with input from a staff dietitian. In some hospitals, the dietitians are responsible for ordering hospital diets. Diets may be changed if and when the patient's condition makes it desirable. The nursing staff often identifies and communicates needed changes in the patient's diet.

WHAT IS A FOOD ALLERGY?

A **food allergy** is a condition that develops when a person is hypersensitive to certain proteins found in food. It is an immune response that can be mildly annoying or severe enough to induce death through **anaphylactic shock** (a life-threatening condition in which the breathing passages can be blocked from inflammation of the airways). Peanuts, tree nuts, seafood, seeds, milk, and eggs can cause anaphylaxis in highly allergic persons and reexposure to such foods presents the risk of life-threatening reactions. All persons who are at risk for food anaphylaxis or who have other severe environmental allergies, such as to bee stings, should have an "epi" pen available. This device is a syringe filled with epenephrine (adrenalin) that helps stop the inflammation process from occurring.

The immune system is designed to destroy harmful foreign substances in the body. With food allergies, the body reacts to certain food proteins as if they were harmful substances. For this immune response to be avoided, the offending foods need to be reduced or entirely eliminated from the diet.

More young children than adults experience food allergies. Infants who are exposed to highly allergenic foods, such as egg whites, may have an increased risk

TABLE 5-4
PROGRESSIVE BASIC HOSPITAL DIETS

CLEAR LIQUID DIET	FULL LIQUID DIET	SOFT DIET*	REGULAR, HOUSE, GENERAL, OR FULL DIET
CHARACTERISTICS			
Temporary diet of clear liquids without residue; nonstimulating, non–gas-forming, non-irritating; 400-500 kcal	Foods liquid at room temperature or lique-fying at body temperature	Normal diet modified in consistency to have limited fiber Liquids and semisolid food; easily digested	Practically all foods Simple, easy-to-digest foods, simply pre-pared, palatably sea-soned; a wide variety of foods and various methods of prepara-tion; individual intoler-ances, food habits, ethnic values, and food preferences considered
ADEQUACY			
Inadequate; deficient in protein, minerals, vita-mins, and kilocalories	Can be adequate with careful planning; ade-quacy depends on liq-uids used If used longer than 48 hours, high-protein, high-calorie supple-ments to be considered	Entirely adequate liberal diet	Adequate and well balanced
USE			
Acute illness and infections Postoperatively Temporary food intolerance To relieve thirst To reduce colonic fecal matter Intolerance for solid food 1- to 2-hour feeding intervals Before certain tests	Transition between clear liquid and soft diets Postoperatively Acute gastritis and infections Febrile conditions 2- to 4-hour feeding intervals	Between full liquid and light or regular diet Between acute illness and convalescence Acute infections Chewing difficulties Gastrointestinal disorders Three meals with or without between-meal feedings	For uniformity and con-venience in serving hospital patients Ambulatory patients Bed patients not requir-ing therapeutic diets

*Because of the trend toward a more liberal interpretation of diets and foods, in some hospitals the soft diet may be com-bined with the light diet, with cooked low-fiber vegetables allowed in place of purées.

TABLE 5-4
PROGRESSIVE BASIC HOSPITAL DIETS—cont'd

CLEAR LIQUID DIET	FULL LIQUID DIET	SOFT DIET*	REGULAR, HOUSE, GENERAL, OR FULL DIET
FOODS			
Water, tea, coffee, coffee substitutes	All liquids on clear liquid diet plus:	All liquids	All foods from the Food Guide Pyramid
Fat-free broth	All forms of milk	Fine and strained cereals	
Carbonated beverages	Soups, strained	Cooked tender and puréed vegetables	
Synthetic fruit juices	Fruit and vegetable juices	Cooked fruits without skin and seeds	
Ginger ale	Eggnog (pasteurized)	Ripe bananas	
Plain gelatin	Plain ice cream and sherbets	Ground or tender meat, fish, and poultry	
Sugar	Junket and plain gelatin dishes	Eggs and mild cheeses	
No milk or fats	Soft custard	Plain cake and puddings	
Orange juice may cause distention	Cereal gruels	Moderately seasoned foods	
Salt, plain hard candy, fruit ices, all fruit juices without pulp	Puréed meat and meat substitutes only; for use in soups only	Enriched white, refined whole-wheat bread (no seeds)	
	Butter, cream, margarine, sugar, honey, hard candy, syrup; salt, pepper, cinnamon, nutmeg, and flavorings; puréed vegetables for use in soups only		
MODIFICATION			
Liberal clear liquid diet includes fruit juices, egg white, whole egg, thin gruels	Consistency for tube feedings: foods that will pass through tube easily	Low residue—no fiber or tough connective tissue; traditional bland—no chemical, thermal, physical stimulants; cold soft—tonsillectomy; mechanical or "dental" soft—requiring no mastication (diced, chopped, mashed foods in place of puréed); light or convalescent diet—intermediate between soft and regular	For a light or convalescent diet, fried foods, rich pastries, foods rich in fats, coarse vegetables, possibly raw fruits and vegetables, and gas-forming vegetables may be omitted

TABLE 5-5
MENU MODIFICATION OF FOOD GROUPS OF THE FOOD GUIDE PYRAMID FOR THERAPEUTIC DIETS

FOOD GROUP	REGULAR	SOFT	LIBERAL BLAND	SODIUM RESTRICTED	LOW FAT	KILOCALORIE RESTRICTED
Breads and cereals	All breads and cereals allowed	All breads and cereals allowed Modify in consistency as needed (milk toast, rice pudding, and so on)	Allowed as tolerated	Avoid instant hot cereals, breads with salted toppings, salted crackers Salt-free products may be used, depending on level of sodium restriction	Avoid products with added fat	Avoid products with added fat
Fruits and vegetables	All fruits and vegetables allowed	Juices, soft, canned, or cooked vegetables and fruits; chop and mash as needed	Allowed as tolerated	Avoid dried fruits with sodium preservatives Avoid high-sodium canned vegetables and juices	Avoid vegetables in cream or cheese sauces	Avoid vegetables in cream or cheese sauces, fruits packed in syrup Limit to amounts prescribed in diet
Milk	All milk and dairy products allowed	All milk and dairy products allowed	Allowed as tolerated	Limit milk depending on level of sodium restriction	Use skim milk and low-fat cheeses	Use skim milk and low-fat cheeses unless calorie level allows use of higher-fat products
Meat	All meat and alternates allowed	Soft, tender, or ground meats plain or in casseroles and soups	No spicy meats and high-fat meats if not well tolerated	Avoid all processed and cured meats	Use lean meats	Use lean meats, limit to amounts prescribed in diet
Fats, sugars, and miscellaneous	Condiments and seasonings as desired Fats, sugar, and alcohol in moderation	Condiments and seasonings as desired Fats, sugar, and alcohol in moderation	*Omit:* Black pepper, chili powder, alcohol, and caffeine-containing beverages	Avoid salt and salt seasonings, salted snack foods, commercially canned soups	Limit use of fats and oils	Limit use of fats, oils, alcohol, and foods high in sugar

of food hypersensitivity. Fortunately many children outgrow their food sensitivities and intolerances. However, millions of Americans suffer from food allergies.

Food allergens and antigens are the proteins or other large molecules from food that induce an immune response. The **immunoglobulin E (IgE) antibody** is produced in response to these "foreign" substances in an attempt to rid the body of them. The IgE causes the typical allergy symptoms. Symptoms affect the skin, nasal passages, and respiratory or gastrointestinal (GI) tract. Hives, diarrhea, nausea, vomiting, cramps, headache, and asthma are common symptoms of food allergy. If the entire circulatory system is affected, shock occurs.

There are two major types of allergic reaction to foods: (1) immediate and (2) late. Immediate reactions are characterized by the rapid appearance of symptoms, often within minutes after the offending food is eaten or upon contact. The immediate allergic response is generally the more severe, and life-threatening, form of allergy. Late reactions are more subtle. Up to 48 hours may elapse between eating the allergenic food and the appearance of symptoms such as nasal congestion.

The foods that most often cause allergic reactions are milk, fish, shellfish, nuts, berries, egg whites, chocolate, corn, wheat, pork, legumes (green peas, lima beans, and peanuts), and some fresh fruits, such as those in the peach family.

Atopic dermatitis is one allergic condition that has a genetic basis, but needs to be provoked by environmental influences. There is some hope that by identifying infants with a high risk for this condition, early avoidance of allergens may prevent its development. This approach should only be taken in consultation with a physician and RD to avoid possible adverse growth and development if food intake is being restricted.

HOW IS A FOOD ALLERGY DIAGNOSED?

Medical Diagnostic Tests

Skin testing involves scratching or puncturing the skin with extracts of food. A skin reaction such as raised bumps around this area may be indicative of an immune response to the causative food extracts. The radioallergosorbent test (RAST) uses a blood sample. Both the skin test and the RAST can be incorrectly interpreted and thus are not considered infallible. The skin test should be performed under medical supervision to avoid or safely treat anaphylactic shock that can ensue.

Nutritional Diagnostic Tests

A detailed allergic history is important in diagnosing and managing food allergy. Specific details of foods, beverages, and medications ingested are recorded with any noted symptoms for a period of 2 to 4 weeks. This close observation may help pinpoint problematic substances in the diet.

Elimination diets are used to determine the causative food allergen. These diets contain a few carefully chosen foods, with common allergens omitted. The elimination diet should be followed for 1 to 2 weeks. An improvement in physical symptoms may indicate that an allergenic food has been eliminated. Foods are slowly and cautiously put back into the diet, one food at a time, for a few days. If no symptoms are noted, another food is added for another couple of days. This procedure is continued to ensure tolerance and to identify those foods that are linked to the redevelopment of allergic symptoms.

HOW ARE FOOD ALLERGIES TREATED?

Once food allergens are identified, a nutritionally adequate diet that eliminates the offending foods needs to be developed. Education is critical. A person may know he or she has a milk allergy, but may not think of all foods made with milk, such as cream soups, margarine with milk solids, cheese, and milk chocolate. Alternative

TABLE 5-6
EGG-FREE DIET

FOOD GROUP	FOODS ALLOWED	FOODS EXCLUDED
Beverages	All plain milks, creams, and buttermilks Cocoa, tea, coffee Carbonated beverages	Eggnogs, malted beverages Beverages "cleared" with egg or shells
Soups	Creamed meat, fish, and vegetable soups prepared without egg (such as egg noodles)	Any soups "cleared" with egg or shells, egg powder, dried egg, and albumin
Protein sources	All plain meats, fish, and poultry (some severely allergic individuals cannot eat the meat of egg-laying chickens) Cheese	All breaded or batter-dipped foods if egg was used in the mix Sausages, croquettes, or loaves using egg as a binding agent
Vegetables	Fresh, frozen, canned, raw, or cooked	None unless combined with egg
Fruit	All fresh, frozen, canned, or dried All juices	None
Breads and cereals	Rye-Krisp, corn pone, beaten biscuits, and plain crackers Any homemade breads without egg Any breakfast cereal Rice Pasta made without egg	Gingerbreads, griddle cakes, muffins, waffles, fancy breads, pretzels, saltines Commercial breads and rolls containing eggs or that have been brushed with egg
Fats	All butters, creams, homemade salad dressings without eggs	All others unless label shows made without egg, albumin, or egg powder
Combination	Any made without egg or egg products	Any made with egg or egg products; avoid biscuit toppings, thickened sauces
Sweets and snacks	Plain fruit-flavored gelatins Fruit pies Ices Cookies, frostings, cakes, and puddings made without eggs Popcorn, nuts, olives, pickles Sugars, hard candy	Prepared mixes for pancakes, cakes, cookies (may contain egg powder), cream-filled pies, meringues, ice cream, sherbet Some commercial candies that contain egg or albumin

Courtesy of the Bureau of Nutrition Services, Office of Mental Retardation and Developmental Disabilities, Albany, NY.

terms for milk protein on the food label—for example, lactalbumin, lactoglobulin, casein, nonfat milk solids, or whey—may not be familiar to the patient. The services of an RD are helpful in patient education and may be required when the patient has multiple food allergies to avoid nutritional inadequacies. Tables 5-6 and 5-7 list common foods to be omitted on the egg-free diet and the milk-free diet.

■ TABLE 5-7
■ MILK-FREE DIET

FOOD GROUP	FOODS ALLOWED	FOODS EXCLUDED
Beverages	Soft drinks Soya milk products Coffee, tea Decaffeinated coffee	All milk and milk-containing beverages
Soups	Any broth-based soup with no milk products	All creamed soups
Protein sources	All fresh meats Kosher luncheon meats, hot dogs, bologna, and salami labeled "Parve" (may be very spicy) All-beef hot dogs All poultry without stuffing All fish Eggs Dried beans, peas Peanut butter	Non-Kosher luncheon meats: bologna, salami, wieners, sausage, meat loaf, cold cuts Poultry with stuffing Meat balls, meat loaves Cheese Yogurt Breaded items that contain milk in batter or bread crumbs made with milk
Vegetables	Any fresh, canned, or frozen vegetables Pasta Rice	All creamed vegetables Any creamed sauces, including au gratin Mashed potatoes (unless made without milk)
Fruit	Any fresh, frozen, or canned fruit or juice	None
Breads and cereals	Rye-Krisp, homemade brands made without milk, rye breads Italian breads	Other baked goods
Fats	Poultry, meat, and pure vegetable fats and oils Dressings made without milk or milk products Margarine (without milk solids)	Butter Cheese Gravy made with milk or cream Any salad dressings containing milk or milk products
Combination	Any made without milk or milk products	Any dishes containing milk or milk products
Sweets and snacks	Plain fruit-flavored gelatin Angel and sponge cakes Fruit ices Jellies and jams Sugars, hard candy	Prepared mixes: waffle, cake, muffin, pancake Puddings, creams Ice cream, sherbet Milk chocolate candy

Courtesy of the Bureau of Nutrition Services, Office of Mental Retardation and Developmental Disabilities, Albany, NY.

Individuals who are sensitive only to wheat products can follow a gluten-restricted diet (see Box 3-2) in which wheat, rye, oats, and barley are omitted. However, the person with a wheat allergy may need to restrict only wheat. Persons with celiac disease and dermatitis herpetiformis (an allergic skin disorder) need to avoid all sources of gluten. Food products with cornmeal or rice flour are acceptable for persons with wheat allergy or gluten intolerance. Cornstarch can be used as a thickening agent. The American Dietetic Association can provide sources for allergy recipes (see Appendix 1). Many commercial products for allergy diets are available. Careful reading of the labels on such products is necessary to detect any specific allergen to be omitted in the diet. Writing to food manufacturers to inquire about possible cross-contamination (such as dusting the food conveyor belt with flour) can be helpful. Often a person who is allergic to one food will be allergic to others in the same food family. For example, someone allergic to peanuts usually cannot eat peas or beans either, simply because they are members of the pea family.

HOW DO FOOD INTOLERANCES DIFFER FROM FOOD ALLERGIES?

Food intolerances do not involve the immune response, but food allergies do. Food intolerances are not life threatening because the immune response is not evoked. Food allergies usually begin in childhood, whereas food intolerances can begin at any age. Food intolerances may have a biologic basis, such as a lack of a digestive enzyme, or a psychologic basis.

The general public often confuses intolerances and allergies, but it is important to know the difference. A person with milk allergy may become seriously ill from any trace of milk; a person with lactose intolerance may be able to tolerate small quantities of milk or low-lactose forms of milk such as yogurt and cheese. See Box 3-1 for a sample lactose-free diet.

WHAT ARE SOME COMMON FOOD INTOLERANCES?

Some food intolerances are well documented, whereas others are not understood or recognized. A common food intolerance that is well known throughout the world is lactose intolerance. A more rare intolerance is sucrose intolerance in which the enzyme sucrase is deficient. See Chapter 3 for further discussion of lactose intolerance and Box 3-1 for a sample diet.

Fat Intolerance

Fat intolerance is often related to pancreatitis and gallstones. Alcoholism is commonly associated with pancreatitis and problems digesting fat. Vegetarians or others who normally follow a low-fat diet often report nausea and indigestion as a result of increased meat or fat intake. These are both physiologic intolerances to fat. A low-fat meal containing up to 15 g of fat should be physiologically tolerated.

Intolerance to Vegetables and Fruits

Intolerances to vegetables and fruits are highly individual. The problem may not be the food as much as the style of eating. Thorough chewing and eating slowly will lessen symptoms of intolerance. Many people avoid legumes (dried beans) because of excessive flatulence. Such people may benefit by slowly increasing amounts eaten. Chewing thoroughly and including adequate fluid in the diet are important. Some people find a commercial enzyme preparation such as Beano™ to be helpful (although persons with an allergy to mold should avoid this product because it is derived from mold). Older persons often find that lettuce causes indigestion or abdominal pain. Again, small amounts of lettuce that are thoroughly masticated may help. Jerusalem artichokes contain a type of carbohydrate that humans cannot digest. Undigested carbohydrate allows bacteria to multiply in the GI tract, which leads to flatulence. Apple skin may be a problem for some people. The cause of intolerance may be a sudden increase in the fiber content of these foods. Gradually increasing the amounts of fruits and vegetables eaten may be beneficial.

Intolerance to Hot, Spicy Foods

An intolerance to hot, spicy foods is often associated with peptic ulcers, pancreatitis, and gallbladder disease. The intolerance may be physical or psychologic in the case of persons who believe they cannot tolerate spicy foods. Intolerance to spicy foods is not diagnostic of peptic ulcers.

WHAT IS NUTRITIONAL SUPPORT?

Nutritional support is the provision of macronutrients (carbohydrate, protein, and fat) to promote healthy weight management and nutritional status. It is used during times of physiologic stress, when the oral intake from standard meals cannot keep pace with the increased metabolic needs of the stress state. An example of this is with AIDS, when kilocalorie needs may be as high as 3500 kcal or more per day because of a fever from an opportunistic infection. The increased need for kilocalories with AIDS will likely be found with other complications such as mouth sores making eating painful and diarrhea causing nutritional intake to be unavailable to the body cells. Nutritional support in this scenario may involve altering the diet to include high-kilocalorie cold beverages to prevent weight loss. The cold temperature would be soothing to the mouth and the beverage would be lactose-free with banana flakes added to help control diarrhea.

The simplest form of nonoral nutritional support is **peripheral parenteral nutrition (PPN)**. This involves intravenous dextrose (a 5% sugar solution—D5W—delivered into a vein of the arm). It is used in addition to oral intake and is often used in conjunction with the delivery of a saline solution to treat dehydration. It can provide only minimal amounts of nutrition because the route of access is a small vein. Therefore although a patient may receive only PPN, he or she must receive it for a limited time and the catheter site should be rotated every 2 to 3 days.

The most complex form of nutritional support is called **total parenteral nutrition (TPN)** or **hyperalimentation**. This form of nutritional support involves feeding complete nutritional needs through large arteries. Hyperalimentation is used when the GI tract is not functioning. The TPN consists of a dextrose solution, such as D50W or D70W. D50W stands for 50% dextrose in water, which provides 1.7 kcal per milliliter of water. A protein solution—and vitamins, minerals, and trace elements in liquid form—is also provided with the dextrose on a daily basis. The protein source is amino acids. Fat emulsions are generally given about twice a week or daily to provide essential fatty acids and supplement the kilocalories provided by carbohydrate (dextrose) and protein (amino acids). A person with TPN sometimes is still able to eat or may do so in the transition to an oral diet.

After total gastrectomy (stomach removal), use of nasojejunal **tube feeding** or a jejunostomy (Figure 5-7) has been found to be well tolerated. The use of **percutaneous endoscopic gastrostomy (PEG) tubes**—a permanent feeding tube surgically implanted through the stomach—has increased with children and

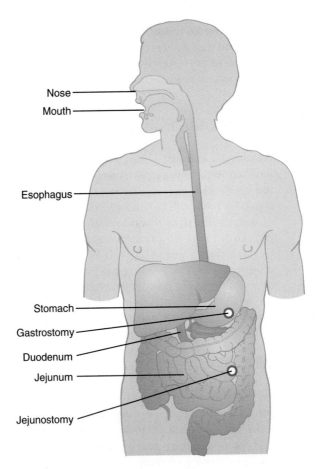

FIGURE 5-7 Tube feeding routes.

adults who have neurologic damage resulting in dysphagia (see Chapter 3). This form of nutrition support provides a major improvement for children requiring long-term tube feeding. However, for children who are likely to return to oral feeding as their main source of nourishment, oral feeding needs to be encouraged whether it is by using a pacifier, drinking water, or eating small amounts of food. It has been found that infants who receive only nasogastric tube feeding for an extended period have significant and persistent difficulty making the transition to oral feeding. These children need to be slowly retrained how to chew and swallow.

WHAT ARE INDICATIONS FOR NUTRITIONAL SUPPORT?

Conditions of **physiologic stress** (a state in which increased amounts of stress-related hormones are present) are created through trauma, surgery, burns, fever, and infections (Table 5-8). Kilocalorie and protein needs can be dramatically increased under such conditions, causing weight loss and loss of muscle mass unless an adequate diet is consumed. Often these conditions cannot be treated through meals alone. Thus medical nutritional support is generally required during times of physiologic stress. Oral intake or **enteral nutrition** through a tube into the GI system is the preferred route. The rule of thumb is "When the gut works, use it."

Nutritional support is essential for anyone who has had an unplanned weight loss of 10% or more within 3 months; shows a significant loss of muscle mass; has a serum albumin level of less than 3 g/dL, a serum transferrin level of less than 150 mg/dL, or both; or is scheduled for major surgery, for example, a total gastrectomy or another procedure in which there is stress and a potential for starvation after surgery.

Recording a patient's food intake will give a fairly accurate estimate of kilocalories and nutrients consumed in relation to weight and other lab assessments. This information can be used to assess whether the patient's nutritional needs can be met orally or if alternative methods of nutritional support should be considered.

Patients with pressure sores and chronic obstructive pulmonary disease will often benefit from nutritional support. Stressful conditions resulting from cancer, surgery, burns, head injury, infections, and fevers often require nutritional support. The opportunistic infections and resulting fever that occur with ARC or full-blown AIDS will require a substantial increase in kilocalorie and protein intake.

AIDS is an example of a chronic illness that requires a total health care team approach. Although nutrition support will be needed to extend life expectancy, there are many issues that will need to be dealt with. Loss of appetite can have biopsychosocial causes. Sores of the mouth and esophagus can make eating painful and difficult. **Thrush** (an infection of the mouth) causes an increased need for kilocalories because of the accompanying fever, as well as a diminished desire to eat. Medications for treatment of AIDS may also cause nausea. Abdominal discomfort and diarrhea associated with malabsorption of food nutrients compound the lack of desire to eat while increasing the need for additional nutrients. Psychologically, **dementia** (deranged mental functioning) can cause such disorientation that the person with AIDS forgets to eat. Depression is common and can reduce a desire to eat. Social isolation is a known aspect of decreased eating and desire to eat.

Whenever possible, the patient should be encouraged to ingest a normal diet by mouth. This is the preferred and most natural method of nutritional support. It has the psychologic advantage of giving the patient control over at least one aspect of treatment. It also provides the physical benefit of promoting continued GI functioning. High-kilocalorie, high-protein foods such as milk shakes, custards, and puddings are often used in conjunction with between-meal feedings.

TABLE 5-8
PHYSIOLOGIC RESPONSES TO STRESS

TYPE OF STRESS	POSSIBLE PHYSIOLOGIC RESPONSE
Surgery	Blood loss, shock, hemorrhage
	Depletion of protein or increase in protein metabolism
	Negative nitrogen balance
	Dehydration
	Edema
	Nausea, vomiting, diarrhea
	Electrolyte imbalance
Fractures of long bones and other trauma	Increase in protein metabolism
	Loss of phosphorus, potassium, sulfur
	Development of osteoporosis because of immobilization and loss of calcium
	Electrolyte imbalance
	Loss of fluids
	Renal failure and uremia
Burns	High loss of nitrogen
	Increased water loss
	Anorexia
	Fluid loss
	Weight loss
	Electrolyte imbalance
	Mineral losses
Infection	Increased metabolism
	Dehydration
	Fever
	Body tissue breakdown
	Nausea and vomiting
	Anorexia
	Poor synthesis of B-complex vitamins related to antibiotics given
	Loss of sodium and potassium if fever is present
Fevers, including those of short and long duration	Increased protein metabolism
	Depletion of body's energy stores
	Lowered sodium, chloride, and potassium levels
	Disturbance of appetite, digestion, and absorption

When more complete nutritional intake is needed, commercial liquid supplements should be used. These liquid supplements include the known vitamins, minerals, and other nutrients essential for health.

WHAT ARE THE METHODS OF DELIVERING NUTRITIONAL SUPPORT TO THE PATIENT?

The techniques for providing the patient with optimal kilocalorie and nutrient requirements range from very simple to complex. Figure 5-8 shows how the type of nutritional support is determined. A patient receives nutritional support by oral feedings, tube feedings, PPN, or TPN, all of which are discussed in the following sections. Providing adequate nutritional support without being too aggressive is a major concern in patient care. One means to help determine kilocalorie needs of critically ill patients is use of the metabolic cart (see Figure 3-3). The metabolic cart measures oxygen intake and carbon dioxide output to best estimate needed kilocalories.

For temporary nutritional support, a small, flexible tube is inserted through the nose and placed either into the stomach (**nasogastric tube**) or beyond the stomach into the duodenum. The latter approach is used when there are concerns about vomiting and **aspiration** (food or liquid entering the lungs). The duodenal or jejunal positioning of the tube is also appropriate at times when stomach emptying may be impaired, such as after surgery. The tube may be left in place for several days and changed on an occasional basis as needed, or the tube may be removed daily and repositioned each night, for example, in the case of home enteral nutritional support.

Long-term enteral nutrition may be required, such as with throat cancer or with neurologic damage that causes swallowing difficulties. Long-term nutritional support is best done with the feeding tube implanted directly into the stomach (a **gastrostomy**) or the jejunum (a **jejunostomy**). The liquid supplement may be provided through gravity, by simply pouring the supplement at a slow rate directly into the tube (this is not recommended for jejunal feedings), or through the use of a pump set at the desired rate of flow. The supplement should not be excessively cold when administered. Possible complications of enteral feeding are listed in Table 5-9, with suggested solutions if problems arise.

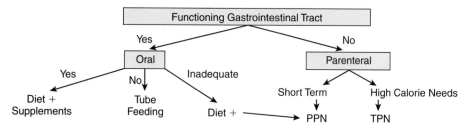

FIGURE 5-8 Determining the type of nutritional support for the patient.

TABLE 5-9
ENTERAL FEEDING COMPLICATIONS AND PROBLEM SOLVING

PROBLEM	CAUSE	PREVENTION/TREATMENT
MECHANICAL		
Aspiration pneumonia	Delayed gastric emptying, gastroparesis Gastroesophageal reflux Diminished gag reflex	Feed beyond the pylorus or ligament of Treitz. Reduce administration rate. Select isotonic or lower-fat formula. Regularly check gastric residuals, tube placement, and abdominal girth. Keep head of bed elevated 30° to 45° during and after feeding. Use small-bore feeding tubes to minimize compromise of lower esophageal sphincter. Keep head of bed elevated 30° to 45° during and after feeding. Initially and regularly check tube placement.
Pharyngeal irritation, otitis	Prolonged intubation with large-bore nasogastric tubes	Use small-bore feeding tubes whenever possible. Consider gastrostomy or jejunostomy sites for long-term feeding.
Nasolabial, esophageal, and mucosal irritation and erosion	Prolonged intubation with large-bore nasogastric tubes Use of rubber or plastic	Use small-caliber feeding tubes made of bicompatible materials. Tape feeding tube properly to avoid placing pressure on the nostril. Consider gastrostomy or jejunostomy sites for long-term feeding.
Irritation and leakage at ostomy site	Drainage of digestive juices from stoma site	Attend to skin and stoma care. Use gastrostomy tubes with retention devices to maintain proper tube placement.
Tube lumen obstruction	Thickened formula residue Formation of insoluble formula-medication complexes	Irrigate feeding tube frequently with clear water or use an enteral pump that provides a water flush. Avoid instilling medications into feeding tubes, when possible. Use liquid forms. Irrigate tubes with clear water before and after delivering medications and formula and after aspirating gastric contents.

▌ TABLE 5-9
▌ ENTERAL FEEDING COMPLICATIONS AND PROBLEM SOLVING—cont'd

PROBLEM	CAUSE	PREVENTION/TREATMENT
GASTROINTESTINAL		
Diarrhea	Low-residue formulas	Rule out non–formula-related causes.
	Rapid formula administration	Select fiber-supplemented formula.
	Hyperosmolar formula	Initiate feedings at low rate.
	Bolus feeding using syringe force	Temporarily decrease rate.
	Hypoalbuminemia	Reduce rate of administration.
	Nutrient malabsorption	Select isotonic formula or dilute formula
	Microbial contamination	concentration and gradually increase
	Disuse atrophy of the GI tract	strength.
	Rapid GI transit time	Reduce rate of administration.
	Prolonged antibiotic treatment or other drug therapy	Select alternate method of administration.
		Use hydrolyzed, peptide-based formulas or parenteral nutrition until absorptive capacity of small intestine is restored.
		Select a hydrolyzed, peptide-based formula that restricts offending nutrients.
		Avoid prolonged hangtimes.
		Use sanitary handling and administration techniques.
		Use enteral nutrition support whenever possible.
		Select fiber-supplemented formula.
		Review medication profile and eliminate causative agent if possible.
Cramping, gas, abdominal distention	Nutrient malabsorption	Select a hydrolyzed formula or one that restricts offending nutrients.
	Rapid, intermittent administration of refrigerated formula	Administer formula by continuous method.
	Intermittent feeding using syringe force	Administer formula at room temperature.
		Advance administration rate according to patient tolerance.
		Reduce rate of administration.
		Select alternate method of administration.
Nausea and vomiting	Rapid formula administration	Initiate feedings at low rate and gradually advance to desired rate.
	Gastric retention	Temporarily decrease rate.
		Select isotonic or dilute formula.
		Reduce rate of administration.
		Select low-fat formula.
		Consider need for postpyloric feeding.
Constipation	Inadequate fluid intake	Supplement fluid intake.
	Insufficient bulk	Select fiber-supplemented formula.
	Inactivity	Encourage ambulation, if possible.

Continued

■ **TABLE 5-9**
■ **ENTERAL FEEDING COMPLICATIONS AND PROBLEM SOLVING—cont'd**

PROBLEM	CAUSE	PREVENTION/TREATMENT
METABOLIC		
Dehydration	Elevated fluid needs or losses of GI fluid and electrolytes	Supplement intake with appropriate fluids. Monitor and intervene to maintain hydration status.
Overhydration	Rapid refeeding Excessive fluid intake	Use a calorically dense formula. Reduce rate of administration, especially in patients with severe malnutrition or major organ failure.
Hyperglycemia	Inadequate insulin production for the amount of formula being given Metabolic stress Diabetes mellitus	Select low-carbohydrate formula. Initiate feedings at low rate. Monitor blood glucose. Use insulin if necessary.
Hypernatremia	Inadequate fluid intake or excessive losses	Assess fluid and electrolyte status. Increase water intake.
Hyponatremia	Fluid overload Syndrome of inappropriate antidiuretic hormone secretion (SIADH) Excessive GI fluid losses from diarrhea, vomiting Chronic feeding with relatively low-sodium enteral formulas as the sole source of dietary sodium	Assess fluid and electrolyte status. Restrict fluids, if necessary. Use diuretics, if necessary. Use a rehydration solution such as EquaLYTE Enteral. Rehydration Solution to replace water and electrolytes. Supplement sodium intake, if necessary.
Hypophosphatemia	Aggressive refeeding of malnourished patients Insulin therapy	Monitor serum levels. Replenish phosphorus levels before refeeding.
Hypercapnia	Excessive carbohydrate loads given patients with respiratory dysfunction and CO_2 retention	Select low-carbohydrate, high-fat formula.
Hypokalemia	Aggressive refeeding of malnourished patient	Monitor serum levels. Provide adequate potassium.
Hyperkalemia	Excessive potassium intake Decreased excretion	Reduce potassium intake. Monitor serum levels.

Fallacy: If diarrhea develops with tube feeding, the feeding must stop immediately.

Fact: The cause of diarrhea may be unrelated to formula use, especially if the formula is isotonic and lactose-free. Other problems should be ruled out such as the presence of hyperosmolar electrolyte solutions or sorbitol in some medications (Table 5-9).

How Is the Type of Liquid Supplement Determined?

Digestion and absorption processes and nutrient needs should be ascertained to determine the type of liquid supplement required. If the person has the ability to digest all nutrients and can absorb all nutrients, any liquid preparation that meets the DRI for the person's kilocalorie needs is appropriate. The kilocalorie needs might dictate the appropriate type of supplement: some supplements are designed for high-kilocalorie needs and other supplements are designed for low-kilocalorie needs. Formulas that provide 2 kcal/mL are useful for the fluid-restricted patient.

Often during times of stress, the body is unable to break down lactose, which results in abdominal distention, bloating, and diarrhea. For this reason, many commercial supplements are lactose-free. Fat malabsorption is also common in many disease states. Medium-chain triglyceride (MCT) oil is another common ingredient in commercial supplements. It does not require bile salts so the fat is more easily absorbed.

A person's condition may require other diet restrictions such as low sodium, low sugar, low protein, or low potassium. There are specially developed formulas for these restrictions or related conditions, such as for kidney disease or diabetes. There are also formula modules that allow the patient to follow a recipe to meet individual needs.

If the patient's GI tract is not fully functioning, a formula containing digested nutrients can be administered. These formulas are referred to as **elemental** or defined formula diets (e.g., Vivonex and Vital). They are commonly used for short bowel syndrome, intestinal malabsorption, and pancreatitis, depending on the severity of the condition. These formulas are absorbed in the upper part of the small intestine. Elemental formulas generally are given via tube feeding, as most patients do not like their taste.

All formulas should be refrigerated once they are mixed or opened to prevent bacterial contamination. Any unused portion of the formula should be discarded after 24 hours.

How Is the Amount or Rate of Flow Determined?

The amount of liquid supplement is determined by assessing the person's need for kilocalories, proteins, fluids, vitamins, and minerals. The rate of flow when a pump is used can be calculated by a mathematical equation to meet the needs. For example, if the person can easily have the pump run for 12 hours and the supplement desired contains 1 kcal/mL, 125 mL per hour for 12 hours would be required to meet 1500 kcal (divide 1500 mL by 12 hours to equal 125 mL per hour). However, this is too high an amount to start. Thus a steady progression in flow rate is recommended, starting at about 50 mL per hour and increasing by about 25 mL every 12 to 24 hours until the desired rate is achieved. Alternatively, the length of time of tube feeding could be increased to allow for a slower rate of delivery while meeting the kilocalorie needs sooner.

If a pump (Figure 5-9) is not used, the flow rate is more difficult to manage; however, management can be achieved using a clamp and timing the flow rate. Manual delivery through a gastrostomy should take at least 15 minutes. To help with tolerance, the solution should not be excessively cold.

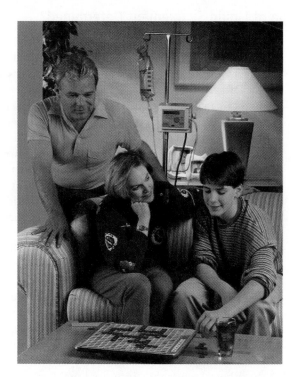

FIGURE 5-9 Tube feeding systems have been developed so that patients are not confined to a hospital bed. Some may even be used in the home. (Used with permission of Ross Products Division, Abbott Laboratories, Columbus, OH. From Tube feeding at home. Ross Products Division, Abbott Laboratories.)

How Are Fluid Needs Determined?

A good rule of thumb is that 1 mL of water is needed for each kilocalorie provided. The actual water content of commercial liquid supplements can be obtained from the manufacturer (see Appendix 2 for phone numbers of the major suppliers), but usually is about 75% to 80% of the total formula volume. Thus the volume of a 2000-kcal solution is generally 2000 mL, but only about 1600 mL of that is actual water content. Water flushes to keep the tube clean are recommended each time a bag of formula is used. The amount of water for this purpose needs to be calculated into the patient's nutritional support regimen. All sources of fluid taken by the patient, including those taken for medication delivery, may need to be considered to avoid fluid overload.

HOW IS NUTRITIONAL SUPPORT MONITORED?

Serum glucose levels need to be monitored at least daily. In any physiologic stress condition, glucose intolerance is common. Because many nutritional support preparations are high in sugar, a patient can easily reach unacceptably high levels of serum glucose. No patient should have a BG level exceeding 200 mg/dL and pregnant women should maintain a BG level less than 120 g/dL at all times (for whole blood measures; plasma glucose meters values are 15% higher). Excess intake of carbohydrate can also elevate serum triglycerides, which should be monitored. Another indicator of excess carbohydrate intake is increased carbon dioxide production. Respiratory therapists can play a role in identifying tolerance to nutrition support. Modifications of supplement use, decreased rate of delivery, or implementation of insulin may be required to avoid hyperglycemia.

The serum albumin level should be monitored for all patients receiving tube feeding or TPN. A low level (less than 3.5 mg/dL) may hinder the patient's ability to absorb the formula. Albumin may then be administered parenterally (intravenously) and the formula should be diluted to one-quarter strength until the desired albumin level is reached (if the formula is isotonic, dilution is not necessary). Blood urea nitrogen (BUN) is a lab value that can indicate how the body is accepting the increased protein intake. A very high level can indicate too much protein in the feeding regimen, but can also be a sign of dehydration or excessive protein breakdown from an inadequate kilocalorie intake. A low BUN level may indicate excess fluid intake, severe malnutrition, or impaired liver function.

Patients receiving tube feedings should be weighed daily to ensure that the patient is receiving adequate kilocalories to promote weight gain. Adequate fluid intake is especially important with formulas containing high amounts of protein so that the kidneys can efficiently excrete nitrogenous waste products. Encouraging the patient to drink fluids, as well as rinsing the tube with water between feedings, will help increase fluid intake. Electrolytes and appropriate nutritional assessment tests should be monitored weekly.

Patients receiving TPN need to have essential trace minerals such as chromium, copper, manganese, molybdenum, selenium, and zinc added to parenteral fluids to prevent the development of deficiency syndromes. Trace-metal monitoring is critical in infants and those on long-term TPN to prevent deficiency or toxicity.

Phlebitis (inflammation of a vein) is a potential complication of PPN, so the infusion site should be closely observed. The nursing staff is called on to pay strict attention to the care of the TPN catheter to avoid **sepsis** (infection) at the site of the catheter, which is one of the more common problems associated with TPN.

WHAT IS THE NUTRITION RECOVERY SYNDROME?

Also referred to as the **refeeding syndrome**, the nutrition recovery syndrome can occur when nutritional support is provided too aggressively, particularly in the malnourished person. As the cells begin to be renourished, they take nutrients from the plasma first. Thus low serum phosphorus levels are common when nutritional support is undertaken and death can result if they become too low. Monitoring lab values is imperative to the safe use of nutritional support. Overestimation of kilocalorie needs can cause the refeeding syndrome. An increase in the heart rate, temperature, and respiration rate may occur.

WHEN IS NUTRITIONAL SUPPORT DISCONTINUED?

Nutritional support should be gradually discontinued whenever the individual starts consuming enough food orally to maintain adequate nutritional intake. Small, frequent feedings are recommended. A low-residue and lactose-free diet may be necessary if diarrhea occurs, as is sometimes the case with patients who have been receiving TPN. If parenteral feedings are withdrawn too rapidly, hypoglycemia may result. Intravenous dextrose can help, or tube feedings may be needed to supplement the oral diet until the patient makes the final adjustment to oral feeding. Kilocalorie intake studies and daily weight records will indicate whether nutritional support can be withdrawn.

WHY ARE FOOD AND DRUG INTERACTIONS CONSIDERED IN THE NUTRITIONAL CARE PLANNING PROCESS?

The health care team must be aware of the many factors that can adversely affect a person's nutritional status, including the effects of drugs on nutrient absorption, excretion, and metabolism, especially when long-term and multiple-drug therapy is necessary. With the vast array of medications used, it is beyond the scope of this text to review specific food-drug interactions. Health care professionals may want to purchase manuals or computer software on food and drug interactions (see Appendix 1 for resources). Children, elderly persons, chronically ill persons, and those with a marginal or inadequate nutrient intake are most susceptible to drug-induced nutritional deficiencies. A good nutritional status and a nutritious diet can reduce this risk. A proper diet can also reduce the risk of any altered effectiveness of drugs. The success of a patient's treatment often depends on the effectiveness of medications. The RD can provide specific dietary instructions to the patient as to when to take medications in relation to meals and which foods, if any, must be avoided. A pharmacist may also need to be consulted for multiple medication regimens.

How Do Drugs Affect Nutrient Absorption?

Drugs may affect absorption of nutrients by damaging the intestinal mucosa, by binding with nutrients, or by decreasing the availability of bile acid, which would inhibit the absorption of the fat-soluble vitamins. Folate absorption is decreased by the use of the antiinflammatory agent sulfasalazine, but rather than the use of folate supplements, a varied and adequate diet should be encouraged.

How Do Food and Nutrients Affect Drug Action?

Food and some beverages, such as coffee or cola drinks, as well as specific nutrients can adversely affect drug action. For example, natural licorice in large quantities can complicate treatment in patients receiving antihypertensive agents because licorice can cause sodium retention, which could result in edema and hypertension.

How Do Food and Vitamin Supplements Affect Drug Action?

Large amounts of vitamin K in a supplement, for example, can reduce the effectiveness of anticoagulants. Tetracycline should not be administered at the same time as a mineral supplement (e.g., calcium) because the absorption of both the minerals and the tetracycline would be inhibited.

How Do Drugs Affect Nutrient Excretion?

Certain drugs such as **diuretics** (medications that cause fluid loss) can deplete potassium (e.g., furosemide or lasix and thiazides). A sodium-restricted diet and potassium-rich foods (see Table 5-10) are often prescribed. Medications that deplete potassium often induce hyperglycemia, resulting in the need to follow a moderate carbohydrate diet. When a diuretic and digitalis are given together, hypokalemia and hypomagnesemia may result and digitalis toxicity must be guarded against. An important thing to remember, however, is that other diuretics such as spironolactone and the newer ACE inhibitors (a type of blood pressure medication) are potassium-conserving, in which case extra dietary potassium is not necessary and may even create a problem. Salt substitutes containing potassium should be avoided when these medications are used.

How Do Drugs Affect Nutrient Metabolism?

Certain drugs bind with enzymes and affect the metabolism of some nutrients. For example, long-term ingestion of pyrimethamine, an antimalarial drug, will likely produce **megaloblastic anemia** (a form of anemia often associated with lack of vitamin B_{12}, or folic acid or folacin) because it antagonizes folacin. Phenobarbital and phenytoin, which are used in the treatment of epilepsy, can

◼ TABLE 5-10
◼ FOODS HIGH IN POTASSIUM

VERY HIGH POTASSIUM SOURCES (>300 mg POTASSIUM)	MODERATELY HIGH POTASSIUM SOURCES (>200 mg POTASSIUM)
Milk, 1 c	Grapefruit, 1 whole
Yogurt, 1 c	Oranges, 1 whole or 4 oz juice
Apricots, 3 whole or 6 halves	Green beans, 1 c
Banana, 1 small	Tomato, 1 whole or ½ c juice
Broccoli, 1 stalk or 1 c cooked	Peanut butter, 2 tbsp
Cantaloupe, 1 quarter	Molasses, 1 tsp blackstrap or 4 tsp "green label"
Carrots, 1 c cooked	
Potatoes, ½ c	
Spinach, ½ c cooked	
Turnips, 1 c cooked	
Winter squash, ½ baked	
Legumes (dried beans and peas), ½ c cooked	

increase bone demineralization. Ingestion of adequate dietary vitamin D should be encouraged to promote the absorption of calcium.

Can Drugs Cause Weight Gain?

Weight gain associated with the use of medications such as steroidal, antihypertensive, and antiinflammatory agents occurs frequently because of sodium and water retention. Other medications, such as some antipsychotic medications, cause an increased appetite with associated weight gain. This interaction may be useful in helping lonely elderly persons regain their appetite to achieve or maintain a healthy weight.

WHAT IS LONG-TERM CARE?

Long-term care consists of a whole group of medical and psychosocial activities and services designed to keep a person as independent as possible for as long as possible. Acute care is undertaken in a hospital setting, whereas long-term care is provided in a variety of settings. Currently, long-term care generally involves placing the patient in a nursing home. Group homes are also commonly used for adults with developmental disabilities. Services brought to the patient such as meals, home-health aide assistance, and public health nursing can help maintain a person's independence.

One approach used in long-term care is characterized by staff performing *for* the resident, resulting in a lack of progress on the part of the patient. In respect to nutrition, the resident who is wheelchair bound may not be allowed independence in wheeling to the dining room or may be fed instead of assisted, even though encouragement, adaptive feeding utensils, and transfer to a regular chair may promote independence. The preferred approach allows the resident to do things for himself or herself, such as ambulating independently to the dining area and self-feeding. The focus is on consumption of a balanced meal, appropriate food consistency, and where and how the meal is consumed. The dining atmosphere, quality of food, and the service provided are all conducive to rehabilitation.

What Are Some Suggestions for Assisting a Patient During Mealtimes?

Attractive food service plays an important role in stimulating the appetite and enjoyment of food. A good appetite is necessary to ensure adequate nutritional intake. Mealtime is often a major event of the day for the patient and every effort must be made to prepare the room and the patient to receive the meal. Brushing teeth or rinsing of the mouth before eating can stimulate appetite. Ensuring availability of dentures for those who wear them is important. Some patients eat better if arrangements can be made for the use of china dishware. Holidays are often a time of sadness for patients in an institutional setting. Using colorful napkins and tray decorations at these times can stimulate the appetite.

The patient's room should be adjusted for adequate, but not glaring, light and a comfortable temperature. If the patient wears glasses, make sure that they are on and are clean. If the patient is blind, the foods should be described before eating begins. Medication for pain or nausea is sometimes recommended for improved meal intake.

Assessment of feeding needs is essential. An eating skills screening form should be completed for individuals at risk, to promote an effective total health care team approach (Figure 5-10). Responsibilities of the various health care disciplines in patient feeding are listed in Table 5-11. Proper positioning is essential for good

---

Eating Skills Screening Form (Sample)

Client Name: _____   Date of Intake: _____

Date of Birth: _____   Age: _____   Sex: _____   Height (in): _____   Weight (lb): _____

General Status of Health: Excellent ☐   Good ☐   Fair ☐   Poor ☐

Position of Individual for Feeding
_____ Upright Unsupported
_____ Upright Supported
_____ Held
_____ Bed/Lying Down

Method of Feeding
_____ Independently spoon feeds
_____ Spoon feeds with assistance
_____ Finger feeds
_____ Fed by caregiver

Present Diet
_____ Blended
_____ Soft
_____ Chopped
_____ Regular
_____ Dietary Restrictions

Sample Daily Intake
(Explain on reverse side, including snacks and schedule.)

Appetite
_____ Good
_____ Fair
_____ Shows preference for certain foods
_____ Allergies

Prior Food Experiences
(Explain on reverse side.)

Alertness
_____ Focuses attention on eating
_____ Responds to presence or absence of food
_____ Responds to environment
_____ Unresponsive or apathetic

Sensory Functions
Intact Impaired
_____ _____ Visual
_____ _____ Auditory
_____ _____ Tactile

Eating Skills
Good Fair Poor
_____ _____ _____ Head/trunk control
_____ _____ _____ Jaw control
_____ _____ _____ Lip closure
_____ _____ _____ Tongue movements
_____ _____ _____ Swallowing
_____ _____ _____ Chewing

Oral Reflexes
_____ Rooting
_____ Suckling
_____ Bite reflex
_____ Hyperactive gag
_____ Hypoactive gag
_____ Tongue thrust
_____ Hypersensitivity around mouth

Motor Deficits Affecting Self-feeding
(Explain on reverse side.)

Dental Care and Status
(Explain on reverse side.)

Sudden and/or Large Weight Change
_____ Loss   _____ Gain

Comments _____
_____
_____
_____

FIGURE 5-10 Sample of an eating skills screening form. (Courtesy of Ross Laboratories, Columbus, Ohio.)

TABLE 5-11
THE TEAM APPROACH TO HEALTH CARE IN FEEDING

HEALTH CARE PROFESSIONAL	RESPONSIBILITY
Dietitian	Meal planning Supervision of food and modified diet preparation Delivery of meals Execution of diet orders Diet modification Nutrition counseling Nutrition assessment
Nurse	Mealtime supervision Proper positioning Charting of food and fluid intake Communication with dietitian and physician regarding acceptance of food served Implementation and integration of total care plan
Occupational therapist	Assessment of oral motor function Instruction of staff on appropriate alignment for feeding Assessment of need for assistive devices Working with client on chewing, swallowing, and other functional skills necessary to achieve feeding independence
Physical therapist	Evaluates mobility deficits Prescribes appropriate feeding activities May assist in evaluating oral motor problems
Speech pathologist	Provides assessment of oral motor functions and recommends appropriate treatment May provide help in solving problems and work with problems of bite reflex and tongue thrust
Psychologist	Evaluates specific behaviors that affect nutrition (such as food stealing, pica behavior, obsessive eating, and bizarre eating habits) and plans ways to manage them
Social worker	Collects social history and demographic data regarding patient and family Summarizes client's financial status and reaction to proposed therapy Provides financial information if needed by client in acquiring funds
Dentist	Provides assessment of patient's dental health (condition of gums, oral structure, and sensitivity related to teeth)
Physician	Identifies feeding problems Requires consultation in writing to appropriate health care professional
Recreational therapist	Provides premeal activities (music for dining, socialization)

Data from Consultant Dietitians in Health Care Facilities: Feeding is everybody's business: a manual for health care professionals involved in feeding programs. Mead Johnson Nutritional Division, Evansville, IN.

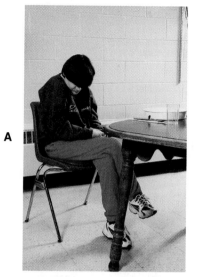
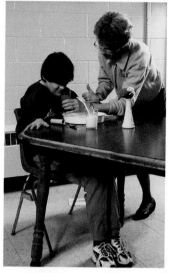

A

B

FIGURE 5-11 **A**, Improper, and **B**, proper positioning at mealtimes.

nutritional intake and avoidance of aspiration of food into the lungs (Figure 5-11). An individual is properly positioned for eating if the following are true:

- The head and upper trunk are as upright as possible.
- The feet are adequately supported.
- The hip and knees are flexed to approximate an 85-degree angle.
- The head is tipped slightly forward.
- The table height is appropriate.
- The arms are centered close to the body.
- The person is seated close to the table.
- Adaptive eating devices may be required (Figure 5-12). Feeding techniques can further help with eating (Table 5-12).

It is important that you, as the person assisting the patient, be relaxed and seated in a comfortable position, when possible. You should engage in pleasant neutral conversation, avoiding discussion of the patient's illness or any criticism of the meal or the patient. This is a good time to teach the patient. Explain the reasons for the various foods offered, especially if the patient does not understand the diet well.

If the patient must be fed, you should alternate one food with another and offer liquids frequently. Provide liquids also whenever they are requested. Open containers, cut meat, and apply condiments if necessary to ensure an adequate intake. If the patient cannot eat a meal or a portion of the meal for valid reasons, such as the meat being too tough, offer to get substitute food (providing the patient's condition warrants it).

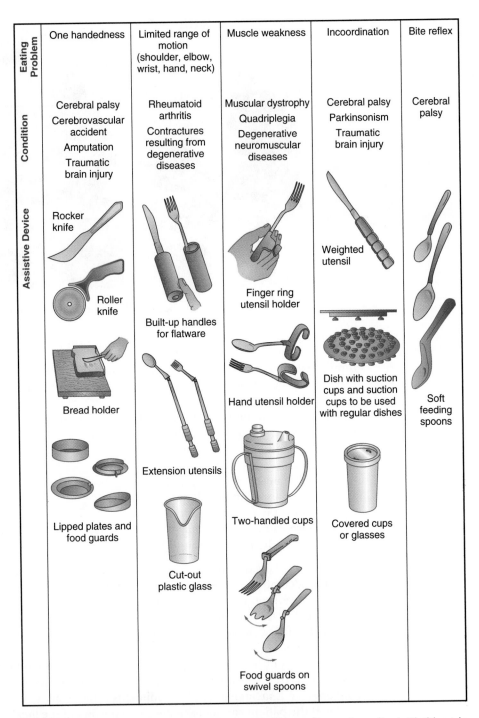

FIGURE 5-12 Assistive devices for eating problems. (From Consultant Dietitians in Health Care Facilities: Feeding is everybody's business: a manual for health care professionals involved in feeding programs. Mead Johnson Nutritional Division, Evansville, IN.)

TABLE 5-12
FEEDING TECHNIQUES FOR RESOLVING AND IMPROVING FEEDING PROBLEMS

POSSIBLE ABNORMAL REFLEX OR PROBLEM	FEEDING TECHNIQUE
ROOTING REFLEX Mouth opens and head turns in the direction of the stimulus when cheeks or lips are touched beyond 3 months of age.	Avoid stimulation to face between swallows or bites, such as wiping face with a cloth.
SUCK-SWALLOW Rhythmical suck and simultaneous swallowing movement that continues as long as stimulus is present.	Occupational therapy program for oral normalization such as mouth and tongue stimulation, lip closure, stroking the throat, and so on. Follow OT program to progress from sucking to chewing. When using stimulation techniques, use firm, deep pressure rather than light pressure, which may tickle or irritate. Gradually increase texture and thickness of food.
TONIC NECK REFLEX Develops at 4 weeks. Stimulated by receptors in the neck, it aids in eye-hand coordination. Position of the arms depends on position of the head.	
ASYMMETRICAL TONIC NECK REFLEX When the head is turned toward the right, the right arm extends outward. If to the left, the left arm extends. Prevents individual from keeping the head in position to be fed and interferes with jaw control. When self-feeding, it prevents proper hand-to-mouth coordination.	Position head and whole body in midline. (Refer to Positioning discussed previously.)
GAG REFLEX Prevents passage of food into the windpipe. Present from birth on through life, although it weakens in later life. In hypertonicity, a gag is elicited by tactile stimulation to the anterior half of the tongue. Caused by hypersensitive tongue, and difficulty in swallowing. In hypotonicity, no gag response occurs regardless of what part of the tongue is prodded.	Gagging is a "yellow light, not a red light." The feeder may think that gagging on a new food means that the individual is not ready for more complicated textures. This may not be so, but just a warning to take things more slowly. To prevent behavioral problems, handle gagging in a very matter-of-fact way. Simply place hand over the child's mouth and close it until he swallows. Be careful to prevent food from entering the windpipe. Keep the head forward. Neck extension can cause aspiration. Tongue stimulation at other than mealtime to decrease hypersensitivity to touch. To control tongue activity, place food on the middle of the tongue with a slightly downward pressure of the spoon. Feeder must be extremely careful in feeding this individual to prevent choking. Feed slowly. Walk the tongue with a tongue depressor or fingers in small steps to the point of gag, then withdraw depressor, close client's mouth, and wait for a swallow.

Information approved by an occupational therapist of Broome Developmental Services, Ithaca, NY.

Continued

POSSIBLE ABNORMAL REFLEX OR PROBLEM	FEEDING TECHNIQUE
BITE REFLEX Rapid rhythmical opening and closing of the jaw as long as the stimulus is present. This reflex is integrated by 4 months.	Use small Xylon spoon when feeding to prevent injury to oral structures. Wait for relaxation before removing spoon (do not try to pull spoon out).
LIP CLOSURE Necessary for removing food from the spoon and for preventing drooling.	Prefeeding stimulation of lips and jaw control in which the index finger is above the upper lip, pulling downward slightly as the spoon is removed. Never scrape food off the spoon with the client's teeth. A spoon with a flat bowl will work better than a deep-bowled spoon. Do not try to scrape any excess food from the lips with the spoon or wipe the client's mouth or chin after every bite. This may give the client the wrong signal to open his mouth rather than keeping it closed to masticate and swallow. Allow for a little messiness while the client learns that the touch of the spoon means that he is to open his mouth and withdrawal of the spoon means he is to close his mouth
TONGUE MOBILITY Used in moving food to the back of the mouth for swallowing and relocating food from the sides of the mouth.	Encourage lip-licking with the tongue by placing something tasty on the lips such as peanut butter. Also place small pieces of cereal between the lips and gums.
DROOLING Caused by ineffective swallowing of saliva. It is evident when there is poor jaw and tongue control and poor lip closure.	The therapist must solve the drooling problem indirectly by correcting the other feeding problems first.
REFUSAL TO EAT SOLID FOOD Hypersensitivity to touch. Dislikes change. May have very tight mouth.	Eliminate canned pureed food. Introduce wide variety of regular table food that has been pureed. Gradually introduce thickened consistency. Then food with general lumpiness such as rice pudding rather than discrete lumps. When introducing vegetables, initially avoid vegetables with an outer shell such as corn, peas, and lima beans.
REFUSAL TO DRINK FROM A CUP Poor coordination to suck-swallow. Previous experience from choking on liquids.	Begin cup drinking by using thickened liquids that flow more slowly and give the client more time to swallow. Alternate spoonfuls of thickened liquid with spoonfuls of client's other food at the meal. Gradually increase the number of spoonfuls of liquid given in succession, but give client enough time to swallow between spoonfuls. Gradually thin down liquid. For example: add apricot nectar to pureed apricots. Then reduce strained fruit gradually until the client is drinking juice alone. Use jaw control to close lips and jaw, and reinforce "normal" swallowing pattern.

WHAT IS THE NURSE'S AND OTHER HEALTH CARE PROFESSIONAL'S ROLE IN NUTRITION COUNSELING AND THE HEALTH CARE SETTING?

To be successful in helping an individual accept a certain dietary regimen, the nurse or other health care professional must display warmth and understanding, establish a rapport, and be positive in approaching the patient. Acknowledging the strengths in the person's diet history is helpful. For example, if the patient consumes breakfast routinely and eats a variety of foods from the food groups of the Food Guide Pyramid (see Chapter 1), the health care professional can build on those important features in the meal pattern and compliment the individual's efforts in making good food choices. Specific problems can be focused on, making it easier to attain realistic goals, such as eating low-salt snacks versus salty ones. Repeated counseling sessions may be necessary for the development of permanent behavioral modification. It is critical for any health care professional to be well informed before appropriate nutritional guidance can be provided. The role of the health care professional is to be positive and supportive in the context of the total health care team. Helping to identify patients at high nutritional risk is a critical role of all health care professionals. Referral to an RD is paramount for complex medical and health issues.

**CHAPTER
STUDY
QUESTIONS
AND
CLASSROOM
ACTIVITIES**

1. Have a class role play with one student serving as a nurse or other health care professional attempting to use active-listening strategies in assessing the needs of a volunteer patient. The "patient" should be from another ethnic background (refer to class activity in Chapter 1 regarding differences in ethnic cultures and food choices). Other class members should critique the role play for good communication techniques and to determine how successfully the nutrition care process was put into practice. The role play might be repeated to cover a number of different ethnic backgrounds.
2. List positive communication messages that promote honest answers to assessment questions.
3. List three possible reasons a person may develop diarrhea while receiving tube-feeding; what solutions might be helpful?
4. What are the different nutrition management concerns for HIV and AIDS? What nutritional monitoring technique should be done on a regular basis?
5. Interview nurses at the local health department to assess what measures are taken to prevent the spread of HIV and AIDS in the community.
6. What are some symptoms of food allergy?
7. What is the difference between food allergy and food intolerance?
8. Plan a day's menu for someone who is allergic to milk.

Case Study

CRITICAL THINKING

The nurse was drawing blood from Tony's arm while the clinic social worker was asking him questions about how he came to be here today. He thought to himself, "Well, you see, it all started with my wife's diagnosis of breast cancer and my having had diabetes for several years and not questioning the void that that sweet, young waitress seemed to fill, if only temporarily, after I unloaded my burdens on her." His actions seemed so logical at the time. In retrospect, he wondered how much his eating poorly, while Maria was in the hospital receiving chemotherapy, contributed to his depression that landed him here today. Now, what did the social worker ask him about how many other sexual partners he had had? Did he tell her the complete story or simply say, "My wife and I married when I was 18, after dating her since we were in grade school. The answer is, two." He really needed to get out of here quickly because he needed to get to the gym, where his personal trainer was going to start him on an exercise program. He needed to get his life back, especially because Maria was okay, even if she did have to have a mastectomy. He didn't want to think about his health anymore, or his diabetes, or whether he had the HIV virus, or not. He said a little prayer of thankfulness for still having his wife and really prayed that this clinic was totally unnecessary.

Critical Thinking Applications

1. Discuss how illness within a family can affect the family functioning.
2. List an example of an open-ended and a close-ended question that the social worker might have used.
3. Discuss the effect that prayer can have on health.
4. Discuss communication strategies for working with an angry or distraught patient.
5. If Tony tests positive for HIV, what nutritional advice would be appropriate?
6. Write a sample nutrition care plan developing goals, interventions, and evaluation means.

Nutritional Assessment and Care Plan

Name: _____ Date: _____
DOB: _____ Age: _____
Diagnoses: _____

Subjective Data

Food habits:

Fluid intake:

Activity level:

Objective Data

Diet order:

Meal pattern:
Breakfast   Lunch   Supper

Consistency:
Medications:

Supplements:

Male/Female:
Bowel/bladder functions:
Weight HX:

Laboratory values:
Weight: _____   Height: _____
Physical indicators:

Meal observations:

Medical factors affecting nutritional status:

Physical limitations:

Problem   **Goal**   **Intervention**

Recommendations:

Signature: _____

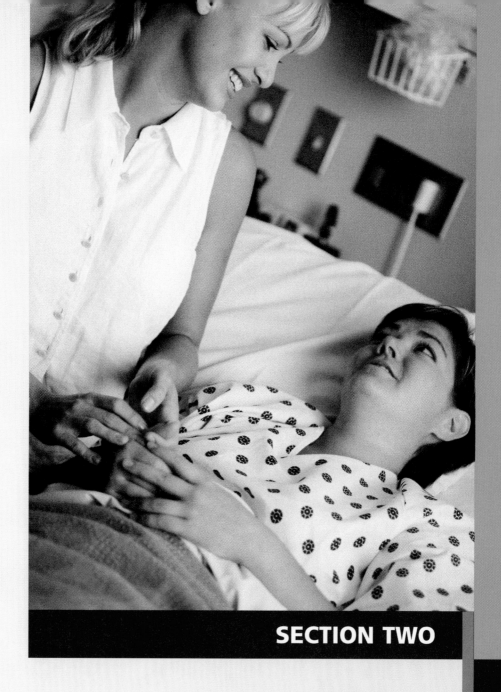

Chronic and Acute Illness

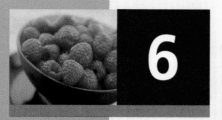

6

The Insulin Resistance Syndrome: The Common Gene

OBJECTIVES

After completing this chapter, you should be able to:

- Describe the insulin resistance syndrome.
- Identify individuals at risk for the insulin resistance syndrome.
- Recognize an appropriate lifestyle plan for managing insulin resistance.
- Explain the application of nutrition labeling in managing insulin resistance.

TERMS TO IDENTIFY

Androgens
Atherosclerosis
C-reactive protein (CRP)
Central obesity
Dyslipidemia
Endometrial hyperplasia
Glucagon
Glycemic index

Gout
Hirsutism
Hyperglycemia
Hyperinsulinemia
Hypertension
Hypoglycemia
Insulin resistance
Leptin

Lipoprotein lipase
Metabolic obesity
Oral glucose tolerance test (OGTT)
Polycystic Ovary Syndrome (PCOS)
Thrifty gene theory
Type 2 diabetes

INTRODUCTION

Only since 1995 has insulin resistance been recognized as a real entity. It was considered just a theory before this time. The insulin resistance syndrome was initially called Syndrome X and is now also referred to as the Metabolic Syndrome per the 1998 World Health Organization (WHO) definition.

As you recall from Chapter 3, food kilocalories are converted to energy in the body cells. Insulin assists in the metabolism of the macronutrients, but is particularly important for the transfer of glucose from the blood into the body cells. When this process is interrupted, there are many potential health problems. The compensating excess production of insulin to override the resistance at the cell level is a major contributor to the adverse health problems associated with insulin resistance.

Insulin resistance describes a condition in certain individuals in which the body cells resist the action of insulin. The means of this resistance is not understood. Some researchers feel this condition has hormonal causes, whereas others feel it is more like a physical barrier composed of excess hydrogen in the cell membranes. It may turn out to be different causes that inhibit the action of insulin, but have the same outcomes as described in this chapter.

The insulin resistance syndrome is often referred to as the common gene theory because it is commonly found—1 of every 4 Americans are estimated to have this syndrome. The rate of insulin resistance in some populations is as high as 60%. Insulin resistance is also called the common gene theory because it is the underlying cause of many chronic health problems. About one third of persons with insulin resistance go on to develop Type 2 diabetes.

There is now a tremendous amount of research taking place to learn more about this syndrome. Section Two of this textbook includes the several health problems caused by the genetic predisposition to insulin resistance. As this section points out, the health problems associated with insulin resistance are only realized through environmental factors, with diet playing a large role.

This chapter provides an overview of the insulin resistance syndrome. Other chapters in this section expand on the specific health problems associated with this syndrome, including central obesity, coronary heart disease, and diabetes, with its resulting effects on the kidneys. Research is expanding on other health conditions associated with the insulin resistance syndrome, such as conditions involving the thyroid gland and certain forms of cancer (see Chapter 11).

WHAT IS THE INSULIN RESISTANCE SYNDROME?

The insulin resistance syndrome is comprised of several correlates or associated health problems, including the following:

- **Central obesity**: carrying weight in the abdomen or a high waist-to-hip ratio (see Chapter 7)
- **Metabolic obesity**: a term used to describe excess abdominal fat when the definition of obesity had not been met

- **Hypertension**: high blood pressure (see Chapter 8)
- **Dyslipidemia**: high levels of triglycerides and low levels of HDL cholesterol (see Chapter 8)
- **Gout**: a condition related to high levels of uric acid (see later in this chapter)
- **Polycystic ovary syndrome (PCOS)**: a clinical diagnosis based on high levels of male hormones, male pattern hair growth, and ovarian cysts (see later in this chapter)
- **Type 2 diabetes**: a condition related to high levels of blood glucose (see Chapter 9)

These conditions are correlated with insulin resistance. There is still debate on cause and effect. Historically, thinking has generally focused on the development of obesity as the cause of insulin resistance (Kim et al., 2000) and its listed correlates. However, recent research shows that insulin resistance has a genetic link only realized through the environment. Environmental factors that worsen insulin resistance are related to the Westernized diet and reduced activity levels. Persons with insulin resistance have been noted to require 10 times as much insulin to control blood glucose levels as compared with other individuals (Reaven, 1999).

Persons with a family genetic predisposition to insulin resistance may be the result of a history of survival through famines. In fact, insulin resistance is often referred to as the **thrifty gene theory** (being thrifty in calorie expenditure; see Chapter 7 for management of obesity related to insulin resistance). It is likely that thousands, if not millions, of years ago before there were restaurants, corner grocery stores, refrigeration, and transportation, many of our ancestors faced continual cycles of famine. Those who did not starve to death in such famines likely had a thrifty gene.

Many of us have the genetic legacies of those survivors, in that persons who inherited the thrifty gene gain body fat easily in times of plenty. They also have a difficult time losing weight. This would have been a survival advantage before a stable food intake could be relied upon, but in current times it results in obesity and Type 2 diabetes (Joffe and Zimmet, 1998).

WHAT ARE THE RISK FACTORS FOR INSULIN RESISTANCE?

One genetic risk factor for insulin resistance is a family history of the correlated conditions listed earlier. Someone who has a strong family history of diabetes, for example, is at higher risk of having insulin resistance.

Although carrying weight in the abdomen is correlated with insulin resistance, there is debate on the best measurement. Some advocate a waist-to-hip ratio greater than 1.0 for men and 0.8 for women. Others suggest it is the total waist measurement that is most important and advocate routine measurements in the health setting (Okosun et al., 1999). A waist size greater than 40 inches for men and 35 inches for women is indicative of central obesity.

Certain population groups are known to have high rates of insulin resistance. The Pima Indians of Arizona have the highest reported occurrence of obesity and non–insulin-dependent diabetes mellitus in the world. This situation developed with the abrupt changes in lifestyle accompanying the rerouting of the Gila River about 100 years ago to provide irrigation waters for California. The prevalence of obesity and diabetes among the Arizona Pimas has increased to epidemic proportions over the past few decades. The Pimas have taught us a lot about the genetic predisposition of insulin resistance, obesity, and diabetes, which environmental factors such as reduced physical activity and changes in diet have brought about over this past century (Weyer et al., 2001).

The epidemic of obesity and diabetes among the Arizona Pimas is in contrast to the low rates among Mexican Pimas (Ravussin et al., 1994). The lower rates of diabetes among the Mexican Pimas is attributed to their higher physical activity levels and maintenance of a more traditional diet.

Native Americans, in general, have a high prevalence of Type 2 diabetes. The Native Americans of Canada have a 40% occurrence rate—in contrast to a virtually undetectable rate less than a century ago—and a tripling of the coronary heart disease rate over the past 20 years (Hegele, 2001). South Pacific Islanders are also at high risk of insulin resistance (Simmons et al., 2001).

Other known groups with high rates of the insulin resistance syndrome include persons with Spanish (i.e., Hispanic and Latino) and South Asian heritage (Kain et al., 2001). Whereas African American children tend to have **hyperinsulinemia** (excess insulin in the blood) and are often insulin resistant (Danadian et al., 1999), Africans have by contrast a relatively low rate of diabetes—about half the rate of Americans at large (Erasmus et al., 2001). This reinforces the hypothesis that genetic predisposition to insulin resistance requires lifestyle factors for the syndrome to be realized.

There is a general trend for higher rates of insulin resistance among persons with heritage from places nearer the equator. There are exceptions to this because insulin resistance is known to occur in all ethnic groups. The author has, in fact, worked with many Irish and Italian Americans with the insulin resistance syndrome.

Aside from groups known to have high rates of insulin resistance, there are other indicators. Children with early onset of puberty or obesity may be at an increased risk for the development of insulin resistance.

One lab value increasingly used to identify those with insulin resistance and hyperinsulinemia is the ratio of fasting glucose levels to fasting insulin levels. It was found that a fasting glucose to insulin ratio less than 7 may serve as an early identification of children at risk for complications of insulin resistance (Silfen et al., 2001). Fasting hyperinsulinemia is a widely used surrogate measure of insulin resistance and predicts Type 2 diabetes in various groups (Weyer et al., 2000).

Another lab value increasingly taken into account is the level of **C-reactive protein (CRP)** (a type of protein found with inflammation). Low-grade chronic inflammation reflected by increased CRP identifies those at risk for Type 2 diabetes and coronary heart disease. Women with Polycystic Ovary Syndrome (PCOS; see section later this chapter) are insulin resistant and have increased risk for Type 2 diabetes and coronary heart disease. Women with PCOS have shown significantly elevated CRP concentrations (Kelly et al., 2001).

Fallacy: A person with a strong family history of diabetes is doomed to develop it himself.

Fact: Studies show that groups at risk of developing diabetes can prevent this condition if there is regular physical activity, maintenance of a healthy weight, and emphasis on foods high in fiber and low in saturated fat.

WHAT IS THE ROLE OF HYPERINSULINEMIA IN THE INSULIN RESISTANCE SYNDROME?

There are still many unanswered questions related to insulin resistance and hyperinsulinemia. Generally speaking, we do know that if the body cells resist the action of insulin, there will be a corresponding rise in insulin production to metabolize blood glucose levels.

A person with a genetic predisposition to insulin resistance tends to have an altered insulin response. With insulin resistance there is often a delayed production of insulin. This can result in a transient state of **hyperglycemia** (high levels of blood glucose). When the body does respond to the hyperglycemia, it is often with excess insulin production over a prolonged period. This hyperinsulinemia can result in symptoms of **hypoglycemia** (low levels of blood glucose; see Chapter 9) if meals are delayed.

Reactive hypoglycemia is a common, but underdiagnosed, medical problem whose pathophysiology is not completely understood. Symptoms may occur years before the onset of diabetes and are likely because of hyperinsulinemia among persons with the insulin resistance syndrome.

The symptoms of hypoglycemia affect the quality of life. However, most persons with hypoglycemia symptoms are not in an immediate health emergency. Severe hypoglycemia requiring medical assistance is usually limited to persons taking insulin or insulin-stimulating medications such as the *sulfonylurea* medications.

It appears that patients with hypoglycemia symptoms have a heightened counterregulatory response. As you may recall from Chapter 3, counterregulatory hormones work opposite of insulin. These hormones correct hypoglycemia by causing the liver to release its stored sugar, called *glycogen*. The symptoms that occur from these hormones, however, can be unpleasant. Altered **glucagon** (a counterregulatory hormone that is the first produced in response to low levels of blood glucose) secretion has been noted in reactive hypoglycemia. Glucagon in excess leads to feelings of nausea. It is likely that impaired glucagon sensitivity and secretion may contribute to *postprandial* (after-meal) hypoglycemia in reactive hypoglycemia (Ahmadpour and Kabadi, 1997). Patients with reactive hypoglycemia may have excess production of adrenal hormomes (Lerman-Garber et al., 2000). Increased adrenalin, also called epinephrine, causes an increased heart rate and physical tremors. It is interesting to note that hypoglycemia was found to be linked to some cases of agitation, requiring emergency room care (Moritz et al., 1999).

Excess insulin levels are found with central obesity. It is still, however, a bit of a chicken-and-egg question. Which came first? Hyperinsulinemia and central obesity are known to worsen insulin resistance. However, it may be the genetic predisposition to insulin resistance that first sets up excess production of insulin. Some health care professionals suggest that hyperinsulinemia encourages the gain of abdominal weight in the first place. This weight gain then reinforces insulin resistance, creating a vicious cycle.

In regard to dyslipidemia (see Chapter 8), it has been clearly shown that the enzyme **lipoprotein lipase** (an enzyme that helps the breakdown of triglycerides) is altered in the presence of hyperinsulinemia. This results in reduced breakdown of triglycerides. Defects in the lipoprotein lipase gene are associated with dyslipidemia in the general population (Samuels et al., 2001). Thus elevated triglyceride levels in the blood are generally associated with hyperinsulinemia, especially if the person also has central obesity. Reduction in hyperinsulinemia generally improves dyslipidemia.

Hypertension is commonly associated with diabetes and has the same pathogenetic mechanism as insulin resistance (Kirpichnikov and Sowers, 2001). There are still unanswered questions regarding the specific mechanism related to hypertension and the underlying cause of insulin resistance. One study found hyperinsulinemia and excess **leptin** (another hormone related to weight) play an

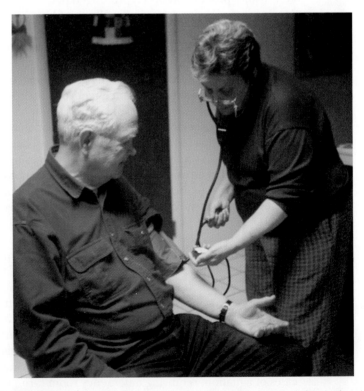

FIGURE 6-1 Hypertension is commonly found with excess abdominal weight.

important role in the development of hypertension in obese patients. Insulin and leptin increase sodium retention and encourage blood vessels to constrict (Hano and Nishio, 2001). In other words, hyperinsulinemia makes the blood vessels less elastic, resulting in hypertension. Other research has not been able to show that hyperinsulinemia causes hypertension. Some new research is indicating that blood pressure increases in an insulin-resistant state (Chen et al., 2001). A person with central obesity and hypertension likely has the insulin resistance syndrome (Figure 6-1).

Hyperinsulinemia is now believed to be related to early heart disease in the form of **atherosclerosis** (buildup of plaque inside the arteries and other blood vessels; see Chapter 8). Although the incidence of heart disease increases with diabetes, the former often precedes the diagnosis of the latter. The presence of insulin resistance is observed many years before the onset of Type 2 diabetes. Insulin resistance at this stage appears to be significantly associated with cardiovascular risk factors (Cefalu, 2001a). Cardiovascular disease usually precedes the diagnosis of diabetes. More than half of individuals with diabetes mellitus die from cardiovascular causes (Wilson et al., 2001).

Hyperinsulinemia is generally found with Type 2 diabetes. The chief problem with Type 2 diabetes is the underlying insulin resistance at the cell level. However, hyperinsulinemia can worsen insulin resistance, making it more difficult for the body to regulate blood glucose levels.

WHAT ARE THE CAUSES OF GOUT, AND HOW IS IT MANAGED?

Gout, the condition of having elevated uric acid levels, is known to occur with insulin resistance. Alcohol consumption, use of diuretics, and excess weight gain may increase the risk of gout attack among patients with high levels of uric acid (Lin et al., 2000).

Recent research shows gout to be a risk factor for heart disease. This is likely because of the role of uric acid in thrombotic tendency (Longo-Mbenza et al., 1999).

A diet low in carbohydrates and high in protein and unsaturated fat has been recommended for persons with gout because they all enhance insulin sensitivity and therefore may promote a reduction in serum uric acid levels (Schlesinger and Schumacher, 2001). This guideline was reinforced with a study that showed weight loss with a 1600-kcal diet consisting of 40% carbohydrate, 30% protein, and 30% fat and replacing refined with complex carbohydrates and saturated with monounsaturated and polyunsaturated fats. Reduced serum levels of uric acid and dyslipidemia occurred with this approach (Dessein et al., 2000).

fact
FALLACY

Fallacy: Comfrey, a type of herb used for treatment of inflammation, is safe to use and can help gout.

Fact: Comfrey contains a natural chemical substance (usually consumed by drinking comfrey tea) that is now recognized to be toxic to the liver and has been banned in Germany and Canada for this reason (Stickel and Seitz, 2000).

WHAT ARE THE CAUSES OF THE POLYCYSTIC OVARY SYNDROME?

The PCOS is related to hyperinsulinemia. In the presence of excess levels of insulin, male type hormones, called **androgens**, may be formed. This results in the masculinization of some women, leading to male-pattern hair loss, excessive body hair (called **hirsutism**), and excessive ovarian cysts. The high levels of male hormones impair ovulation and lead to disrupted menstrual cycles and infertility. It is the most common cause of menstrual disorders (Loverro et al., 2001).

The underlying cause of PCOS is primarily related to insulin resistance and hyperinsulinemia. At least 50% of patients with PCOS are obese (Hoeger, 2001). Women with PCOS are at high risk for impaired glucose tolerance and Type 2 diabetes. This is especially true of minority women. A 2-hour **oral glucose tolerance test (OGTT)** (a test that involves the use of a standard amount of carbohydrates, such as 50 g, followed by postprandial measurement of glucose levels) is advised for screening women with PCOS at high risk of diabetes rather than fasting glucose levels alone (Legro, 2001). An increased potential for **endometrial hyperplasia** (thickening of the endometrial layer of the uterus) and malignancy is associated with PCOS and underscores the need for prompt identification and treatment. Attention to endometrial thickness (measured by transvaginal sonogram) and elevated insulin levels (measured by fasting plasma insulin) can improve clinical surveillance of both conditions (Elliott et al., 2001). The prevalence of the mother's menstrual irregularity and the incidence of the father's premature balding and hypertension were significantly higher in women with PCOS (Mao et al., 2000).

Fallacy: Children instinctively know how to make food choices to stay healthy.

Fact: Children need the guidance of adults in selecting foods. The insulin resistance syndrome includes many chronic diseases such as obesity, heart disease, and high blood pressure that can start in childhood as a result of poor food choices. Using the Food Guide Pyramid to teach children to eat more high fiber plant foods, such as vegetables, fruits, and legumes (beans), is appropriate.

HOW CAN THE INSULIN RESISTANCE SYNDROME BE MANAGED?

Many populations with traditional ethnic eating habits do not have the health problems associated with the insulin resistance syndrome. However, many populations at risk for insulin resistance develop the syndrome when the diet and lifestyle changes to a more Westernized one. It has been shown in numerous examples that the insulin resistance syndrome does not occur in physically active groups that choose a diet relatively low in fat and sugar (Pavan et al., 1999).

In short-term studies, adoption of a traditional diet of many different cultures is associated with reduction in metabolic abnormalities found with insulin resistance. One study found about one-third fewer cases of the insulin resistance syndrome among those who followed the traditional high-fiber Pima Indian diet versus a typical Westernized diet (Williams et al., 2001).

Preventing the development of obesity seems to be critical in preventing the insulin resistance syndrome, although the genetic predisposition to insulin resistance is inherited. See Chapter 7 for more on the prevention and management of obesity.

It was found that the **glycemic index** (estimation of the effect of food on blood sugar levels) may influence outcome in terms of cardiovascular risk and risk of metabolic syndrome diseases (Frost and Dornhorst, 2000). The glycemic index is discussed more fully in Chapter 9.

Research has shown improved sensitivity to insulin with light to moderate (½ to 1 drink daily) alcohol intake (Bell et al., 2000). However, as discussed earlier in the text (see Chapter 3), this advice is only appropriate for those individuals who already drink and are not predisposed to alcoholism.

Fallacy: Juice contains less sugar than soda pop.

Fact: Juice contains as much total sugar as does soda pop. The sugar in juice is primarily fructose, whereas the sugar in soda pop is sucrose or high-fructose corn syrup, but they all are simple sugars and will raise blood sugar levels. For persons with insulin resistance, this tends to promote hyperinsulinemia, which may encourage the insulin resistance syndrome.

WHAT MEDICAL METHODS OF MANAGING INSULIN RESISTANCE ARE THERE?

Metformin (Glucophage) is a medication for persons with diabetes. It is specifically aimed at managing insulin resistance. As described earlier, the exact physiology of insulin resistance is not understood. Thus the manner in which glucophage works to reduce insulin resistance is not known, either. Still, this insulin-sensitizing medication presents a promising treatment for PCOS, offering metabolic and gynecologic benefits for women who have this syndrome. All of the evidence to date suggests that metformin is a safe drug to administer to women who may become pregnant (Iuorno and Nestler, 2001). Estrogen is also reported to improve carbohydrate metabolism, including reducing insulin resistance, in healthy women (Cefalu, 2001b). Other medications exist to control insulin resistance and more are expected to be developed.

WHAT IS THE ROLE OF THE NURSE OR OTHER HEALTH PROFESSIONAL IN THE PREVENTION AND MANAGEMENT OF THE INSULIN RESISTANCE SYNDROME?

The nurse or other health professional should be aware of the common occurrence of the insulin resistance syndrome. At least 1 of every 4 persons is at risk for insulin resistance. Health care professionals need to be aware of the correlates of the insulin resistance syndrome, such as central obesity and hypertension.

Prompt identification of at-risk individuals can help to prevent early heart disease and diabetes. Referral to a dietitian who is also a certified diabetes educator may be in order for a thorough assessment and identification of dietary risk factors to prevent development of the insulin resistance syndrome.

A general area in which all health care professionals can help manage insulin resistance is by helping to control the food environment. This might entail offering low-sugar beverages, such as seltzer water or diet soda, at social events. For snacks, one could offer high-fiber, low-carbohydrate vegetable trays with either a dip low in total fat or at least low in saturated fat, such as a mayonnaise-based dressing or a bean-based dip such as hummus.

CHAPTER STUDY QUESTIONS AND CLASSROOM ACTIVITIES

1. If you are working with an individual who has central obesity and hypertension, is this individual at risk of diabetes?
2. Ask students to raise their hands if they have experienced symptoms of hypoglycemia that are resolved with food, such as feeling weak, shaky, or irritable.
3. Ask students to raise their hands if they have heritage that puts them at risk for insulin resistance: Native American, Spanish, African, or Asian. Poll students with a family history of insulin resistance correlates who have a genetic heritage different from those named. Estimate the percentage of students in class who are at risk for the insulin resistance syndrome. Students should not be made to feel obligated to share family health history.
4. Assess the following menu for the questions below:

Breakfast	Lunch	Dinner
Banana	Hot dog on roll	Cheeseburger
Corn flakes	Mustard and relish	French fries
Whole milk	Chocolate chip cookies	Coleslaw
Sugar	Coke	Milkshake
Toast, butter, and jelly		

Judge these meals according to the Food Guide Pyramid.

Identify the foods or beverages high in sugar and saturated fat.

What suggestions would you make to this menu to lower the risk of developing the insulin resistance syndrome?

Case Study

Tony was sitting in his doctor's office. He seemed to be spending a lot of time in health-related activities—visiting the health clinic, working out at the gym, and now seeing his doctor. Turn 50 and you fall apart, he thought. He needed to review his medications with the doctor. He had gotten the phone call that the doctor wanted to see him because his triglycerides had gone very high and he was thinking of putting him on more medication. Tony thought he already had too many meds, with two for high blood pressure, one for gout, and two for his diabetes. He felt like telling the doctor to set up the appointment to have his stomach stapled because he had been told over and over that if he could only lose weight, his health problems might go away. At least I don't have AIDS, he thought to himself. He was also concerned about his son's growing weight problem. He hoped he was not destined to have the same health problems. Time for a family meeting, he thought to himself.

Critical Thinking Applications

1. What underlying health condition does Tony have that contributes to his weight problem, high blood pressure, high triglycerides, and gout?
2. With Tony's son's growing weight problem, is he at risk for developing diabetes? What can he do to help prevent diabetes?
3. What nutritional advice might you give Tony and his family to help manage their health?
4. Bring sample food and beverage labels to class that might be of help to Tony and his family. Compare grams of carbohydrate, fiber, protein, and saturated fat content.

REFERENCES

Ahmadpour S, Kabadi UM: Pancreatic alpha-cell function in idiopathic reactive hypoglycemia. Metabolism. June 1997; 46(6):639-643.

Bell RA, Mayer-Davis EJ, Martin MA, D'Agostino RB Jr, Haffner SM: Associations between alcohol consumption and insulin sensitivity and cardiovascular disease risk factors: the Insulin Resistance and Atherosclerosis Study. Diabetes Care. November 2000; 23(11):1630-1636.

Cefalu WT: Insulin resistance: cellular and clinical concepts. Exp Biol Med (Maywood). January 2001; 226(1):13-26.

Cefalu WT: The use of hormone replacement therapy in postmenopausal women with Type 2 diabetes. J Womens Health Gend Based Med. April 2001; 10(3):241-255.

Chen W, Srinivasan SR, Elkasabany A, Ellsworth DL, Boerwinkle E, Berenson GS: Combined effects of endothelial nitric oxide synthase gene polymorphism (G894T) and insulin resistance status on blood pressure and familial risk of hypertension in young adults: the Bogalusa Heart Study. Am J Hypertens. October 2001; 14(10):1046-1052.

Danadian K, Balasekaran G, Lewy V, Meza MP, Robertson R, Arslanian SA: Insulin sensitivity in African American children with and without family history of Type 2 diabetes. Diabetes Care. August 1999; 22(8):1325-1329.

Dessein PH, Shipton EA, Stanwix AE, Joffe BI, Ramokgadi J: Beneficial effects of weight loss associated with moderate calorie/carbohydrate restriction, and increased proportional intake of protein and unsaturated fat on serum urate and lipoprotein levels in gout: a pilot study. Ann Rheum Dis. July 2000; 59(7):539-543.

Elliott JL, Hosford SL, Demopoulos RI, Perloe M, Sills ES: Endometrial adenocarcinoma and polycystic ovary syndrome: risk factors, management, and prognosis. South Med J. May 2001; 94(5):529-531.

Erasmus RT, Blanco E, Okesina AB, Matsha T, Gqweta Z, Mesa JA: Prevalence of diabetes mellitus and impaired glucose tolerance in factory workers from Transkei, South Africa. S Afr Med J. February 2001; 91(2):157-160.

Frost G, Dornhorst A: The relevance of the glycaemic index to our understanding of dietary carbohydrates. Diabet Med. May 2000; 17(5):336-345.

Hano T, Nishio I: Treatment of hypertension in the patients with obesity. Nippon Rinsho. May 2001; 59(5):973-977. [Article in Japanese.]

Hegele RA: Genes and environment in Type 2 diabetes and atherosclerosis in aboriginal Canadians. Curr Atheroscler Rep. May 2001; 3(3):216-221.

Hoeger K: Obesity and weight loss in polycystic ovary syndrome. Obstet Gynecol Clin North Am. March 2001; 28(1):85-97, vi-vii.

Iuorno MJ, Nestler JE: Insulin-lowering drugs in polycystic ovary syndrome. Obstet Gynecol Clin North Am. March 2001; 28(1):153-164.

Joffe B, Zimmet P: The thrifty genotype in Type 2 diabetes: an unfinished symphony moving to its finale? Endocrine. October 1998; 9(2):139-141.

Kain K, Catto AJ, Grant PJ: Impaired fibrinolysis and increased fibrinogen levels in South Asian subjects. Atherosclerosis. June 2001; 156(2):457-461.

Kelly CC, Lyall H, Petrie JR, Gould GW, Connell JM, Sattar N: Low-grade chronic inflammation in women with polycystic ovarian syndrome. J Clin Endocrinol Metab. June 2001; 86(6):2453-2455.

Kim JY, Nolte LA, Hansen PA, Han DH, Ferguson K, Thompson PA, Holloszy JO: High fat diet–induced muscle insulin resistance: relationship to visceral fat mass. Am J Physiol Regul Integr Comp Physiol. December 2000; 279(6):R2057-R2065.

Kirpichnikov D, Sowers JR: Diabetes mellitus and diabetes-associated vascular disease. Trends Endocrinol Metab. July 2001; 12(5):225-230.

Legro RS: Diabetes prevalence and risk factors in polycystic ovary syndrome. Obstet Gynecol Clin North Am. March 2001; 28(1):99-109.

Lerman-Garber I, Valdivia Lopez JA, Flores Rebollar A, Gomez Perez FJ, Antonio Rull J, Hermosillo AG: Evidence of a linkage between neurocardiogenic dysfunction and reactive hypoglycemia. Rev Invest Clin. November-December 2000; 52(6):603-610.

Lin KC, Lin HY, Chou P: The interaction between uric acid level and other risk factors on the development of gout among asymptomatic hyperuricemic men in a prospective study. J Rheumatol. June 2000; 27(6):1501-1505.

Longo-Mbenza B, Luila EL, Mbete P, Vita EK: Is hyperuricemia a risk factor of stroke and coronary heart disease among Africans? Int J Cardiol. September 30, 1999; 71(1):17-22.

Loverro G, Vicino M, Lorusso F, Vimercati A, Greco P, Selvaggi L: Polycystic ovary syndrome: relationship between insulin sensitivity, sex hormone levels, and ovarian stromal blood flow. Gynecol Endocrinol. April 2001; 15(2):142-149.

Mao W, Li M, Zhao Y: Study on parents phenotypes in women with polycystic ovary syndrome. Zhonghua Fu Chan Ke Za Zhi. October 2000; 35(10):583-585. [Article in Chinese.]

Moritz F, Bauer F, Boyer A, Lemarchand P, Kerleau JM, Moirot E, Navarre C, Muller JM: Patients in a state of agitation at the admission service of a Rouen hospital emergency department. Presse Med. October 9, 1999; 28(30):1630-1634. [Article in French.]

Okosun IS, Cooper RS, Prewitt TE, Rotimi CN: The relation of central adiposity to components of the insulin resistance syndrome in a biracial U.S. population sample. Ethn Dis. Spring-Summer 1999; 9(2):218-229.

Pavan L, Casiglia E, Braga LM, Winnicki M, Puato M, Pauletto P, Pessina AC: Effects of a traditional lifestyle on the cardiovascular risk profile: the Amondava population of the Brazilian Amazon. Comparison with matched African, Italian and Polish populations. J Hypertens. June 1999; 17(6):749-756.

Ravussin E, Valencia ME, Esparza J, Bennett PH, Schulz LO: Effects of a traditional lifestyle on obesity in Pima Indians. Diabetes Care. September 1994; 17(9):1067-1074.

Reaven GM: Insulin resistance: a chicken that has come to roost. Ann N Y Acad Sci. November 1999; 892:45-57.

Samuels M, Forbey K, Reid J, Abkevich V, Bulka K, Wardell B, Bowen B, Hopkins P, Hunt S, Ballinger D, Skolnick M, Wagner S: Identification of a common variant in the lipoprotein lipase gene in a large Utah kindred ascertained for coronary heart disease: the -93G/D9N variant predisposes to low HDL-C/high triglycerides. Clin Genet. February 2001; 59(2):88-98.

Schlesinger N, Schumacher HR Jr: Gout: can management be improved? Curr Opin Rheumatol. May 2001; 13(3):240-244.

Silfen ME, Manibo AM, McMahon DJ, Levine LS, Murphy AR, Oberfield SE: Comparison of simple measures of insulin sensitivity in young girls with premature adrenarche: the fasting glucose-to-insulin ratio may be a simple and useful measure. J Clin Endocrinol Metab. June 2001; 86(6):2863-2868.

Simmons D, Thompson CF, Volklander D: Polynesians: prone to obesity and Type 2 diabetes mellitus but not hyperinsulinanemia. Diabet Med. March 2001; 18(3):193-198.

Stickel F, Seitz HK: The efficacy and safety of comfrey. Public Health Nutr. December 2000; 3(4A):501-508.

Weyer C, Hanson RL, Tataranni PA, Bogardus C, Pratley RE: A high fasting-plasma insulin concentration predicts Type 2 diabetes independent of insulin resistance: evidence for a pathogenic role of relative hyperinsulinemia. Diabetes. December 2000; 49(12):2094-2101.

Weyer C, Vozarova B, Ravussin E, Tataranni PA: Changes in energy metabolism in response to 48 h of overfeeding and fasting in Caucasians and Pima Indians. Int J Obes Relat Metab Disord. May 2001; 25(5):593-600.

Williams DE, Knowler WC, Smith CJ, Hanson RL, Roumain J, Saremi A, Kriska AM, Bennett PH, Nelson RG: The effect of Indian or Anglo dietary preference on the incidence of diabetes in Pima Indians. Diabetes Care. May 2001; 24(5):811-816.

Wilson SH, Kennedy FP, Garratt KN: Optimisation of the management of patients with coronary heart disease and Type 2 diabetes mellitus. Drugs Aging. 2001; 18(5):325-333.

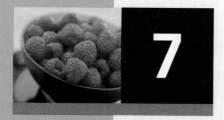

7 Obesity and Healthy Weight Management

OBJECTIVES

After completing this chapter, you should be able to:

- Describe obesity and discuss its prevention and treatments.
- Recognize healthy weight management practices.
- Relate the importance of physical activity to healthy weight management.

TERMS TO IDENTIFY

Aerobic exercise	Hyperphagia	Neuropeptides
Anaerobic exercise	Hyperplasty	Obesity
Body Mass Index (BMI)	Hypertrophy	Overweight
Dawn phenomenon	Hypothalamus	Satiety
Desirable weight	Lipogenesis	Underweight
Energy balance	Mitochondria	
Fad diet	Morbid obesity	

INTRODUCTION

There are many theories, but few easy solutions, to the obesity epidemic developing around the world. The simple thinking of reduced caloric intake and increased energy expenditure is not an easy solution for many persons. Ultimately this equation is correct, but there is a wide range of individual needs and abilities to follow this simple wisdom.

The low-fat mantra, which began in the 1980s, was aimed at an easy reduction of caloric intake by the general public. The thinking was that because fat has over twice the kilocalories per gram weight of either carbohydrate or protein, weight loss would easily follow with a low-fat diet. However, a false illusion was created: many consumers feel that a nonfat food can be freely consumed. The kilocalories of sugar and carbohydrate are often overlooked.

Many consumers, in their frustration at lack of weight loss on the low-fat diets, turn to low-carbohydrate diets. Rather than focusing on the concentrated kilocalories of sugar, many follow diets that advocate a virtual ban on all foods containing a substantial amount of carbohydrates—including many vegetables and fruits. Some restrict their caloric intake by skipping meals or following liquid diets. Others follow very intricate meal planning with precise percentages of protein, fat, and carbohydrate for all their meals. Still others limit carbohydrates in the day, saving most of their carbs for the night meal. Some individuals refuse to make food choices and so are able to rely on the rigidness of a **fad diet** (a diet that promises quick weight loss and an easy cure).

Unfortunately, in today's society, extreme behaviors are often encouraged. This is certainly true with athletic competition and weight control. Aiming for very low body fat and high lean muscle mass percentages can be detrimental to health if not done in a sensible manner. Anorexia and bulimia have increasingly become problems of our athletic youth and young adults—see Chapters 13 and 14 for more on eating disorders and sports nutrition throughout the lifespan. On the other hand, today's focus on super-sized food portions in restaurants contributes to overeating. Restaurants offer very large portions to justify their high food costs. However, the cost of operating the food service establishment is related to overhead and staffing costs—not food costs. Consumers are merely being misled when they think that large portions are a bargain.

All persons, whether overweight or not, benefit from a diet that contains a wide variety of foods to ensure an adequate nutrient intake. Energy needs depend on the percentage of lean body tissue present and the level and duration of activity performed. Optimum health and performance are usually promoted by a diet with 45% to 60% of kilocalories supplied by complex carbohydrates, up to 20% by protein, and no more than 35% by fat, with ample water to prevent dehydration.

The smallest amount of carbohydrate a person should ingest is about 100 g daily (40% of a 1000-kcal diet). Six meals with about 15 g of carbohydrates each, with emphasis on high soluble-fiber foods such as legumes, oatmeal, or barley is low enough in carbohydrates for even the most insulin-resistant person (see Chapter 6). In this author's experience, most persons lose weight with 30 g of carbohydrate in each of six meals, with an upper limit of 200 g daily. Higher protein intake may be appropriate if from fish—there is long-term data showing safety from consuming a large amount of fish, as with the traditional Inuit Indian and Alaskan diets. Increased intake of other protein sources, beyond 20% of kcals, are more likely to induce health problems such as cancer and cannot be advocated at this time. Up to 40% of caloric intake from fat may be acceptable if the emphasis is on monounsaturated fats such as olive oil and most nuts. This has been noted in the health of persons following a traditional Mediterranean diet. An increased intake of omega-3 fatty acids from fatty fish is also associated with health.

Because there is no one genetic makeup, no one diet can be expected to address the needs of all individuals. Assessment of current nutritional intake and family health history can help determine the best course of action to slow weight gain among those who are moderately overweight and help reverse the problem of obesity.

It still comes back to the basic premise of less food and more exercise. Weight loss will usually occur by adhering to that premise. It is extremely rare that a person cannot lose weight; achieving sustainable weight loss is another matter. This chapter explores the different types of weight loss theories and approaches and suggests strategies that best result in permanent weight loss. It is written from the wealth of experience the author has in helping patients to lose and maintain weight loss.

Fallacy: A person with central obesity should avoid all carbohydrate foods.

Fact: It is true that many persons with the insulin resistance syndrome have better outcomes on a lower-carbohydrate diet. Most, however, do well with 40% to 50% or less than 200 g of carbohydrates for a 1500-kcal diet. Following a very low-carbohydrate diet (fewer than 100 g) can be potentially harmful because of concomitant reduction in vitamins, minerals, and phytochemicals, which are all found in carbohydrate-rich plant foods, which are important to long-term health. Milk, another natural source of carbohydrates, should be included to help prevent osteoporosis. Emphasis on legumes, greens, and other low-carbohydrate vegetables, with moderate amounts of whole grains and fruit, low-fat or skim milk, and lean meats such as fish and chicken, is the foundation of a healthy diet. These foods can be worked into a lower-carbohydrate meal plan appropriate to meeting both weight loss and long-term health goals. Spreading carbohydrates out over the course of the day is particularly helpful for some with insulin resistance and hyperinsulinemia. Everyone can lose weight on about 15 g of carbohydrates in six small meals; it is a bit like putting a handful of twigs on the fire all day long. Small, frequent meals "rev up" the metabolism and promote weight loss.

WHAT ARE THE RATES OF OVERWEIGHT AND OBESITY?

Current incidence rates of obesity are about 20% to 25% in American adults and 15% to 20% in Europeans (Kromhout et al., 2001). The number of individuals who are either overweight or obese is even higher: an estimated 55% of U.S. adults are overweight or obese (Wofford et al., 1999).

Regions where obesity was once thought impossible are now showing the effects of excess caloric intake. One survey in Taiwan noted a dramatic weight increase among schoolchildren from 1980 to 1994 (Chu, 2001).

WHAT STANDARDS ARE USED TO DETERMINE DESIRABLE WEIGHT?

Achieving a weight that is conducive to physical health and psychologic health is part of healthy weight management. **Desirable weight**, however, may be higher than ideal body weight according to predetermined weight-for-height charts. For this reason, the term *healthy weight* is increasingly gaining acceptance. Other factors such as age, general health status, and potential for achieving and maintaining weight loss are considered when determining desirable weight.

Aiming for an unrealistic weight that cannot be permanently maintained is not a healthy goal. Generally, a 10% weight loss for the overweight person is feasible and can have a significant effect on health. Slow weight loss of approximately ½ to 1 lb per week is more likely to be permanent and therefore falls within the boundaries of healthy weight management.

The term **overweight** refers to an excess of body weight 10% greater than the standard, whereas **obesity** is used to describe an excess of body *fat*. Although weight alone does not indicate the degree of body fat, an individual is still classified by many health professionals as obese if weight is 20% or more than the standard weight for height; **morbid obesity** is excess of 30% of the standard weight. A person is **underweight** if he or she is 10% below recommended weight for height.

The **Body Mass Index (BMI)** is considered one of the simpler tools that more accurately determine appropriate body weight. The BMI has replaced an older standard, the *Metropolitan Life Height and Weight Tables* because of inherent shortcomings such as ethnic bias and emphasis on death statistics rather than health problems. The BMI is now the preferred standard of determining appropriate body size. Its formula was developed over a hundred years ago by a mathematician named Quetelet. As only a mathematician can, he realized that dividing a person's weight in kilograms by the square of the height in meters (kg/m^2) gives a better sense of body proportion. A healthy BMI is between 21 and 25 with an upper limit of 27—see Appendix 12 for a nomogram version of the BMI. A BMI under 30 may be acceptable if there are no health problems. A BMI of 30 equates to being 20% overweight, which constitutes obesity. Morbid obesity refers to a BMI greater than 40 (30% overweight). Someone who is underweight has a BMI of less than 19. A BMI of 15 equates to 20% underweight, which is a dangerously low level that could result in death.

Other Body Fat Measurements

More precise methods of determining body fat percentage include the following:

- Skinfold measurements taken at different body sites
- The bioelectric impedance machine, which sends an imperceptible electric current through the body
- Underwater weighing (usually done only at research centers)

WHAT ARE THE CAUSES OF OBESITY?

The causes of obesity are numerous, complex, and not thoroughly understood. Generally speaking, obesity occurs as a result of long-term positive **energy balance** for individual needs. In other words, weight gain occurs when caloric intake exceeds expenditure (Table 7-1) over an extended period. Many factors can affect energy balance in an individual: eating habits, cooking methods, family customs, emotional problems, peer pressure, food advertising, and food availability all have influence on caloric intake, whereas factors such as age, gender, heredity, body composition, occupation, and exercise habits all affect energy expenditure.

There are indications of genetic susceptibility to obesity. However, the environment seems to allow the genetic predisposition to be realized. Obesity, high blood pressure, and elevated insulin and triglyceride levels are all effects of the insulin resistance syndrome.

It is well recognized that hyperinsulinemia occurs with central obesity. What is up for debate is whether the obesity leads to hyperinsulinemia or vice versa. Persons with genetic risk for insulin resistance seem to be more prone to weight gain. This helps explain the pattern of family obesity among those with a family history of diabetes. Others feel the increased amount of insulin is simply a marker for the degree of obesity. It is a chicken-and-egg question. Which came first? This question often separates believers in the low-fat diets from believers in the low-carb diets. Neither belief has been adequately studied.

The Thrifty Gene Theory

Some population groups may have survived over the centuries because of an ability to preserve body mass during times of famine and to gain body mass easily during times of plenty. This ability would have been particularly important, historically speaking, in the hunter-gatherer lifestyle, which was dominant before agricultural development, and is referred to as having the thrifty gene. This theory helps to explain the occurrence of the insulin resistance syndrome and development of central obesity when there is exposure to conditions associated with a Westernized lifestyle (increased food intake and reduced physical activity).

Hyperinsulinemia

Some researchers believe that hyperinsulinemia, as found with the insulin resistance syndrome, is the cause of obesity. One study found that **hyperphagia** (high

■ **TABLE 7-1**
■ **KILOCALORIES EXPENDED PER HOUR FOR VARIOUS TYPES OF ACTIVITIES**

TYPE OF ACTIVITY	KCAL/HR*
SEDENTARY ACTIVITIES Reading, writing, eating, watching TV or movies, listening to radio, sewing, playing cards; typing, office work, and other activities done while sitting that require little or no arm movement or that require moderate arm movement; and activities done while sitting that require more vigorous arm movement	0-100
LIGHT ACTIVITIES Preparing and cooking food, doing dishes, dusting, handwashing small articles of clothing, ironing, walking slowly, personal care, miscellaneous office work and other activities done while standing that require some arm movement, and rapid typing and other activities done while sitting that are more strenuous	110-160
MODERATE ACTIVITIES Making beds, mopping and scrubbing, sweeping, light polishing and waxing, laundering by machine, light gardening and carpentry work, walking moderately fast, other activities done while standing	0-240
VIGOROUS ACTIVITIES Heavy scrubbing and waxing, handwashing large articles of clothing, hanging out clothes, stripping beds, other heavy work, walking fast, bowling, golfing, gardening	250-350
STRENUOUS ACTIVITIES Swimming, playing tennis, running, bicycling, dancing, skiing, playing football	350 and more

*From U.S. Department of Agriculture: Food and Your Weight. Home and Garden Bulletin No. 74. Washington, DC. A range of caloric values is given for each type of activity to allow for differences in activities and in persons. Of the sedentary activities, for example, typing uses more kilocalories than watching TV. Some persons will use more kilocalories in carrying out either activity than others; some persons are more efficient in their body actions than are others. Values closer to the upper limit of a range will give a better picture of kilocalorie expenditures for men and those near the lower limit a better picture for women.

food intake) leads to hyperinsulinemia, which stimulates **lipogenesis** (formation of body fat) among Zucker rats, which are commonly used in studies of obesity (Unger and Orci, 2001). Another study further reinforced this theory by showing that overweight men developed hyperinsulinemia after eating a high-carbohydrate meal. Lipogenesis was associated with fasting serum glucose and insulin concentrations (Marques-Lopes et al., 2001). Fructose, the sugar found in fruit, has been found to cause substantial insulin resistance and hyperinsulinemia in both lean and obese rats (Suga et al., 2000). A hypothesis espoused by Ginny Huszagh, MNS, RD, is that adipose tissue (body fat) is less insulin resistant than is lean tissue (muscle). This helps explain why a person with insulin resistance and concomitant hyperinsulinemia tends to gain body fat easily.

Fallacy: Aspartame, or Nutrasweet, causes obesity and is a poison.

Fact: The brand-name sugar substitute Nutrasweet is made up of two amino acids: aspartic acid and phenylalanine. The controversy over health has to do with how these two amino acids are joined together, which is how the sweet flavor results. The compound that joins the amino acids together is similar to methyl alcohol, which in large amounts is clearly a poison. However, just as with alcohol, the liver is able to metabolize this compound safely. Only in extremely large amounts is there a possible health risk. The caution on the labels regarding phenylalanine is related to those persons with PKU, a congenital metabolic problem. There is a theory yet unproven that the sensation of sweetness by the taste buds induces insulin production. Because debate continues as to whether obesity causes hyperinsulinemia, it cannot be said that Nutrasweet causes obesity. For someone who is concerned about this sweetener, other choices can be made, such as drinking water or seltzer and choosing low-sugar foods or foods with alternative sweeteners such as Splenda; see Chapter 9 for more on sugar substitutes.

Other Hormonal Imbalances

Numerous hormones are related to adiposity levels. Insufficient levels of the thyroid hormones T3/T4 cause a decrease in basal metabolic rate that can lead to weight gain. A deficiency in growth hormone leads to increased levels of body fat. Increased cortisol levels may promote lipogenesis, in part, as a result of concomitant increase in insulin levels. Cortisol is correlated significantly with the depth and duration of hypoglycemia (Nye et al., 2001).

The Fat Cell Theory

During childhood, excess caloric intake can result in an increased number of fat cells (**hyperplasty**). Enlargement of these fat cells (**hypertrophy**) can occur at any age, but especially after puberty. Once a fat cell is created, it exists for life. Therefore when an obese person loses weight, fat cells do not disappear, they only shrink. A person with hyperplastic obesity is believed to have more trouble losing weight and an increased likelihood of regaining any lost weight.

Leptin

Leptin is a hormone that is believed to be involved in body weight regulation and that may serve to promote **satiety** (the satisfied feeling after eating). Leptin acts within the **hypothalamus** (a portion of the brain) to alter the levels of several **neuropeptides** (molecules found in brain tissue such as endorphins). The altering of neuropeptides is believed to regulate food intake. Leptin further decreases the lipogenic activity of insulin (Rohner-Jeanrenaud, 1999). Recent studies in ob/ob mice, which lack circulating leptin, have shown dramatic reductions in food intake and body weight after leptin treatment. However, animals that developed obesity, hyperglycemia, and hyperinsulinemia have also developed *hyperleptinemia* (high levels of leptin in the blood). The implication is that obese persons may be resistant to leptin at the cellular level. Thus more research is needed to verify the role of leptin in the prevention and management of obesity. One study found inappropriate leptin secretion or disposal was associated with failure to maintain weight loss in obese men in a behavior modification weight loss program (Naslund et al., 2000).

Medications

Cortisol has been implicated as a cause of obesity. Reactivation of the medication cortisone into cortisol in subcutaneous adipose tissue may exacerbate obesity (Rask et al., 2001). The second-generation antipsychotics were found to induce weight gain to a larger extent than that of traditional neuroleptics with schizophrenia. Health care professionals need to be aware of the problem of weight gain associated with some antipsychotic medications (Kurzthaler and Fleischhacker, 2001).

Fallacy: Obesity is caused by lack of willpower.

Fact: Many overweight persons do not consume a total amount of kilocalories in excess of what their thinner counterparts consume. There may be metabolic differences between the obese and the thin person such that the obese person may be better able to conserve kilocalories consumed. More research is needed to fully establish the metabolic differences contributing to obesity.

WHAT ARE SOME PREVENTION STRATEGIES FOR OBESITY?

Preventing obesity is far easier to achieve than correcting it. Strategies should begin in childhood because obesity tracks from childhood into adulthood (Maffeis and Tato, 2001). Helping children to accept a variety of plant-based foods such as legumes, vegetables, and fruits is of critical importance. Placing positive emphasis on low-calorie plant-based foods can encourage children's acceptance of them. Rather than saying "yum" to dessert, say it to vegetables and fruits. See Chapter 13 for more ideas on promoting positive food associations among children. Furthermore, higher intakes of calcium and monounsaturated fat have been associated with lower body fat assessments in preschool children (Carruth and Skinner, 2001).

Fast-food restaurants need to serve more high-fiber foods as our busy lifestyles increasingly promote eating outside the home. Increased fiber sources might include bean-based soups and a variety of vegetables and fruits. Children need to eat more than French fries to establish an adequate vegetable intake.

The history of Native Alaskans sheds some light on the role of fats versus carbohydrates in the development of obesity. Incidence of being overweight among

Native Alaskans is significantly higher than was found even 25 years ago. It has been noted that those who maintained a diet of indigenous carbohydrate and protein foods, including seal oil, were less likely to develop obesity and diabetes over this time frame (Murphy et al., 1995). Indigenous carbohydrate foods in Alaska consist of such foods as reeds that grow in the brief summer months, seaweed, and the few other high-fiber, plant-based foods that can grow in the extreme cold climate. Historically, carbohydrate intake was very low—about 5% of total nutrient intake. In the days of old, Alaskans certainly did not say, "Oh, I'd better throw out this seal blubber because it has too much fat." The traditional Native Alaskan diet was composed primarily of protein and fat. Research performed as recently as the 1950s shows that starvation was the chief health problem, not obesity. This reinforces the belief that not all fats are equal in respect to obesity. Seal oil is high in the unsaturated fat omega-3. The change in dietary fat to more saturated fats, including hydrogenated fats, and increased intake of refined carbohydrate foods are implicated in the growing obesity problem of Native Alaskans.

The debate on the ideal protein intake is intensified by one study of preschool children that found a high-carbohydrate meal was consumed in greater amount than a high-protein meal and provided a significantly greater observed caloric intake (Araya et al., 2000). This supports the notion that a high-carbohydrate diet may lead to weight gain.

Promotion of physical activity is critical in the prevention of obesity. When people had to forage for their food, they expended energy. Our sedentary lifestyles in combination with an increased intake of simple carbohydrates and saturated fat appears to be the driving force behind the development of obesity. School-based physical education needs to be a priority to stop the epidemic of childhood obesity. Involvement in sports can play an important role in encouraging children to be physically active. Everyone can take the stairs and not the elevator. Dancing is a fun form of physical activity at any age.

Childhood weight gain involves many issues. It is paramount to have the child maintain a positive self-esteem and to feel empowered to make appropriate food choices. Parents can assist by promoting vegetables, fruits, whole grains, and other high-fiber foods such as legumes to promote satiety while facilitating appropriate growth and development of the young child. Lean meats and use of unsaturated fats as found in nuts and peanut butter may be of further help to control hunger and limit caloric intake. Limiting the availability of foods high in saturated fat and sugar within the home can be helpful. This helps to avoid food battles by removing the stimulus.

Beverages are often the issue behind a child's excess weight gain. A child who consumes a liter of soda pop or juice is taking in over ½ c of pure sugar, which equates to over 400 kcal that can cause a weight gain of almost 1 lb per week if these kilocalories are in excess of the child's needs. Parents and other caregivers should promote water as a beverage with fruit juice and milk intake appropriate to the Food Guide Pyramid.

These and other strategies can be used throughout life. The benefit of spreading caloric intake over many small meals rather than a few large meals for control of blood glucose, serum lipids, and body fat has been known for many years. The importance of small, frequent meals has even been found in livestock. Veal calves fed by bucket were often found to develop insulin resistance and hyperglycemia during fattening. These problems were resolved when the calves were fed in six or more portions during a 16-hour period from an automatic feeder, as compared with twice daily from a bucket (Kaufhold et al., 2000). Eating rapidly is also associated with obesity (Kral et al., 2001). Thus eating small, frequent meals at a slow pace will likely help prevent or manage obesity.

These strategies, once started in childhood, can continue into adulthood. If the adult has learned to like a variety of plant-based, high-fiber foods and sugar-free drinks such as water, obesity is less likely to occur as caloric requirements decrease from having a sedentary job or being incapacitated from illness or from aging. It is often too late to start this process after obesity has already set in.

All health professionals need to keep an open mind that we do not yet have all the answers to the puzzle of the obesity epidemic. Consequently, we need to assess individual nutritional intake and hunger levels and plan accordingly rather than simply handing out preprinted diet sheets. Individuals with a family history of diabetes or other indicators of the insulin resistance syndrome need more guidance than simply being told not to eat fat. It is especially helpful for these individuals to emphasize high-fiber foods, limit concentrated sweets, and include moderate amounts of unsaturated fats, especially the monounsaturated and omega-3 fatty acid sources. Using food labels can be helpful to indicate the amount of fiber and unsaturated fats in foods. Referral to a registered dietitian is often appropriate. For individuals with insulin resistance, referral to a registered dietitian who is also a certified diabetes educator or one well versed in diabetes management may be most helpful.

WHAT IS A SUCCESSFUL WEIGHT LOSS PLAN?

Promoting successful long-term weight loss is difficult. The health care professional, as well as the obese patient, often sets up unrealistic goals. One guideline to defining successful weight loss is the intentional loss of at least 10% of initial body weight and keeping it off for at least 1 year. This guideline allows at least 20% of overweight or obese persons to be considered successful with their weight loss. Once these successful individuals have maintained a weight loss for 2 to 5 years, the chances of longer-term success greatly increase (Wing and Hill, 2001). In the commercial weight loss program Weight Watchers, nearly half of the group studied maintained a weight loss of 5% or more and about 1 of 5 maintained a loss of 10% or more (Lowe et al., 2001).

Typically, successful weight loss plans help incorporate high-fiber foods to promote satiety and follow the adage of dietitians that "all foods can fit." An overly restrictive diet is generally setting a person up for weight loss failure in the long run.

It is imperative that all health professionals reinforce a slow, steady rate of weight loss to promote long-term weight management. There should be enough protein and fat in the diet to promote satiety. Lifetime habits, not short-term diets, should be promoted. The only exceptions to this are if the individual's life is at risk because of sleep apnea or if surgery is imperative for a rapid loss of body fat. Rapid weight loss needs to be medically supervised.

WHAT ARE SOME TREATMENT STRATEGIES FOR OBESITY?

Obesity Treatments

The majority of all obese persons can be categorized as mildly obese; that is, less than 30% heavier than the ideal. For these mildly obese individuals, the comprehensive treatment plan includes some basic components: (1) a nutritionally adequate eating plan; (2) physical activity; and, as needed, (3) behavior modification and (4) cognitive behavioral therapy.

Extreme morbid obesity has been treated with various surgical techniques, such as gastric bypass and stapling, jaw wiring, fat suctioning, and modified fasting. These treatments have had limited success and are not currently routinely recommended unless there is a high mortality risk from the obesity.

Food intake for any individual attempting to lose weight should meet the body's needs for all nutrients, but not for caloric intake. It takes a deficit of about 500 kcal per day to lose 1 lb of fat in 1 week because 3500 kcal equates to 1 lb of body fat. For safe and permanent weight loss, an individual should lose a maximum of 1 to 2 lbs per week. This is a much slower weight loss than most people are willing to accept because the media continually advertise quick weight loss approaches. Persons with a history of diet failures or weight cycling may be more accepting of a slow weight loss approach, having learned firsthand that rapid weight loss is not maintained in the long run.

Because of the way the body uses fuel from carbohydrate, fat, and protein, rapid weight loss will compel the body to use protein (muscle) instead of fat for energy. Rapid weight loss is therefore highly undesirable because it decreases muscle mass, which will lower the requirements for caloric intake. Weight cycling can change the body's composition so that muscle percentage decreases (with each dieting attempt) and body fat percentage increases (regain of mostly body fat with each failed dieting attempt).

Experience has shown that to lose weight at an optimal ½ to 1 pound per week, most women need to consume about 1200 kcal per day; men will lose this amount with an intake of about 1500 to 1800 kcal per day. These levels may vary, however. Too much emphasis on kilocalories can be counterproductive. Reducing fat and sugar intake and learning to eat based on internal hunger cues rather than for other reasons can go a long way toward normalizing intake and weight management. Vitamin and mineral supplementation should be included when energy intake is less than 1200 kcal per day. Before embarking on any weight loss program, an individual should be examined by a physician. The dieting plan should also be individualized and flexible and referral to a registered dietitian can allow for an individualized meal plan. See Box 7-1 for general dieting tips.

Review of the literature suggests that weight loss is independent of diet composition. Kilocalorie restriction is the key variable associated with weight reduction

■ **BOX 7-1**
■ **DIETING TIPS**

1. Eat regularly, choosing foods relatively low in fat and sugar.
2. Chew thoroughly and slowly.
3. Stop eating when the stomach is comfortably full.
4. Make diet changes that can be maintained for life; quick fixes are counterproductive for healthy weight management.
5. Wait 15 minutes before having second helpings.
6. Include exercise for healthy weight management.
7. To deal with the perceived need to "clean your plate," remember that excess food goes either to waste or to the waist.
8. When faced with an indulgence, ask yourself, "How will I feel tomorrow if I don't eat this food today?" Give yourself permission to eat if feelings of deprivation may arise.
9. When ready to give up on dieting efforts, remember Ann Landers' quote: "The difference between a successful person and an unsuccessful person is that the successful person never stops trying."
10. For individualized meal-planning tips, consult a registered dietitian, the expert in nutrition.

in the short term (Kennedy et al., 2001). Individual needs, however, need to be taken into account. The bottom line is that individuals can lose weight on either a diet low in carbohydrates or in fat because these nutrients are both good sources of kilocalories. A person who fights excessive hunger may benefit from a higher fat level because of the satiety aspect of delayed digestion and hormonal effect that fat provides. Many people are now afraid to eat fat, but health care professionals can help to dispel the myth that all fats are fattening. Sound meal planning is still important for long-term health.

Fallacy: Skipping meals is a good way to lose weight.

Fact: Studies have shown that eating three to six meals a day is the best and most healthful approach. Skipping meals tends to suppress the metabolism (the rate at which kilocalories are burned) and can lead to overeating later in the day.

The Food Exchange System

The Food Exchange System is a tool used in reducing caloric intake. Originally developed by the American Diabetes Association and the American Dietetic Association, the system aims to control carbohydrate and caloric intake in the management of diabetes (see Appendix 9). It can also be used for weight management alone. Richard Simmons' famous Deal-A-Meal card system is based on the exchanges. Weight Watchers has also used this system in the past. However, it is often too complicated and does not teach the recognition of internal cues of hunger and satiety.

TABLE 7-2

THE FOOD GUIDE PYRAMID AS A HEALTHY WEIGHT LOSS PLAN

FOOD GROUP	SERVING SIZE	COMMENTS
Bread, cereal, rice, and pasta group (6-11 servings)*	1 slice of bread 1 oz of ready-to-eat cereal (check labels: 1 oz = ¼ to 2 c, depending on cereal) ½ c of cooked cereal, rice, or pasta ½ hamburger roll, bagel, English muffin 3-4 plain crackers (small)	Count each serving of starch as 80 to 100 kcal Based on carbohydrate content and kilocalories, count dry vegetables (potatoes) and sweet vegetables (sweet corn, sweet peas, and sweet winter squash) as a starch
Vegetable group (3-5 servings)*	1 c of raw leafy vegetables ½ c of other vegetables, cooked or chopped raw ¾ c of vegetable juice	One serving of vegetables is about 25 kcal Vegetables that are low in carbohydrate and kilocalories are high in water content and are not sweet
Fruit group (2-4 servings)*	1 medium apple, banana, orange, nectarine, peach ½ c of chopped, cooked, or canned fruit ¾ c of fruit juice	One serving of fruit is about 60-100 kcal Fruits that are dry (bananas) or are in portions greater than ½ c contain more kilocalories
Milk, yogurt, and cheese group (2-3 servings)*	1 c of milk or yogurt 1 ½ oz of natural cheese 2 oz of processed cheese	1 c of skim milk contains about 80 kcal 1% milk has 100 kcal, 2% 125 kcal, and whole milk, 170 kcal 2 oz of full-fat cheese contains 200 kcal
Meat, poultry, fish, dry beans, eggs, and nuts group (2-3 servings)*	2-3 oz of cooked lean meat, poultry, or fish (1 oz of meat = ½ c of cooked dry beans, 1 egg, or 2 tbsp of peanut butter)	1 oz of most meat contains 75 kcal Lean meat contains 50 kcal/oz and high-fat meat contains 100 kcal/oz 1 tbsp peanut butter contains 100 kcal and is counted as 1 oz of meat in the Exchange System 1 oz = ¼ c; 3 oz is the size of a deck of cards

*Recommended number of servings per day.

The Food Guide Pyramid

Although the Food Guide Pyramid was not directly developed as a weight loss plan, it can be used as such. The minimum number of servings contain as little as 1200 kcal if only lean meats and skim milk and no added fats or sugars are consumed (Table 7-2). The diet can safely be further reduced to 1000 kcal if five servings of low-carbohydrate vegetables are consumed instead of fruits because most vegetables have fewer than half the kilocalories of fruit for similar nutritional value. This needs to be based on individual acceptance of nutrient-dense vegetables such as greens, broccoli, and Brussels sprouts (which all provide both vitamins A and C). Such a restrictive diet may lead to nutritional deficiencies if followed long term or if food choices are not made wisely. The upper limit of recommended servings of the Food Guide Pyramid contains about 2000 kcal, which may be adequately low for an overweight, but active, man.

Table 7-3 shows how a normal 3000-kcal diet, which may be needed with an active adolescent teenager, can be modified to give one family member a 1200-kcal diet without preparing separate meals. Some items are omitted, some are served in smaller portions, and some are served in modified form—for example, skim milk instead of whole milk or coffee black instead of with cream and sugar.

Food Labels

Reading food labels can be a good way to help plan meal goals. A low-fat meal is defined as 15 to 20 g of fat or less. Snacks might be planned around 3 g of fat or less. Daily protein intake should be at least 60 g with a low caloric intake. Carbohydrate content of food is also included on labels. The total carbohydrate value listed on food labels is the sum of the amounts of sugar and fiber, which are indicated separately, as well as the amount of starch, which is generally not listed separately. Weight loss can usually be achieved with a daily intake of 40 to 50 g of fat and 150 to 200 g of carbohydrate (fiber may be subtracted from the carbohydrate number on food labels because it is virtually indigestible and contributes little in terms of kilocalories). Labels can be used by those individuals who want to count their kilocalories.

Fallacy: If the food label states 0 g of fat, the food may be eaten freely.

Fact: The low-fat message has been very successful—almost too successful, in some cases. It is possible to have too low an intake of fat and an absolute minimum of 20 to 30 g per day should be promoted for overall health and well-being. In the quest to achieve a low-fat diet, many have forgotten about carbohydrates and, specifically, sugar. Pointing out that 4 g of sugar equates to 1 tsp can be an eye-opener to many. About a handful (½ c) of jelly beans or other pure-sugar candies, which contains about 100 g of sugar at 4 kcal/g, equates to about 400 kcal.

High in Fiber, Low in Fat

Emphasizing foods with a high satiety and low caloric value allows individuals to trust their natural hunger and satiety cues. This can be a commonsense and easy weight loss plan for many individuals. An increase in either soluble or insoluble fiber intake increases postprandial satiety and decreases subsequent hunger.

■ TABLE 7-3
■ MODIFIED 3000-KILOCALORIE DIET

1200 KILOCALORIES		3000 KILOCALORIES	
BREAKFAST			
Orange juice	½ c	Orange juice	½ c
Soft-cooked egg	1 egg	Soft-cooked egg	1 egg
Whole wheat toast	1 slice	Bacon	2 medium strips
Butter or margarine	1 tsp	Whole wheat toast	2 slices
Skim milk	1 c	Butter or margarine	2 tsp
Coffee (black), if desired	1 c	Whole milk	1 c
		Coffee	1 c
		Cream	1 tbsp
		Sugar	1 tbsp
LUNCH			
Sandwich:		Sandwich:	
Enriched bread	2 slices	Enriched bread	3 slices
Boiled ham	1 ½ oz	Boiled ham	3 oz
Mayonnaise	2 tsp	Mayonnaise	2 ½ tsp
Mustard	free	Mustard	free
Lettuce	1 large leaf	Lettuce	2 large leaves
Celery	1 small stalk	Celery	1 small stalk
Radishes	4 radishes	Radishes	4 radishes
Dill pickle	½ large	Dill pickle	½ large
Skim milk	1 c	Whole milk	1 c
		Tomato soup with milk	1 c
		Apple	1 medium
DINNER			
Roast meat	3 oz	Roast meat	4 oz
Rice, converted	½ c	Rice, converted	⅔ c
Spinach	¾ c	Spinach, buttered	¾ c
Lemon	¼ medium	Lemon	¼ medium
Salad:		Salad:	
Peaches, canned	1 half peach	Peaches, canned	2 halves
Cottage cheese	2 tbsp	Cottage cheese	2 tbsp
Lettuce	1 large leaf	Lettuce	1 large leaf
		Rolls, enriched	2 small
		Butter or margarine	1 tsp
		Plain cake, iced	1 piece, 3 × 3× 2 in
BETWEEN-MEAL SNACK			
Apple	1 medium	Saltines	4
		Peanut butter	2 tbsp
		Whole milk	1 c

From U.S. Department of Agriculture: Food and Your Weight. Home and Garden Bulletin No. 74. Washington, DC.

Studies indicate that consumption of an additional 14 g of fiber daily for more than 2 days is associated with a 10% decrease in caloric intake and loss of body weight of about 1 lb per month—just by eating more fiber (Howarth et al., 2001). The Weight Watchers program now uses a point system. Foods high in fiber and low in fat are counted as having fewer points than foods low in fiber and high in fat.

Behavior Modification

Behavior modification involves assisting the obese individual in identifying the personal eating behaviors that have been promoting weight gain and maintaining obesity. Many may know how much food they should eat, but have eating habits not conducive to change. Once these habits have been recognized, various techniques can be used to minimize their effects or remove them from the environment. For example, a person may have become conditioned to eat a high-fat snack upon returning home after work. The change might be to a lower-calorie snack or a smaller portion. The goal might also be to learn to eat more slowly. For another person, it might be to drink beverages low in sugar. For another it might be to learn methods of stress management other than turning to food. Many older adults who lived through the Great Depression find it exceedingly difficult to leave food on their plates. Strategies to prepare more appropriate food portions or order them at restaurants might be helpful. By focusing on small, gradual behavioral changes, the individual learns to gain control of eating behaviors, with the goal of permanently changing poor habits.

Medications and Supplements

Many individuals want a quick fix to promote weight loss. The following research is described to show current thinking. It should be remembered that there are no long-term data supporting the safety of any diet aid. Past experience indicates extreme caution should be undertaken. The use of supplements should always be reviewed with a physician. Refer back to Chapter 4 for quality concerns about the largely unregulated supplement industry.

Having said that, some studies do show results with certain supplements. One study found that loss of body fat was significantly greater with chromium intake, yet muscle mass was maintained. This, however, was in conjunction with a modest dietary and exercise regimen. No significant adverse effects were found from the ingestion of 600 μg of niacin-bound chromium daily over 2 months (Crawford et al., 1999). The herbal mixture of ma huang and guarana was found to promote significantly greater short-term weight and fat loss than no treatment. Dry mouth, insomnia, and headache were the adverse symptoms reported most frequently by the herbal product. There is some association with these herbal products and stroke and death. The authors recommend long-term safety studies (Boozer et al., 2001). Many trials have demonstrated statistically significant weight loss with the medication called *orlistat*. However, it is felt that the difference may not always be of clinical significance. Possible adverse effects should be taken into account when prescribing orlistat, particularly gastrointestinal effects (O'Meara et al., 2001).

Fallacy: Eating carbohydrates only at night is a good weight loss plan.

Fact: The only scientific evidence supporting this weight loss approach is that we are the most insulin resistant upon rising. This is called the **dawn phenomenon** and generally results in an increased need for insulin. Therefore including a smaller amount of carbohydrates at breakfast may be helpful for those with insulin resistance. There is no evidence, however, that this phenomenon is a factor for individuals without insulin resistance and, by lunchtime, there is no evidence that carbohydrates should be avoided even by those who are insulin resistant.

WHAT ARE THE RATIONALES FOR THE VARIOUS POPULAR DIETS?

The current popular diets can be summarized based on their rationales. The following is a brief synopsis of these diet approaches.

The Very Low–Fat Diets

Very low–fat diets are aiming their approach at the concentrated kilocalories of fat. Fat has 9 kcal/g weight, as compared with 4 kcal/g weight of carbohydrate and protein. As an extreme example, ½ c pure fat is well over 1000 kcal. By comparison, even ½ c sugar is only 400 kcal. Even better, ½ c of most vegetables has only 25 kcal. Thus, although sugar has fewer kilocalories than fat, it is still a concentrated source of kilocalories. So it is indeed possible to lose weight on a very low–fat diet, but because fat also helps with the feeling of satiety, such a diet often leaves dieters hungry and dissatisfied. This approach has also caused many individuals to be afraid of eating any fat. This is a health problem in that essential fatty acid deficiency can occur, resulting in hair loss and endocrine problems. Also, a very low–fat diet is inherently high in carbohydrates, which may lead to increased heart disease for a person with insulin resistance and hyperinsulinemia.

The Very Low–Carbohydrate Diets

Very low–carbohydrate diets have sprung from the belief, substantiated by growing research, that insulin induces the gain of body fat. However, the consumer who follows this type of diet shares the extremist view that all carbohydrate foods are bad, which can lead to very poor diets. Because carbohydrate is primarily found in plant-based foods, these diets can set a person up for vitamin and mineral deficiencies. Some may argue that such a diet is sufficient as long as the person following it takes a vitamin and mineral supplement. However, it has been estimated that there are at least 100 phytochemicals (refer back to Chapter 4) yet to be discovered. Even arsenic is now considered essential for health, but it is much wiser to get it from plant-based foods than from a supplement because arsenic in excess is a known poison (watch the old movie *Arsenic and Old Lace* if you were not aware of this). If someone follows the guidelines for managing Type 2 diabetes (see Chapter 9), there will be a reduction in insulin needs while still meeting the requirements of a healthy diet.

Liquid Diets

A variety of liquid diets are available on local grocery store shelves and are often promoted by physician's offices and hospitals. Such diets can be appropriate for someone whose life is in imminent danger and needs to lose weight quickly, but they should always be followed under physician supervision. This author has worked with persons who have actually gained weight with liquid diets. These products have a relatively high glycemic index and can cause hyperinsulinemia in persons with insulin resistance. A liquid diet may work for the individual who tends to eat large portions. The prepackaged portion and convenience of consumption may be helpful. However, there are many prepackaged or smaller portioned foods also readily available.

Food Restrictive Diets

There are many versions of food restrictive diets. A popular one has been the cabbage soup diet. Granted, there is absolutely nothing wrong with eating cabbage soup. However, there is a whole variety of vegetable-based soups that are low in kilocalories. The thinking behind these restrictive diets is that overweight persons cannot control their food intake. With limitations on what foods may be consumed, the rationale is that they will eat less. This is particularly true after eating cabbage day in and day out for weeks on end.

The Low-Glycemic Diets

The low-glycemic diets can be very appropriate. The thinking behind these diets is that high-glycemic meals (those which are high in simple sugars and low in fat) set a person up for hyperinsulinemia with a rise and fall in blood glucose levels, leading to hunger. There is an element of truth to this approach. However, these diets are often very complex, with specific ratios of protein and fat to carbohydrates. The complexity can leave the person dependent on preplanned menus that can be very inconvenient in the real world. The basic message of including high-fiber foods, such as vegetables, legumes, fruits, or whole grains, in a diet with some lean meat or other protein source and moderate amounts of unsaturated fat, such as oil and vinegar on a salad, serves the same purpose and is a bit easier to follow.

Prepackaged Foods Diets

These programs can be useful for short-term weight loss. However, weight gain often occurs after the individual has grown weary of the foods or the program closes its doors. These types of commercial programs often seek other forms of revenue from their consumers, such as selling vitamins and minerals or other supplements touted to promote weight loss. These are often very expensive programs that do not have long-term success rates. Consumers can save a lot of money and develop long-term food habits simply by purchasing prepackaged foods from their local grocery store. Better yet, save even more money by making these same foods from scratch. There is nothing magical about cooking low-cal foods. It can be as easy as filling half a cantaloupe with low-fat cottage cheese and serving it with minestrone and a slice of whole-grain toast dipped in garlic and olive oil. Yummy, low-cal, easy, and delicious!

WHAT IS THE ROLE OF PHYSICAL FITNESS IN HEALTHY WEIGHT MANAGEMENT?

Physical Fitness

The first and most obvious reason that exercise is important for weight management is that it burns kilocalories. The duration and intensity of the activity, as well as the weight of the individual performing it, are all factors that affect just how many kilocalories are expended (see Table 7-1).

Activity is also important because it causes more kilocalories to be expended even *after* the exercise is finished. Research shows that physical activity can increase the metabolic rate for as long as 24 hours after the activity ceases. This is especially true of aerobic exercise.

Regular involvement in exercise goes even further in the quest to prevent and manage obesity. It has to do with the functioning of body cells. **Mitochondria** are the parts of body cells that act like furnaces to burn our food kilocalories through the process of oxidation. Regular exercise leads to a greater muscle mitochondrial content (Hood et al., 2000). Endurance training causes basic changes in mitochondrial function, which may contribute to a higher basal metabolic rate (Tonkonogi, et al., 2000). Over 90% of energy is spent in muscle cells. Oxygen and fuel substrates (carbohydrates and lipids) ultimately converge in muscle mitochondria (Hoppeler and Weibel, 2000).

Regular exercise, either alone or in combination with dietary modification, can have an important role in weight management. Exercise is a necessary component of daily living, but one that is often forgotten. Exercise will help do the following:

- Decrease body fat while helping to preserve and tone muscle tissue
- Manage mental stress
- Increase energy levels
- Provide a sense of control over health and lifestyle
- Control appetite

The amount of exercise recommended for persons with health problems will depend on the physician's advice. Generally, walking and swimming are safe

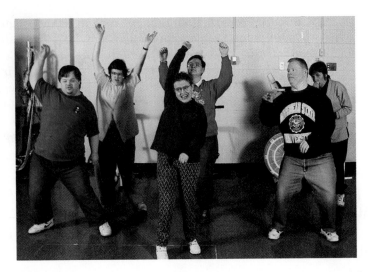

FIGURE 7-1 Clients exercising in a simple dance routine to promote weight loss.

exercises for all persons. Those who are bedridden (see Figure 14-2) or are in wheelchairs can use upper arm exercises to help maintain muscular strength and health. Individuals of all abilities will generally enjoy some form of dancing as a means to increase physical activity (Figure 7-1).

Aerobic Versus Anaerobic Exercise for Weight Management

Aerobic exercise is any exercise that requires more air (just like the term sounds: "air-o-bic"). This type of activity tends to use the highest percentage of body fat for fuel, thus promoting the most beneficial weight loss. Aerobic exercise involves large muscle groups and builds cardiovascular endurance. Aerobic exercise includes cycling, jogging, walking briskly, soccer, basketball, cross-country skiing, rowing, and dancing. When such activity is performed continuously for at least 20 minutes 3 to 5 times per week, there is considerable benefit for weight management and cardiovascular health. Achieving goals through athletic events has the additional reward of an increased sense of well-being (Figure 7-2). Those persons not able to be involved with endurance levels of activity can still benefit with even 5 minutes here or there, which is better than no exercise and can encourage a person to slowly increase physical activity.

Anaerobic exercise means exercise without air. Weight training is an example of anaerobic exercise; it will produce an increase in lean body mass, which will indirectly help weight management because more energy is required to maintain muscle than adipose tissue. In the short term, muscle development can be associated with weight gain, but this is a healthy gain and is often accompanied by a loss of inches related to body fat. (A pound of muscle takes up less space than a

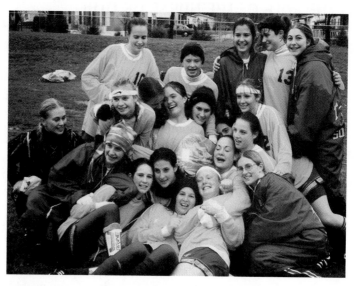

FIGURE 7-2 Team spirit soars after winning a regional varsity soccer game.

pound of fat because it is denser; thus weight loss may not occur, even though inches decrease.)

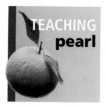

TEACHING **pearl**

A good analogy for the effect of aerobic exercise in patient education is that of a fire in a fireplace that is going out. You can say, "When you blow on the fire, giving it more air, it burns faster. And although we do not have fire in our stomachs, we still use air (oxygen) to burn our food kilocalories. Aerobic exercise causes us to take in more oxygen, so we burn food kilocalories faster."

Other Benefits of Exercise

Exercise is associated with improved blood sugar control for the person with diabetes, reduced blood pressure, increased amounts of good HDL cholesterol, and improved bone density. Weight-bearing exercise can slow down bone loss after menopause.

Exercise-Associated Problems

It is wise to seek medical clearance before embarking on an exercise program. This is particularly true for persons with diabetes who have complications. Diabetic neuropathy can affect the ability of the heart rate to increase during times of exercise. This is a problem because the body cannot increase the flow of blood and oxygen to the working body cells.

WHAT IS THE ROLE OF THE NURSE OR OTHER HEALTH CARE PROFESSIONAL IN PROMOTING HEALTHY WEIGHT AND PHYSICAL ACTIVITY?

The Dietary Guidelines for Americans, the Food Guide Pyramid, and food labels are excellent tools that the health professional can use effectively in teaching individuals to make good food choices for maintaining physical fitness and wellness.

The nurse or other health care professional can assist persons of all ages in identifying appropriate weight for health and effective means to achieve changes in body composition. The health care professional can assess if an individual is following a fad diet and whether there is a risk of nutrient imbalances. Reviewing the knowledge base of effective and healthy weight loss or obesity prevention is appropriate. It is imperative that health care professionals keep an open mind to the variety of approaches used in managing weight and health. Listening to the patient's account of prior weight loss attempts and current practices can go a long way in establishing a trusting relationship. Referral to a registered dietitian is in order when a patient expresses frustration at the inability to lose weight. The dietitian can often identify the problem and help develop effective strategies. Outpatient dietitians or those in private practice are often the ones who specialize in long-term weight loss support and consulting.

CHAPTER STUDY QUESTIONS AND CLASSROOM ACTIVITIES

1. Determine your BMI (see Appendix 12).
2. Two slices of whole-wheat bread contain 30 g of carbohydrates, 6 g of protein, and 2 g of fat. How many kilocalories do the two slices contain?
3. How might you advise a family to plan meals to meet the needs of all its members—overweight adults and growing children? Should you suggest separate meals? Why or why not?
4. Plan a 1200- to 1500-kcal diet pattern appropriate for weight loss.
5. How many grams of carbohydrates equate to 500 to 600 kcals?
6. How does exercise help with weight management?
7. Compare the macronutrient content of a commercial weight loss drink with a can of soda pop and a half-pint carton of milk. Describe the differences and similarities. Discuss the pros and cons of the drinks. Compare the caloric value of the drink with that of a meal consisting of a turkey sandwich, $\frac{1}{2}$ c carrot sticks, and a half-pint of low-fat (1%) milk; refer to Appendix 5 as needed.

Case Study

CRITICAL THINKING

Anna had been going to a weight loss support group and was now adding up her points for the day. She thought that the doughnut offered at the office meeting, which she thoroughly enjoyed, was going to add up to a lot of points. No fiber in doughnuts and way too much fat. But it had tasted good and she would eat more sensibly later. She did wish, however, that the office stock of goodies was not sitting right next to her desk. She had a hard enough time keeping her weight under control and then all this food sitting, looking right at her. She looked out the window to get her mind off food. She would eat the piece of fruit she brought to work later, before going to aerobics class. After aerobics class, she planned to go to her parents' house because her dad wanted to have a family discussion aimed at helping her younger brother stop his weight gain.

Critical Thinking Applications

1. What commercial weight loss program uses a point system?
2. Discuss Anna's philosophy that she could make up for the doughnut later in the day. Look up the fat, carbohydrate, and caloric content in a typical doughnut (see Appendix 5). What might she do to counter the kilocalories of the doughnut later in the day?
3. Discuss experiences among the class regarding workplace eating issues. Brainstorm strategies to resolve workplace eating problems.
4. Why might Anna feel the need to eat before her aerobics class?
5. How might a family support or inhibit weight management?

REFERENCES

Araya H, Hills J, Alvina M, Vera G: Short-term satiety in preschool children: a comparison between high protein meal and a high complex carbohydrate meal. Int J Food Sci Nutr. March 2000; 51(2):119-124.

Boozer CN, Nasser JA, Heymsfield SB, Wang V, Chen G, Solomon JL: An herbal supplement containing Ma Huang-Guarana for weight loss: a randomized, double-blind trial. Int J Obes Relat Metab Disord. March 2001; 25(3):316-324.

Carruth B, Skinner J: The role of dietary calcium and other nutrients in moderating body fat in preschool children. Int J Obes Relat Metab Disord. April 2001; 25(4):559-566.

Chu NF: Prevalence and trends of obesity among school children in Taiwan—the Taipei Children Heart Study. Int J Obes Relat Metab Disord. February 2001; 25(2):170-176.

Crawford V, Scheckenbach R, Preuss HG: Effects of niacin-bound chromium supplementation on body composition in overweight African American women. Diabetes Obes Metab. November, 1999; 1(6):331-337.

Hood DA, Takahashi M, Connor MK, Freyssenet D: Assembly of the cellular powerhouse: current issues in muscle mitochondrial biogenesis. Exerc Sport Sci Rev. April 2000; 28(2):68-73.

Hoppeler H, Weibel ER: Structural and functional limits for oxygen supply to muscle. Acta Physiol Scand. April 2000; 168(4):445-456.

Howarth NC, Saltzman E, Roberts SB: Dietary fiber and weight regulation. Nutr Rev. May 2001; 59(5):129-139.

Kaufhold JN, Hammon HM, Bruckmaier RM, Breier BH, Blum JW: Postprandial metabolism and endocrine status in veal calves fed at different frequencies. J Dairy Sci. November 2000; 83(11):2480-2490.

Kennedy ET, Bowman SA, Spence JT, Freedman M, King J: Popular diets: correlation to health, nutrition, and obesity. J Am Diet Assoc. April 2001; 101(4):411-420.

Kral JG, Buckley MC, Kissileff HR, Schaffner F: Metabolic correlates of eating behavior in severe obesity. Int J Obes Relat Metab Disord. February 2001; 25(2):258-264.

Kromhout D, Bloemberg B, Seidell JC, Nissinen A, Menotti A: Physical activity and dietary fiber determine population body fat levels: the Seven Countries Study. Int J Obes Relat Metab Disord. March 2001; 25(3):301-306.

Kurzthaler I, Fleischhacker WW: The clinical implications of weight gain in schizophrenia. J Clin Psychiatry. 2001; 62 Suppl 7:32-37.

Lowe MR, Miller-Kovach K, Phelan S: Weight-loss maintenance in overweight individuals one to five years following successful completion of a commercial weight loss program. Int J Obes Relat Metab Disord. March 2001; 25(3):325-331.

Maffeis C, Tato L: Long-term effects of childhood obesity on morbidity and mortality. Horm Res. 2001; 55 Suppl 1:42-45.

Marques-Lopes I, Ansorena D, Astiasaran I, Forga L, Martinez JA: Postprandial de novo lipogenesis and metabolic changes induced by a high-carbohydrate, low-fat meal in lean and overweight men. Am J Clin Nutr. February 2001; 73(2):253-261.

Murphy NJ, Schraer CD, Thiele MC, Boyko EJ, Bulkow LR, Doty BJ, Lanier AP: Dietary change and obesity associated with glucose intolerance in Alaska Natives. J Am Diet Assoc. June 1995; 95(6):676-682.

Naslund E, Andersson I, Degerblad M, Kogner P, Kral JG, Rossner S, Hellstrom PM: Associations of leptin, insulin resistance, and thyroid function with long-term weight loss in dieting obese men. J Intern Med. October 2000; 248(4):299-308.

Nye EJ, Grice JE, Hockings GI, Strakosch CR, Crosbie GV, Walters MM, Torpy DJ, Jackson RV: The insulin hypoglycemia test: hypoglycemic criteria and reproducibility. J Neuroendocrinol. June 2001; 13(6):524-530.

O'Meara S, Riemsma R, Shirran L, Mather L, ter Riet G : A rapid and systematic review of the clinical effectiveness and cost-effectiveness of orlistat in the management of obesity. Health Technol Assess. 2001; 5(18):1-81.

Rask E, Olsson T, Soderberg S, Andrew R, Livingstone DE, Johnson O, Walker BR. Tissue-specific dysregulation of cortisol metabolism in human obesity. J Clin Endocrinol Metab. March 2001; 86(3):1418-1421.

Rohner-Jeanrenaud F: Neuroendocrine regulation of nutrient partitioning. Ann N Y Acad Sci. November 18, 1999; 892:261-271.

Suga A, Hirano T, Kageyama H, Osaka T, Namba Y, Tsuji M, Miura M, Adachi M, Inoue S: Effects of fructose and glucose on plasma leptin, insulin, and insulin resistance in lean and VMH-lesioned obese rats. Am J Physiol Endocrinol Metab. April, 2000; 278(4):E677-E683.

Tonkonogi M, Krook A, Walsh B, Sahlin K: Endurance training increases stimulation of uncoupling of skeletal muscle mitochondria in humans by non-esterified fatty acids: an uncoupling-protein-mediated effect? Biochem J. November 1, 2000; 351 Pt 3:805-810.

Unger RH, Orci L: Diseases of liporegulation: new perspective on obesity and related disorders. FASEB J. February 2001; 15(2):312-321.

Wing RR, Hill JO: Successful weight loss maintenance. Annu Rev Nutr. 2001; 21:323-341.

Wofford MR, Andrew ME, Brown A, King D, Pickett RA, Stevens J, Wyatt S, Jones DW: Obesity hypertension in the atherosclerosis risk in communities cohort: implications of obesity guidelines. J Clin Hypertens (Greenwich). July 1999; 1(1):27-32.

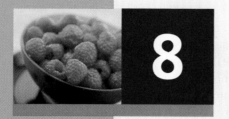

8 Cardiovascular Disease

OBJECTIVES

After completing this chapter, you should be able to:

- Identify risk factors related to the development of cardiovascular disease.
- Describe medical nutrition therapy for cardiovascular disease and hypertension.
- Describe how the management of the dyslipidemia found in conjunction with the insulin resistance syndrome differs from management of low-density lipoprotein cholesterol.
- Describe appropriate foods to prevent or manage cardiovascular disease.
- Describe the role of the nurse or other health care professional in the prevention and management of cardiovascular disease.

TERMS TO IDENTIFY

Adult Treatment Panel III
   (ATP III)
Arteriosclerosis
Atherosclerosis
Cardiovascular disease (CVD)
Cerebrovascular accident
   (CVA)
Congestive heart failure
   (CHF)
Coronary heart disease
   (CHD)
Coronary thrombosis

Dietary Approaches to Stop
   Hypertension (DASH) diet
Dyslipidemia
Edema
Free radicals
High-glycemic index
High-glycemic load
Homocysteine
Hypercholesterolemia
Hyperlipidemia
Hypertension
Hypertriglyceridemia

Lipids
Morbidity
Mortality
Myocardial infarction (MI)
National Cholesterol
   Education Program (NCEP)
Plant stanols
Therapeutic Lifestyle
   Changes (TLC) diet
Thrombosis
Trans fatty acids
Triglycerides

INTRODUCTION

Most people do not worry about heart disease. **Cardiovascular disease (CVD)**, also known as **coronary heart disease (CHD)** or more simply heart disease, kills more people than all forms of cancer combined and is still the leading cause of death for Americans, both men and women. The good news is that there has been progress in preventing the **mortality** (death) and **morbidity** (effects of disease) of heart disease. The proportion of Americans with high cholesterol has continued to drop, in part because of better screening and interventions.

Although some individuals are not prone to CHD, most people will benefit from dietary changes that lower the total fat content to about 30% and saturated fat to less than 10%. However, other factors related to cultural food choices and genetic heritage play a role in CHD risk. For example, in the southeastern United States the occurrence of heart disease and stroke and the rates of congestive heart failure (CHF) and renal failure are the highest in the country (Jones et al., 1999).

Individual guidance should complement the general guidelines to allow for specific needs; for example, guidelines can be adjusted to suit frail, elderly persons or terminally ill patients who may need to rely on high-fat foods for adequate kilocalorie intake. For everyone, attempts to lower the risk of CHD should not take precedence over sound nutritional intake. Meat, milk, and cheese are still important to one's diet; however, moderation and an emphasis on low-fat and low-sodium alternatives can result in a healthy balance.

WHAT ARE THE TYPES OF CARDIOVASCULAR DISEASE?

Cardiovascular disease relates to the heart and the entire vascular system. Thus **hypertension** (high blood pressure), **cerebrovascular accident (CVA)** or, more commonly, stroke, and **arteriosclerosis** (hardening of the arteries) are all examples of CVD. In diseases of the heart, one or several parts of the heart may be damaged, such as the heart muscle or the valves.

What Is Atherosclerosis?

Atherosclerosis is a complex disease of the arteries; it is a form of arteriosclerosis. The passageways through the arteries become roughened and clogged with fatty deposits so that blood cannot flow freely, like clogged sink pipes (Figure 8-1). Atherosclerosis is thought to be a cause of heart attack (**coronary thrombosis, myocardial infarction [MI]**, or coronary) and CVA.

WHAT ARE LIPOPROTEINS AND THEIR DIFFERENT FORMS AND EFFECT ON CARDIOVASCULAR DISEASE?

High-density lipoprotein (HDL), low-density lipoprotein (LDL), and very low-density lipoprotein (VLDL) are all forms of cholesterol found in the blood. **Lipids** is a term used to describe all forms of fat found in the blood. Chylomi-

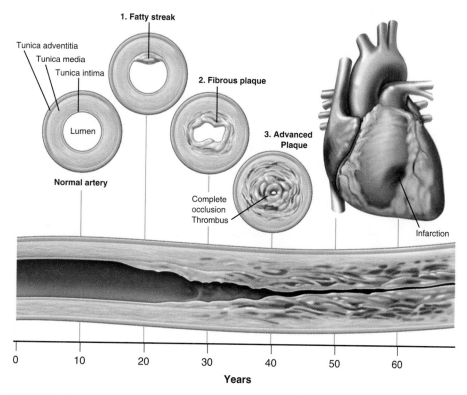

FIGURE 8-1 Natural progression of atherosclerosis. (From Harkreader H. Fundamentals of nursing: caring and clinical judgment, ed 1, Philadelphia: WB Saunders, 2000.)

crons are another form of lipoprotein. The VLDL is the main carrier of **triglycerides** (a type of blood fat) synthesized in the body. The HDL, which has more protein than does LDL or VLDL, is believed to allow more cholesterol to be taken from the body's cells, resulting in greater transport and removal of cholesterol through the liver. **Hypercholesterolemia** refers to elevated serum LDL cholesterol. **Hyperlipidemia** is the term used to describe a combination of high levels of LDL cholesterol and triglycerides. **Dyslipidemia**, as discussed in Chapter 6, refers to high levels of triglycerides with low levels of HDL cholesterol.

High-density lipoproteins have been termed the *good* lipoproteins or fats. In fact, research has shown that individuals with more HDLs have less heart disease. Recent clinical trials in patients with CHD indicate that increasing low levels of HDL cholesterol significantly reduces the occurrence of heart attack and stroke in patients whose only lipid abnormality was low HDL (Boden and Pearson, 2000). An easy way to remember the role of HDL is to think *H* for *housecleaner* because a high level of HDL seems to keep blood vessels and arteries clean.

The total cholesterol number is the mathematical sum of the HDL plus the LDL plus one fifth of the triglyceride level (if triglycerides are less than 400). This will be noted if the phrase "calculated LDL" is used on the lab report.

Treatment goals vary depending on the differing levels of these lipids. Referral to a registered dietitian should take place to review an individual's particular needs, especially if there are multiple risk factors for CVD.

WHAT ARE THE RISK FACTORS FOR CARDIOVASCULAR DISEASE?

The 2001 guidelines developed by the **Adult Treatment Panel III (ATP III)** is a set of recommendations by the **National Cholesterol Education Program (NCEP)** of the National Heart, Lung, and Blood Institute to reduce CHD by lowering cholesterol levels. These recommendations include the following risk factors:

1. Elevated LDL cholesterol (less than 100 mg/dL is the optimal goal)
2. Cigarette smoking
3. Hypertension: blood pressure of 140/90 mm Hg or greater, or on antihypertensive medication
4. Low HDL cholesterol (less than 40 mg/dL)
5. Family history of premature CHD
6. Cardiovascular disease in male first degree relative younger than 55
7. Cardiovascular disease in female first degree relative younger than 65
8. Age (men 45 years or older; women 55 years or older)
9. Diabetes
10. Multiple metabolic risk factors (insulin resistance or metabolic syndrome)

High-density lipoprotein cholesterol greater than 60 mg/dL counts as a negative risk factor; its presence removes one risk factor from the total count.

How Is the Metabolic or Insulin Resistance Syndrome Related to Cardiovascular Disease?

As you recall from Chapter 6, the metabolic or insulin resistance syndrome is a diagnosis made by correlates. The primary correlates—central obesity, hypertension, dyslipidemia, and Type 2 diabetes (see Chapter 9)—are all risk factors for CVD. Multiple risk factors, as found in the insulin resistance syndrome, further increase risk for CVD and call for intensified risk management to lower CVD risk.

Insulin resistance generally promotes hyperinsulinemia (excess insulin in the blood). Hyperinsulinemia is gaining acceptance as a cause of atherosclerosis because it is believed to alter the lining of the blood vessels enhancing plaque build-up. Although more research is needed to confirm the role of hyperinsulinemia, this theory does help explain why CVD often precedes the diagnosis of diabetes. **Hypertriglyceridemia** (excess triglycerides in the blood) has recently been confirmed as having a role in CVD. The cut-off point for elevated triglycerides has been lowered from 200 to 150 mg/dL because of newer research on the CVD risk.

In only half of the CVD cases the causes related to the risk factors are hypertension, cigarette smoking, and elevated total and LDL cholesterol levels

(Hughes, 2000). For this reason, research continues on other strategies to reduce CVD risk.

The following is a list of some of the emerging risk factors of the ATP III guidelines and the basis for the consideration of risk:

- Homocysteine
- Prothrombotic factors
- Proinflammatory factors
- Impaired fasting glucose

High levels of **homocysteine**, a sulfur-containing amino acid, are an important risk factor for CVD, including stroke. It is interesting to note that homocysteine may also play a role in neurodegenerative disorders (see Chapter 14) and that most anticonvulsants raise homocysteine levels (Diaz-Arrastia, 2000). Thus a person using anticonvulsant medication for management of seizures may be at increased risk of CVD.

Homocysteine has been shown to contribute to the plaque formation found in atherogenesis. One study found that this plaque build-up and other changes were significantly decreased with dietary supplementation of folate and vitamins B_6 and B_{12}, which lowered levels of homocysteine in the blood (Hofmann et al., 2001). The homocysteine levels of persons who used vitamin B supplements, including riboflavin, were about 20% lower than were those of persons who did not. Further, high levels of homocysteine were associated with alcohol intake, caffeine intake, the number of cigarettes smoked, and antihypertensive medication use (Jacques et al., 2001). Low-dose vitamin B_6 further lowers fasting plasma homcysteine in persons who have good folate and riboflavin status. This suggests that any program aimed at the treatment or prevention of high levels of homocysteine should include vitamin B_6 supplementation (McKinley et al., 2001).

Although persons who follow a vegetarian diet often have low intakes of cholesterol and saturated fat, recognizing that there is an increased risk for high levels of homocysteine is important. This was true with over half of persons following a vegan diet, over 25% in other vegetarians, and only 5% among nonvegetarians. Higher amounts of vitamin B_{12} and folate are required when there is low intake of methionine (an amino acid found in small amounts in plant-based foods). Intake of vitamin B_{12} is low in the vegan diet unless supplementation is used. Thus high levels of homocysteine in the blood can occur with a vegetarian diet related to vitamin B_{12} deficiency (Krajcovicova-Kudlackova et al., 2000).

Thrombosis is the formation of clots. Clots can be stationary when attached to the walls of blood vessels, but can later dislodge and plug a smaller blood vessel. Eighty percent of patients with diabetes mellitus die from a thrombosis. This is, in part, caused by the enhanced activation of platelets and clotting factors seen in diabetes (Carr, 2001). Excess risk for thrombosis is associated with hyperinsulinemia and glucose intolerance (Meigs et al., 2000). Glucose intolerance is also referred to as impaired fasting glucose and is considered a risk factor for CVD.

As discussed in Chapter 6, C-reactive protein (CRP) is receiving a great deal of interest as a marker for a number of health issues, including CVD. Inflammatory processes are believed to contribute to CVD. The C-reactive protein is a marker of inflammation and has been found to be a risk factor of CVD. The correlation of CRP and CVD is noted in one study involving Asian Indians. This population was found to have high levels of CRP (Chambers et al., 2001). Further, Asian Indians are known to have an increased risk of CVD. Thus controlling the inflammation process can lower CRP levels and may lower CVD risk. Including the omega-3 fats from cold-water fish is known to reduce inflammation and to reduce CVD risk (discussed in a later section).

Are There Other Risk Factors for Cardiovascular Disease?

Oxidation of LDL cholesterol is thought to play a key role in the development of atherosclerosis. When the body cells use oxygen in the metabolism of energy, it is not a clean process. **Free radicals** are formed through oxidation. The free radicals cause damage at the cell level. This reinforces the importance of a good diet that includes foods rich in antioxidants.

Obesity is one of the risk factors of atherosclerosis and obesity is related to LDL oxidation. Weight loss is associated with less oxidation of LDL cholesterol (Vasankari et al., 2001).

Can Excess Iron in the Diet Cause Cardiovascular Disease?

Some researchers have hypothesized that, compared with men, women are at a decreased risk of heart disease because menstruation lowers their iron stores, which in turn may limit the oxidation of lipids. After menopause, women do have an increased rate of heart disease. The role that iron plays in the development of heart disease is still, however, in the theory stage. Because iron-deficiency anemia is a known health problem, caution should be exercised in decreasing iron intake in the diet.

Individuals at risk of high serum iron levels, such as those with hemochromatosis (see Chapter 4) should be advised to avoid iron. For the general public, avoidance of iron is not yet recommended. However, those with low risk of anemia may benefit by avoiding excess iron. Vitamin and mineral supplements designed for men and older adults are formulated to be lower in iron because of their low risk of anemia.

Some studies have shown that increased iron stores are associated with increased cardiovascular events. Increased iron stores may play a role in the development of CVD by increasing lipoprotein oxidation. Individuals carrying the hereditary hemochromatosis mutation may be at increased risk of CVD (Rasmussen et al., 2001). One study of men who donated blood did not support the theory that reducing iron stores lowers CVD risk (Ascherio et al., 2001). However, levels of body iron stores (serum ferritin) do rise with age after adolescence in men and menopause in women. To date, there have been insufficient studies to disprove the iron and CVD theory (Zacharski et al., 2000).

What Are Risk Factors and Prevention Strategies for Strokes?

There are a variety of risk factors for stroke, including hypertension, diabetes, obesity, and lack of physical activity. New strategies for stroke prevention have been identified, including encouragement of a diet high in vegetables, fruits, whole grains, and omega-3 fatty acids. Control of homocysteine levels and moderate alcohol consumption further help prevent stroke (Jeerakathil and Wolf, 2001).

What Are Safe Blood Cholesterol Levels?

The levels set by the NCEP coordinating committee indicate that total cholesterol should be less than 200 mg/dL. The NCEP also indicates that LDL should optimally be less than 100 mg/dL, triglycerides less than 150 mg/dL, and HDL greater than 40 mg/dL with the goal being more than 60 mg/dL to best help prevent CVD. Cholesterol levels that are very low (less than 150 mg/dL) are controversial as being a risk factor to health.

The guidelines of the NCEP now recommend that adults aged 20 years and older have their total and HDL measured. If the total cholesterol is 200 mg/dL or more, or the HDL is less than 40 mg/dL, a complete lipoprotein profile is advised (including the LDL cholesterol and triglyceride levels).

Fallacy: My grandfather lived to be 100 and ate eggs and bacon daily; therefore I do not have to worry about heart disease.

Fact: Individuals who subscribe to the preceding idea need to be reminded that heredity also comes from the grandmother's side of the family, as well as from both parents. Careful questioning often reveals some form of CVD risk in the family's history, even if it is not heart disease specifically. A person might also be exposed to other risk factors that did not affect previous generations of his or her family, such as cigarette smoking, diabetes, or low levels of physical activity.

HOW IS CARDIOVASCULAR DISEASE PREVENTED AND TREATED BY DIET CHANGES?

The great degree of variation in the cause of CVD should be recognized by now. Individual risk factors play a role in determining the best course of action with specific dietary guidelines.

For persons with only hypercholesterolemia, and no other risk factors for CVD, the advice is somewhat straightforward: limit saturated fat and cholesterol, referred to as the Step I and Step II diets of the American Heart Association (AHA). The Step I diet limits saturated fat to 10% of kilocalories and cholesterol to 300 mg (see Box 8-1 for sample menu). The Step II level is used if the Step I diet is not adequate to achieve lipid goals or there is preexisting CVD. The Step II diet limits

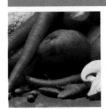

BOX 8-1
ONE-DAY
SAMPLE
MENU FOR
A STEP I DIET
(APPROXI-
MATELY
2000 KCAL)

BREAKFAST
grapefruit half
1 c oatmeal
1 slice whole-wheat toast
2 tsp natural peanut butter

8 oz skim milk
coffee
2 tsp brown sugar or jelly

LUNCH
turkey sandwich:
   3 oz turkey (no skin)
   2 slices bread
   tomato slices

½ c coleslaw made with 1 tsp
   mayonnaise dressing
small apple
iced tea with lemon

AFTERNOON SNACK
8 oz low-fat yogurt

¼ c almonds

SUPPER
3 oz pork tenderloin
1 c brown rice
½ c spinach sautéed in 2 tsp
   olive oil and garlic

½ c carrots with lemon juice
1 c tossed salad with 1 tbsp Italian
   dressing
8 oz skim milk

EVENING SNACK
3 c low-fat popcorn

saturated fat to less than 7% of kilocalories and cholesterol to 200 mg. For persons with the insulin resistance or metabolic syndrome, the ATP III guidelines advocate the **Therapeutic Lifestyle Changes (TLC)** diet (Table 8-1). The TLC Diet is similar to the Step II diet with the additional recommendation of limiting carbohydrate to 50% to 60% of total kilocalories and up to 35% fat with emphasis on monounsaturated fat. The TLC diet also advocates increased fiber, especially soluble fiber. **Plant stanols** (now found in some margarines) are also advocated if lipid levels are not improved with initial diet changes.

For persons who have multiple risk factors for CVD, medical nutrition therapy becomes very complex. Referral to a dietitian is often the best course of action to identify and plan the therapeutic approach. Use Figure 8-2 as a practice model to follow in implementing the TLC for someone with the insulin resistance or metabolic syndrome.

There continues to be debate on optimal amounts of cholesterol in the diet. The ATP III guidelines advocate less than 200 mg of cholesterol daily. This contrasts to other findings that suggest that consumption of up to one egg per day (about 225 mg of cholesterol, depending on the size of the egg) is unlikely to have substantial effect on the risk of CVD or stroke among healthy men and women. There has been noted, however, an apparent increased risk of CVD associated with higher egg consumption among diabetic participants, which war-

TABLE 8-1

ATP III GUIDELINES FOR THERAPEUTIC LIFESTYLE CHANGES (TLC) DIET

NUTRIENT COMPOSITION OF TLC DIET	
NUTRIENT	**RECOMMENDED INTAKE**
Saturated fat	Less than 7% of total calories
Polyunsaturated fat	Up to 10% of total calories
Monounsaturated fat	Up to 20% of total calories
Total fat	25%-35% of total calories
Carbohydrate	50%-60% of total calories
Fiber	20-30 grams per day
Protein	Approximately 15% of total calories
Cholesterol	Less than 200 mg/day
Total calories (energy)	Balance energy intake and expenditure to maintain desirable body weight/prevent weight gain

NEW FEATURES OF ATP III
MORE INTENSIVE LIFESTYLE INTERVENTION (TLC)
Therapeutic diet lowers saturated fat and cholesterol intakes to levels of previous Step II Adds dietary options to enhance LDL reduction • Plant stanols/sterols (2 grams per day) • Viscous (soluble) fiber (10-25 grams per day) Increased emphasis on weight management and physical activity

National Heart, Lung, and Blood Institute: Adult Treatment Panel guidelines for therapeutic lifestyle changes (TLC) diet. Washington DC, 2001, The National Institutes of Health.

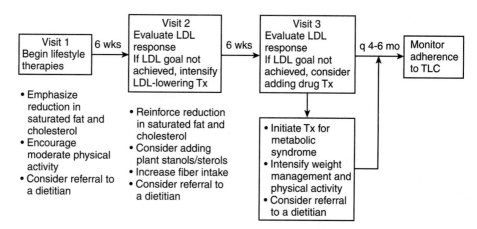

FIGURE 8-2 A model of steps in therapeutic lifestyle changes (TLC) diet. (From National Heart, Lung, and Blood Institute, 2001.)

rants further research (Hu et al., 1999). Reduction in cholesterol and egg intake is also warranted for persons with very high LDL levels.

The debate on dietary cholesterol's effect on CVD is further disputed with research found with a group of Chinese, the Hakka, who have low rates of CVD. The major foods of the Hakka people are rice, fish, vegetables, and fruits; they have a wide use of soybeans and an extensive consumption of visceral organs. The rich source of trace minerals in organ meats is believed to protect the Hakka against CVD (Liu and Li, 2000). Organ meats, however, are also very high in cholesterol content.

As stated earlier, the optimal level of fat intake becomes more challenging in the management of the insulin resistance syndrome. For these individuals, control of blood glucose and management of hyperinsulinemia is critical. One study looking at this question noted that a diet high in saturated fat (20%) induced the highest levels of insulin after an oral glucose tolerance test. This was compared with a diet rich in monounsaturated fatty acids (38% total fat with 22% monounsaturated fat). The high monounsaturated fat diet allowed the lowest levels of fasting blood glucose, insulin, and free fatty acids as compared with either the high saturated fat diet or the Step I diet. In addition, systolic and diastolic blood pressure was higher with the Step I diet. Thus a diet rich in monounsaturated fats is the most beneficial in regard to carbohydrate metabolism and blood pressure (Salas et al., 2000). The ATP III guidelines now recommend 25% to 35% of kilocalories as fat with up to 20% in the monounsaturated form (refer to Table 8-1). Table 8-2 shows the equivalent amount of fat based on 30% of various kilocalorie levels and how to calculate this percentage.

The higher fat guidelines are reinforced in another study that found minimal lipid formation with higher fat diets (more than 30%). It has also been shown that in persons consuming nuts, there is decreased risk of CVD (Almario et al., 2001). Most nuts are low in saturated fat, but are high in the unsaturated fats.

The additional factor of glycemic index also plays a role. A low-fat diet containing 10% fat that was also high in complex carbohydrate had comparable results to a high-fat diet (Hudgins, 2000). Thus individualization of dietary treatment is appropriate. If a person chooses to follow a very low-fat diet, emphasis should be on high-fiber foods. The high-monounsaturated fat diet is still optimally high in fiber content as well.

Both **high-glycemic index** meals (those that significantly raise the blood glucose levels) and a high total carbohydrate intake, referred to as a **high-glycemic load**, have been related to risk of CHD. Findings from a nationally representative sample of adults in the United States suggest that high dietary glycemic index and high-glycemic load are associated with a lower concentration of plasma HDL cholesterol (Ford and Liu, 2001).

A high-glycemic index meal is one that is high in simple carbohydrates (sugars and starch as found in white flour or processed grain products) that raise blood glucose levels. Starch, as found in white flour pasta and white bread were formerly referred to as complex carbohydrates. These types of starches are now recognized to have similar blood glucose effect as simple sugars. Liquid sugars, such as found in juice and soda pop, have the highest glycemic index. A complex

TABLE 8-2
RECOMMENDED TOTAL FAT FOR VARIOUS KILOCALORIE LEVELS

KILOCALORIE LEVEL	TOTAL RECOMMENDED FAT (30%)
1200	40 g
1500	50 g
1800	60 g
2100	70 g
2400	80 g
2700	90 g
3000	100 g

To calculate percentage of fat of total kilocalories:

1. Multiply total kilocalories by percentage of fat (0.30 used above), which yields the number of kilo-calories to be contributed by fat.
2. Divide the number of kilocalories of fat by 9 to determine the total grams of fat.

To calculate the percentage of total kilocalories of a given amount of fat:

1. Multiply grams of fat by 9 to equal kilocalories contributed by fat.
2. Divide kilocalories from fat by total kilocalories to determine the percentage.

An easier way to calculate the recommended number of grams of fat is to divide the total kilocalories by 30. For example:

$$\frac{1800 \text{ kilocalories}}{30} = 60 \text{ g of fat}$$

Use the exchange list system (see Appendix 9) for an easy method to calculate fat content from a given menu. Foods not listed in the exchange list will generally be listed in a food composition table from which fat content can be determined (see Appendix 5).

carbohydrate food is one that is high in fiber, such as with legumes and vegetables. Fruits and whole grains have less fiber, in comparison to carbohydrate content, than do legumes and vegetables. They can still, however, play a positive role in prevention of CVD.

Evidence that vegetables and fruits may protect against CHD is accumulating. However, the constituents of vegetables and fruits responsible for this protective effect have not been determined (Eichholzer et al., 2001). Results suggest an inverse association between vegetable intake and risk of CVD. The data support current dietary guidelines to increase vegetable intake for the prevention of CVD (Liu et al., 2001).

Intake of antioxidant nutrients, which are found in high amounts in vegetables and fruits, has been shown to be associated with reduced risk of atherosclerosis. There are a variety of antioxidants found in plant-based foods. Generally speaking, those with color such as carrots, blueberries, and spinach are high in antioxidants. One interesting study found that consumption of ginger extract significantly reduced the development of atherosclerotic lesions. This was, at least in part, caused by a lower oxidization of LDL cholesterol (Fuhrman et al., 2000).

The use of antioxidant vitamin supplements is sometimes advocated to reduce CVD risk; however, receiving these vitamins via foods will also increase the intake of fiber and naturally occurring phytochemicals, which may be important as well. Plant-based foods high in antioxidants, trace minerals, and naturally occuring phytochemicals and fiber continue to be the first line approach to preventing and treating CVD with low saturated fat and moderate monounsaturated and cholesterol intake. Although increased dietary intakes of vitamin E are associated with a reduced cardiovascular risk, the clinical results of recent studies evaluating the effect of vitamin E supplementation have generally been disappointing (Carpentier, 2000).

The CRP, as discussed in Chapter 6, is receiving increased attention as a predictor of a variety of health problems, including CVD. One study found that both nondrinkers and heavy drinkers had higher CRP concentrations than did moderate drinkers. In view of the association of CRP with the risk of CHD, an anti-inflammatory action of alcohol could contribute to the link between moderate consumption and lower cardiovascular mortality (Imhof et al., 2001). However, great caution should be taken concerning alcohol promotion for cardioprotective purposes (Hemstrom, 2001). Recall from the earlier review of alcohol that we are not able, at this time, to identify individuals at risk for alcoholism. The best advice for those who do drink is to do so in moderation for CVD protection.

Where Is Cholesterol Found?

There are two main sources of cholesterol. One is the body's natural production of cholesterol in the liver, in the gastrointestinal tract, and in almost all body cells that have a nucleus. This natural cholesterol production is affected by diet. Saturated fats tend to increase the production of cholesterol and unsaturated fats tend to have the opposite effect. Intake of cholesterol in the diet has little effect on the body's own natural cholesterol production, although it may impair the ability of the body to clear LDL from the blood.

The second source of cholesterol is the food we eat. Remember that cholesterol is found only in animal products and specifically in animal fat and organ meats. Skim milk and egg whites, although both animal products, have no measurable fat and therefore no significant amount of cholesterol. Plant fats such as peanut butter do not contain any cholesterol. Reducing the solid, saturated fat in the diet now appears to be more important than reducing dietary cholesterol intake. For persons with the insulin resistance syndrome, replacement kilocalories for saturated fat should be monounsaturated fats, as found in most nuts, olives, and avocados or omega-3 fatty acids found in cold-water fish. For persons with no risk factors for insulin resistance, the saturated fat can be replaced with carbohydrate, although the ones high in fiber are still preferable for a number of reasons.

What Are Omega-3 Fatty Acids and What Is Their Significance in Preventing Cardiovascular Disease?

The most unsaturated form of fat found in foods is referred to as omega-3 fatty acids. This form of fat is prevalent in cold-water fish and other foods such as flaxseed and dark green, leafy vegetables.

Omega-3 fats are known to reduce blood levels of triglycerides and thus are recommended in the control of CVD. These fats also reduce the inflammation process of the body and tend to reduce the clotting time of the blood. A study looking at changes in triglyceride levels with fish consumption, versus with weight loss, versus with fish consumption in conjunction with weight loss, found that triglycerides fell 29% with fish consumption, but 26% with weight loss. However, there was an amazing 38% drop in triglycerides with both fish consumption and weight loss. Further, one form of HDL cholesterol, HDL(2), increased by 24% (Mori et al., 1999).

Greenland Eskimos, who have a low incidence of atherosclerosis, have a high intake of the omega-3 type of fat through consumption of almost 1 lb of fish daily. This reinforces, once again, that not all fats are bad for our health.

The cardioprotective effect of omega-3 fatty acids is so great that the AHA is now recommending that everyone consume fatty fish at least twice weekly or, if this is simply impossible, to take omega-3 fatty acid supplements. An alternative that some do not object to is to take cod liver oil. One teaspoon of cod liver oil is the equivalent of eating 5 oz of fish and contains about 500 mg eicopentenoic (EPA) and decohexanoic (DHA)—the forms of omega-3 fats. One to two teaspoons of cod liver oil weekly will meet the guideline set forth by the AHA to eat fatty fish twice weekly. Supplement use should be reviewed with the person's physician to avoid excess intake because of the anticlotting aspect of omega-3 fatty acids.

Older adults may recall the routine intake of sardines and herring or the use of cod liver oil. Many of the younger generations have not had this exposure to fish, which may increase their risk for CVD later in life. Given the benefits of omega-3 fatty acids, we should start to help our children, if not ourselves, learn to like fish. Advice to eat more tuna fish is generally well accepted. Albacore tuna is relatively high in omega-3 fatty acids. (See Chapter 13 for tips on helping children learn to eat new foods.)

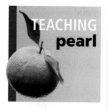

TEACHING pearl

The following is a fun scenario to describe when you're explaining omega-3 fatty acids as being found in cold-water fish. Review the fact that saturated fats, as found in butter, always get very hard at cold temperature. Now, have the person picture what would happen to fish living in the cold arctic waters if their body fat was saturated. Obviously, the fish would become solid and not be able to swim. Omega-3 fatty acids have the ability to remain soft at very cold temperatures, allowing the fish to swim and survive in the frigid waters.

What Are Trans Fatty Acids and What Is Their Effect on Cardiovascular Disease?

Vegetable oils that have the element hydrogen added to them turn the oils into solid fats. Hydrogenated fats are referred to as **trans fatty acids**. In the last 10 years or so, the adverse health effect of hydrogenated fats has been recognized. However, the ability to precisely measure the saturated fat equivalent of the man-made hydrogenated fats is still being developed. Whether or not we can quantify the exact amount, solid fats are considered to be acting as saturated fats. One explanation for the increased CVD with trans fatty acids is that they decrease HDL cholesterol (de Roos et al., 2001). The estimated amount of trans fatty acids will be added to the saturated fat number currently found on food labels.

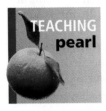

TEACHING pearl

For anyone born before 1942, you will likely get a good chuckle from them if you ask if they recall putting yellow food coloring in margarine. During the 1940s, it was recognized that adding the element hydrogen to liquid vegetable oils turned the oil into solid fat. When margarine came to the market, you had to mix in your own coloring. It was a fond experience by the children at that time to have this task—a bit like playing with Play-doh.™ Thus margarine and Crisco™ shortening did not exist before the 1940s.

What Is the Connection between Cardiovascular Disease and Fiber?

There is growing evidence that dietary fiber may play a role in preventing and controlling CVD. As noted in Chapter 2, the water-soluble fibers—pectins from fruits, gums from legumes, and the water-soluble fiber in oat grain—appear to be effective in reducing serum cholesterol levels. The benefits of soluble fiber are so impressive that daily consumption has been advised, whether it comes from oat bran, brown rice, legumes, barley, or other sources. (See Appendix 6 for fiber content of foods.)

Soluble fiber is believed to lower LDL cholesterol through its absorptive role: it absorbs bile salts, which are essential for proper digestion. Because the liver is forced to make more bile salts, it is so busy doing this that it does not have time to produce the LDL.

Soluble fiber is further recognized to contribute to low-glycemic index meals and thus helps to promote normal blood glucose and insulin levels.

Foods high in soluble fiber and insoluble fiber further help reduce CVD as these foods are high in trace minerals and antioxidants.

What Are Plant Stanols?

Plant stanols or stanyl esters are substances now being added to some margarines. They have been shown to lower levels of cholesterol, in part by decreasing the intestinal absorption of cholesterol. There is some concern that the reduced absorption of cholesterol by stanols may also reduce the absorption of other nutrients. To date, they have not been found to significantly decrease absorption of fat-soluble vitamins or beta carotene (Relas et al., 2001).

Depending on dose, plant stanol ester treatment has been shown to reduce serum cholesterol levels by 10% to 33%. Lowered serum cholesterol levels were also a result of reduced secretion of VLDL cholesterol (Volger et al., 2001).

How Can Dietary Intake of Saturated Fat and Cholesterol Be Controlled?

1. Eat no more than one egg yolk per day or no more than four egg yolks a week for those with diabetes or who have shown the need for lower cholesterol intake.
2. Moderate the use of shrimp and limit organ meats for those who have shown the need for lower cholesterol intake.
3. Use fish, skinless chicken and turkey, and veal in most of the meat meals for the week; use moderate-sized portions (3 oz of meat equals the size of a deck of cards) of beef, lamb, pork, and ham less frequently. Substitute low-fat protein foods such as legumes for meat regularly (e.g., red beans and rice or tofu and vegetable stir-fry). Legumes are also very high in soluble fiber.
4. Choose lean cuts of meat, trim visible fat, and discard the fat that cooks out of the meat. Removing the skin from a piece of chicken eliminates about 1 tsp of fat.
5. Avoid deep-fat frying or use an oil that is low in saturated fats (peanut and canola oil are monounsaturated fats) when frying is done.
6. Restrict the use of fatty luncheon and variety meats such as sausage and salami.
7. Instead of butter and cooking fats that are solid or completely hydrogenated, emphasize liquid vegetable oils, such as olive oil and soft or liquid margarines. Cooking with other liquids such as wine, water, broth, or fruit juice will help reduce the fat content of meals.
8. Instead of whole milk and cheeses made from whole milk and cream, use skim or low-fat (1%) milk and low-fat or part-skim milk cheeses.
9. Use more plant foods in place of animal foods. For example, fill up on legumes and vegetables rather than meat. Think of meat as a side dish rather than as the main dish.
10. When shopping, look for food labels with less than 15 g of fat for a meal and less than 3 g of fat for a snack. The level of saturated fat should be less than one third of the total amount of fat per day. An acceptable level of sodium per meal is 800 mg; snack foods should have less than 200 mg of sodium per serving with the daily goal less than 2400 mg of sodium.

WHAT IS THE ROLE OF EXERCISE IN THE MANAGEMENT OF CARDIOVASCULAR DISEASE?

Exercise is a well-known component of weight control. Because obesity is associated with other risk factors found in the development of CVD, exercise should be an integral aspect in both the prevention and the treatment of CVD. Physical activity, including moderate-intensity exercise such as walking, is associated with substantial reduction in risk of stroke. The more exercise, the greater the response noted (Hu et al., 2000).

In addition, regular aerobic exercise (any exercise that makes a person take in more air, such as a brisk walk) is associated with increased levels of

HDL cholesterol and decreased levels of LDL cholesterol and it has been recommended that patients with low HDL levels be encouraged to exercise. One study suggests that regular endurance exercise training may be particularly helpful in men with low HDL, elevated triglycerides, and abdominal obesity (Couillard et al., 2001). This level of exercise is generally considered to be at least 30 minutes of exercise that significantly raises the heart rate at least 3 to 4 times weekly.

Among women with diabetes, increased physical activity, including regular walking, is associated with substantially reduced risk for cardiovascular events (Hu et al., 2001). However, particularly for someone with long-standing diabetes, consultation with a physician before engaging in exercise is advised.

WHAT IS HYPERTENSION AND WHAT IS ITS RELATION TO CARDIOVASCULAR DISEASE?

Hypertension is an elevation of the blood pressure to greater than normal levels, which is generally considered to be more than 140/90 mmHg (the top number is the systolic pressure and the bottom number is the diastolic pressure). Among persons with other CVD risk factors, such as diabetes, the goal for blood pressure is less than 130/85 mmHg. Hypertension damages blood vessels and the lining of arteries. This damage impedes adequate circulation and enhances the build-up of plaque. Hypertension is a common and powerful contributor to all of the major CVDs, including coronary disease, stroke, peripheral artery disease, renal disease, and heart failure. One study noted that in women greater than 45 years of age, 60% of Caucasian women and 79% of African American women have hypertension (Caulin-Glaser, 2000).

What Are the Causes of Hypertension?

Of persons with hypertension, 80% also have other insulin resistance risk factors. This percentage is significant because 1 out of 4 Americans are estimated to have insulin resistance, based on Framingham Study data (Kannel, 2000). The underlying insulin resistance with hyperinsulinemia found in adults, with or without diabetes, is generally believed to increase sodium retention. Because sodium draws fluid, pressure builds up within the cardiovascular system, leading to high blood pressure. Further, hyperinsulinemia promotes hypertension because of the sympathetic overstimulation of the blood vessels. This overstimulation has been referred to as making the walls of blood vessels stiff. Hyperinsulinemia may be a contributing factor to sympathetic nervous stimulation associated with weight gain (Masuo et al., 2000).

In persons with insulin resistance, exercise training is a therapeutic approach that lowers blood pressure, in part by correcting hyperinsulinemia (Kohno et al., 2000). Reducing insulin production via reduced carbohydrate intake may further reduce the incidence of hypertension for those individuals with insulin resistance and the resulting hyperinsulinemia.

What Dietary Treatments Are Used for the Control of Hypertension?

Because obesity is a predisposing factor in hypertension, a low-kilocalorie diet is often prescribed to reduce weight. Although this is the ideal solution, it can be difficult to achieve. However, stabilizing the weight of one who has been experiencing a steady weight gain may achieve the desired outcomes of an improved lipid profile and reduced blood pressure.

Sodium restriction is often recommended. Further adjustments in protein and fluids and sodium intake are made if there is concurrent kidney disease. Sodium restriction improves the effectiveness of diuretic therapy.

Patients who take potassium-depleting diuretics are advised to increase their potassium intake to replenish what is lost in the increased urine volume. Bananas and orange juice are frequently recommended for their potassium content, but many foods are high in potassium. Most fresh vegetables (especially dark green, leafy ones), most fruits, legumes, milk, and fresh meats are good sources of potassium (see Table 5-10) and add only a small amount of sodium to the diet. Physicians should be consulted before using a potassium substitute for salt; individuals on ACE inhibitors should not use salt substitutes containing potassium.

Blood pressure is controlled by increasing the intake of minerals such as potassium, magnesium, and calcium (Resnick et al., 2000). Among adolescents at risk for hypertension, blood pressure was lower in those with higher intakes of a combination of nutrients, including potassium, calcium, magnesium, and vitamins derived from fruits, vegetables, and low-fat dairy products (Falkner et al., 2000).

A diet low in sodium, alcohol, and protein is associated with lower systolic blood pressure. Potassium intake is associated with both lower systolic and diastolic blood pressure (Hajjar et al., 2001). Findings confirm that among older adults there is a significant relationship overall between systolic blood pressure and mortality over 6 years of follow-up in both whites and African Americans. Diastolic pressure was a risk factor for whites only (Blazer et al., 2001).

A low-saturated fat and high-soluble fiber intake may also lower blood pressure, probably through reduced insulin resistance. The **Dietary Approaches to Stop Hypertension (DASH) diet** is similar to the Food Guide Pyramid, but with increased emphasis on vegetables and fruits (4 to 5 servings of each) and whole grains. The DASH diet also advocates inclusion of nuts and legumes. This approach promotes increased intake of potassium, calcium, and magnesium while promoting decreased intake of sodium. Exercise, alcohol reduction, and weight loss have further significant blood pressure lowering effects (Miller et al., 1999).

What Are the Purposes and Indications for Sodium-Controlled Diets?

There are several reasons for restricting sodium intake (see Chapter 4 to review information on this mineral). The indications for restricting sodium intake include the following:

1. Hypertension (to relieve elevated or high blood pressure)
2. **Congestive heart failure (CHF)** (a condition in which the heart cannot pump blood adequately)

3. **Edema** (a condition of fluid build up, which can be treated by helping the body to eliminate sodium and fluids)
4. Renal disorders with edema
5. Adrenocorticotropic hormone and cortisone therapy
6. Cirrhosis of the liver with ascites (a disease often caused by alcoholism, but also derived from other causes)
7. The Dietary Guidelines for Americans of 2400 mg of sodium per day

What Is a Sodium-Restricted Diet?

A sodium-restricted diet is a normal adequate diet with a modified sodium content, from a very low amount of 1000 to 3000 mg.

An average diet prepared in the kitchen with some commercially prepared foods, foods salted during cooking, and some salt added at the table provides about 3000 to 7000 mg of sodium daily. (These numbers should not be confused with salt intake—sodium composes 40% of salt. One teaspoon of salt contains about 2000 mg of sodium.) For therapeutic purposes, sodium intake may vary from 1000 mg daily to 2000 mg or more. Diets in which sodium is limited were formerly called low-salt diets, when salt was omitted only in the preparation of food, and salt-free diets, when it was not allowed either in cooking or at the table. Such diets are now named in terms of the level of sodium restriction, the most usual being the 2000 to 4000 mg sodium diet (mild restriction), the 1000 mg sodium diet (moderate), and the 500 mg sodium diet (very strict and seldom used). Table 8-3 shows the differences among sodium-restricted diets for different sodium levels. See Chapter 4 for more information on sodium.

Although the initial elimination of salt from the diet is very difficult for a person used to its taste, the taste for salt can be unlearned. Use of spices, herbs, lemon juice, or vinegar can help enhance the taste appeal of food while the preference for salt is changing.

WHAT IS THE ROLE OF DRUG THERAPY IN THE MANAGEMENT OF CARDIOVASCULAR DISEASE?

Drug therapy certainly has a place in the management of CVD. However, because all medications have potential negative side effects, medical nutrition therapy, such as the AHA Step I Diet or the TLC Diet, should be the first step in CVD management. If hypercholesterolemia does not respond to medical nutrition therapy as provided by a registered dietitian, several medications may be prescribed that are used in conjunction with medical nutrition therapy for the greatest effect. The level of elevated lipids also dictates the drug of choice, as some medications lower total cholesterol and LDL cholesterol, whereas others lower triglyceride levels.

The role of hormone replacement therapy for postmenopausal women to prevent CVD is currently being debated. Previous research had shown that estrogen helped prevent CVD, but newer research shows no significant effect among women with established CHD (Bittner, 2000).

TABLE 8-3
SODIUM-RESTRICTED DIETS

FOODS	2-4 g SODIUM	1 g SODIUM
Milk	3 c milk or yogurt, no processed cheese; natural cheese (1 oz) can replace 1 c milk; free use of low-sodium cheese	2 c milk or yogurt; up to 1 oz natural cheese can be substituted for 1 c milk; free use of low-sodium cheese
Meat and meat substitutes	Limited use of processed meats; free use of fresh meat	No processed meat; use salt-free canned tuna; limited use of regular peanut butter; free use of low-sodium peanut butter
Breads and cereals	Avoid breads and crackers with salt topping; regular bread may be used in normal amounts; free use of low-sodium bread and cereal products; avoid canned soups and vegetables and cereals with added salt	Up to 2 slices regular bread may be used or 1 serving regular processed cereal; free use of low-sodium breads and cereals
Vegetables and fruits	All fresh, frozen, and dried; all canned fruit but limited use of canned vegetables; free use of low-sodium canned vegetables; no salted products such as potato chips or French fries	Use only low-sodium canned vegetables; limited use of naturally high-sodium vegetables (beets, carrots, celery, spinach); free use of all others
Condiments:		
Sweets		
Brown sugar	Free use	Free use
Table sugar	Free use	Free use
Honey	Free use	Free use
Jams and jellies	Free use	Free use
Maple syrup	Free use	Free use
Molasses	Free use	Free use
Sauces:		
Catsup	Limited use	Use low-sodium
Mayonnaise	Limited use	Use low-sodium
Mustard	Limited use	Use low-sodium
Soy sauce	Limited use	Use low-sodium
Worcestershire sauce	Limited use	Not allowed
Butter/margarine	Limited use	Use low-sodium
Other:		
Cooking oil	Free use	Free use
Vinegar	Free use	Free use
Spices:		
Natural	Free use	Free use
Salt-based	Limited use	Not allowed
Lemon	Free use	Free use
Horseradish	Free use	Limited use
Salt	Very limited use (few sprinkles)	Use salt substitute (physician approval)

WHAT IS THE ROLE OF THE NURSE OR OTHER HEALTH CARE PROFESSIONAL IN THE PREVENTION AND CONTROL OF CARDIOVASCULAR DISEASE?

The nurse and other health care professionals are important team members in the fight against CVD. A large body of evidence reinforces the belief that nutritional changes can lower the risk of CVD. Yet many individuals either are not aware of how to make appropriate dietary changes to help prevent CVD or believe that the cost of change is greater than the results accrued. The nurse has the opportunity through direct patient contact to assess the reasons that various individuals may not be following the general CVD reduction guidelines.

A health care professional can assess whether lack of knowledge is the reason for poor dietary compliance by saying, "You probably have heard about cholesterol and saturated fat in television commercials, but are you aware of which foods contain high amounts?" Sometimes a negative attitude or belief may be the reason for not making dietary changes. To assess this, a good question would be, "How do you feel about all the talk concerning cholesterol?"

Through positive reinforcement of steps taken, no matter how small, and referral to appropriate services, the nurse and other health care professionals can play a key role in reducing this society's primary health risk.

CHAPTER STUDY QUESTIONS AND CLASSROOM ACTIVITIES

1. Interview family members regarding personal family history of CVD and hypertension. Use Figure 8-3 to determine your personal risk factors for heart disease.
2. List traditional ethnic foods from your family's meals (those your grandparents ate or those that are currently consumed); which foods do you like to eat that are low in saturated fat and high in soluble fiber?
3. Collect samples of vegetable oils, including at least one that is predominantly a saturated fat, one that is a monounsaturated, and one that is a polyunsaturated fat, and refrigerate all of them. Compare textures to determine the degree of solidity. Which ones are cardioprotective?
4. Taste-test low-sodium food products. Compare these foods with different seasonings, such as spices, herbs, lemon, and jelly.
5. List 20 everyday foods and then read food labels of these foods to determine saturated fat and sodium content.
6. Evaluate your family's saturated fat intake according to food labels. Does your family eat foods that contain trans fatty acids? What are some alternatives?
7. What could you recommend for a lunch for someone who is employed at a construction work site and has dyslipidemia and hypertension? What could you recommend for a dessert for such a person?

H   E   A   R   T

Everyone plays the game of health whether he wants to or not. What is your score? Add up the numbers in each category that most nearly describe you.

Heredity	1 No known history of heart disease	2 One relative with heart disease over 60 years	3 Two relatives with heart disease over 60 years	4 One relative with heart disease under 60 years	6 Two relatives with heart disease under 60 years
Exercise	1 Intensive exercise, work, and recreation	2 Moderate exercise, work, and recreation	3 Sedentary work and intensive recreational exercise	5 Sedentary work and moderate recreational exercise	6 Sedentary work and light recreational exercise
Age	1 10-20	2 21-30	3 31-40	4 41-50	6 51-65
Lb	0 More than 5 lb below standard weight	1 ±5 lb standard weight	2 6-20 lb overweight	4 21-35 lb overweight	6 36-50 lb overweight
Tobacco	0 Nonuser	1 Cigar or pipe	2 10 cigarettes or fewer per day	4 20 cigarettes or more per day	6 30 cigarettes or more per day
Habits of eating fat	1 0% No animal or solid fats	2 10% Very little animal or solid fats	3 20% Little animal or solid fats	4 30% Much animal or solid fats	5 40% Very much animal or solid fats

Your risk of heart attack:
4-9 Very remote	16-20 Average	26-30 Dangerous
10-15 Below average	21-25 Moderate	31-35 Urgent danger—reduce score!

Other conditions—such as stress, high blood pressure, and increased blood cholesterol—detract from health and should be evaluated by your physician.

FIGURE 8-3 Risk factors in heart disease. (Courtesy of the School of Public Health, Loma Linda University, Loma Linda, Calif.)

8. Bring some family recipes to class. Assess whether these recipes contribute to heart disease because they are high in saturated fat, or sodium, or both. How could the recipes be modified to lower the fat and sodium content?

9. Assess your diet needs on the National Heart, Lung, and Blood Institute web page (www.nhlbi.nih.gov/chd/).

CRITICAL THINKING

Case Study

Well, now I am having a stress test, Tony thought to himself. He had stress all right: stress from all these doctors, tests, health problems, and too much to do at work to be leaving, once again. "But," he said to himself, "I could have a grandson soon." His new daughter-in-law had announced she was pregnant. He then reminded himself that he wouldn't mind another granddaughter either. His doctor had decided that he was at high risk for a heart attack, or worse, he could be left paralyzed from a stroke. This was because he had diabetes, high blood pressure, high triglycerides, and was overweight. He decided he would just have to get used to taking care of himself better because he did want to be around for a long time. He had done a lot over the years, thanks to his first dietitian back home who had taught him about carbohydrate counting to control his diabetes. Slipping from good eating habits was so easy, though.

Critical Thinking Applications

1. List Tony's risk factors for CVD.
2. How might a health care professional promote or lessen Tony's stress level?
3. What is the level and type of fats that may help prevent CVD for Tony? List some examples.
4. Describe the type of diet that Tony should be following.

REFERENCES

Almario RU, Vonghavaravat V, Wong R, Kasim-Karakas SE: Effects of walnut consumption on plasma fatty acids and lipoproteins in combined hyperlipidemia. Am J Clin Nutr. July 2001; 74(1):72-79.

Ascherio A, Rimm EB, Giovannucci E, Willett WC, Stampfer MJ: Blood donations and risk of coronary heart disease in men. Circulation. January 2, 2001; 103(1):52-57.

Bittner V: Hormone replacement therapy in clinical cardiology. Cardiol Rev. January-February 2000; 8(1):57-64.

Blazer DG, Landerman LR, Hays JC, Grady TA, Havlik R, Corti MC: Blood pressure and mortality risk in older people: comparison between African Americans and whites. J Am Geriatr Soc. April 2001; 49(4):375-381.

Boden WE, Pearson TA: Raising low levels of high-density lipoprotein cholesterol is an important target of therapy. Am J Cardiol. March 1, 2000; 85(5):645-650.

Carpentier Y: Atherosclerosis and micronutrients. Rev Med Brux. September 2000; 21(4):A363-A366. [Article in French.]

Carr ME: Diabetes mellitus: a hypercoagulable state. J Diabetes Complications. January-February 2001; 15(1):44-54.

Caulin-Glaser T: Primary prevention of hypertension in women. J Clin Hypertens (Greenwich). May, 2000; 2(3):204-209.

Chambers JC, Eda S, Bassett P, Karim Y, Thompson SG, Gallimore JR, Pepys MB, Kooner JS: C-reactive protein, insulin resistance, central obesity, and coronary heart disease risk in Indian Asians from the United Kingdom compared with European whites. Circulation. July 10, 2001; 104(2):145-150.

Couillard C, Despres JP, Lamarche B, Bergeron J, Gagnon J, Leon AS, Rao DC, Skinner JS, Wilmore JH, Bouchard C: Effects of endurance exercise training on plasma HDL cholesterol levels depend on levels of triglycerides: evidence from men of the health, risk factors, exercise training and genetics (heritage) family study. Arterioscler Thromb Vasc Biol. July 2001; 21(7):1226-1232.

de Roos NM, Bots ML, Katan MB: Replacement of dietary saturated fatty acids by trans fatty acids lowers serum HDL cholesterol and impairs endothelial function in healthy men and women. Arterioscler Thromb Vasc Biol. July 2001; 21(7):1233-1237.

Diaz-Arrastia R: Homocysteine and neurologic disease. Arch Neurol. October 2000; 57(10):1422-1427.

Eichholzer M, Luthy J, Gutzwiller F, Stahelin HB: The role of folate, antioxidant vitamins and other constituents in fruit and vegetables in the prevention of cardiovascular disease: the epidemiological evidence. Int J Vitam Nutr Res. January 2001; 71(1):5-17.

Falkner B, Sherif K, Michel S, Kushner H: Dietary nutrients and blood pressure in urban minority adolescents at risk for hypertension. Arch Pediatr Adolesc Med. September 2000; 154(9):918-922.

Ford ES, Liu S: Glycemic index and serum high-density lipoprotein cholesterol concentration among US adults. Arch Intern Med. February 26, 2001; 161(4):572-576.

Fuhrman B, Rosenblat M, Hayek T, Coleman R, Aviram M: Ginger extract consumption reduces plasma cholesterol, inhibits LDL oxidation and attenuates development of atherosclerosis in atherosclerotic, apolipoprotein E-deficient mice. J Nutr. May 2000; 130(5):1124-1131.

Hajjar IM, Grim CE, George V, Kotchen TA: Impact of diet on blood pressure and age-related changes in blood pressure in the US population: analysis of NHANES III. Arch Intern Med. February 26, 2001; 161(4):589-593.

Hemstrom O: Per capita alcohol consumption and ischaemic heart disease mortality. Addiction February 2001; 96 (Suppl 1):S93-S112.

Hofmann MA, Lalla E, Lu Y, Gleason MR, Wolf BM, Tanji N, Ferran LJ Jr, Kohl B, Rao V, Kisiel W, Stern DM, Schmidt AM: Hyperhomocysteinemia enhances vascular inflammation and accelerates atherosclerosis in a murine model. J Clin Invest. March, 2001; 107(6):663-664.

Hu FB, Stampfer MJ, Colditz GA, Ascherio A, Rexrode KM, Willett WC, Manson JE: Physical activity and risk of stroke in women. JAMA. June 14, 2000; 283(22):2961-2967.

Hu FB, Stampfer MJ, Rimm EB, Manson JE, Ascherio A, Colditz GA, Rosner BA, Spiegelman D, Speizer FE, Sacks FM, Hennekens CH, Willett WC: A prospective study of egg consumption and risk of cardiovascular disease in men and women. JAMA. April 21, 1999; 281(15):1387-1394.

Hu FB, Stampfer MJ, Solomon C, Liu S, Colditz GA, Speizer FE, Willett WC, Manson JE: Physical activity and risk for cardiovascular events in diabetic women. Ann Intern Med. January 16, 2001; 134(2):96-105.

Hudgins LC: Effect of high-carbohydrate feeding on triglyceride and saturated fatty acid synthesis. Proc Soc Exp Biol Med. December 2000; 225(3):178-183.

Hughes S: Novel risk factors for coronary heart disease: emerging connections. J Cardiovasc Nurs. January 2000; 14(2):91-103.

Imhof A, Froehlich M, Brenner H, Boeing H, Pepys MB, Koenig W: Effect of alcohol consumption on systemic markers of inflammation. Lancet. March 10, 2001; 357(9258):763-767.

Jacques PF, Bostom AG, Wilson PW, Rich S, Rosenberg IH, Selhub J: Determinants of plasma total homocysteine concentration in the Framingham offspring cohort. Am J Clin Nutr. March 2001; 73(3):613-621.

Jeerakathil TJ, Wolf PA: Prevention of strokes. Curr Atheroscler Rep. July, 2001; 3(4): 321-327.

Jones D, Basile J, Cushman W, Egan B, Ferrario C, Hill M, Lackland D, Mensah G, Moore M, Ofili E, Roccella EJ, Smith R, Taylor H: Managing hypertension in the southeastern United States: applying the guidelines from the Sixth Report of the Joint National Committee on Prevention, Detection, Evaluation, and Treatment of High Blood Pressure (JNC VI). Am J Med Sci. December 1999; 318(6):357-364.

Kannel WB: Risk stratification in hypertension: new insights from the Framingham Study. Am J Hypertens. January 2000; 13(1 Pt 2):3S-10S.

Kohno K, Matsuoka H, Takenaka K, Miyake Y, Okuda S, Nomura G, Imaizumi T: Depressor effect by exercise training is associated with amelioration of hyperinsulinemia and sympathetic overactivity. Intern Med. December 2000; 39(12):1013-1019.

Krajcovicova-Kudlackova M, Blazicek P, Babinska K, Kopcova J, Klvanova J, Bederova A, Magalova T: Traditional and alternative nutrition—levels of homocysteine and lipid parameters in adults. Scand J Clin Lab Invest. December 2000; 60(8):657-664.

Liu S, Lee IM, Ajani U, Cole SR, Buring JE, Manson JE: Intake of vegetables rich in carotenoids and risk of coronary heart disease in men: the Physicians' Health Study. Int J Epidemiol. February 2001; 30(1):130-135.

Liu XQ, Li YH: Epidemiological and nutritional research on prevention of cardiovascular disease in China. Br J Nutr. December 2000; 84 (Suppl 2):S199-203.

Masuo K, Mikami H, Ogihara T, Tuck ML: Weight gain-induced blood pressure elevation. Hypertension. May 2000; 35(5):1135-1140.

McKinley MC, McNulty H, McPartlin J, Strain JJ, Pentieva K, Ward M, Weir DG, Scott JM: Low-dose vitamin B_6 effectively lowers fasting plasma homocysteine in healthy elderly persons who are folate and riboflavin replete. Am J Clin Nutr. April 2001; 73(4):759-764.

Meigs JB, Mittleman MA, Nathan DM, Tofler GH, Singer DE, Murphy-Sheehy PM, Lipinska I, D'Agostino RB, Wilson PW: Hyperinsulinemia, hyperglycemia, and impaired hemostasis: the Framingham offspring study. JAMA. January 12, 2000; 283(2):221-228.

Miller ER Jr, Erlinger TP, Young DR, Prokopowicz GP, Appel LJ: Lifestyle changes that reduce blood pressure: implementation in clinical practice. J Clin Hypertens (Greenwich). November 1999; 1(3):191-198.

Mori TA, Bao DQ, Burke V, Puddey IB, Watts GF, Beilin LJ: Dietary fish as a major component of a weight-loss diet: effect on serum lipids, glucose, and insulin metabolism in overweight hypertensive subjects. Am J Clin Nutr. November 1999; 70(5):817-825.

Rasmussen ML, Folsom AR, Catellier DJ, Tsai MY, Garg U, Eckfeldt JH:A prospective study of coronary heart disease and the hemochromatosis gene (HFE) C282Y mutation: the atherosclerosis risk in communities (ARIC) study. Atherosclerosis. February 15, 2001; 154(3):739-746.

Relas H, Gylling H, Miettinen TA: Acute effect of dietary stanyl ester dose on post-absorptive alpha-tocopherol, beta-carotene, retinol and retinyl palmitate concentrations. Br J Nutr. February 2001; 85(2):141-147.

Resnick LM, Oparil S, Chait A, Haynes RB, Kris-Etherton P, Stern JS, Clark S, Holcomb S, Hatton DC, Metz JA, McMahon M, Pi-Sunyer FX, McCarron DA: Factors affecting blood pressure responses to diet: the Vanguard study. Am J Hypertens. September 2000; 13(9):956-965.

Salas J, Lopez Miranda J, Jansen S, Zambrana JL, Castro P, Paniagua JA, Blanco A, Lopez Segura F, Jimenez Pereperez JA, Perez Jimenez F, Pereperez JA: The diet rich in mono-unsaturated fat modifies in a beneficial way carbohydrate metabolism and arterial pressure. Med Clin (Barc). February 26, 2000; 114(7):249.[Article in Spanish.]

Vasankari T, Fogelholm M, Kukkonen-Harjula K, Nenonen A, Kujala U, Oja P, Vuori I, Pasanen P, Neuvonen K, Ahotupa M: Reduced oxidized low-density lipoprotein after weight reduction in obese premenopausal women. Int J Obes Relat Metab Disord. February 2001; 25(2):205-211.

Volger OL, van der Boom H, de Wit EC, van Duyvenvoorde W, Hornstra G, Plat J, Havekes LM, Mensink RP, Princen HM: Dietary plant stanol esters reduce VLDL cholesterol secretion and bile saturation in apolipoprotein e*3-leiden transgenic mice. Arterioscler Thromb Vasc Biol. June 2001; 21(6):1046-1052.

Zacharski LR, Chow B, Lavori PW, Howes PS, Bell MR, DiTommaso MA, Carnegie NM, Bech F, Amidi M, Muluk S: The iron (Fe) and atherosclerosis study (FeAST): a pilot study of reduction of body iron stores in atherosclerotic peripheral vascular disease. Am Heart J. February 2000; 139(2 Pt 1):337-345.

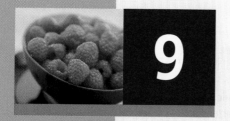

9 Diabetes Mellitus

OBJECTIVES

After completing this chapter, you should be able to:

- Describe the different types of diabetes mellitus.
- Describe the symptoms and clinical findings of diabetes mellitus.
- Relate the nutritional management of diabetes mellitus to the Dietary Guidelines for Americans and the Food Guide Pyramid.
- Explain differences in the nutritional management of the various forms of diabetes.
- Describe the importance of the self-monitoring of blood glucose.
- Explain the role and special concerns of exercise in diabetes management.
- Describe the role of health care professionals in facilitating the nutritional aspects of diabetes management.

TERMS TO IDENTIFY

Acanthosis nigricans
Albuminuria
Antibodies
Autoimmune disease
Autonomic neuropathy
Beta cells
Carbohydrate counting
Certified Diabetes Educator (CDE)
Counterregulatory hormones

Dawn phenomenon
Diabetes mellitus
Diabetic coma
Diabetic retinopathy
Endocrinology
15:15 rule
1500 rule
Food exchange lists
GAD antibodies
Gastroparesis

Gestational diabetes mellitus (GDM)
Glucagon
Glycated
Glycemic index
Glycogenolysis
Glycosuria
Hemoglobin
Hemoglobin$_{1c}$ (HbA$_{1c}$)
Honeymoon period

Continued

INTRODUCTION

Tremendous strides have been made in our understanding of the pathophysiology and management of diabetes since the outcomes of the Diabetes Control and Complications Trial (DCCT) study were released in 1993. Progress in cellular metabolism and gene identification has further contributed to a better understanding of diabetes. As science and technology continue to advance, there will be further developments in the prevention of both diabetes and its associated complications. This is an exciting time to be practicing in this field of **endocrinology** (the study of hormones).

As you may recognize by now, diabetes is generally the final outcome of the insulin resistance syndrome. At least, this is true for Type 2 diabetes, formerly referred to as adult-onset diabetes. Once a person is no longer capable of producing large amounts of insulin to compensate for the resistance at the cell level, the result is **hyperglycemia**, or high blood glucose (BG).

Type 2 diabetes is reaching epidemic proportions worldwide. This is related to changing lifestyles and diets with increased rates of obesity and decreased physical activity. Historically, juvenile-onset diabetes, now referred to as Type 1 diabetes, was distinguished by age. This is no longer the case. Type 2 diabetes now accounts for about one third of all cases of diabetes among children. Type 2 diabetes is occurring in all population groups, especially in ethnic minorities and among youth, is an emerging public health problem (Fagot-Campagna et al., 2000).

All health care professionals, especially nurses, should become thoroughly versed in the management of diabetes. Very few people know that diabetes is related to heart disease, stroke, kidney disease, hypertension, blindness, and nerve damage with circulation problems. Health care professionals can play a vital role in educating the public about diabetes, especially those at risk of developing diabetes. Prevention is the ultimate goal.

WHAT ARE THE BASIC FACTS ABOUT DIABETES MELLITUS?

The Latin derivation of the term **diabetes mellitus** means simply, "sweet urine." Diabetes, commonly referred to by the public as "having sugar," is a serious metabolic disorder related to the utilization of carbohydrate and its end product, glucose (blood sugar). The metabolism of protein and fat is affected by diabetes as well. According to the American Diabetes Association, diabetes affects approximately 16 million individuals in the United States, or 5% of the total population and up to 15% of the elderly population. Of the 1 in 20 Americans who have diabetes, only about half know they have it. Mortality statistics of diabetes are underrated because most people with diabetes die from related causes such as heart disease.

In 1997, the American Diabetes Association released updated criteria to two fasting plasma glucose (FPG) levels of 126 mg/dL or greater to diagnose diabetes. This level of FPG has been found equivalent to the 200 mg/dL value in the oral glucose tolerance test for diagnosis. It is recommended that screening for diabetes should start at age 45 and be repeated every 3 years in persons without risk factors and earlier and more often in those with risk factors, such as family history or other insulin resistance correlates (Gavin, 1998). Screening for Type 2 diabetes is important because of its slow and gradual development, which is often asymptomatic.

ETIOLOGY

Type 1 Diabetes

Type 1 diabetes is an **autoimmune disease**. Simply said, an autoimmune disease occurs when a person's immune system gets confused and starts attacking itself. In the case of Type 1 diabetes, the **beta cells**, which produce insulin in the pancreas, are attacked by the body's immune system. This may be verified by serum lab tests for **antibodies** (the part of the immune system that is mobilized for destruction of perceived foreign invaders in the body). The destruction causes eventual loss of all insulin production.

The peak age of Type 1 diabetes onset is during puberty, but it can occur at any age. Winter months are a peak time of onset of Type 1 diabetes. It is believed that the body's exposure to a viral illness can precipitate the development of the autoimmune process in susceptible individuals. The onset of this type of diabetes is usually sudden and severe. The person with Type 1 diabetes has most, if not all, of the clinical signs and symptoms at the time of diagnosis that will be discussed in following sections.

Persons with Type 1 tend to have few relatives with diabetes, but do have the genetic predisposition for its development. Persons with Type 1 diabetes often have family members with other forms of autoimmune diseases. Higher rates of Type 1 diabetes are generally found among persons with family heritage from northern latitudes. Type 1 diabetes is relatively rare in relation to Type 2 diabetes, occurring in about 5% to 10% of all cases of diabetes.

Figure 9-1 shows the differences between Type 1 and Type 2 diabetes. Verifying the existence of diabetes autoimmune markers is sometimes used to distinguish Type 1 diabetes from Type 2 diabetes. However, one study found almost one third of children with newly diagnosed Type 2 diabetes had positive **GAD antibodies** (an antibody specific to diabetes). Absence of diabetes autoimmune markers is not a prerequisite for the diagnosis of Type 2 diabetes in children and adolescents (Hathout et al., 2001).

The GAD antibody is just one of many antibodies the body is capable of producing. Antibodies are produced when the body perceives a foreign substance, to attack and destroy the substance. The GAD antibody specifically targets the insulin-producing cells of the pancreas, ultimately causing the cessation of insulin production.

Type 2 Diabetes

Type 2 diabetes, previously referred to as non–insulin-dependent diabetes mellitus (NIDDM), is chiefly caused by insulin resistance at the cell level. Type 2 diabetes is no longer correctly referred to as NIDDM because of the confusion surrounding the term. The confusion began when a person with Type 2 diabetes started taking insulin. This did not mean that the person went from being a NIDDM to an insulin-dependent (IDDM). To prevent further confusion, the American Diabetes Association officially dropped the NIDDM versus IDDM classification and prefers the numerical designation of Type 1 for autoimmune diabetes and Type 2 diabetes for all nonautoimmune forms of diabetes.

There are varying amounts of insulin production in Type 2 diabetes: high, normal, or low. A person with Type 2 diabetes who is underproducing insulin is generally thin and sometimes referred to unofficially as Type 1½. Typically, a person with Type 2 diabetes is actually overproducing insulin and has the associated central obesity. It is the insulin resistance at the cell level that can allow both hyperglycemia and hyperinsulinemia.

Heredity plays a critical role in the development of Type 2 diabetes. Persons with this form of diabetes generally have many family members with a history of diabetes and the other correlates of the insulin resistance syndrome. The genetic predisposition and incidence of Type 2 diabetes increase in persons whose ancestors are from regions nearer the equator, with the highest prevalence being among persons of African, Native American, Asian, Pacific Island, and Southern European heritage, such as the Hispanic population. Asian Indians have a high rate of diabetes, but low rates of obesity. They do, however, have high **waist-to-hip ratios (WHR)** (waist measurement divided by hip measurement) with high levels of insulin resistance and hyperinsulinemia.

There is a great deal of evidence that links a more Westernized lifestyle (a low-fiber, high-fat, and high-sugar diet with low levels of physical activity) with the development of Type 2 diabetes. However, the genetic predisposition toward diabetes must be present before diet and obesity can cause diabetes.

There are a variety of environmental elements that allow the genetic predisposition to insulin resistance to be realized as Type 2 diabetes. For example, an

	Insulin-Dependent	Non–Insulin-Dependent
Gender:	Males and females	Increased rate among females.
Ethnicity:	Increased rates among persons with Northern European heritage.	Increased rate among persons with heritage from equatorial countries (highest rates found with Native American, Hispanic, African American, Asian, Pacific Islander, Mediterranean).
Age of Onset:	Generally under 30 years with peak onset before puberty.	Generally over 40 years, although the genetic predisposition is inherited and onset may be seen at younger ages.
Weight:	Usually normal or underweight; unintentional weight loss often precedes diagnosis.	Usually overweight, but may be of normal weight.
Treatment:	Insulin injections necessary to prevent death. Food and exercise have to be balanced with insulin injections.	Weight loss is usually the first goal. Reduction of sugar and fat and increase of fiber (soluble) helpful. Oral hypoglycemic agents or insulin or both may be necessary for good blood sugar management but are not necessary to prevent imminent death. Exercise important.
Beta Cell* Functioning:	Totally absent (no insulin is produced) after the "honeymoon period": residual insulin is produced for about 1 year after diagnosis.	Excess insulin production usually evident (hyperinsulinemia), but due to insulin resistance at the cell level, there is relative insulin insufficiency. Insulin production may also be normal or below normal.

*Beta cells are found in the pancreas.

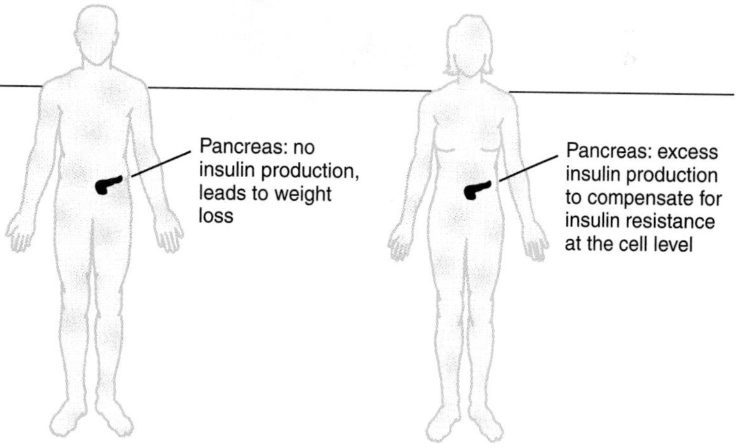

Pancreas: no insulin production, leads to weight loss

Pancreas: excess insulin production to compensate for insulin resistance at the cell level

FIGURE 9-1 Differences between Type 1 and Type 2 diabetes mellitus.

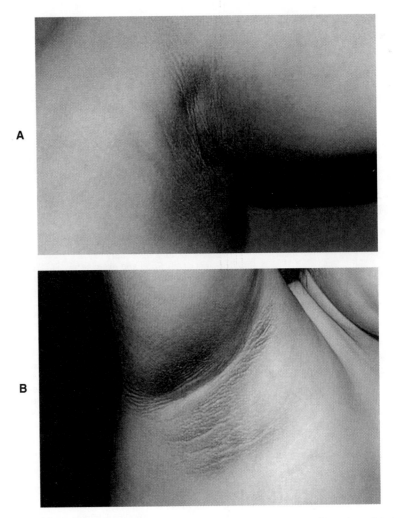

FIGURE 9-2 Acanthosis nigricans. (From Callen JP, Greer KE, Paller AS, and Swinyer LJ: Color atlas of dermatology, ed 2, Philadelphia, 2000, WB Saunders.)

increased risk for Type 2 diabetes in male and female smokers has been associated with insulin resistance (Ostgren et al., 2000). One study found that the lower the intake of vegetables and fruits, the greater the likelihood of the development of diabetes (Ford and Mokdad, 2001).

A skin condition called **acanthosis nigricans** (Figure 9-2) is a risk factor for diabetes. In this condition there is a thickening of the skin, usually in the body folds, which takes on a gray, brown, or black pigmentation. Hyperinsulinemia and central obesity are also risk factors for diabetes. A study in New Mexico found the estimated prevalence of hyperinsulinemia among middle school students was about 9%. A total of 47% of students who had acanthosis nigricans were obese and had hyperinsulinemia. Screening for acanthosis nigricans is an easily performed, noninvasive method for identifying adolescents at risk for Type 2 diabetes (Mukhtar et al., 2001).

MANAGEMENT OF DIABETES

Type 1 Diabetes

Without insulin, life cannot exist. In the days before the discovery of injectable insulin, persons with Type 1 diabetes simply wasted away from malnourishment. It is for this reason that Type 1 diabetes is an IDDM form of diabetes. Control is accomplished only through insulin injection with structured meals and exercise. Persons taking insulin are best advised to consult with **Certified Diabetes Educators (CDEs)**(health care professionals who specialize in diabetes management and are required to pass an exam every 5 years to prove continued proficiency) on insulin adjustment.

An inadequate amount of insulin leads to ketoacidosis quickly and makes a person very ill. **Ketoacidosis** is an acidic state caused by a rapid breakdown of body fat. During the first year after diagnosis of Type 1 diabetes, there may be a temporary period of insulin production before the beta cells completely exhaust their production. This is referred to as the **honeymoon period**. Thus a person with newly diagnosed Type 1 diabetes may find that he or she needs little or no insulin after early treatment of hyperglycemia. Patients should be forewarned that this situation will change as the honeymoon period comes to an end.

Because onset typically begins in childhood, management issues become complex. The complete lack of natural insulin production makes the balancing of food and exercise with insulin injection a challenge. Regular BG monitoring is required for optimal health. There is great stress on the family to care for a child with diabetes. Sibling relationships can suffer. Diabetes summer camp programs, in which acceptance of the disease and management strategies are emphasized, can be very helpful for families.

Type 2 Diabetes

Among persons at risk for diabetes, it was found that the risk of diabetes was reduced by over half with weight loss of about 10 lbs with reduced intake of fat and saturated fat and increased intake of fiber and physical activity (Tuomilehto et al., 2001). Consumption of low-fat dairy products is associated with lower incidence and mortality of Type 2 diabetes and lower blood pressures (Schrezenmeir and Jagla, 2000). Improvements in the quality of diet and level of activity, without actual weight loss, often allows normal glucose levels to be realized.

A person with Type 2 diabetes who uses insulin for good BG management may be able to decrease or discontinue insulin treatment eventually if there is good dietary and exercise management. An oral diabetes medication, metformin, brand name Glucophage, may also be used in Type 2 diabetes, with or without insulin. Metformin has been shown to improve glycemic control without weight gain. If insulin is already being used and metformin is added, about one-third less insulin is required by injection (Fritsche et al., 2000).

Reduction of stressors such as infection, burns, and surgery is also important for BG management without having to rely on injected insulin. Thus a person with Type 2 diabetes may need temporary use of insulin while hospitalized for surgery or during times of illness.

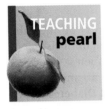

TEACHING pearl

The analogy of a coal stove is useful to explain insulin resistance and can further be related to the coal and shovel for insulin needs. Consider each body cell to be a microscopic coal stove. Thus we are made up of millions of furnaces waiting to use the carbon found in carbohydrate foods for our fuel source (you may recall that mitochondria within the cells act like furnaces). The insulin acts as the shovel to put the carbon (coal), into the body cells (coal stoves) so that it can be used for energy.

If the door on the coal stove does not open easily, it is difficult to get the coal inside the stove. This is like insulin resistance at the cell level, generally found with Type 2 diabetes. In regard to the coal stove, if the door cannot be opened, there is no way to get the coal inside. Consequently, the fire will go out. In relation to the body cells, if glucose cannot easily enter, the body simply makes more insulin in an attempt to force the fuel inside.

In Type 2 diabetes small, frequent, carbohydrate meals (like several small shovels of coal over the course of the day) are more efficiently burned for fuel. This allows the glucose levels to even out, preventing both hyperglycemia from small meals and hypoglycemia by including snacks between meals.

In the case of Type 1 diabetes, the doors of the body cells may open up, but there is no shovel to move the coal. Hence insulin by injection, like the coal shovel, is required to move the fuel. However, if there is a very small shovel and a very large bucket of coal, it will be a long time before the fuel level is back to normal. Alternatively, if there is a very large shovel, but a small bucket of coal, the fuel is going to run out quickly. In regard to glucose, **hypoglycemia** (low BG level) can occur if there is too much insulin (too large of a shovel) in relation to low carbohydrate intake (small bucket of coal). For Type 1 diabetes management this is described as the insulin-to-carbohydrate ratio (big shovel for a big bucket; small shovel for a small bucket of coal).

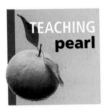

TEACHING pearl

Another useful analogy is to refer to hyperinsulinemia as "an army of insulin." In other words, if one soldier cannot get into the fort, you call out an army. Use of insulin by a person with Type 2 diabetes is like calling in the navy as well. By reducing insulin resistance, a person with Type 2 diabetes can send the navy home or may potentially be able to stop insulin by injection. This is not true for Type 1 diabetes, except in the honeymoon phase.

Maturity Onset Diabetes of Youth

This form of diabetes is just now beginning to be understood. **Maturity onset diabetes of youth (MODY)** is a form of diabetes that develops in younger adults, but is similar to Type 2 diabetes. It may or may not require insulin therapy. In practical terms, there are no set criteria for the diagnosis of MODY. An endocrinologist may use clinical judgment to make this diagnosis. The bottom line is whatever works to keep BG levels normalized is appropriate. The major distinction of MODY versus Type 1 diabetes is that Type 1 will always require insulin use in the long run. This form of diabetes may or may not require insulin.

Impaired Fasting Glucose (Impaired Glucose Tolerance)

Although impaired glucose tolerance (IGT) has been referred to in the past as borderline diabetes, it is now a diagnosis, based on lab values. An oral glucose tolerance test may be used to diagnose IGT. An alternative, **impaired fasting glucose (IFG)**, is diagnosed when FPG is greater than 110 mg/dL (diabetes being two fasting blood glucose [FBG] values greater than 126 mg/dL). Treatment remains the same as that for Type 2 diabetes (see the following sections).

Gestational Diabetes

Gestational diabetes mellitus (GDM) is a temporary form of diabetes that occurs during the latter part of pregnancy. It is often found in women with a family history of Type 2 diabetes and thus is generally related to the genetic predisposition to insulin resistance. Because it occurs after fetal development (see Chapter 12), the risk for birth defects is different than for a woman who has Type 1 or preexisting Type 2 diabetes. There is virtually no difference in pregnancy outcomes for a woman who has GDM or Type 1 or Type 2 diabetes, as compared with a woman without diabetes, if near normal BG is achieved before conception and maintained at near normal levels throughout the pregnancy. Increased placental hormones produced during the latter stages of pregnancy, which work counter to insulin (see the section on counterregulatory hormones), are the primary cause of GDM.

Weight loss is not an appropriate goal for the woman with gestational diabetes because of the growth needs of the developing fetus. Diet control focuses on slow but steady weight gain, avoidance of concentrated sugar sources (because they are high in carbohydrate content), and frequent, small, balanced meals. A prescribed kilocalorie-restricted diet is generally unnecessary and can even be harmful unless the patient understands that the kilocalorie restriction is for control of weight gain, not for weight loss.

The blood sugar goals during pregnancy are very strict (the goal for all BG levels, including postprandial, are less than 120 mg/dL. However, if a plasma glucose meter is used, this equates to a 15% high value or 135 mg/dL 2 hours after meals). Self-monitoring of blood glucose (SMBG) is essential, as is checking for morning urine ketones. Occasionally a woman with GDM will require insulin to maintain good control of blood sugar levels. The detection of ketones may signal the need for more carbohydrates (such as when a woman with GDM tries too aggressively to lower carbohydrates in an attempt to avoid the use of insulin). If the need for carbohydrates to prevent ketone formation results in hyperglycemia, insulin will be required until the time of delivery. See Chapter 12 for more information on diabetes and pregnancy.

Reactive Hypoglycemia

In **reactive hypoglycemia**, excess carbohydrates cause the body to produce too much insulin. However because the overproduction of insulin is delayed, the BG level first rises too high and then falls too quickly (Figure 9-3 shows the difference between hyperglycemia and hypoglycemia). This form of glucose intolerance may be a precursor to the development of diabetes.

Reactive hypoglycemia is characterized by serum glucose levels that fall in the range of 50 to 60 mg/dL, with symptoms of hypoglycemia (Box 9-1) that are relieved by eating. The symptoms progress as the BG level falls or when it reaches a low level. Persons with uncontrolled diabetes may experience feelings of hypoglycemia at normal levels of BG until their body has time to adjust to a lower, more normal level of BG.

The person with reactive hypoglycemia needs to eat small amounts of carbohydrates (about 30 to 50 g) frequently (every 3 hours). Including a protein

BOX 9-1
COMMON SYMPTOMS THAT SIGNAL HYPOGLYCEMIA

Weakness
Mental confusion
Headache
Clammy skin
Physical tremors
Rapid heart beat
Double or blurred vision

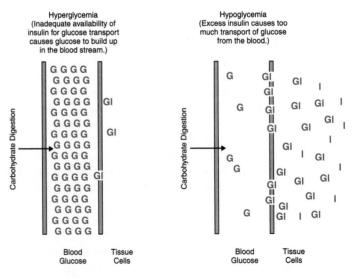

FIGURE 9-3 Hyperglycemia and hypoglycemia.

source with meals and snacks helps to maintain appropriate BG levels because it slows carbohydrate digestion, causing only minimal stimulation of insulin secretion (Box 9-2 lists high-protein snack ideas). The need for protein to be included with the carbohydrate is based on individual symptoms. Caffeine and alcohol may exacerbate the symptoms of hypoglycemia because of their effect on liver glycogen and **glycogenolysis** (the breakdown of glycogen into glucose).

WHAT ARE THE SYMPTOMS AND CLINICAL FINDINGS OF DIABETES?

The warning signs of diabetes are unusual thirst; frequent urination; abnormal hunger; sudden weight loss (which usually indicates Type 1 diabetes, but can also occur in Type 2 diabetes with severe hyperglycemia); skin disorders, infections such as vaginal yeast infection, and delayed wound healing; blurred vision; and unexplained weakness and fatigue.

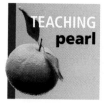

TEACHING pearl

A good assessment question to ask a patient is whether he or she has to get up in the middle of the night to use the bathroom and how often. Persons with undiagnosed diabetes are often relieved to hear they can again expect an uninterrupted night's sleep with improved BG control. This can motivate patients to adhere to medical nutrition therapy and exercise prescriptions.

BOX 9-2
HIGH-PROTEIN SNACK IDEAS FOR REACTIVE HYPOGLYCEMIA*

Graham cracker with peanut butter
Apple or banana slices with peanut butter
Celery with peanut butter
Part-skim cheese and crackers
Nuts and raisins (small amount of raisins)
Low-fat cottage cheese and fruit
Unsweetened fruit juice and cheese
Half sandwich (meat, peanut butter, or cheese)
Hard-cooked egg and small glass of low-fat milk
Hot cereal with melted peanut butter
Cold cereal with bite-sized chunks of peanut butter and low-fat milk
Half of a bagel and light cream cheese
Parmesan muffin (English muffin with liquid margarine or olive oil and parmesan cheese—fresh grated parmesan is delicious)
Half a cantaloupe stuffed with low-fat cottage cheese

*Regular meals should be reduced in portion sizes to compensate for the added kilocalories consumed through snacks. Regular meals also need to be balanced, including a protein source and excluding large quantities of concentrated sweets. Snacks should be consumed about 2 to 3 hours after regular meals.

Hyperglycemia

Hyperglycemia is associated with the complications of diabetes. It also causes many of the symptoms of diabetes. Blurred vision can be caused when excess sugar in the eye changes the shape of the lens. Infections increase with hyperglycemia because the body's immune system does not work as efficiently. There are conditions under which the body's BG levels rise normally, such as stress of infection, illness, or surgery. Postprandial hyperglycemia may be an independent risk factor for the development of diabetic complications (Palumbo, 2001). **Retinopathy** (a disease of the eye) and **nephropathy** (a disease of the kidneys) were directly related to higher FPG (greater than 126 mg/dL) or 2-hour plasma glucose (greater than 200 mg/dL) which identifies those at high risk of microvascular disease and mortality (Gabir et al., 2000).

Glycosuria

One way the body tries to lower blood sugar is to flush it out the kidneys, which results in **glycosuria** (glucose in the urine). Frequent urination and thirst are often associated with hyperglycemia. The level of blood sugar generally has to rise unacceptably high (more than 180 mg/dL) before glucose is detected in the urine. This is referred to as the **renal threshold**. Thus glycosuria tests are generally not recommended except as an easy screening test and for those persons who refuse, or are unable, to test blood sugars.

Ketonuria

Without insulin, carbohydrates are unavailable for energy utilization. Instead, the body calls on fat as an energy source. Under normal conditions, the liver breaks down small amounts of fatty acids to form ketones. These ketones are further metabolized for energy. In uncontrolled diabetes, ketone production exceeds utilization. The excess is excreted in the urine. This is known as **ketonuria**. If the excess ketones are not removed adequately, the condition known as ketoacidosis develops. In ketoacidosis, the blood pH changes to a more acidic level, which can cause death. Treatment should be prompt and hospitalization will be needed if blood becomes too acidic. This condition generally occurs in Type 1 diabetes, but it can also occur in persons with Type 2 diabetes who are producing large amounts of counterregulatory or stress hormones, such as with infection or surgery.

Dehydration

The excess fluid loss associated with high levels of BG causes water to be taken from body tissues. This can result in dehydration if water is not replaced and blood sugar controlled. Dehydration with concentrated amounts of glucose in the blood can cause a condition known as **hyperglycemic hyperosmolar nonketotic syndrome (HHNK)**. This condition is commonly found in elderly patients, in whom diabetes is much more prevalent and in whom there is a diminished sensation of thirst because of the aging process. Because dehydration of the brain can occur, many elderly patients with HHNK have a history of lethargy, sleepiness, and confused state lasting from several days to weeks before progressing into a coma. Dehydration and HHNK are easily treated if caught in the early stages. All older patients, but especially those with diabetes, should be taught the importance of adequate water intake even when they are not thirsty.

Polydipsia and Polyuria

Increased thirst, known as **polydipsia**, is experienced as the body senses the need to replace excess fluids lost from frequent urination (**polyuria**). This is an attempt by the body to remove excess ketones and glucose.

Polyphagia

Increased appetite, known as **polyphagia**, is the body's response to the need for energy. However, this need is not being satisfied because carbohydrates are not available for energy. This can be another sign that a person has undiagnosed diabetes. A health care professional should inquire about a person's appetite and whether it has changed. Polyphagia may cause weight gain.

Weight Loss

Because the sugar is staying in the blood and is not used for energy, a feeling of fatigue, hunger, and weight loss can be associated with hyperglycemia. Glucose that does not enter the body cells is excreted in the urine with excess ketones. Both represent wasted energy sources. Weight loss results because the energy demand exceeds available sources. This is more likely to happen with Type 1 diabetes or in severe cases of Type 2 diabetes in which there is insufficient or no insulin production.

WHAT ARE MEASURES OF GOOD DIABETES MANAGEMENT?

Self-Monitoring of Blood Glucose

Self-monitoring of blood glucose (SMBG) is a form of treatment in the sense that the patient can take responsibility for diabetes management. Self-monitoring consists of taking a drop of blood and placing it on a strip that is inserted into a BG meter. Several types of meters are available, as are automatic lancet devices. Patients should be given information on available meters so that they can select the one that best suits their needs. Recommended times to test BG levels include before meals and 1 to 2 hours postprandially to identify responses to carbohydrate content and other meal factors such as time of day (breakfast will often raise BG more than meals consumed at other times of the day because of the dawn phenomenon, discussed later). This is referred to as **pattern management** because patterns may be noted that give an indication of when hyperglycemia or hypoglycemia may be predicted based on SMBG and food and activity records.

Typically, a meal can be expected to raise the blood sugar by 40 to 50 points. With a fasting blood sugar level of 100 mg/dL, an ideal meal should keep the blood sugar level to about 150 mg/dL. If the blood sugar level goes higher than this, it indicates either excess carbohydrates in the meal, per individual needs, or a need for medication.

The advantage of SMBG is the knowledge and flexibility it affords in diabetes management. Less guesswork is involved and SMBG allows the diabetic patient greater objectivity in decision making to prevent both hyperglycemia and hypoglycemia.

Alternatives to finger sticks for BG monitoring do exist. Increasingly, persons with diabetes are using their forearm to measure glucose levels. A continuous glucose sensor has been developed that works by having a biosensor inserted just below the surface of the skin. Eventually this system will be designed to "talk" with an insulin pump, thus serving as an artificial pancreas. Other devices and means to monitor glucose levels continue in the development stage.

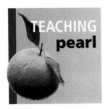

TEACHING pearl

Questions such as "How do I adjust my diet and insulin for exercise?" or "Can I eat a piece of birthday cake safely?" can be addressed through SMBG. For example, a person might find that a half piece of birthday cake with his or her evening meal may raise blood sugar to an acceptable level. If blood sugar goes above 200 mg/dL two hours after eating the cake, the person might consider not eating more.

Ketone Checks

All persons with diabetes should know about ketones. Ketones form from the breakdown of body fat when there is inadequate insulin, inadequate carbohydrate, or both. For women with GDM, ketones should be checked daily upon rising in the morning. Individuals with Type 1 diabetes should test for ketones whenever their blood sugar is over 240 mg/dL on two or more occasions or when they are ill. Ketones are particularly important to assess during illness, when the likelihood of elevated BG and dehydration occurs. Symptoms of nausea, vomiting, and deep labored breathing may be signs of impending ketoacidosis. Ketonuria (ketones in the urine) is treated with insulin (medical guidance needs to be sought) and increased water intake with moderate amounts of carbohydrate. If ketone production is acutely elevated, hospitalization will be required.

What Is Hemoglobin A₁c and What Is Its Role in Diabetes Management?

Most people know that hemoglobin is a component of the red blood cells used to carry oxygen throughout the body. The amount of **hemoglobin A₁c (HbA₁c)**, a subfraction of hemoglobin, measures the attachment of glucose to hemoglobin (see Figure 9-4 for correlations between HbA₁c and average BG). The glycated proteins (body proteins attached permanently to glucose) are believed to

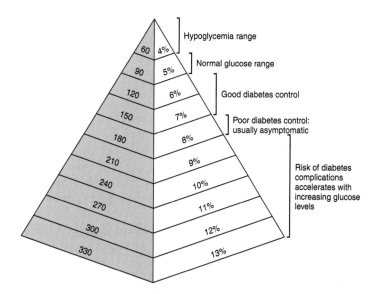

FIGURE 9-4 Hemoglobin A_{1c} and average BG goals.

be a major cause of complications of diabetes. Frequent daily BG measurement, using a BG meter, is still important both to measure hypoglycemia and to assess the amount of carbohydrate per meal or per insulin unit that is appropriate for good BG management.

Testing for HbA_{1c} is recommended every 3 months because the hemoglobin molecule lives for about 3 months. This test provides the average glucose readings over a 3-month period. The goal is to see improvement, or lowering, in HbA_{1c} levels and to maintain a normalized level of HbA_{1c} (less than 7%), thereby reducing long-term diabetic complications. Persons with retinopathy (a form of eye disease, discussed later) are advised to attain a reduction of no more than 2 percentage points per year in HbA_{1c} because of concerns that the retinopathy may worsen and possibly result in blindness if BG levels are treated too rapidly.

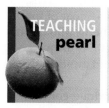

TEACHING
pearl

The glycosylation of protein found in body cells can be described as body cells being carmelized. Envisioning carmelized apples may help a person recognize this is not a healthy situation.

Lipid Screening

Lipid (blood fat) abnormalities go hand in hand with poor control of diabetes. An increased level of BG is believed to contribute to these abnormalities, with insulin resistance and hyperinsulinemia. A high level of triglycerides (more than

150 mg/dL) with an associated low level of high-density lipoprotein cholesterol (less than 40 mg/dL) is generally found in persons with uncontrolled Type 2 diabetes. The cholesterol and low-density lipoprotein cholesterol may or may not be elevated. However, even if the LDL cholesterol is normal, there is a tendency toward small, dense LDL particles that are more likely to cause cardiovascular disease. There is usually improvement in the blood lipids as diet, weight, and BG levels are improved. Medication is sometimes needed as well.

Albuminuria Screening

All patients with diabetes mellitus should have their urine tested for albumin. Persons who have had Type 1 diabetes for more than 5 years and all persons with Type 2 diabetes should be tested annually because the person may have had diabetes for many years before the diagnosis. **Albuminuria** (albumin in the urine) is associated with advancing kidney disease and should be treated aggressively with ACE inhibitors (a form of blood pressure medication). Once **macroalbuminuria** (very large amounts of albumin in the urine) occurs, a moderate protein intake of 0.8 g of protein per kilogram of body weight is advised, with reduction in sodium intake (2 g of sodium are generally adequate) if the person has concomitant hypertension.

WHAT IS INTENSIVE INSULIN MANAGEMENT?

The term intensive insulin management was coined during the DCCT in 1993, when it was first proven and reported that achieving near normal BG reduced diabetes complications by upwards of 75% in persons with Type 1 diabetes. These results were found by achieving average BG levels of less than 155 mg/dL. To achieve this level of BG control safely, without increased risk for severe hypoglycemia or hyperglycemia, the study participants were taught to give insulin in three daily injections (to try to imitate how Mother Nature provides insulin) or by insulin pump. It is now recommended that insulin injection be more frequent in an attempt to better mimic the way insulin is normally produced. Normally the body produces small amounts around the clock with increased amounts each time we eat a meal containing carbohydrate. The goal of intensive insulin therapy is the normalization of blood sugar. All patients who use insulin should know when the peak time of action for their insulin is likely to occur. This knowledge will allow them to plan a meal or snack and avoid exercise at these times.

By additionally altering insulin dose based on the carbohydrate content of meals, more stable and desirable BG levels can be achieved. **Carbohydrate counting** is a form of medical nutrition therapy whereby a person with diabetes can learn how to adjust short-acting insulin (called "Regular" or "R" or Humalog, "Lispro" insulin) based on the person's varying intake of carbohydrate. See Box 9-3 for an easy method to estimate carbohydrate content of plant-based foods based on level of water, level of sweetness, and density.

BOX 9-3
CARBOHYDRATE COUNTING

GRAINS AND STARCHY VEGETABLES (15 G OF CARBOHYDRATES)
3 c popcorn
1 c puffed cereals
½ c pasta, *dry vegetable* (potato, beans) or *sweet vegetable* (corn, peas, winter squash)
1 slice bread or 1 oz equivalent (½ c)
⅓ c rice
¼ c *dry/sweet vegetable* (yams or "sweet potato")

FRUITS (15 G OF CARBOHYDRATES)
1 c high water-content fruits (melon and berries)
½ c *most fruits*
¼ c most dried fruits
½ banana
⅛ c dry/sweet fruits (raisins or dried banana chips)

MILK (~15 G OF CARBOHYDRATES)
1 c milk or yogurt (unsweetened)

LOW-CARBOHYDRATE VEGETABLES (5 G OF CARBOHYDRATES)
1 c raw vegetables (high in water/low in sweetness)
½ c cooked vegetables (high water/low sweetness)
(Do not count carbohydrates unless = 15 g or more)

CONCENTRATED CARBOHYDRATE SOURCES
1 tsp sugar = 4 g of carbohydrates
½ c sugar = 95 g of carbohydrates
1 tbsp flour = 5 g of carbohydrates
½ c flour = 45 g of carbohydrates

What Is Insulin and How Is It Produced?

Insulin is a hormone that is produced in the beta cells of the **islets of Langerhans** found in the **pancreas**; it is produced in response to hyperglycemia. Because insulin is composed of protein, oral intake of insulin is not possible because it would be digested before being used. Thus persons taking oral diabetes medication are not taking insulin, but rather are using the medication to help their own natural insulin production work more effectively (such people are diagnosed as having Type 2 diabetes because they are producing insulin).

Insulin allows BG into body cells where it can be burned for energy. The body will normally produce small amounts of insulin at all times because it is needed to metabolize carbohydrates for the continual energy necessary to sustain life. This type of background insulin, used in Type 1 diabetes management, will be

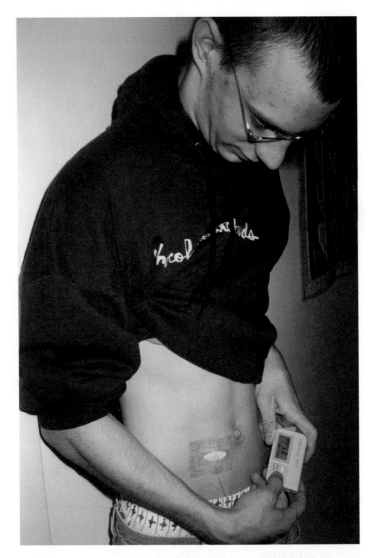

FIGURE 9-5 Mature adolescents can easily work with an insulin pump.

referred to as either the "basal rate" with insulin pumps (Figure 9-5) or the "long-acting" insulin types used with injections such as NPH insulin. Larger amounts of meal-related insulin are normally produced in the pancreas in relation to carbohydrate consumption. Thus "meal bolus insulin," using short-acting insulins, is now being used in relation to the carbohydrate content of the meals in both the insulin pump and by injection with a syringe. This is referred to as the **insulin-to-carbohydrate ratio**, which is usually 1:15—1 unit of short-acting regular insulin is given for every 15 g of carbohydrate. Individuals using this approach need to work closely with CDEs and registered dietitians to verify their individual ratio (which can range from a low of 1:3 to a high of 1:30 or higher for children) before they start adjusting their insulin dose on their own.

A new form of long-acting insulin, called glargine, brand name Lantus, is hoped to help replace NPH or Ultralente insulin that both have **peak action** times (when the insulin works at its peak or most rapid time of action). Lantus is essentially peakless and works for about 24 hours; it is generally advised to be injected at bedtime.

The short-acting insulin Humalog is generically referred to as Lyspro because the amino acids lysine and proline are switched in the insulin molecule. This form of short-acting insulin works very rapidly because the insulin tends not to form hexamer crystals and is able to get into the bloodstream more quickly. The result is that Lyspro (Humalog) insulin enters the bloodstream in 5 to 15 minutes (versus 30 minutes with the "R" short-acting insulin), has a peak action time of 1 hour (versus 2-3 hours with regular short-acting insulin), and is totally cleared from the body in about 3 to 5 hours. One study demonstrating the effectiveness of Humalog insulin noted that supper-time use, as compared with "R" insulin, allowed improved postprandial BG levels and significantly lower occurrence of night-time hypoglycemia (Zinman, 2000). Persons changing from "R" insulin to Humalog insulin need to be alerted to different peak action times and to symptoms of ketonuria.

How Is Insulin Prescribed?

Only health care professionals licensed to prescribe can alter insulin doses. Other health care professionals can advise a person with diabetes to seek medical opinion on dose changes as noted by review of SMBG records. Dosage changes might also be considered if specific guidelines have been reviewed with the person's physician, such as when a dietitian might advise a particular insulin dose based on verified insulin to carbohydrate ratios. Generally a long-acting insulin (such as NPH or "N" insulin) is given in the morning and at bedtime, and short-acting, regular or "R" or Humalog insulin is given at breakfast and dinner. The person with Type 2 diabetes who is not able to produce enough insulin to compensate for the cell's insulin resistance may be given a long-acting insulin in one to two injections.

Insulin pumps (see Figure 9-5) only use the short-acting "R" or Humalog insulin. Persons transferring to a pump will likely need about 75% of their usual dose of insulin, which is generally divided with half for the basal rate and half for the meal bolus needs. For example, a person on 60 units of insulin by injection will need about 45 units on the pump (75%). About half of this dosage is given in the basal rate (22 units divided by 24 hours or 0.9 units given per hour via the insulin pump). The other half is used to cover mealtime carbohydrates, based on the insulin-to-carbohydrate ratio the individual requires.

The amount of hourly basal insulin needed in insulin pumps is tested to verify that the BG level remains stable. The basal rate can be slowly increased or decreased by about 0.1 unit per hour based on individual needs. Often an increased basal rate is needed to cover the dawn phenomenon (discussed later) with lower basal rates for other times of the day. A temporary increase in basal rate may be needed during times of illness. Once basal rates are set correctly, the person using the pump can safely have a great deal of flexibility in timing of meals and amounts eaten if the insulin-to-carbohydrate ratio is accurately determined and applied.

Insulin pump therapy is increasingly being used for Type 1 diabetes because it allows for flexibility in lifestyle and improved management of glucose. It is also used for women with diabetes during pregnancy. Women who began pump therapy in pregnancy were highly likely to continue pump use after delivery and preferred the flexibility that this treatment allowed (Gabbe et al., 2000).

How Is the Insulin-to-Carbohydrate Ratio Determined?

By using SMBG records, the effect of a given amount of carbohydrates consumed for the number of units of short-acting or regular insulin given can be determined. The goal is for the BG to rise no higher than about 50 points (mg/dL) after meals. Generally 1 to 2 hours after meals will be the highest BG level, except if Humalog insulin is used, in which case the peak BG is noted in about 45 minutes after meals. After 4 to 5 hours, if the BG level ends up where it started before the meal (give or take 20 to 30 points), simple math tells you the outcome. For example, if these BG goals are achieved and 45 g of carbohydrates were consumed in a meal with 3 units regular insulin given, the ratio is 1:15. This needs to be repeated more than once to verify it is correct because many variables will affect BG levels.

Persons with Type 2 diabetes generally look at the total amount of carbohydrates consumed per meal that allow for these same goals. By reducing postprandial hyperglycemia, HbA$_{1C}$ goals can be better achieved with reduction in complications of diabetes. Controlling postprandial BG excursions may further allow for decreased use of insulin or oral diabetes medications.

What Is the 1500 Rule?

The **1500 rule** is an estimate that is used to determine expected point drop of BG per unit of insulin. This formula is used for additional insulin needed to correct hyperglycemia. It replaces the old sliding-scale insulin regimen. The 1500 rule is used by counting up the usual amount of total units of insulin (including both long-acting and short-acting insulins) and dividing the number of total units of insulin into the number 1500. If a person is using the short-acting insulin Humalog, the total daily units of insulin is divided into the number 1800. For example, a person who takes 100 units of insulin will have an expected BG point drop of 18 points per 1 unit of Humalog insulin. Or, if the total number of daily units of insulin is 30 units, the expected point drop for each additional unit of insulin is 60 points (1800 ÷ 30 units = 60 point drop). This can be applied to correct hyperglycemia, but needs to be done with medical guidance to assess the cause of the hyperglycemia. A potentially fatal result can occur unless the person understands the effect of insulin for his or her individual needs.

What Other Hormones Are Involved in Diabetes Management?

Several **hormones** (chemicals produced by the body that regulate body functioning) act in concert to regulate BG levels. Insulin, produced in the pancreas, is the only hormone that lowers BG levels. Many hormones act to raise glucose levels, the most important being glucagon, epinephrine (also called adrenalin), cortisol, and growth hormone. These are called **counterregulatory hormones** because they work in an opposite manner to insulin. Any deviation in the balance of these hormones will cause fluctuations in BG levels.

Abnormal levels of counterregulatory hormones can have a variety of effects that relate to good health. For example, there is an increased rate of depression with diabetes related to excess levels of cortisol (Weber et al., 2000). Because cortisol interferes with the use of insulin, elevated glucose levels can occur. The impaired insulin sensitivity and resultant hyperinsulinemia are also related to depression (Okamura et al., 2000).

The **Somogyi effect** may be noted with an increased production of the counterregulatory hormones in response to hypoglycemia. The implication is that hyperglycemia often follows hypoglycemia. In other words, a low blood sugar count is often followed by high blood sugar. This effect can be noted when patients record their BG levels. Explaining the Somogyi effect to patients who are on insulin is important because they may try to correct hyperglycemia with more insulin. Taking more insulin starts a roller-coaster effect on BG. If the Somogyi effect can be determined, a decreased insulin dose may best stop further hyperglycemia. This is because the underlying cause of hypoglycemia is being corrected and the body will stop producing the excess in counterregulatory hormones.

The **dawn phenomenon** occurs commonly for both types of diabetes and is related to increased production of cortisol and growth hormone (both counterregulatory hormones) in the early morning hours. It is believed that the body produces these hormones to wake up. The consequence is that the morning BG will rise, even without eating. Further, a person with Type 2 diabetes or GDM may require smaller amounts of carbohydrates at breakfast to prevent postprandial hyperglycemia. The person with Type 1 diabetes may require a different insulin-to-carbohydrate ratio at breakfast than at other meals, or those on insulin pumps may require a higher basal rate of insulin in the early morning hours.

Persons taking insulin should be prescribed a glucagon kit that a family member or co-worker can be taught to use if the person with diabetes becomes unconscious from severe hypoglycemia. **Glucagon** is a counterregulatory hormone normally produced by the body in response to hypoglycemia, but a person who is receiving insulin by injection may also need glucagon by injection. When a person is unconscious or unable to swallow because his or her nerves have lost their energy source, oral intake of carbohydrate or sugar is not recommended. The glucagon kit contains a syringe with sterile water that is mixed in a vial with a glucagon tablet and injected after being dissolved. The person receiving the medication should be rolled on his or her side in case of vomiting.

WHAT ARE THE CAUSES, SYMPTOMS, AND TREATMENT OF HYPOGLYCEMIA?

Either insulin or certain **oral hypoglycemic agents** (also called diabetes pills) can cause the blood sugar to drop below a point at which the body can function. Symptoms of hypoglycemia when no diabetes medication is being taken are not life threatening and generally can be resolved naturally, through the release of stored glycogen in the liver. In the presence of excess alcohol in the blood, the breakdown of glycogen is impaired, which may result in hypoglycemia.

Individuals with hypoglycemia may begin to perspire; they may experience hunger and nervousness; their skin may become pale, cold, and clammy; and they may experience mental confusion, physical tremors, weakness, headache, rapid heart beat, numbness in the tongue, and double or blurred vision (see Box 9-1). Hypoglycemia also alters mood states, for example, inducing depression and anxiety that may be persistent with recurrent episodes of severe hypoglycemia (Strachan et al., 2000).

When symptoms of hypoglycemia are noted, the blood sugar level should be checked to verify hypoglycemia. However, not all individuals with diabetes experience these symptoms, especially children, elderly persons, or persons who have frequent episodes of hypoglycemia. The latter can be resolved by meticulous prevention of hypoglycemia for at least 2 weeks. Modest amounts of caffeine increase the symptoms of hypoglycemia in patients with Type 1 diabetes (Watson et al., 2000). The health professional or close family member should suspect hypoglycemia, and treat it accordingly, when a diabetic child becomes unusually quiet or fretful or when the adult diabetic patient becomes weak or faint. A physician should be consulted if the cause is not readily apparent or if hypoglycemia occurs frequently.

The treatment for a person who can swallow is to give 15 g of a rapid-acting carbohydrate source, such as 4 oz of orange juice, 4 tsp of sugar mixed in water, or three to four glucose tablets (Box 9-4). Liquid sources of sugar will correct hypoglycemia the most quickly. The carbohydrate has to get through the stomach before it can significantly affect blood sugar levels. The blood sugar should be rechecked in 15 minutes and the procedure repeated until the blood sugar returns to normal. This is referred to as the **15:15 rule**. For severe hypoglycemia, the amount of carbohydrate may be increased to 30 g of carbohydrate because every 15 g of carbohydrate only raises the BG level up to 50 points (mg/dL). Squeezing cake icing or honey inside the cheek is appropriate only if the person is alert enough to swallow.

A person may or may not need a follow-up snack to maintain glucose levels in the normal range after correcting hypoglycemia with the 15:15 rule. With experience in using SMBG, a person may better gauge the necessity of having a snack. As a general guideline, if the next meal will be several hours later, such as in the middle of the night, it may be beneficial to have a more substantial snack (half of a sandwich).

If the person becomes unconscious, glucagon can be injected or an intravenous solution of glucose may be administered in the hospital or ambulance

BOX 9-4
PORTIONS FOR DIETARY TREATMENT OF HYPOGLYCEMIC EPISODES IN CONSCIOUS PERSONS

15 G CARBOHYDRATE
3 oz apple juice
4 oz orange juice
5 oz regular soda pop
4 tsp honey
4 tsp sugar
¼ c sherbet

30 G CARBOHYDRATE
6 oz apple juice
8 oz orange juice
10 oz regular soda pop
8 tsp honey
8 tsp sugar
½ c sherbet

The 15:15 rule: Check blood sugar; if low (less than 70 mg/dL) treat with 15 g of carbohydrates. Recheck blood sugar in 15 minutes; if still low repeat with another 15 g of carbohydrates. If the blood sugar is severely low (less than 50 mg/dL) treat with 30 g of carbohydrates and recheck in 15 minutes.

setting. Long-term treatment includes diet, activity, insulin modification (the chart on page 284 shows factors that raise or lower BG levels), or education to help prevent future episodes

Hypoglycemia can result in a severe headache, sometimes referred to as a diabetic headache. This may be caused by the release of histamine from either hypoglycemia or dehydration. The basal ganglia (located in each hemisphere of the brain) can release high amounts of histamine as needed for many central nervous system functions (Brown et al., 2001). Increase in hypothalamic histamine release may be a response to loss of glucose as a fuel source. Histamine may be involved in the regulation of energy metabolism in the brain (Oohara et al., 1994).

WHAT IS THE NUTRITIONAL MANAGEMENT OF DIABETES?

Meal Planning

Balanced meals are helpful in the management of diabetes and in the promotion of health. This is true for anyone with insulin resistance, whether or not the person has diabetes.

Pure carbohydrate meals will raise the blood sugar level faster because carbohydrates are digested in 1 hour or less. Including at least a small amount of protein or unsaturated fat with a meal or snack will slow down the process of digestion, thereby limiting its affect on blood sugar and staving off hunger. A meal containing protein and fat generally is considered to have a low-glycemic index. Although the macronutrient carbohydrate has the greatest effect on postprandial BG levels, a diet rich in plant foods will provide a variety of trace minerals and phytochemicals. In particular, legumes, nuts, whole grains, vegetables, and fruits contain naturally occuring phytochemicals and have other natural antioxidants that have been associated with the protection and treatment of chronic diseases including diabetes, heart disease, and hypertension.

In the past, meals were planned using **food exchange lists**. It is important to be aware of this type of meal planning, but carbohydrate counting is a simpler, and thus more effective, meal plan approach. The complete exchanges take into account the protein, fat, and carbohydrate content of foods, which makes meal planning more complicated than needed because carbohydrates have the greatest effect on BG levels. In the food exchange system there is a similar carbohydrate content in the food groups. A person who has learned the food exchange system in the past will find it an easy transition to carbohydrate counting. One serving of any food may be exchanged for another serving in the same list. The full exchange list is shown in Appendix 9. It is important that the diet be individually planned to facilitate patient compliance, thus dissemination of preplanned diet guides is not in the best interest of persons with diabetes.

Fallacy: A person with diabetes needs to learn the Exchange System and the number of kilocalories in food.

Fact: Health professionals who continue to instruct persons with diabetes only on the Exchange System or who place them on a specific kilocalorie diet are doing a disservice to the person. This is outdated guidance. It is much easier for a person to learn the effect of meals on postprandial BG levels, which empowers the person to understand the connection between carbohydrate and BG outcomes. Institutions that provide diabetic meals should base the meals on the carbohydrate content, not on preset kilocalorie levels. Keeping carbohydrates consistent in meals such as 50 g per meal works well for most persons with diabetes. Those who do SMBG can verify how strict or how flexible they can be with meals, and adjust carbohydrate portions accordingly. Persons taking insulin can learn how to match insulin use to carbohydrate intake via SMBG, otherwise called an insulin-to-carbohydrate ratio. See the section on Carbohydrate Counting on next page.

Kilocalories

The amount of kilocalories needed by a person with diabetes should be the same as for a person without diabetes. Adjustments in kilocalories may be necessary to maintain or attain normal body weight and can be made as necessary. Generally, 20 to 30 kcal per kilogram adult body weight is adequate to maintain weight. A 500-kcal reduction from this level should result in a weekly weight loss of 1 lb. The person with Type 2 diabetes is more likely to need to lose weight, whereas the person with Type 1 diabetes is more likely to need to gain weight, especially at the time of diagnosis. Many individuals are not math-oriented. Fortunately, there are many strategies to achieve weight goals (refer back to Chapter 7) that are not related to counting kilocalories. Individual assessment of learning needs and health goals is important before providing nutritional guidance.

Carbohydrate Counting

Carbohydrates are now recognized to be the prime factor in producing meal-related hyperglycemia. The recommended allowance for carbohydrate is generally 50% to 60% of total kilocalories. For an obese woman with gestational diabetes, a carbohydrate restriction of 35% to 40% of kilocalories may be recommended (Major et al., 1998). For the person with Type 1 diabetes, the amount of carbohydrate is based on preferences because the insulin dose can match the carbohydrate intake. Of the total carbohydrate intake, high-fiber foods should be included. Sugar may be tolerated in small quantities and should be counted as part of total grams of carbohydrates in a meal. Four grams of sugar, as listed on food labels, is the same as 1 tsp of sugar. Individuals can determine the effect of table sugar, or sucrose, on their BG level through the use of SMBG. It was found in the DCCT study that the total amount of carbohydrate, versus the type, had the biggest effect on BG levels.

In carbohydrate counting, the person with diabetes learns how many carbohydrates are in foods (see Box 9-3) and aims for a regular amount, such as 50 g with each meal for the person with Type 2 diabetes or based on insulin-to-carbohydrate ratios for the person with Type 1 diabetes. The SMBG is imperative to determine individual needs for carbohydrate.

Fiber promotes normal BG levels after meals by slowing the time of digestion. The recommendation for fiber intake remains the same for persons with diabetes as for the general public: 25 g of fiber for persons requiring 2000 kcal. The recommendation of the Dietary Guidelines for Americans for increased fiber is beneficial not only for the general public, but also for the person with diabetes in particular. A goal of 20 to 30 g of fiber should be promoted, with particular emphasis on legumes and other sources of soluble fiber such as greens and other vegetables, fruits, and grains with a gummy texture.

Although dietary goals for the general public recommend the consumption of three servings of whole grains per day, average consumption in the United States is less than one serving per day. Increasing whole-grain intake in the population can result in improved glucose metabolism and can delay or reduce the risk of developing Type 2 diabetes mellitus (Hallfrisch et al., 2000).

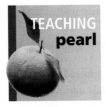

You might say to a person that the old adage "oatmeal sticks to the ribs" is absolutely true. This food can be helpful when a person is trying to prevent his or her postprandial BG level from rising too high. Legumes are also very high in soluble fiber. The Italian phrase "beans and greens" further helps a person remember which foods are high in soluble fiber.

For a person with long-standing diabetes, **gastroparesis** (a form of paralysis of the stomach caused by damage to the nerves leading to its muscles) can occur. A person with gastroparesis may benefit with less insoluble fiber, as found in the skin and seeds of plant-based foods. Insoluble fiber has a crunchy texture. A person with gastroparesis will still benefit with soluble fiber sources because the fiber easily dissolves in the liquid content of the digestive tract.

Sugar substitutes (Table 9-1) are not always preferable. Sugar alcohols, such as sorbitol and xylitol, are often found in dietetic foods; they contain similar kilocalories per gram and can cause the BG levels to rise and thus should not be considered *free foods*. In addition, excess intake may lead to diarrhea. Saccharin, aspartame (NutraSweet), acesulfame-K, and a new sugar-substitute sucralose (Splenda) have no appreciable kilocalorie content in amounts commonly consumed, but may be used in foods that contain other sources of kilocalories, such as fat. These foods may give a person with diabetes the false perception that if the food is sugar-free it is also kilocalorie-free. Fructose, or fruit sugar, has similar effects on BG as other sugars and should be considered as part of the total carbohydrate intake.

Fallacy: Although persons with diabetes need to avoid sugar, they can eat honey without a problem.

Fact: Honey is composed of glucose and fructose, two simple sugars, and as such cannot safely be used freely. Occasional and moderate use, especially by a person who practices SMBG, may be appropriate.

Carbohydrate Distribution

Carbohydrates should be distributed among the meals and snacks according to individual need. A person with insulin resistance generally benefits with about 30 to 50 g of carbohydrates per meals and snacks. On occasion, for a person who has very severe insulin resistance, the guidelines are 15 g of carbohydrates in each of six meals for a total of about 100 g of carbohydrates. The individual guidelines are based on premeal and postmeal BG excursions, or the amount of carbohydrate required to raise the glucose less than 50 points (mg/dL). Individual BG patterns can determine whether snacks are really necessary. A bedtime snack containing carbohydrates for the person with Type 1 diabetes whose BG level is less than 100 mg/dL is generally advised. Distributing carbohy-

TABLE 9-1
NUTRITIVE AND NONNUTRITIVE SWEETENERS*

NAME	COMPOSITION	SOURCES
NUTRITIVE SWEETENERS		
Glucose	Monosaccharide	Found in blood as the end product of starch digestion Occurs naturally in fruit
Fructose	Monosaccharide	Found in fruit and honey
Sucrose	Disaccharide composed of glucose and fructose	Commonly known as table sugar and widely used in commercial foods
Lactose	Disaccharide composed of glucose and galactose	Found in milk and unfermented milk products[†]
Maltose	Disaccharide composed of two glucose molecules	Produced during brewing and bread making; also made commercially
Honey	Mainly fructose and glucose	Made from plants by honeybees
Maple syrup	Primarily sucrose	Made by boiling off the liquid found in sap of mature sugar maple trees
Corn syrup	Composed of glucose molecules of different chain lengths	Produced from cornstarch
High-fructose corn syrup	Contains 40%-100% fructose	Produced enzymatically from cornstarch
Molasses	Contains 50%-75% sucrose	Produced during the processing of table sugar
Sorbitol, mannitol, xylitol	Sugar alcohols	Found naturally in fruit and used as a sugar substitute
Aspartame	Methyl ester of two amino acids: phenylalanine and aspartic acid (aspartate)	Commonly known as NutraSweet and widely used in low-sugar food products; kilocalories are insignificant because small amounts are used because it is intensely sweet—180-220 times as sweet as sucrose
NONNUTRITIVE SWEETENERS		
Saccharin	Organic compound	Originally banned in 1977 after being implicated as causing bladder tumors in rats fed high doses; currently available as a sugar substitute
Cyclamate	Available as cyclamic acid, calcium cyclamate, and sodium cyclamate	Banned since 1969 after evidence showed it as a possible cancer-causing agent in rats; Food and Drug Administration may reconsider its use given more studies on its safety
Acesulfame postassium	Compound that is not metabolized	Approved by Food and Drug Administration in 1988; now used in a wide variety of foods and beverages. 200 times sweeter than sugar. Referred to as acesulfame K on food labels
Sucralose	Compound made from sugar, but not metabolized	Known as Splenda®; used in all types of foods and beverages. Can be used in cooking and baking. 600 times sweeter than sugar

*Nutritive sweeteners are those that provide kilocalories; nonnutritive sweeteners are entirely free of kilocalories because they are not metabolized.
†Lactose as found in milk is not harmful to diabetic individuals.

drates throughout the day will help prevent both hypoglycemic and hyperglycemic reactions.

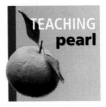

The carbohydrate content of a piece of cake can be determined by looking at the food label of the cake and frosting container based on the portion consumed. A homemade cake can be estimated for carbohydrate content knowing that ½ c of flour contains 45 g of carbohydrates and ½ c of sugar contains 95 g of carbohydrates (see Box 9-3). The amount of carbohydrates found in a given recipe can thus be calculated for the portion consumed. You can estimate the carbohydrate content of any piece of cake based on its level of sweetness. If a piece of cake is about the size of ½ c, it has to have at least 15 g of carbohydrates from the flour (½ c grain-based food is about 15 g of carbohydrates). Depending on the level of sweetness the cake may range from about 30 g carbohydrates (such as a piece of ginger bread type cake) to usually about 50 g of carbohydrates. The cake cannot have 100 g because that would approximate pure sugar, which cake is not.

Protein

The percentage of kilocalories derived from protein should be 10% to 15% with a maximum of 20%. This allows the individual with diabetes from 1 to 1.5 g of protein per kilogram of body weight, which should be appropriate. A level of protein intake at 0.8 g of protein per kilogram body weight or less may be desirable to control kidney disease.

One concern related to protein intake is the fat associated with protein foods. It has been well established that saturated fat as found in red meat and in whole-fat milk products, such as cheese, worsens insulin resistance. One study looked at different types of protein foods and their effect on insulin resistance. It was noted that codfish protein prevents obesity-induced muscle insulin resistance with a high-fat diet. This was in contrast to the high-fat diet with casein (milk protein) that led to severe insulin resistance (Lavigne et al., 2001).

Fat

Fat intake should be individualized based on weight needs, cholesterol levels, and BG needs. For the person with Type 2 diabetes, a high-carbohydrate, low-fat diet can increase blood triglyceride levels, whereas a diet high in monounsaturated fat, but low in saturated fats, can be helpful (Berry, 1997). The omega-3 fatty acids suppress the inflammatory process. The importance of omega-3 fatty acids in immune function has been corroborated by many clinical trials in which patients show improvement when given fatty acid supplementation (Pompeia et al., 2000). The message to eat fish, especially coldwater, fatty fish which are rich in omega-3 fats, should be promoted. This includes codfish, albacore tuna, salmon, herring, sardines, mackerel, blue fish, lake trout, and smelt.

Fallacy: Diabetic individuals must give up the foods they love.

Fact: The rule of moderation applies to both the general public and the diabetic individual in achieving the goal of good nutritional intake. Moderate amounts of all foods are acceptable. All food consists of carbohydrates, proteins, fats, or a combination, and therefore can be worked into the exchange list system. The potential problem with this approach is individual definitions of moderation. Assessment of weight control and SMBG are two methods that can indicate whether moderation is truly moderate. A referral to a registered dietitian is strongly advised to educate persons with diabetes about how to make appropriate changes in their diets and to help manage their diabetes.

Vitamins and Minerals

Vitamins and minerals are essential to the metabolism of energy, which has direct bearing on diabetes as a metabolic disorder. Ultimately, the ideal means to achieve adequate intake of the variety of essential vitamins and minerals is through minimally processed plant-based foods, lean meats, and low-fat milk products.

When there is inadequate intake of vitamins and minerals the metabolism of glucose is diminished. This is true with thiamin and biotin deficiency leading to IGT (Bender, 1999). There is protection against the development of diabetes with whole grains, which provide dietary magnesium (Meyer et al., 2000). The germ portion of the whole grain is rich in a variety of vitamins and minerals that can be protective against diabetes. Pancreatic beta cell death can be prevented or delayed by vitamin B_3, copper, and vitamin E, which are all found in the germ portion of whole grains (Adeghate and Parvez, 2000).

There is some evidence of a higher need for certain vitamins. This is related to the loss of minerals from polyuria or as induced by diuretics such as magnesium. Dark green leafy vegetables, legumes, whole grains, and fish are rich sources of magnesium. A diabetic state can lead to a vitamin B_6-deficiency, in part caused by a magnesium deficiency (Okada et al., 1999). Vitamin B_6 is found in large amounts in liver and whole grains.

Generally speaking, a person with diabetes may take a multivitamin and mineral supplement if good sense is used in the dose (100% to 200% of the DRI) and quality assurance of the supplement is confirmed (refer back to Chapter 4). Very large doses of vitamins and minerals or use of herbs can have a pharmacologic effect and should only be used in conjunction with the advice of a physician.

Can a Person with Diabetes Drink Alcoholic Beverages?

Mixed drinks, liqueurs, and sweet wines should be avoided because of the high content of simple sugars. Beer, hard liquor mixed with water or diet soda, and dry wine may be tolerated in limited quantities, but should be consumed only after consultation with the patient's physician and dietitian.

It is important that the patient eat food containing carbohydrates when having alcohol because alcohol can induce hypoglycemia. Alcohol, in moderation, enhances the action of insulin. However, if alcohol is consumed in conjunction with increased physical activity, the person needs to be alert to symptoms of hypoglycemia. Alcohol intake decreases glucagon significantly, so the person is less able to naturally correct for hypoglycemia (Rasmussen et al., 2001). The person with diabetes should tell a companion that he or she has diabetes in case hypoglycemia develops while drinking alcohol. Hypoglycemia has been mistaken for intoxication. A drink of orange juice would be recommended if a person with diabetes appears inebriated.

How Can a Person with Diabetes Eat at Restaurants?

Restaurant eating poses no problem if there is adequate selection. Simple foods without gravy or other sauces may be desirable and sweets should be avoided or included as part of the meal carbohydrate. Portions might also be controlled by ordering a couple of appetizers rather than the entree, which generally is inappropriately large for persons trying to control their weight and blood sugar. Dessert might be shared with a friend. Eating on the road can be a particular challenge. Low-carbohydrate snack foods might be packed for dealing with the "munchies," whereas other snacks containing carbohydrates are essential for the person taking insulin or other diabetes medication when regular mealtimes may be difficult or impossible to achieve. Persons with Type 1 diabetes need to be instructed on how to make alternative choices of food based on carbohydrate content. The use of carbohydrate counting can allow for a close approximation of the carbohydrate content of foods (refer back to Chapter 2). Many fast food restaurants now make available the nutritional content of their food selections (see Appendix 4).

WHAT IS THE GLYCEMIC INDEX OF FOOD?

Not all carbohydrate foods cause BG levels to rise equally. This is primarily related to the time of digestion and consistency of the meal. Sources of liquid carbohydrate foods, such as juice, raise the BG quickly (which is desirable when treating hypoglycemia). In other words, liquid carbohydrate sources pour through the stomach and rapidly enter the bloodstream. Foods that contain soluble fiber generally leave the stomach slowly because of the gummy texture of these foods. The speed with which food raises BG is referred to as the glycemic index of food. Thus carbohydrate sources that are liquid have a high glycemic index, whereas carbohydrate foods high in soluble fiber, such as legumes, have a relatively low glycemic index. It is generally known that legumes and greens have a lower glycemic index than do root vegetables and grains. High-fiber foods have a lower glycemic index than do low-fiber foods. Foods that are highly processed and easier to digest leave the stomach more quickly and can be described as having a high-glycemic index. For example, cold processed cereal will often raise the BG more rapidly than does oatmeal. Bagels, which are boiled before they are baked, tend to have a high-glycemic index. By using SMBG, persons with diabetes can determine their own glycemic index to foods.

Protein foods that are low in carbohydrates have a lower glycemic index. Fats have the lowest glycemic index. Thus cheese would not be expected to significantly raise the blood sugar, but it is discouraged because of its high saturated fat content and its contribution to insulin resistance and heart disease. Low-fat cheeses are appropriate if the sodium is taken into account.

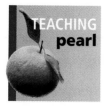

TEACHING **pearl** — To help patients understand glycemic index, you might use the analogy of a gas tank and engine of a car. Liquid sources of carbohydrates, such as juice, soda pop, and even milk, will pour through the stomach quickly or essentially flood the engine. Carbohydrates high in soluble fiber or combined in meals containing proteins and fats, leave the stomach more slowly, or stay in the tank for a longer time.

WHAT IS THE ROLE OF EXERCISE IN DIABETES MANAGEMENT?

Exercise is an integral component of treatment in Type 2 diabetes. It is a factor in weight control and has been found to lower BG levels to the point of reducing or eliminating the need for oral hypoglycemic agents or insulin. The improvement in glucose tolerance and insulin sensitivity induced by endurance or resistance training generally deteriorates within three days of the last exercise session (Albright et al., 2000). All persons, whether diabetic or not, benefit with physical activity to maintain good cardiovascular health.

Because of potential nerve damage from long-standing diabetes, medical input should be sought before engaging in exercise. For example, the heart rate response to exercise may be impaired. This could result in oxygen deprivation if the activity is too strenuous. Children and adults who are on insulin may need to lower their insulin dose while increasing their carbohydrate intake if their physical activity level is greatly increased over usual amounts.

In Type 1 diabetes with a ketotic or hyperglycemic state (when BG level is greater than 240 to 300 mg/dL) exercise can actually increase glucose levels further. This is primarily because insulin is a prerequisite for glucose usage in exercising muscles. Hyperglycemia is generally indicative of insufficient insulin availability. Exercise should be avoided unless BG levels are under control. Even the patient with well-controlled Type 1 diabetes, however, needs to achieve a balance between the extra energy demands of exercise and diet and insulin. The general rule of thumb is to eat at least 15 g of carbohydrates for every 1 hour of exercise as based on weight and intensity of exercise (Table 9-2) to decrease the amount of insulin, or both, and to avoid exercising at the times that insulin is acting at peak levels. These guidelines help prevent the development of severe hypoglycemia, which is caused by excess insulin in relation to the amount of BG available.

The SMBG is a valuable tool for determining the best way to adjust diet and insulin before, during, and after exercise. Increased amounts of carbohydrates

TABLE 9-2
GRAMS OF CARBOHYDRATE USED PER HOUR BASED ON WEIGHT AND EXERCISE

ACTIVITY	GRAMS OF CARBOHYDRATE USED PER HOUR (BASED ON AN INDIVIDUAL'S WEIGHT)		
	100 LB	150 LB	200 LB
Walking (3 mph)	14	21	28
Jogging (5 mph)	30	45	60
Running (7 mph)	52	77	103
Running (9 mph)	69	103	138
Bicycling (5 mph)	13	20	27
Bicycling (10 mph)	30	45	60
Bicycling (15 mph)	52	77	103
Swimming (20 yd/min)	24	36	48
Swimming (50 yd/min)	58	87	117
Gardening (light)	8	12	16
Golf (with golf cart)	9	14	19
Mopping floors	12	18	24
Lawn mowing (power, pushing)	13	19	25
Bowling	13	19	25
Golf (pulling cart)	13	20	27
Scrubbing floors	17	25	33
Softball	17	25	33
Badminton	19	28	37
Horseback riding (trot)	19	28	37
Square dancing	19	28	37
Roller skating	19	28	37
Tennis (doubles)	19	28	37
Volleyball	19	28	37
Raking leaves or hoeing	20	30	40
Ice skating or roller skating	23	34	45
Mini trampoline	23	35	47
Digging a garden	23	35	47
Ice skating (10 mph)	23	35	47
Chopping wood	23	35	47
Dancing (disco)	24	36	48
Mowing (hand mower)	25	38	51
Tennis (singles)	25	38	51
Dancing (square)	29	44	59
Waterskiing	29	44	59
Snow shoveling	30	45	60
Digging ditches	31	46	62
Rock climbing	31	46	62
Dancing (fast step)	31	46	62
Downhill skiing	33	50	67
Basketball (pickup)	39	58	77
Squash	40	60	80
Soccer	40	60	80
Basketball (vigorous)	44	65	87
Racquetball (singles)	60	90	120
Cross-country skiing (6 mph)	70	105	140

From MiniMed Inc., Sylmar, CA.

may need to be consumed for up to 24 hours while the body replenishes its glycogen stores and allows for stable BG.

WHAT ARE COMPLICATIONS OF DIABETES?

Insulin Reaction and Diabetic Coma

Insulin reaction (or insulin shock) occurs when more insulin is injected than is needed. Box 9-4 describes nutritional management of a conscious person. Insulin shock can result from omitting foods from the diet, increasing activity and exercise (which burns more kilocalories than normal), or making an error in insulin injection in relation to exercise. The result is hypoglycemia, a lowering of the BG level. The onset is usually sudden. If the hypoglycemia is not treated promptly, the diabetic patient becomes mentally confused and disoriented. If this situation is prolonged, seizures, unconsciousness, and death can result. All family members should have supplies on hand and know how to inject glucagon to raise blood sugar for an unconscious person. (Glucagon, as discussed earlier, is a counterregulatory hormone that acts to release stored glycogen from the liver, thereby providing a blood sugar source; it is available with a physician's prescription.) Medical services should be sought in the case of insulin shock to help prevent another occurrence.

Diabetic coma is a potential result of ketoacidosis, which is discussed earlier in this chapter. In this condition, the BG level becomes elevated and glycosuria and ketonuria occur. The person experiences drowsiness, lethargy, and sometimes nausea with vomiting. The skin becomes hot and dry. There is a fruity odor to the breath (acetone). Breathing is deep and labored. Death can result if the patient is not treated promptly with insulin and fluids. Hospitalization is required.

Heart Disease

Deaths among persons with diabetes are highly related to cardiovascular disease. Up to 80% of diabetic patients die of macrovascular complications, including coronary artery disease, stroke, and peripheral vascular disease. Numerous studies in patients with Type 2 diabetes have shown the benefits of aggressive treatment of blood pressure and lipids (Spanheimer, 2001). The American Diabetes Association recommends that physicians measure blood lipids and treat associated problems as a primary intervention to reduce the risk of cardiovascular disease among persons with diabetes. The goals of blood pressure are more conservative for a person with diabetes. The American Diabetes Association advises a blood pressure goal of less than 130/80 mm Hg. Refer back to Chapter 8 for management of cardiovascular disorders.

Kidney Disease

Persons with Type 1 diabetes are at particular risk for kidney disease caused by damage to small blood vessels. Kidney disease occurs more frequently in Type 2 diabetes because there are many more persons with this type of diabetes. The

DCCT study found that maintaining good blood sugar control will greatly lessen the risk of kidney disease.

Eating protein in more moderate portions is appropriate—almost no one needs more than 6 oz of meat per day—but it only becomes necessary when there is severe kidney damage, as with macroalbuminuria. Aside from the protein found in meat, the type of fat it contains is important. Omega-3 fatty acids found in cold-water fish and fish oil have been shown to lower blood pressure and triglyceride levels in humans.

Controlling blood pressure is critical to preserving kidney functioning. Regular blood pressure screening is necessary and antihypertensive therapy, particularly the use of ACE inhibitors, helps preserve the functioning of the kidneys when there is mild hypertension with **glycated** albumin (glucose attached to the protein, as in this case the albumin) as found with hyperglycemia. Borderline hypertension needs to be treated aggressively in persons with diabetes to preserve kidney function.

Eye Disease

Diabetic retinopathy (a disease of the back of the eye where visual images are conveyed to the brain) occurs in about half of all persons who have had diabetes for more than 10 years and in about 80% of all persons who have had diabetes for more than 25 years. Controlling blood sugar levels significantly lowers the risk of retinopathy, according to the DCCT study. Hypertension should also be controlled. Regular eye exams, at least annually, with special tests to monitor for retinopathy are necessary to save vision. Treatment is available today that can preserve the sight of most persons with diabetes.

Nerve Disease

Nerve disease can occur at any location of the body, but typically affects peripheral nerves (such as those in the feet and legs) and the autonomic nervous system (comprising the nerves that send unconscious messages to the body, such as in the stomach, heart, or intestines). Problems with peripheral nerves (**peripheral neuropathy**) in the feet can cause burning, pain, and, if severe, no feeling at all. It is paramount for persons with peripheral nerve problems of the feet to follow meticulous foot care. This can help prevent foot infections, which could lead to amputation. Any sign of a problem should immediately be taken care of by a physician or **podiatrist** (foot doctor).

Problems with the autonomic nervous system are referred to as **autonomic neuropathy**. This condition is generally believed to be caused by prolonged hyperglycemia, of many years standing. Gastroparesis is an outcome of autonomic neuropathy. Partial paralysis of the nerves leading to the muscles of the stomach results in diminished movement of food through the stomach. This can be a cause of unexplained hypoglycemia because blood sugar levels can be raised only when food leaves the stomach. When this condition is suspected, a dye test is administered to determine the amount of time it takes for the food to leave the stomach. There is medication for this condition.

Exercise may be discouraged for a person with autonomic neuropathy because the heart may not be able to speed up to increase the oxygen intake. Other conditions related to autonomic neuropathy include silent heart attacks (no pain associated with a MI), **orthostatic hypertension** (high blood pressure caused by standing erect), absence of sweating that can result in dry and cracked skin, and impotence.

Another form of autonomic neuropathy affects the ability of the body to produce glucagon and epinephrine in response to low BG. This is referred to as **hypoglycemic unawareness** because symptoms of hypoglycemia—shakiness, rapid heartbeat, and so on—will not be felt. Hypoglycemic unawareness does not directly cause autonomic neuropathy.

It is now known that frequent hypoglycemia leads to hypoglycemic unawareness, unrelated to autonomic neuropathy. It appears that the body adapts to continued bouts of hypoglycemia, perceiving hypoglycemia as normal. By having a person meticulously avoid hypoglycemia, for as little as 2 weeks, the body readapts to higher levels of glucose, and the person can have a return of hypoglycemia symptoms. Having symptoms is useful to prevent severe hypoglycemia that can induce permanent brain damage.

Dental Health

The incidence of dental caries is reduced with good BG control in diabetes. Saliva production may be diminished, especially with dehydration that occurs with severe hyperglycemia. Because saliva neutralizes the acid formation in the mouth, severe periodontal disease can develop with uncontrolled diabetes. Periodontal disease often starts at puberty among children with diabetes. Persons with diabetes should receive oral hygiene instruction and visit a dentist at least twice a year (Iughetti et al., 1999).

Times of Illness

The need for insulin increases when a person is acutely ill, even if there is a diminished intake of food. To prevent excess production of ketones, the person with Type 1 diabetes must maintain adequate insulin injections and carbohydrate intake (a minimum of 15 g of carbohydrate per hour or 30 to 50 g of carbohydrates every 3 to 4 hours) and contact a physician immediately when illness occurs.

The quality of the diet is less important than the quantity of carbohydrate consumed during severe illness; thus the intake of simple sugars such as those found in regular ginger ale may be recommended. Sipping juice or soft drinks throughout the day may be helpful when the intake of food is greatly diminished, as during an illness. To prevent the loss of needed electrolytes, which can result from vomiting and diarrhea, orange juice should be consumed for potassium and soup for sodium. Sports drinks or other commercial drinks containing electrolytes may also be consumed to provide sodium and potassium. Adequate intake of fluid sources, without carbohydrates to manage hyperglycemia, is imperative because dehydration compounds the undesirable effect of hyperglycemia and ketonuria.

WHAT COUNSELING STRATEGIES CAN NURSES AND OTHER HEALTH PROFESSIONALS USE IN DIABETES MANAGEMENT?

The nurse or other health professional needs to determine real needs versus perceived needs of persons who have already learned to live with diabetes. People sometimes believe their diabetes is under control because they feel healthy. Others may be in denial, feeling unable to cope with the demands of having diabetes. Positive verbal reinforcement for any attempt at control is always useful. Beyond that, the nurse can help patients to identify their perceived needs in relation to diabetes management, can make referrals as appropriate (for example, to the physician, dietitian, or diabetes support group), and can advocate gradual changes (small steps) in the control of diabetes. Simply being empathetic about the frustrations and challenges that are likely to be encountered by the individual with diabetes is an important role of the health care professional.

Another area to assess is the patient's knowledge of the physiology of diabetes mellitus—such knowledge is necessary for effective decision making in diabetes management. Does the individual have a basic understanding of what makes BG levels increase or decrease (see the following list)? Does the individual have the skills to determine what course of action is most appropriate for the various situations likely to be encountered, such as for differing food intake or physical activity levels? Does he or she have the ability to follow through by making adjustments in diet, insulin administration, or activity? Is the person able to accept the reality of having diabetes mellitus and to take responsibility for its control? How does the person's environment (social, economic, and so on) reinforce or inhibit diabetes management? By identifying areas of strength for positive reinforcement and areas of need for referral or personal assistance, the nurse or other health care professional can have an integral and valuable role in facilitating the potential for full and productive lives in individuals with diabetes mellitus.

Factors Lowering Blood Sugar Levels:
Weight loss or reduced intake of food
Exercise*
Diabetes medication

Factors Raising Blood Sugar Levels:
Weight gain or increased food intake
Excess carbohydrate intake
Excess saturated and total fat intake
Mental or physical stress
Steroids, beta-blockers, diuretics
Infections and illness
Dawn phenomenon

*If there is insufficient insulin in the body, exercise will raise blood sugar levels. If BG levels are consistently elevated above 240 mg/dL or in cases of ketonuria, exercise should be postponed until diabetes is better controlled.

CHAPTER
STUDY
QUESTIONS
AND
CLASSROOM
ACTIVITIES

1. Bring some convenience food labels into class. How can they be calculated into a diabetic person's diet?

2. Self-monitor your BG levels using Chemstrips (strips which are visually read rather than using a BG meter) for at least 1 day, before meals and 2 hours postprandially. Maintain a record of your eating habits, including amounts eaten and times of meals and time and duration of activities. Based on this experience, discuss in class how you feel about advocating SMBG for all individuals with diabetes.

3. Determine what changes, if any, you would have to make if you were diagnosed as having diabetes. Could you consistently follow a low-fat, low-sugar meal plan? How would you feel if you had to reduce the amount of sweets and greasy foods in your diet?

4. Describe why a person with hyperglycemia is at increased risk of heart disease and kidney disease.

5. Become a member of the American Diabetes Association (for about $28 per year) and receive its monthly publication, "Diabetes Forecast." Each publication contains a feature story about a person with diabetes with other informative articles.

6. If a person with Type 1 diabetes takes NPH insulin at 7:00 AM, what time will the insulin peak? If this person begins to feel shaky at 3:00 PM, what should he or she do?

7. Knowing that milk contains about 15 g of carbohydrates per cup and that the form of carbohydrate in milk is lactose, calculate how many teaspoons of sugar equivalent it contains.

8. Determine if the following individual is likely to experience hypoglycemia:

   Insulin-to-carbohydrate ratio (1 unit of insulin to 15 g of carbohydrate): 1:15
   Total units of insulin daily (*Hint:* 1500 rule): 45 units
   Premeal BG: 175 mg/dL
   Meal insulin dose: 10 units regular insulin
   Meal carbohydrate consumed (*Hint:* Insulin-to-carbohydrate ratio): 60 g

9. Role-play in class a person who refuses to take control of diabetes, who has a HbA_{1C} of 10% (average BG of 240 mg/dL). One student should role-play the nurse or other health care professional; the second student can role-play the person with diabetes. Discuss as a class the nurse's communication style and approach. Was it effective? How else might the situation be handled?

Case Study

Now she had diabetes, Rita thought to herself. First her son and now her. She did not recall any history of diabetes in the family. She had battled high blood pressure for years, but did not think she would ever get the diagnosis of diabetes. When she thought about it, however, she recalled her granddaughter had diabetes when she was pregnant the second time. The diabetes, however, went away after the birth of her great-granddaughter. She thought, "Sure seems odd how the younger generation has more health problems."

Her own grandparents, who had been born in Italy, had lived until they were well into their 90s and were amazingly healthy and active up until the last few years. Rita was sure the change in eating habits were related. Her own parents had grown up eating very little meat, but lots of beans and greens from Pasta Fazule, a bean and pasta soup, and an amazing assortment of vegetables including spinach, artichokes, and fennel. She even recalled eating what she thought of as a weed with her grandmother going outside in the warm weather to pick it from the back fields. Burdock, if she recalled the name correctly. Now all they seemed to eat as a family was meat and potatoes—usually French fries or pasta with lots of cheese and tomato sauce. She decided they would all benefit returning to the old-style Italian way of eating and use olive oil to cook with and not so much butter and cheese.

Critical Thinking Applications

1. What risk factors predisposed Rita to diabetes?
2. How might you advise Rita on food choices to control diabetes and hypertension?
3. What benefit would there be changing to olive oil?
4. Describe the benefits of eating more vegetables and less meat and cheese in preventing or managing diabetes.

REFERENCES   Adeghate E, Parvez SH: Nitric oxide and neuronal and pancreatic beta cell death. Toxicology. November 16, 2000; 153(1-3):143-156.

Albright A, Franz M, Hornsby G, Kriska A, Marrero D, Ullrich I, Verity LS: American College of Sports Medicine position stand: exercise and type 2 diabetes. Med Sci Sports Exerc. July 2000; 32(7):1345-1360.

Bender DA: Optimum nutrition: thiamin, biotin and pantothenate. Proc Nutr Soc. May 1999; 58(2):427-433.

Berry EM: Dietary fatty acids in the management of diabetes mellitus. Am J Clin Nutr. October 1997; (4 Suppl):991S-997S.

Brown RE, Stevens DR, Haas HL: The physiology of brain histamine. Prog Neurobiol. April 2001; 63(6):637-672.

Fagot-Campagna A, Pettitt DJ, Engelgau MM, Burrows NR, Geiss LS, Valdez R, Beckles GL, Saaddine J, Gregg EW, Williamson DF, Narayan KM: Type 2 diabetes among North American children and adolescents: an epidemiologic review and a public health perspective. J Pediatr. May 2000; 136(5):664-672.

Ford ES, Mokdad AH: Fruit and vegetable consumption and diabetes mellitus incidence among U.S. adults. Prev Med. January 2001; 32(1):33-39.

Fritsche A, Schmulling RM, Haring HU, Stumvoll M: Intensive insulin therapy combined with metformin in obese type 2 diabetic patients. Acta Diabetol. March 2000; 37(1):13-18.

Gabbe SG, Holing E, Temple P, Brown ZA: Benefits, risks, costs, and patient satisfaction associated with insulin pump therapy for the pregnancy complicated by type 1 diabetes mellitus. Am J Obstet Gynecol. June 2000; 182(6):1283-1291.

Gabir MM, Hanson RL, Dabelea D, Imperatore G, Roumain J, Bennett PH, Knowler WC: Plasma glucose and prediction of microvascular disease and mortality: evaluation of 1997 American Diabetes Association and 1999 World Health Organization criteria for diagnosis of diabetes. Diabetes Care. August 2000; 23(8):1113-1118.

Gavin JR 3rd: New classification and diagnostic criteria for diabetes mellitus. Clin Cornerstone. 1998; 1(3):1-12.

Hallfrisch J, Facn, Behall KM: Mechanisms of the effects of grains on insulin and glucose responses. J Am Coll Nutr. June 2000; 19(3 Suppl):320S-325S.

Hathout EH, Thomas W, El-Shahawy M, Nahab F, Mace JW: Diabetic autoimmune markers in children and adolescents with type 2 diabetes. Pediatrics. June 2001; 107(6):E102.

Iughetti L, Marino R, Bertolani MF, Bernasconi S: Oral health in children and adolescents with IDDM—a review. J Pediatr Endocrinol Metab. 1999; 12(5 Suppl 2):603-610.

Lavigne C, Tremblay F, Asselin G, Jacques H, Marette A: Prevention of skeletal muscle insulin resistance by dietary cod protein in high fat-fed rats. Am J Physiol Endocrinol Metab. July 2001; 281(1):E62-E71.

Major CA, Henry MJ, De Veciana M, Morgan MA: The effects of carbohydrate restriction in patients with diet-controlled gestational diabetes. Obstet Gynecol. 1998; 91:600-604.

Meyer KA, Kushi LH, Jacobs DR Jr, Slavin J, Sellers TA, Folsom AR: Carbohydrates, dietary fiber, and incident type 2 diabetes in older women. Am J Clin Nutr. April 2000; 71(4):921-930.

Mukhtar Q, Cleverley G, Voorhees RE, McGrath JW: Prevalence of acanthosis nigricans and its association with hyperinsulinemia in New Mexico adolescents. J Adolesc Health. May 2001; 28(5):372-376.

Okada M, Shibuya M, Yamamoto E, Murakami Y: Effect of diabetes on vitamin B6 requirement in experimental animals. Diabetes Obes Metab. July 1999; 1(4):221-225.

Okamura F, Tashiro A, Utumi A, Imai T, Suchi T, Tamura D, Sato Y, Suzuki S, Hongo M: Insulin resistance in patients with depression and its changes during the clinical course of depression: minimal model analysis. Metabolism. October 2000; 49(10):1255-1260.

Oohara A, Yoshimatsu H, Kurokawa M, Oishi R, Saeki K, Sakata T: Neuronal glucoprivation enhances hypothalamic histamine turnover in rats. J Neurochem. August 1994; 63(2):677-682.

Ostgren CJ, Lindblad U, Ranstam J, Melander A, Rastam L: Skaraborg: Hypertension and Diabetes Project. Associations between smoking and beta-cell function in a nonhypertensive and nondiabetic population. Hypertension and Diabetes Project. Diabet Med. June 2000; 17(6):445-450.

Palumbo PJ: Gycemic control, mealtime glucose excursions, and diabetic complications in type 2 diabetes mellitus. Mayo Clin Proc. June 2001; 76(6):609-618.

Pompeia C, Lopes LR, Miyasaka CK, Procopio J, Sannomiya P, Curi R: Effect of fatty acids on leukocyte function. Braz J Med Biol Res. November 2000; 33(11):1255-1268.

Rasmussen BM, Orskov L, Schmitz O, Hermansen K: Alcohol and glucose counterregulation during acute insulin-induced hypoglycemia in type 2 diabetic subjects. Metabolism. April 2001; 50(4):451-457.

Schrezenmeir J, Jagla A: Milk and diabetes. J Am Coll Nutr. April 2000; 19(2 Suppl):176S-190S.

Spanheimer RG: Reducing cardiovascular risk in diabetes. Which factors to modify first? Postgrad Med. April 2001; 109(4):26-30, 33-36.

Strachan MW, Deary IJ, Ewing FM, Frier BM: Recovery of cognitive function and mood after severe hypoglycemia in adults with insulin-treated diabetes. Diabetes Care. March 2000; 23(3):305-312.

Tuomilehto J, Lindstrom J, Eriksson JG, Valle TT, Hamalainen H, Ilanne-Parikka P, Keinanen-Kiukaanniemi S, Laakso M, Louheranta A, Rastas M, Salminen V, Uusitupa M: Finnish Diabetes Prevention Study Group. Prevention of type 2 diabetes mellitus by changes in lifestyle among subjects with impaired glucose tolerance. Comment in: N Engl J Med. May 3, 2001; 344(18):1390-1392

Watson JM, Jenkins EJ, Hamilton P, Lunt MJ, Kerr D: Influence of caffeine on the frequency and perception of hypoglycemia in free-living patients with type 1 diabetes. Diabetes Care. April 2000; 23(4):455-459.

Weber B, Schweiger U, Deuschle M, Heuser I: Major depression and impaired glucose tolerance. Exp Clin Endocrinol Diabetes. 2000; 108(3):187-190.

Zinman B: Basal insulin replacement and use of rapid-acting insulin analogues in patients with type 1 diabetes. Endocr Pract. January 2000; 6(1):88-92.

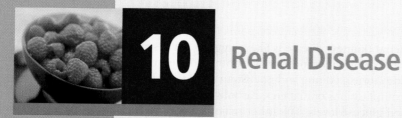

10 Renal Disease

OBJECTIVES

After completing this chapter, you should be able to:

- Describe the basic functions of the kidneys.
- Identify the clinical symptoms and serum parameters of renal disease.
- Describe the principles of nutritional management, including the control of disease and promotion of good nutritional status.
- Describe the role of the nurse and other health care professionals in the management of renal disease.

TERMS TO IDENTIFY

Albumin
Albuminuria
Anuria
Azotemia
Blood urea nitrogen (BUN)
Carnitine
Chronic renal failure (CRF)
Continuous ambulatory peritoneal dialysis (CAPD)
Creatinine
Edema

End-stage renal disease (ESRD)
Erythropoietin
Glomerular filtration rate (GFR)
Hematuria
Hemodialysis
Hypercalciuria
Hypoalbuminemia
Hypotension
Microalbuminuria

Nephrons
Nephrotic syndrome
Oliguria
Osteomalacia
Osteoporosis
Positive nitrogen balance
Proteinuria
Renal insufficiency
Renal osteodystrophy
Uremia

INTRODUCTION

Managing renal (kidney) disease is like a juggling act. Usually not just one, but several nutritional components need to be controlled. Because of clearance problems, protein, phosphorus, sodium, and potassium need to be limited. If renal disease results from complications of diabetes, carbohydrate intake needs to be managed to control blood glucose levels. The other major source of kilocalories—fat intake—needs to be maintained at a level that allows for slow weight loss or weight stabilization without promoting hypercholesterolemia. However, once a person with renal disease begins dialysis, the restrictions are often reversed to compensate for the excess losses incurred. Managing renal disease is complex and difficult for the patient and the entire health care team. But renal failure and the need for dialysis may be lessened or even prevented if the patient is willing and able to control the diverse, interrelated dietary factors that allow for a normal nutritional balance.

WHAT ARE THE FUNCTIONS OF THE KIDNEYS?

Kidneys have three basic functions: (1) excreting waste material, (2) reabsorbing important body constituents, and (3) helping to maintain proper metabolism and hormonal balance. Their most widely known function is to filter body wastes, including drugs and toxins. This filtering process occurs in the **nephrons**, of which there are more than 1 million (Figure 10-1). For renal disease patients,

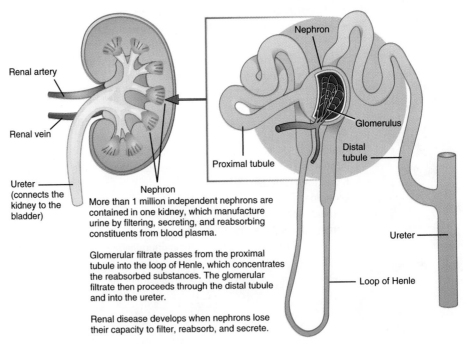

FIGURE 10-1 Anatomy of a kidney.

medications need to be adjusted to reflect diminished clearance through the kidneys. Persons on insulin therapy may need a lower dose of insulin when the kidneys fail because insulin remains in the body longer as the kidneys lose their filtering ability.

Selective reabsorption of nutrients as necessary is another basic function of the kidneys that serves an important role in maintaining the acid-base balance (pH level) and the balance of various body constituents. Thus kidneys help maintain appropriate levels of water, electrolytes, nitrogen, fixed acids, bicarbonates, and other body constituents through the two functions of excretion of wastes and reabsorption of important nutrients.

The third and least well-known function of kidneys is their role in the maintenance of metabolism and hormonal balance. The kidneys convert the inactive form of vitamin D from foods and sun exposure into the active form. They also produce the enzyme *renin*, which affects systemic blood pressure, and the hormone **erythropoietin**, which stimulates red blood cell production by the bone marrow. Figure 10-1 illustrates the composition of the kidneys.

HOW IS RENAL DISEASE DIAGNOSED?

The general criteria for diagnosing renal disease center around the functions of the normal kidney. Given that kidneys excrete excess nitrogen, protein, electrolytes, water, and other substances, tests for abnormal levels of these constituents provide an indication of whether renal disease is present and, if so, how severe it is. Renal disease progresses along a continuum (Table 10-1). Clinical manifestations of renal disease include **hematuria** (blood in the urine), **albuminuria** (**albumin**, a form of protein, found in the urine), **azotemia** (nitrogen in the blood), hypertension, edema, **hypoalbuminemia** (low levels of albumin in the blood), hyperlipidemia, and **proteinuria** (protein in the urine). Lack of urinary

TABLE 10-1
STAGES OF CHRONIC RENAL DISEASE

STAGE	THERAPEUTIC DIETARY MEASURES
Glomerulonephritis	Restrict protein until kidney function improves; restrict sodium if hypertension or edema present; may be self-limiting or proceed to more severe renal disease
Nephrotic syndrome	May need to compensate for protein losses as a result of albuminuria; mild sodium restriction if edema present (3 g/day)
Diminished reserve	May need to control for hypertension with sodium restriction
Renal insufficiency	Restrict protein, fluid, and electrolytes with adequate caloric intake required; level of dietary control based on renal functioning
Renal failure	Begin dialysis; diet needs to compensate for losses from dialysis; phosphorus restriction still needed
Uremia	Kidney transplant unless uremia can be controlled through more frequent dialysis or stricter dietary control

excretion (**anuria**) and decreased urinary output (**oliguria**) suggest renal obstruction, which may lead to irreversible renal damage.

Specific serum indicators routinely used for assessing the degree of renal failure and response to dietary control are the **blood urea nitrogen (BUN)** level and **creatinine** (a nitrogenous compound formed in muscle), albumin, potassium, phosphorus, sodium, and calcium determinations. The **glomerular filtration rate (GFR)** also gives an indication of how fast the kidneys are functioning in excreting wastes. A normal GFR is 125 ml per minute. Initial indication of kidney stress is an elevated GFR. A person with an elevated GFR will usually be placed on an ACE inhibitor (a type of blood pressure medication) which helps preserve kidney functioning. A GFR less than 25 to 30 ml per minute is equated with **renal insufficiency**; less than 15 ml per minute is associated with uremia. **Uremia** is associated with high creatinine levels of over 5 mg/dL; normal creatinine concentration is less than 1.5 mg/dL; and over 10 mg/dL will require dialysis to preserve life. One test used to determine renal functioning is the collection of a 24-hour urine test. This allows the measurement of the GFR. A different version of this 24-hour urine test that allows similar assessment of renal functioning is the spot urine protein-creatinine ratio. A urine protein-creatinine clearance ratio of 0.26 represents normal, whereas a ratio of 3.20 indicates nephrotic proteinuria (Chitalia et al., 2001).

WHAT ARE SOME TYPES AND CAUSES OF RENAL DISORDERS AND THEIR NUTRITIONAL TREATMENT?

Acute Renal Failure

Acute renal failure (ARF) occurs when there is a sudden decrease in the GFR. Oliguria (reduced production of urine to less than 500 ml per 24 hours) may occur with ARF. Depending on the cause, ARF may be short-lived and may require no nutritional intervention. If the patient goes on to develop uremia (a toxic build up of protein by-products in the blood, causing such problems as nausea and vomiting) and other problems such as fluid or electrolyte imbalances, nutritional care becomes a primary treatment. **Chronic renal failure (CRF)** is a term used to describe the long-term condition of renal insufficiency.

Nephrotic Syndrome

Nephrotic syndrome involves loss of the glomerular barrier to protein in the nephron (see Figure 10-1). Protein is thus lost in the urine, which is called **microalbuminuria** (small amounts of albumin in the urine). The amount of protein lost in the urine can be measured. A small amount is called microalbuminuria when the lab value is between 20 and 200 μg per minute. A higher amount of protein lost in the urine is referred to as *macroalbuminuria*.

The loss of protein in the urine in turn causes a decreased serum albumin level, or low levels of protein in the blood. A decreased serum albumin level leads to **edema** (fluid retention). Nutritional care is aimed at improving protein status. A higher protein intake is likely warranted. One indication that enough protein has been restored to the body is the **positive nitrogen balance**. This is the amount of protein needed in the diet to allow for tissue growth; that is, intake of protein that exceeds output. A positive nitrogen balance will help promote a normal serum albumin level and correction of the edema. Adequate caloric intake is required to ensure protein is used for anabolic (growth) reasons.

Another means to correct microalbuminuria is to treat underlying hypertension because microalbuminuria is associated with high blood pressure (Bakris, 2001). Because hypertension is related to the insulin resistance syndrome, dietary measures to manage insulin resistance may be of further help. Such measures include avoiding excess sodium, limiting saturated fat, and moderating carbohydrate content by emphasizing high-soluble fiber foods spread out over the day in several small meals. Increased physical activity may also be warranted.

Nephrotic syndrome may also be related to oxidation of LDL cholesterol partly because of antioxidant deficiency (Posadas-Sanchez et al., 2001). Research supports the need for the inclusion of a variety of plant-based foods that can provide antioxidant vitamins and minerals.

How Much Protein Is Needed to Achieve a Positive Nitrogen Balance?

The amount of protein recommended to achieve a positive nitrogen balance is based on individual needs. In the past, patients were routinely given double the recommended protein intake (1.5 g/kg body weight, compared with the normal recommendation of 0.8 g/kg). The amount needed is reflected in lab values and diminishing edema.

As described above, a calculation can be made to verify a positive nitrogen balance. This calculation will, however, not be precise if the exact amount of the protein intake is not known. The assessment of nitrogen balance is intake minus loss. The amount of the nitrogen intake (through diet) must be greater than what is lost through urine and other body losses to have enough protein for building purposes (anabolism).

How Is Edema Treated in Nephrotic Syndrome?

Because the cause of edema in nephrotic syndrome is secondary to hypoalbuminemia, typical treatment of edema (low-sodium diet and diuretic medications) does not apply. The underlying hypoalbuminemia and subsequent edema will be corrected rather by achieving a positive nitrogen balance through increased protein utilization, which in turn is achieved by an adequate kcaloric intake. Thus a high-protein, high-calorie diet can help correct the edema associated with nephrotic syndrome.

Sodium should be restricted only mildly (about 3 g per day) because further reductions can cause **hypotension** (abnormally low blood pressure). Hypoalbuminemia causes a low blood volume, which would be exacerbated with a very low sodium intake (less than 2 g per day).

Nephritic Syndrome

Nephritic syndrome includes a group of inflammatory diseases of the kidney, specifically of the glomerulus (see Figure 10-1). A term used to describe this condition is *glomerulonephritis*, or simply *nephritis*. Hematuria, hypertension, and mild loss of renal function are common. This condition most commonly follows a streptococcal infection and usually lasts only for a short time, allowing for complete recovery. However, it can develop into chronic nephrotic syndrome (as described above) or end-stage renal disease (ESRD) (see later section).

What Dietary Changes Are Made with Nephritic Syndrome?

No routine dietary changes are made for nephritic syndrome except to maintain health during the inflammation stage. Alterations in protein intake should be based on serum lab values. Mild restrictions of protein and potassium may be indicated. Sodium restriction of 2 to 3 g per day would be appropriate to control hypertension.

Hypertension-Associated Renal Disease

This form of renal disease is thought of as distinct from diabetic nephropathy. However, as hypertension and diabetes are both related to the insulin resistance syndrome, there may be common underlying pathophysiology.

Renal disease caused by hypertension is a major cause of **end-stage renal disease (ESRD)** in the United States. Smoking has been found to be a risk factor in the development of ESRD for patients who have severe essential hypertension (Regalado et al., 2000). The incidence of ESRD caused by hypertension is five times greater in African Americans than in white Americans (Kotchen et al., 2000).

One study found that a 5% weight loss in obese patients reduced blood pressure and urinary albumin excretion rate. This was attributed to decreased insulin resistance with diminished hyperinsulinemia (Ohashi et al., 2001).

Diabetic Nephropathy

Diabetes-related nephropathy is a common cause of ESRD. A person with diabetes for 25 years has a 25% to 40% risk of developing ESRD. The stages of damage leading to ESRD begin with microalbuminuria, and if diabetes and blood pressure are treated early and aggressively, the development of renal disease can be delayed if not halted.

Prevention of diabetic nephropathy includes control of blood glucose and blood pressure (Parving et al., 2001). One study noted that even if high blood pressure is managed, hyperglycemia still causes rapid GFR decline in Type 2 diabetes (Nosadini et al., 2000). Another study found that aggressive antihypertensive treatment in Type 1 diabetic patients can induce remission and regression of diabetic nephropathy. The best outcome, however, still involves lowered blood pressure with reduced albuminuria and better glycemic control (Hovind et al., 2001). The Modification of Diet in Renal Disease (MDRD) study strongly suggests that blood pressure should not be higher than 130/85 mm Hg in patients with CRF and lower than 125/75 mm Hg in patients with CRF and proteinuria above 1 g per day (Rossert and Ronco, 2001).

Treatment of ESRD becomes complicated because hypertension and dyslipidemia (elevated triglycerides and low HDL cholesterol) are usually found in association with diabetes. Managing diabetic nephropathy is very complex. Medical nutrition therapy as provided by a dietitian is critical when trying to balance the nutritional demands of diabetes, hypertension, hypercholesterolemia, and renal disease. In 2001, registered dietitians became providers recognized by the Medicare program (see Chapter 15) for predialysis renal disease and for diabetes mellitus.

How Is the Diet Modified in Chronic Renal Failure?

There is controversy regarding the ideal amount of protein in slowing the progression of CRF. However, it has been shown that a low protein intake reduces renal death by about 40% compared with high protein intake (Fouque et al., 2001).

The National Kidney Foundation Clinical Practice Dialysis Outcomes Quality Initiative (DOQI) guidelines state that predialysis patients with CRF should receive 0.60 to 0.75 g/kg body weight per day of protein. For stable maintenance hemodialysis patients, the recommended protein intake is 1.2 g/kg per day, and for chronic peritoneal dialysis patients, 1.2 to 1.3 g/kg per day. Alternatives to this have been suggested in some research: for predialysis patients, an intake of 0.8 g/kg per day; for those on maintenance hemodialysis, an intake of 0.9 to 1.0 g/kg per day; and for chronic peritoneal dialysis patients, 1.0 to 1.1 g/kg per day (Lim and Flanigan, 2001). The higher amount of protein needed during dialysis is necessary because of the protein loss that occurs when blood is filtered.

Although the precise amount of protein restriction is subject to debate, any reduction in protein intake by a person with CRF will likely be of help. Specific recommendations for protein intake are based on the individual's nutritional assessment as determined by the physician and registered dietitian in conjunction with the patient's desire or perceived ability to follow a set protein restriction.

See Box 10-1 for sample menu of a 60-g protein diet, which is commonly prescribed; high-sugar, high-fat foods and beverages are included to show how caloric intake might be increased. Emphasis on monounsaturated or omega-3 fatty acids can provide adequate caloric intake without adverse effects on diabetes, hypertension, or hypercholesterolemia. The goal of maintaining adequate body weight is necessary to maintain a positive nitrogen balance with appropriate levels of serum albumin.

If high levels of serum potassium occur, a 1500- to 2000-mg limit on potassium intake is appropriate. A normal diet may contain as much as 3000 to 8000 mg because potassium is widely distributed in foods (meats, fruits, whole-grain breads and cereals, and dark green leafy vegetables). Cooking water and the juices from canned fruits and vegetables should be discarded because potassium is water-soluble. Box 10-2 lists foods low in sodium, potassium, and phosphorus.

A low-protein diet will simultaneously restrict phosphorus because phosphorus is found with high-protein foods. A phosphorus intake of 600 to 1200 mg

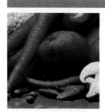

**BOX 10-1
SAMPLE
MENU FOR
A 60-GRAM
PROTEIN DIET**

BREAKFAST

½ c cranberry juice
½ c cream of wheat cereal
2 slices toast
2 tsp butter

2 tsp honey
1 c whole milk
2 tsp sugar
¾ c coffee

LUNCH

2 oz tuna salad
2 slices toast
½ c carrot sticks
6 slices cucumber with leaf lettuce

Italian salad dressing
½ c pineapple rings
1 tsp sugar
1 c Kool-Aid

SUPPER

Pear and peach halves on lettuce
   served with ¼ c cottage cheese
1 c pasta in olive oil and garlic sauce
½ c green beans
1 c whole milk

2 tsp butter
1 dinner roll
1 high-sugar, low-protein popsicle
1 tsp sugar

should maintain desirable levels. Phosphate binders can be used as well, but are now generally avoided because of possible aluminum toxicity. The use of calcium carbonate can decrease serum phosphorus while increasing serum calcium. Excess calcium should be avoided; a maximum intake of 2000 mg is generally advised.

Fluids are also restricted for patients with kidney failure; a balance between intake and output must be achieved. The general guideline is 500 to 1000 ml (about 2 to 4 cups) plus the amount lost in daily urine production and other body fluids such as with perspiration. For example, if the patient has a daily urine and fluid output of 1000 ml, the recommended fluid intake would range from 1500 to 2000 ml per day; if there is anuria (no urine output), the fluid restriction would be 500 to 1000 ml per day. Thus the amount of fluid lost through urinary output needs to be estimated individually before recommended daily amounts can be determined.

Sodium is usually restricted in patients with CRF as well. A typical restriction is 2000 mg per day. The amount of sodium permitted is based on lab values and fluid retention.

Enteral liquid supplements have been developed to assist in providing amino acids (for protein) and kilocalories while contributing low levels of the electrolytes sodium and potassium (see Appendix 8). These products need to be considered part of the total dietary intake. They may serve as an alternative to diet or as a supplement to meet the medical nutrition therapy prescription. If kidney function continues to deteriorate to ESRD, dialysis or kidney transplantation may be required.

BOX 10-2
FOODS FOR MANAGEMENT OF RENAL DISEASE*

≤50 MG SODIUM, POTASSIUM, AND PHOSPHORUS
Fruits
Cranberry juice cocktail, ≤2 c
Lemonade, ≤1 c
Sugars
Granulated, ≤8 c
Hard candy, ≤1 ½ lb
Jelly beans, ≤5 c
Marshmallows, ≤3 ½ oz
Jam, ≤2 tbsp
Jelly, ≤3 tbsp
Fats
Cooking oil (vegetable), unlimited
Lard, unlimited
Salt-free margarine, ≤1 c
Salt-free butter, ≤1 c

≤100 MG SODIUM, POTASSIUM, AND PHOSPHORUS
Fruits and Vegetables
Blueberries, ≤½ c
Grapes, ≤½ c
Lettuce, ≤½ c
Watermelon, ≤½ c
Sugars
Honey, ≤½ c
Alcohol
Beer, ≤12 oz
Table wine, ≤4 oz

*Refer to food composition table (Appendix 5). Specific dietary advice should be given in conjunction with a registered dietitian and a physician. Foods contributing >2 g protein in common portions are not included.

WHAT ARE THE DIFFERENT TYPES OF DIALYSIS?

Dialysis is generally begun when a patient's creatinine level exceeds 10 to 12 mg/dL and the BUN is above 100 mg/dL. This is indicative of ESRD. Dialysis has become commonplace since the U.S. Congress passed legislation allowing federal funds to be used for the procedure. Kidney transplants were also covered in this legislation, which was passed in 1972.

There are two forms of dialysis, both of which have the goal of maintaining and balancing protein, electrolytes (potassium and sodium), and fluid levels. The traditional form is **hemodialysis**, which generally requires a renal patient to travel to a dialysis unit several times a week. For several hours the patient's blood is extracted and filtered through a dialysis solution. The dialyzed blood is then returned through the patient's venous system.

Fallacy: With dialysis, the patient with renal disease need not restrict food intake.

Fact: It is true that to compensate for incurred losses, some of the dietary restrictions are reversed during hemodialysis (e.g., protein, potassium, and sodium for the normotensive patient), but in general there are still restrictions. In fact, the frequency and duration of hemodialysis can be reduced when strict dietary controls are followed. For patients using dialysis, a more liberal dietary intake may be possible.

Continuous ambulatory peritoneal dialysis (CAPD) was developed to improve the quality of life for the dialysis patient in that it does not require attachment to a machine. It entails filling the abdominal cavity with dialysis fluid, which has a high glucose content. The dialysis fluid then absorbs toxins from the blood. After several hours, the dialysis fluid is drained, and fresh dialysis fluid is reinserted. This form of dialysis can also be performed intermittently, usually during sleep.

WHAT ARE SOME NUTRITIONAL RENAL TRANSPLANT ISSUES?

Steroids are required to prevent rejection by the body of new kidneys. Steroid-induced weight gain can occur in conjunction with kidney transplants. Lowering caloric intake may be prescribed, but it should still be high enough to ensure a positive nitrogen balance, which is important for healing and maintaining a healthy immune system.

Hypertension is common after renal transplantation and associated with graft failure in children and adults (Mitsnefes et al., 2001). A moderate sodium intake may be warranted.

WHAT ARE SOME NUTRITIONAL COMPLICATIONS ASSOCIATED WITH RENAL DISEASE OR ITS TREATMENT?

Nutrient Deficiencies

Survival of 20 years or more is now common in patients with ESRD because of improvement in dialysis techniques and kidney transplantation. However, patients treated with hemodialysis for a long time tend to become malnourished from inadequate caloric intake and micronutrient deficiencies (Chazot et al., 2001). About 40% of patients undergoing maintenance dialysis suffer from varying degrees of protein-energy malnutrition (Mehrotra and Kopple, 2001). Protein-calorie malnutrition can occur after 2 to 3 years of following a low-protein diet (0.58 g/kg per day). However, with adequate caloric intake (31 kcal/kg body weight per day), a low-protein diet can be safe (Bernhard et al., 2001).

A high level of serum homocysteine is a risk factor for cardiovascular disease and is found in all patients with ESRD (Dierkes et al., 2001). Homocysteine levels may be reduced by folic acid and vitamins B_{12} and B_6. Supplementation is likely required because a low-protein, low-potassium diet will automatically reduce intake of these vitamins.

Food restrictions in low-protein, low-potassium diets can be compounded by food dislikes or intolerances and can predispose the person with renal disease to ingest an inadequate amount of nutrients. However, even with caution, the risk of vitamin and mineral deficiency is inherent in the restrictive diet. It is prudent for renal patients to have a water-soluble vitamin supplement that approximates the Dietary Reference Intakes (DRIs) (see the inside back cover). Vitamin D supplementation is generally required to treat ESRD. However, the recommendation for vitamin and mineral supplementation should take place in conjunction with physician consultation.

Carnitine, produced in the kidneys, is a substance that oxidizes fatty acids, primarily of the heart and skeletal muscle. Deficiency of carnitine becomes an issue for long-term hemodialysis patients because of decreased availability of lysine, methionine, vitamin C, niacin, vitamin B_6, and iron to synthesize this substance.

Intravenous L-carnitine treatment can lessen fatigue and improve peak exercise capacity in hemodialysis patients (Brass et al., 2001). Because vitamin C is involved in carnitine production and its levels are reduced in patients with uremia, vitamin C depletion may contribute to cramps associated with hemodialysis. It has been found that short-term supplementation with vitamin E (in 400-mg doses) and vitamin C (in 250-mg doses) is safe and effective in reducing hemodialysis-related cramps (Khajehdehi et al., 2001).

Lipid Abnormalities

Patients with ESRD are at high risk for cardiovascular disease and dyslipidemia (Saltissi et al., 2001). Complications of atherosclerosis are the usual cause of death in patients with CRF. Folic acid (at 15 mg per day), vitamin B_6 (150 mg per day), and vitamin B_{12} (1 mg per week) have favorable effects (Naruszewicz et al., 2001). High levels of triglycerides and lipid oxidation are likely important risk factors for cardiovascular disease. Supplementation of vitamin E, an antioxidant vitamin, may be necessary (Galli et al., 2001). The high triglyceride levels that occur with CRF can be treated with a low-sugar, high-fiber diet with moderate amounts of unsaturated fat. Small amounts of sugar may be tolerated as part of a moderate carbohydrate intake.

Renal Osteodystrophy

Renal osteodystrophy consists of a group of bone diseases resulting from the effects of CRF, such as poor bone development in children, **osteomalacia** (soft bones), and **osteoporosis** (brittle bones). Specifically, renal osteodystrophy is caused by a combination of high serum phosphorus levels, low serum calcium levels, and altered parathyroid function. Close monitoring and adherence to a controlled diet can help prevent or delay these complications.

Anemia

Problems with erythropoietin production may lead to diminished production of red blood cells and a form of anemia that is unresponsive to iron supplementation; however, causes of iron deficiency should be ruled out before deciding not to treat with increased iron intake. Providing erythropoietin via blood transfusion may be warranted. Achieving target hemoglobin levels of 11 to 12 g/dL and optimizing iron balance should improve clinical outcomes and increase patient quality of life (Besarab, 1999).

WHAT ARE THE SPECIAL CONSIDERATIONS FOR TREATING CHILDREN WITH RENAL DISEASE?

Children with renal disease have been noted to have stunted growth. Children with CRF may also have a disturbance in the calcium-phosphorus balance, resulting in insufficient availability of calcium for bone growth. Once phosphorus levels are under control, the calcium and vitamin D intake can be increased to help promote bone growth. One study found that recombinant human growth hormone treatment for 1 year resulted in a significant increase in both growth rate and bone strength (Van Dyck et al., 2001).

Making mealtime fun for children is important for good nutritional intake. Liquid supplements designed for renal management can be given popular names such as "Barney Milkshake" for young children. Health care professionals interacting with children should try to make foods sound appealing, provide small portions frequently, and arrange for favorite foods.

WHAT ARE CAUSES AND NUTRITIONAL MANAGEMENT OF KIDNEY STONES (NEPHROLITHIASIS)?

The prevalence of nephrolithiasis in Western countries continues to increase. High sodium, animal protein, sugar intake, and low calcium intake are implicated (Colussi et al., 2000). There are several forms of kidney stones, each with its own medical or nutritional treatment.

The best way to prevent kidney stones is an adequate fluid intake ($1\frac{1}{2}$ to 2 L or more per day), in that it helps to keep the urine dilute, which helps to prevent crystals that lead to stone formation. Once a stone has formed, treatment may best be decided after a chemical analysis of the stone. The most common form of stone is calcium oxalate.

A low incidence of kidney stones has been noted in Greenland Eskimos, which has been attributed to the high intake of oily fish and the omega-3 fatty acid. One study suggests that the omega-3 fatty acid, eicosapentanoic acid (EPA), reduces urinary calcium, which may explain the reduced risk of calcium stone formation with cold-water fish consumption (Yasui et al., 2001).

Calcium Oxalate Stones

The most common form of kidney stones are calcium oxalate or phosphate stones. Calcium oxalate stones come in many forms. Medical input is necessary to determine nutritional intervention and some calcium stones even require medical or surgical intervention.

Oxalate restriction should be considered for calcium oxalate stone formers, especially those with excess levels of urine oxalate (Assimos and Holmes, 2000). A registered dietitian should be consulted for such a diet because foods high in oxalate (legumes and nuts, dark green leafy vegetables, berries, and citrus fruits) are very nutritious. A diet aimed at controlling oxalate stone formation needs to be evaluated for adequacy.

Moderate intake of either beef or plant protein is equally effective in reducing calcium oxalate kidney stone risk (Massey and Kynast-Gales, 2001). Increased oral calcium may be involved in the prevention of calcium oxalate-rich stones because of the ability of calcium to bind with the oxalate (Williams et al., 2001), which lowers the risk of stone formation.

Even if **hypercalciuria** (high levels of calcium in the urine) is noted to be the cause of stone formation, treatment with a low-calcium diet may not be appropriate. Only one type of hypercalciuria will improve on a low-calcium diet. The calcium restriction is now more moderate—in the range of 800 to 1200 mg of calcium per day. A mild sodium restriction (4 to 5 g per day) can decrease urinary calcium levels in another form of hypercalciuria.

Cranberry juice has been recommended for patients with recurrent urinary tract infections; however, cranberry juice has a moderately high concentration of oxalate. Neither cranberry juice nor cranberry concentrate tablets should be consumed by persons at risk of nephrolithiasis (Terris et al., 2001). The avoidance of cranberry juice should be discussed with a physician. In some cases, cranberry juice may be warranted to prevent upper urinary tract infections and to maintain the alkalinity of the urine.

Uric Acid Stones

Limiting protein to about 50 g per day meets basic body needs and is useful for treating uric acid stones. Emphasis on milk instead of meat, eggs, and legumes for protein will help prevent acidic urine. Increased consumption of fruit (except cranberries, plums, and prunes) and decreased consumption of bread products may also help to prevent acidic urine.

Cystine Stones

Cystine stones require a high fluid intake (greater than 4 L per day). Following the diet to avoid acidic urine may also help prevent future formation of cystine stones.

Struvite Stones

Struvite stones are not managed nutritionally. They are usually seen in women and require long-term antibiotic therapy with surgical or ultrasonic stone removal.

Fallacy: A person with kidney stones should follow a low-calcium diet.

Fact: Only recently it has been found that calcium restriction may be counter-productive for a person with kidney stones. Kidney stone formation now appears to be more related to oxalate intake. Oxalate is found in beets, chocolate, nuts, rhubarb, spinach, strawberries, tea, and wheat bran. Megadoses of vitamin C also contribute oxalate. The best course appears to be to avoid excess oxalate and protein while including the recommended amount of milk and increasing the intake of potassium and water.

HOW DO THE DIETARY GUIDELINES RELATE TO MANAGEMENT OF RENAL DISEASE?

Although healthy persons are typically advised to avoid sugar and fat, their consumption may become mandatory for the renal patient to maintain adequate kilocalorie intake without contributing protein and electrolytes. The recommendation to increase sugar and fat may be met with resistance because of long-standing attempts to control health. It should be pointed out that omega-3 fatty acids can actually protect against kidney disease (Brown et al., 2000).

A variety of vegetables and fruits are important for the inclusion of antioxidant vitamins and minerals that can protect against cardiovascular disease associated with renal disease. However, a balance is in order for those with CRF because of the high potassium content of most vegetables and fruits.

Reduced sodium and moderate protein intakes are recommended especially for persons with renal disease. Alcohol may contribute a significant source of kilocalories, but should be avoided. Maintenance of ideal body weight applies to the renal patient and to the general population.

WHAT IS THE ROLE OF THE NURSE AND OTHER HEALTH CARE PROFESSIONALS IN THE MANAGEMENT OF RENAL DISEASE?

The nurse should be aware that nutritional treatment of kidney stones should not be taken lightly. Dietary changes may not be necessary and restrictions can cause nutritional inadequacy and hardship for the patient. Nutritional advice should be made only in consultation with the patient's physician.

A patient with chronic renal disease has difficult decisions to make. Life expectancy with CRF or ESRD can be extended, but only at the expense of an impaired quality of life. Stress on other family members will likely occur. As a consequence, a patient with newly diagnosed CRF can be expected to experience typical grief reactions—denial and anger first, with the need for information and acceptance of responsibility for management of the disease appearing only later.

Through a sensitive approach and strong communication and listening skills, the health care professional can begin to determine what grief stage the patient with renal disease has reached and develop an appropriate plan of action, with referrals as a cornerstone of therapy: a referral to a social worker might be indicated if the patient is exhibiting anger or denial; a referral to a dietitian is imperative when the patient is ready to accept responsibility for dietary control; additionally, a referral to a nurse at a dialysis center is beneficial in regard to dialysis issues such as the control of dry mouth. The nurse can further help the renal patient to identify the available options and the advantages and disadvantages of each. Finally, the health care professional can help convince the patient that life is inherently valuable irrespective of the diminished quality.

For the patient who has begun to take responsibility for the control of chronic renal disease, the health care professional can help serve as a reality tester. The person with renal disease cannot make drastic long-term dietary changes easily and thus should be verbally rewarded for the attempts made, reassured that mistakes and overindulgences will happen, and encouraged not to give up the fight.

CHAPTER STUDY QUESTIONS AND CLASSROOM ACTIVITIES

1. What foods can the patient with renal disease generally consume freely, in moderate amounts, and in restrictive amounts?
2. Why does the patient with CRF need to restrict protein, electrolytes, and fluid?
3. What causes uremic symptoms to develop?
4. Record a 24-hour diet recall on yourself. Calculate the amount of protein, phosphorus, sodium, and potassium in your diet.
5. As a class, visit a dialysis unit. Arrange to have a nurse, a dietitian, and if possible, a patient with renal disease consult with the class on the dietary control of renal disease as it pertains to dialysis.

Case Study

CRITICAL THINKING

Little Dove thought to herself about how she had survived dialysis so far and was now a great-grandmother to two wonderful little girls. However, she felt like there was a family curse: she had battled diabetes for years and was very upset to learn that her grandson's wife had developed gestational diabetes. She hoped none of her family would have to follow her into kidney failure. She wondered if her great-grandchildren would be at increased risk of diabetes and kidney disease because diabetes was found on both sides of the family. Not a day passed that she did not pray to have her family spared the complications of diabetes.

She got her mind back to the matters at hand. The waitress was looking at her funny. She ordered the small cheeseburger and small order of fries. It was better than the super-size portions. That amount of protein and potassium could make her deathly ill before she got back to the dialysis unit on Wednesday. She also asked for a glass of water with her meal, although she really would have liked a nice cold milkshake. That, however, was out of the question in her attempt to control her blood sugar and kidney disease.

Critical Thinking Applications

1. How much potassium, protein, and carbohydrate would Little Dove have if she had consumed a 16 oz milkshake? If her weight is 150 lbs, how much protein and potassium per day would be advised?
2. What alternative beverage could Little Dove have that is low in potassium and sugar?
3. Why does she need to go to the dialysis unit? What kind of renal disease does she have?
4. How would your life be affected if you had to go to a dialysis unit on a regular basis?
5. What measures might protect Little Dove's offspring from developing diabetes and renal disease?

REFERENCES   Assimos DG, Holmes RP: Role of diet in the therapy of urolithiasis. Urol Clin North Am. May 2000; 27(2):255-268.

Bakris GL: Microalbuminuria: What is it? Why is it important? What should be done about it? J Clin Hypertens (Greenwich). March 2001; 3(2):99-102.

Bernhard J, Beaufrere B, Laville M, Fouque D: Adaptive response to a low-protein diet in predialysis chronic renal failure patients. J Am Soc Nephrol. June 2001; 12(6):1249-1254.

Besarab A: Iron and cardiac disease in the end-stage renal disease setting. Am J Kidney Dis. October 1999; 34(4 Suppl 2):S18-S24.

Brass EP, Adler S, Sietsema KE, Hiatt WR, Orlando AM, Amato A: Intravenous L-carnitine increases plasma carnitine, reduces fatigue, and may preserve exercise capacity in hemodialysis patients. Am J Kidney Dis. May 2001; 37(5):1018-1028.

Brown SA, Brown CA, Crowell WA, Barsanti JA, Kang CW, Allen T, Cowell C, Finco DR: Effects of dietary polyunsaturated fatty acid supplementation in early renal insufficiency in dogs. J Lab Clin Med. March 2000; 135(3):275-286.

Chazot C, Laurent G, Charra B, Blanc C, Vovan C, Jean G, Vanel T, Terrat JC, Ruffet M: Malnutrition in long-term haemodialysis survivors. Nephrol Dial Transplant. January 2001; 16(1):61-69.

Chitalia VC, Kothari J, Wells EJ, Livesey JH, Robson RA, Searle M, Lynn KL: Cost-benefit analysis and prediction of 24-hour proteinuria from the spot urine protein-creatinine ratio. Clin Nephrol. June 2001; 55(6):436-447.

Colussi G, De Ferrari ME, Brunati C, Civati G: Medical prevention and treatment of urinary stones. J Nephrol. November-December 2000; 13 Suppl 3:S65-S70.

Dierkes J, Domrose U, Bosselmann KP, Neumann KH, Luley C: Homocysteine-lowering effect of different multivitamin preparations in patients with end-stage renal disease. J Ren Nutr. April 2001; 11(2):67-72.

Fouque D, Wang P, Laville M, Boissel JP: Low-protein diets for chronic renal failure in nondiabetic adults (Cochrane Review). Cochrane Database Syst Rev. 2001; 2:CD001892.

Galli F, Varga Z, Balla J, Ferraro B, Canestrari F, Floridi A, Kakuk G, Buoncristiani U: Vitamin E, lipid profile, and peroxidation in hemodialysis patients. Kidney Int. February 2001; 59 Suppl 78:S148-S154.

Hovind P, Rossing P, Tarnow L, Smidt UM, Parving HH: Remission and regression in the nephropathy of Type 1 diabetes when blood pressure is controlled aggressively. Kidney Int. July 2001; 60(1):277-283.

Khajehdehi P, Mojerlou M, Behzadi S, Rais-Jalali GA: A randomized, double-blind, placebo-controlled trial of supplementary vitamins E, C, and their combination for treatment of haemodialysis cramps. Nephrol Dial Transplant. July 2001; 16(7):1448-1451.

Kotchen TA, Piering AW, Cowley AW, Grim CE, Gaudet D, Hamet P, Kaldunski ML, Kotchen JM, Roman RJ: Glomerular hyperfiltration in hypertensive African Americans. Hypertension. March 2000; 35(3):822-826.

Lim VS, Flanigan MJ: Protein intake in patients with renal failure: comments on the current NKF-DOQI guidelines for nutrition in chronic renal failure. Semin Dial. May-June 2001; 14(3):150-152.

Massey LK, Kynast-Gales SA: Diets with either beef or plant proteins reduce risk of calcium oxalate precipitation in patients with a history of calcium kidney stones. J Am Diet Assoc. March 2001; 101(3):326-331.

Mehrotra R, Kopple JD: Nutritional management of maintenance dialysis patients: why aren't we doing better? Annu Rev Nutr. 2001; 21:343-379.

Mitsnefes MM, Omoloja A, McEnery PT: Short-term pediatric renal transplant survival: blood pressure and allograft function. Pediatr Transplant. June 2001; 5(3):160-165.

Naruszewicz M, Klinke M, Dziewanowski K, Staniewicz A, Bukowska H: Homocysteine, fibrinogen, and lipoprotein(a) levels are simultaneously reduced in patients with chronic renal failure treated with folic acid, pyridoxine, and cyanocobalamin. Metabolism. February 2001; 50(2):131-134.

Nosadini R, Velussi M, Brocco E, Bruseghin M, Abaterusso C, Saller A, Dalla Vestra M, Carraro A, Bortoloso E, Sambataro M, Barzon I, Frigato F, Muollo B, Chiesura-Corona M, Pacini G, Baggio B, Piarulli F, Sfriso A, Fioretto P: Course of renal function in Type 2 diabetic patients with abnormalities of albumin excretion rate. Diabetes. March 2000; 49(3):476-484.

Ohashi H, Oda H, Ohno M, Watanabe S. Weight reduction improves high blood pressure and microalbuminuria in hypertensive patients with obesity. Nippon Jinzo Gakkai Shi. May 2001; 43(4):333-339. [Article in Japanese.]

Parving HH, Hovind P, Rossing K, Andersen S: Evolving strategies for renoprotection: diabetic nephropathy. Curr Opin Nephrol Hypertens. July 2001; 10(4):515-522.

Posadas-Sanchez R, Posadas-Romero C, Zamora-Gonzalez J, Hernandez-Ono A, Banos-Marhaber G, Campos ON, Pedraza-Chaverri J: LDL size and susceptibility to oxidation in experimental nephrosis. Mol Cell Biochem. April 2001; 220(1-2):61-68.

Regalado M, Yang S, Wesson DE: Cigarette smoking is associated with augmented progression of renal insufficiency in severe essential hypertension. Am J Kidney Dis. April 2000; 35(4):687-694; 767-769.

Rossert J, Ronco P: How to slow the progression of chronic renal insufficiency. Rev Prat. February 28, 2001; 51(4):378-384. [Article in French.]

Saltissi D, Morgan C, Knight B, Chang W, Rigby R, Westhuyzen J: Effect of lipid-lowering dietary recommendations on the nutritional intake and lipid profiles of chronic peritoneal dialysis and hemodialysis patients. Am J Kidney Dis. June 2001; 37(6):1209-1215.

Terris MK, Issa MM, Tacker JR: Dietary supplementation with cranberry concentrate tablets may increase the risk of nephrolithiasis. Urology. January 2001; 57(1):26-29.

Van Dyck M, Gyssels A, Proesmans W, Nijs J, Eeckels R: Growth hormone treatment enhances bone mineralisation in children with chronic renal failure. Eur J Pediatr. June 2001; 160(6):359-363.

Williams CP, Child DF, Hudson PR, Davies GK, Davies MG, John R, Anandaram PS, De Bolla AR: Why oral calcium supplements may reduce renal stone disease: report of a clinical pilot study. J Clin Pathol. January 2001; 54(1):54-62.

Yasui T, Tanaka H, Fujita K, Iguchi M, Kohri K: Effects of eicosapentaenoic acid on urinary calcium excretion in calcium stone formers. Eur Urol. July 2001; 39(5):580-585.

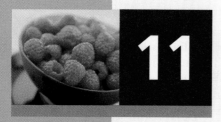

11 Cancer: Nutrition Prevention and Treatment

CHAPTER TOPICS

Introduction
Definition of Cancer
Causes of Cancer and Lifestyle Recommendations to Reduce Cancer Risk
The Effect of Cancer on Nutritional Status
Nutrient Needs and Goals during Treatment
Common Dietary Problems and Solutions
The Role of the Nurse or Other Health Care Professional in Nutritional Counseling
   for Cancer Prevention and Treatment

OBJECTIVES

After completing this chapter, you should be able to:

- Describe cancer prevention strategies.
- Explain how cancer and its treatments affect nutritional status.
- Identify the eating problems associated with cancer and possible solutions.
- Explain why nutritional needs must be met during cancer treatment.
- Describe the role of the nurse in counseling the patient for the prevention or management of cancer.

TERMS TO IDENTIFY

Anorexia	Chemotherapy	Oncology
Cancer	Dysgeusia	Radiation therapy
Cancer cachexia	Esophagitis	Systemic

INTRODUCTION

Another chronic illness associated with the insulin resistance syndrome and an aging population is cancer. Westernized lifestyles contribute to chronic illness with decreased levels of physical activity and the associated rise in the obesity rate. Cancer of the colon and rectum continues to be a major cause of death and illness in people over 50 years of age (Semmens and Platell, 2001). Obesity increases the risk of developing colon cancer, whereas physical activity reduces that risk (Hardwick et al., 2001).

Obesity has also been associated with endometrial cancer (Anderson et al., 2001) and further increases risk of prostate cancer mortality (Rodriguez et al., 2001) and risk of breast cancer after menopause, regardless of family history (Hirose et al., 2001).

Much is known about reducing risk of cancer. The best advice to give the public regarding preventive nutritional practices is to follow the dietary guidelines that emphasize moderation, balance, and variety, with emphasis on plant foods (whole grains, legumes, vegetables, and fruits), monounsaturated fats, and lean meats, such as fish and chicken. This chapter explores current knowledge regarding the prevention of cancer; discusses nutritional goals for the cancer patient; and explains how cancer treatment affects nutritional needs.

WHAT IS CANCER?

Cancer is characterized by the uncontrolled growth and spread of abnormal cells, which continue to reproduce until they form a mass of tissue known as a *tumor.* A *malignant* tumor interrupts body functions and takes away the food and blood supply from normal cells. Cancers develop in various sites and require different methods of management. **Oncology** is the study and the sum of knowledge of tumors.

WHAT ARE THE CAUSES OF CANCER AND HOW CAN ONE REDUCE CANCER RISK?

The role of diet in the development of cancer continues to be studied by the scientific community. There is strong evidence that saturated fat increases the incidence of cancer. Saturated fat is associated with development of prostate cancer and shorter survival after diagnosis (De la Taille et al., 2001). As discussed in earlier chapters, saturated fat worsens insulin resistance and can lead to hyperinsulinemia. The role of hyperinsulinemia in the development of cancer risk is now being recognized.

In assessing family health history, one often finds a history of cancer associated with a history of obesity, heart disease, or diabetes. Recent studies have shown that hyperinsulinemia and abdominal obesity, which are recognized as markers of insulin resistance, are also risk markers for several forms of cancer.

Studies have shown an increase in breast cancer risk among women who have elevated plasma levels of testosterone, which is generally associated with obesity and chronic hyperinsulinemia (Kaaks, 2001).

Insulin and insulin-like growth factors can stimulate growth of colorectal cells, which is related to cancer risk. Refined carbohydrates have been suggested to play a detrimental role in the causation of colorectal cancer (Franceschi et al., 2001). Fasting and 2-hour postprandial hyperinsulinemia are associated with liver cancer (Balkau et al., 2001). There is a link between pancreatic cancer and diabetes mellitus. Furthermore, patients with elevated serum glucose 1 hour after an oral glucose challenge were found to have an increased risk of developing pancreatic cancer (DeMeo, 2001). Thus a reduced carbohydrate intake may help prevent some forms of cancer, particularly for individuals or families with the insulin resistance syndrome.

Most polyunsaturated fats are now also felt to increase cancer risk because of their tendency to oxidize (see Figure 2-4). The exception is the form of polyunsaturated fat known as omega-3 fatty acids, which appear to be strongly protective against cancer.

One way to decrease the intake of saturated and polyunsaturated fats is to limit the total fat intake. However, because the monounsaturated fats found in olive oil and the omega-3 fatty acids found in cold-water fish appear at least neutral if not protective against cancer, the Mediterranean-style diet is an alternative to low-fat diets in the battle against cancer and other chronic illnesses such as heart disease and diabetes.

The traditional Canadian and Alaskan Native American diet includes a high intake of omega-3 fatty acids from cold-water fish. The eicosapentanoic acid (EPA) form of omega-3 has been noted to decrease tumor formation (Petrik et al., 2000). Consumption of cold-water fish might reduce the risk of prostate cancer: one study noted that men who eat fish in at least moderate amounts have a two- to threefold lower rate of prostate cancer than those who do not eat fish (Terry et al., 2001). Reduced rates of skin cancer are associated with the omega-3 fatty acids, ducosahexanoic acid (DHA) and EPA, which are found in cold-water fish. The omega-6 fatty acids, such as arachidonic acid, as found in the fat of beef and pork, reportedly promote increased risk of skin cancer (Liu et al., 2001).

Postmenopausal overweight women have an increased risk of breast cancer. The risk of breast cancer was significantly increased in women who had gained weight or used estrogen replacement therapy (Jernstrom and Barrett-Connor, 1999). Additionally, concentrated phytoestrogen supplements appear to have estrogen-like actions in the breast and may interfere with breast cancer treatment. However, consumption of foods rich in phytoestrogens, such as vegetables, grains, and legumes, should be encouraged (Murkies et al., 2000).

A diet rich in antioxidant vitamins and minerals, as found in a variety of cruciferous vegetables (broccoli, spinach, cabbage, and brussels sprouts), legumes, fruits, whole grains, and green tea has long been associated with reduced cancer risk (Abdulla and Gruber, 2000). One interesting study found that inadequate consumption of vitamin C-containing vegetables and fruits increases risk of infection by *H. pylori*, a common form of bacteria, and is associated with gastric cancer (Brown, 2000). Another study found that women who consumed a large amount of foods containing lutein (dark green leafy vegetables) had a 40% lower risk of ovarian cancer (Berton et al., 2001).

Two fat-soluble vitamins are associated with reduced cancer risk. Vitamin D has been associated with cancer prevention (Guyton et al., 2001) and vitamin E foods and supplements are related to rates of lower bladder cancer, the fourth leading type of cancer in men in the United States (Michaud et al., 2000).

It is well known that excess sun exposure can cause skin cancer. Less well known is that the sun damages DNA, the basic structure of our genes. Dietary deficiencies can also adversely affect DNA structure. A deficiency of the micronutrients folic acid, vitamin B_{12}, vitamin B_6, niacin, vitamin C, vitamin E, iron, or zinc has been found to mimic radiation damage to deoxyribonucleic acid (DNA). This knowledge helps explain why those persons who consume the least amount of fruits and vegetables have about twice the cancer rate for most types (Ames, 2001).

Inadequate intake of *lycopene* (a phytochemical that is red) from cooked tomatoes is the strongest known dietary risk factor for prostate cancer. Thus increased tomato intake can decrease prostate cancer risk. Insulin-like growth factor 1 (IGF-1) also seems to be related to the development of prostate cancer (Mucci et al., 2001).

Insoluble fiber is believed to lower cancer risk in part because it moves food through the gastrointestinal tract faster. This rapid transit of food through the intestines decreases the amount of time carcinogens are in contact with the gastrointestinal mucosa. However, high levels of trace minerals are also found in foods containing fiber. Researchers looking at cancer risk and prevention are increasingly recognizing a multitude of factors that allow complex cellular actions. Thus the fact that eating a variety of low-processed foods reduces cancer risk is likely related to the complexity of nutrients found in such foods. High-fiber foods also have a low glycemic index, which helps to avoid hyperinsulinemia.

Maintaining or returning to more traditionally ethnic eating is important for a number of population groups to prevent chronic illnesses such as cancer. Antioxidants (found in dark green leafy vegetables and deep orange vegetables and fruits), vitamin E (found in nuts and the germ portion of grains such as wheat germ), and vitamin C (found in citrus fruits and dark green leafy vegetables) appear to protect against this disease.

Environmental factors such as excess alcohol intake and cigarette smoking are also linked to the development of cancer, especially that of the gastrointestinal tract and lungs. Low salt intake is associated with reduced cancer rates. The same holds true for limiting foods cooked at high heat, such as barbecued foods. Using tin foil on a barbecue grill reduces the exposure of foods to smoke from meat drippings on hot coals.

Individuals with a family history of cancer should be particularly careful to follow guidelines for cancer prevention. Although a genetic basis for cancer risk is known, prevention can nevertheless be promoted by following certain guidelines:

1. Eat a variety of high-fiber plant-based foods.
2. Limit saturated and polyunsaturated fats.

3. Include foods with monounsaturated or omega-3 fats such as nuts and fish.
4. Avoid sugar-based drinks.
5. Avoid excess intake of alcohol.
6. Limit salty foods.
7. Avoid excess intake of foods cooked at high temperature.
8. Include regular exercise.
9. Maintain a healthy weight.
10. Do not smoke or chew tobacco.

Fallacy: Drinking orange juice reduces the risk of cancer.

Fact: This is an overly simplistic statement that, when put into practice, can actually increase cancer risk among persons with insulin resistance. To help prevent the development of hyperinsulinemia, fresh fruits and vegetables are advisable. Eating an orange is preferable to drinking juice because juice is often consumed in excess amounts. One orange equates to 4 oz of juice. A person who drinks a 12-oz serving of juice is consuming the equivalent of $\frac{1}{4}$ c sugar. Even though this is fructose, not sucrose, excess will promote hyperinsulinemia and cancer risk. Vegetable juices are lower in sugar content.

HOW DO CANCER AND CANCER TREATMENT AFFECT THE NUTRITIONAL STATUS OF THE HOST?

As cancer progresses in the patient, the appetite and food consumption are likely to decrease, resulting in a form of malnutrition and emaciation commonly called **cancer cachexia**. Figure 11-1 shows the pathways that contribute to cancer cachexia. The characteristics of cachexia include weakness, loss of appetite (**anorexia**), metabolic and hormonal abnormalities, a reduction in lean body mass, and a progressive loss of vital functions.

Cachexia may develop for several reasons. An altered sense of taste (**dysgeusia**), a lack of energy, a feeling of fullness, nausea and vomiting, food aversions, altered metabolism, and malabsorption of nutrients are commonly noted in cancer patients, even before therapy begins. Cancer cachexia is characterized by loss of skeletal muscle protein reserves. The omega-3 fatty acid EPA has been found to help prevent loss of skeletal muscle proteins in cancer cachexia (Whitehouse et al., 2001).

Side effects of treatment often add to the patient's discomfort. Chewing and swallowing problems, a sore mouth, **esophagitis** (inflammation of the esophagus), and decreased saliva production may occur, but most of these conditions will cease when treatment is finished. Metabolites, which are chemical substances produced by the tumor, may have an anorexia-inducing effect on the *hypothalamus,* that portion of the brain believed to regulate hunger and satiety.

Among the most common taste changes are a lowered threshold for bitterness and an elevated threshold for sweetness. This may account for the common

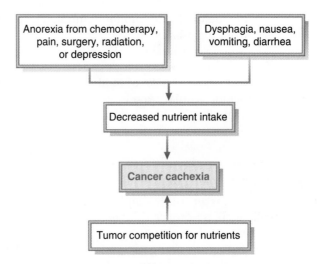

FIGURE 11-1 Cancer cachexia.

aversion to meat and the difficulty in tasting sweet foods. Extra sugar on fruits and cereals is a frequent request of cancer patients. Thresholds for tasting sour and salty foods tend to increase as well.

What Are the Nutritional Problems Resulting from Cancer Treatment?

Cancer is usually treated by surgery, radiation, and chemotherapy, used alone or in combination. Each form of treatment imposes nutritional risks on the patient. Depending on the site of radiation treatment or surgical removal of cancerous areas, there will be different effects on nutritional status. If radiation treatment is near the oral cavity, for example, inflammation can occur that makes eating painful. Dry mouth can occur from damage to the salivary glands. Inadequate saliva production inhibits consumption of dry foods and can therefore allow rapid development of dental decay (see Chapter 13 for more on dental health). If radiation treatment occurs near the abdominal area, digestion and absorption of food nutrients will be adversely affected. Nausea, vomiting, and diarrhea are common side effects of this treatment. Such a person may benefit from a low-lactose diet or more aggressive nutritional support (see Chapter 5).

Surgery

Surgery is used in the treatment of cancer in an attempt to remove tumors or alleviate symptoms (e.g., obstruction of the intestinal tract). The nutritional problems that may develop depend on the type of procedure performed. Providing optimal nutrition may require dietary modifications based on the patient's abil-

■ **TABLE 11-1**
■ **SURGICAL PROCEDURES REQUIRING POSTOPERATIVE DIETARY MODIFICATIONS**

PROCEDURE	NUTRITIONAL PROBLEMS	DIETARY MODIFICATIONS
Radical neck resection	Inability to chew or swallow	Nasogastric tube feeding
Gastrectomy	"Dumping syndrome"	Small frequent meals, liquids between meals, restrict concentrated carbohydrates
Small bowel resection	Diarrhea, malabsorption	Elemental diet
Ileostomy; colostomy	Fluid and electrolyte imbalances	Replacement of fluids and electrolytes

ity or inability to consume, digest, and absorb nutrients. See Table 11-1 for a summary of surgical procedures requiring dietary modification.

Radiation

Radiation therapy (application of radioactive material) to the head, neck, thorax, esophagus, and abdomen can cause acute eating problems. For example, dry mouth, sore throat, severe dental and gum destruction, and altered taste and smell sensations may develop after radiation to the head and neck. Swallowing difficulty (*dysphagia*) and esophagitis often result from radiation to the thorax, and when the abdomen is irradiated, malabsorption of many nutrients occurs if the damage to the gastrointestinal tract is severe. If damage is less severe, gastritis, nausea, vomiting, and diarrhea may result.

Chemotherapy

Chemotherapy is the use of drugs to cure or control cancer. It is **systemic**, meaning that it can affect the entire body rather than just a part of it. The drugs interfere with cells as they divide. Normal cells and cancer cells are affected, and when cells in the gastrointestinal tract are affected, diarrhea, constipation, or poor absorption of nutrients may occur. However, these side effects are only temporary because the gastrointestinal tract cells replace themselves every 3 days. Chemotherapy drugs cause nausea and vomiting. Steroids that cause water retention and bloating are sometimes used. After treatment, these conditions disappear and the patient's nutritional status improves. Steroids used in chemotherapy may require the use of dietary sodium and carbohydrate restrictions because of fluid retention and high serum glucose levels. The side effects experienced during chemotherapy treatments may make it difficult for the patient to consume the optimal amounts of nutrients.

Weight gain is a common problem among breast cancer patients who receive chemotherapy. The evidence suggests the weight gain is the result of reduced physical activity. Exercise, especially resistance training in the lower body, is advised to prevent weight gain among these women (Demark-Wahnefried et al., 2001).

What Are the Reasons for Preventing Weight Loss in the Cancer Patient?

Excess weight loss contributes to loss of muscle and body proteins. Because immune factors are protein-based, excess weight loss encourages opportunistic infections. Thus maintenance of body weight during the treatment of cancer can best increase chance of survival.

The diet of the cancer patient must supply enough protein, fat, carbohydrates, vitamins, minerals, and fluids to meet the increased energy demands of a high metabolic rate to prevent weight loss, to rebuild body tissues, and to promote a sense of well-being during treatment. Individual assessment of caloric intake and weight stabilization will give insight into a particular patient's needs. Nutritionally complete liquid supplements in addition to meals are often needed to ensure adequate nutritional intake. As much as 3000 kcal and 100 g of protein or more may be necessary to prevent tissue breakdown and weight loss (see Chapter 5 for more information on nutritional support). It should be noted, however, that there is debate about which cancer patients will benefit from total parenteral nutrition (TPN).

Why Does Weight Loss Occur in the Cancer Patient?

Decreased caloric intake, increased caloric expenditure (from energy demands of the tumor), or a combination of the two, as well as decreased glucose tolerance and altered protein metabolism, all play a role in weight loss. Reduced gastrointestinal function with diminished movement of food from the stomach causes the individual to feel full too soon and further diminishes the appetite.

In conditions of stress (see Chapter 5), increased amounts of counterregulatory hormones that inhibit the action of insulin are produced. This results in gluconeogenesis (production of blood glucose from protein). Increased breakdown of proteins in the muscle of the cancer patient causes a loss of amino acids, resulting in muscle weakness and wasting. The ability to preserve muscle mass during periods of reduced food consumption is diminished in persons with cancer. Thus loss of muscle and protein stores is common for them.

What Are the Nutritional Goals of the Cancer Patient?

The intake of all vitamins and minerals should at least meet the Daily Reference Intakes (DRI). (See the inside back cover.) Individual needs must be assessed carefully because radiation, chemotherapy, and surgery impose nutritional risks (see common dietary problems and solutions later in the chapter). Fluids are especially important to replace losses from fever, diarrhea, and vomiting and to aid the kidneys in the removal of waste products that result from cancer treatment. The following are nutritional goals during cancer treatment:

1. Preventing weight loss (a short-term goal)
2. Achieving and maintaining normal weight (a long-term goal)
3. Replacing nutritional losses from side effects of treatment (i.e., fluid and electrolyte losses from vomiting, diarrhea, and malabsorption)
4. Providing adequate amounts of kilocalories, protein, carbohydrates, fat, vitamins, and minerals

Fallacy: The high-fiber, low-fat macrobiotic diet will cure cancer.

Fact: The macrobiotic diet is low in kilocalories and cannot support the high energy and nutrient needs of the cancer patient. Weight loss leading to cachexia would likely result; therefore this diet is not recommended.

COMMON DIETARY PROBLEMS AND SOLUTIONS

Fatigue: Prepare easy meals such as scrambled eggs, toast, and canned fruit
Eat a good breakfast when the patient usually has more energy
Use frozen or canned foods
Drink commercial liquid supplements, milkshakes, or pasteurized eggnog

Altered Taste: Try lemon juice or vinegar on vegetables
Emphasize cold foods such as ice cream and pudding; keep cans of fruit in the
    refrigerator
Experiment with spices and marinades for meat
Add bacon bits for flavor

No Appetite: Include snacks; emphasize small, frequent meals
Include high-calorie drinks such as sherbet blended with juice or milkshakes
Keep sugar-based candy by bedside (brush teeth first; rinse mouth with water
    regularly)

Nausea and Vomiting: Use antiemetic medications before meals (at least ½ hour
    before eating)
Avoid fatty foods
Avoid concentrated sweets; salty foods may be better tolerated
Sip liquids slowly
Avoid reclining directly after meals; use propped pillows in bed
Avoid foods with a strong odor

Sore Mouth or Throat: Eat soft foods
Add gravy, butter, or sauces to dry foods
Avoid very salty, spiced, or acidic foods
Use a straw for beverages
Have a physician prescribe artificial saliva

Diarrhea: Avoid lactose-containing beverages and foods
Use commercial drinks that are lactose-free
Avoid roughage; emphasize soluble-fiber foods, such as oatmeal and split pea
    soup

Constipation: Increase water and fiber intake
Include walking if possible, or leg-lifts if bedridden

WHAT IS THE ROLE OF THE NURSE OR OTHER HEALTH CARE PROFESSIONALS IN NUTRITIONAL COUNSELING FOR CANCER PREVENTION AND TREATMENT?

All health care professionals can promote the guidelines to reduce the risk of developing cancer. This entails speaking with individuals about their personal habits. Many changes can be made in the nutritional environment. Restaurants might be encouraged to use olive oil for dipping bread rather than serving only butter or solid margarines. Advising schools to offer an array of vegetables and fruits will help children develop a taste for high-fiber foods. Helping to provide high-fiber foods and low-sugar beverages at social functions will encourage individuals to make better choices.

The nurse plays an important role in helping the cancer patient cope with difficulties in eating that may arise. For those suffering from nausea and vomiting, for example, nurses can assess the need for antiemetic medications.

Nurses should establish a good relationship with patients before explaining why it is important to eat well. They should be sensitive when giving advice on how to promote optimum nutrition at a time when patients may be feeling poor physically, emotionally, and psychologically. Nurses need to have a total health care team approach to identify the problems leading to poor nutritional status and to implement a plan of action to improve the nutritional status of their patients.

Cancer patients in the home need encouragement to take advantage of the good days, when favorite and well-tolerated nutritious foods can be prepared in advance, frozen or refrigerated, and heated and served later at mealtime. An effort should then be made to provide a pleasant meal environment.

Nurses have the primary responsibility in caring for patients in the home setting. They must learn about patients' true nutritional needs and know when to consult a dietitian or to personally counsel patients wisely to provide comfort as long as possible. Good nutritional status in cancer patients is of utmost importance because it greatly influences the effectiveness of therapy and their overall comfort. Visiting nurses, doctors, dietitians, and volunteers are often active in *hospice care* (a program for the terminally ill, including cancer patients) and assist in dealing with the last stages of life in the home setting, as discussed in Chapter 15.

CHAPTER STUDY QUESTIONS AND CLASSROOM ACTIVITIES

1. Describe a diet that reduces the risk of developing cancer.
2. Name some of the factors contributing to cancer cachexia.
3. What are some of the nutritional problems imposed by cancer treatments? What dietary modifications are necessary?
4. Why is it important to individualize the diet of the cancer patient?

Case Study

Maria had finished receiving radiation and chemotherapy for her breast cancer. Now she was battling not only the weight she had gained during the treatment, but also her fear that the cancer might return. She had done a lot of reading on the prevention of cancer and was feeling quite confused at the moment. She had heard from a co-worker that she should not be eating fruit if she wanted to lose weight. However, everything she read about cancer prevention suggested increased consumption of fruits and vegetables. She decided to call her husband's dietitian to ask about the best approach to weight loss and prevention of cancer relapse.

Critical Thinking Applications

1. What advice would you give Maria to lose weight while eating more fruits and vegetables to help prevent relapse of cancer?
2. What other nutrition advice would be appropriate for Maria?
3. Can it be assumed that Maria's weight gain was from eating more food than usual? What other reason could there be?

REFERENCES

Abdulla M, Gruber P: Role of diet modification in cancer prevention. Biofactors. 2000; 12(1-4):45-51.

Ames BN: DNA damage from micronutrient deficiencies is likely to be a major cause of cancer. Mutat Res. April 18, 2001; 475(1-2):7-20.

Anderson KE, Anderson E, Mink PJ, Hong CP, Kushi LH, Sellers TA, Lazovich D, Folsom AR: Diabetes and endometrial cancer in the Iowa women's health study. Cancer Epidemiol Biomarkers Prev. June 2001; 10(6):611-616.

Balkau B, Kahn HS, Courbon D, Eschwege E, Ducimetiere P: Hyperinsulinemia predicts fatal liver cancer but is inversely associated with fatal cancer at some other sites: the Paris Prospective Study. Diabetes Care. May, 2001; 24(5):843-849.

Berton ER, Hankinson SE, Newcomb PA, Rosner B, Willet WC, Stampfer MJ, Egan KM: A population-based case-control study of carotenoid and vitamin A intake and ovarian cancer (United States). Cancer Causes Control. January 2001; 12(1):83-90.

Brown LM: *Helicobacter pylori:* epidemiology and routes of transmission. Epidemiol Rev. 2000; 22(2):283-297.

De la Taille A, Katz A, Vacherot F, Saint F, Salomon L, Cicco A, Abbou CC, Chopin DK: Cancer of the prostate: influence of nutritional factors. General nutritional factors. Presse Med. March 24, 2001; 30(11):554-556. [Article in French.]

Demark-Wahnefried W, Peterson BL, Winer EP, Marks L, Aziz N, Marcom PK, Blackwell K, Rimer BK: Changes in weight, body composition, and factors influencing energy balance among premenopausal breast cancer patients receiving adjuvant chemotherapy. Comment in: J Clin Oncol. May 1, 2001; 19(9):2367-2369; 2381-2389.

DeMeo MT: Pancreatic cancer and sugar diabetes. Nutr Rev. April 2001; 59(4):112-115.

Franceschi S, Dal Maso L, Augustin L, Negri E, Parpinel M, Boyle P, Jenkins DJ, La Vecchia C: Dietary glycemic load and colorectal cancer risk. Ann Oncol. February 2001; 12(2): 173-178.

Guyton KZ, Kensler TW, Posner GH: Cancer chemoprevention using natural vitamin D and synthetic analogs. Annu Rev Pharmacol Toxicol. 2001; 41:421-442.

Hardwick JC, Van Den Brink GR, Offerhaus GJ, Van Deventer SJ, Peppelenbosch MP: Leptin is a growth factor for colonic epithelial cells. Gastroenterology. July 2001; 121(1):79-90.

Hirose K, Tajima K, Hamajima N, Takezaki T, Inoue M, Kuroishi T, Miura S, Tokudome S: Association of family history and other risk factors with breast cancer risk among Japanese premenopausal and postmenopausal women. Cancer Causes Control. May 2001; 12(4):349-358.

Jernstrom H, Barrett-Connor E: Obesity, weight change, fasting insulin, proinsulin, C-peptide, and insulin-like growth factor-1 levels in women with and without breast cancer: the Rancho Bernardo Study. J Womens Health Gend Based Med. December 1999; 8(10):1265-1272.

Kaaks R: Plasma insulin, IGF-I and breast cancer. Gynecol Obstet Fertil. March 2001; 29(3):185-191. [Article in French.]

Liu G, Bibus DM, Bode AM, Ma WY, Holman RT, Dong Z: Omega-3 but not omega-6 fatty acids inhibit AP-1 activity and cell transformation in JB6 cells. Proc Natl Acad Sci U S A. June 19, 2001; 98(13):7510-7515.

Michaud DS, Spiegelman D, Clinton SK, Rimm EB, Willett WC, Giovannucci E: Prospective study of dietary supplements, macronutrients, micronutrients, and risk of bladder cancer in U.S. men. Am J Epidemiol. December 15, 2000; 152(12):1145-1153.

Mucci LA, Tamimi R, Lagiou P, Trichopoulou A, Benetou V, Spanos E, Trichopoulos D: Are dietary influences on the risk of prostate cancer mediated through the insulin-like growth factor system? BJU Int. June 2001; 87(9):814-820.

Murkies AL, Teede HJ, Davis SR: What is the role of phytoestrogens in treating menopausal symptoms? Med J Aust. November 6, 2000; 173 Suppl:S97-S98.

Petrik MB, McEntee MF, Johnson BT, Obukowicz MG, Whelan J: Highly unsaturated (n-3) fatty acids, but not alpha-linolenic, conjugated linoleic or gamma-linolenic acids, reduce tumorigenesis in Apc(Min/+) mice. J Nutr. October 2000; 130(10):2434-2443.

Rodriguez C, Patel AV, Calle EE, Jacobs EJ, Chao A, Thun MJ: Body mass index, height, and prostate cancer mortality in two large cohorts of adult men in the United States. Cancer Epidemiol Biomarkers Prev. April 2001; 10(4):345-353.

Semmens JB, Platell C: Bowel cancer. Positive expectations for improvements in outcomes. Aust Fam Physician. June 2001; 30(6):539-545.

Terry P, Lichtenstein P, Feychting M, Ahlbom A, Wolk A: Fatty fish consumption and risk of prostate cancer. Lancet. June 2, 2001; 357(9270):1764-1766.

Whitehouse AS, Smith HJ, Drake JL, Tisdale MJ: Mechanism of attenuation of skeletal muscle protein catabolism in cancer cachexia by eicosapentaenoic acid. Cancer Res. May 1, 2001; 61(9):3604-3609.

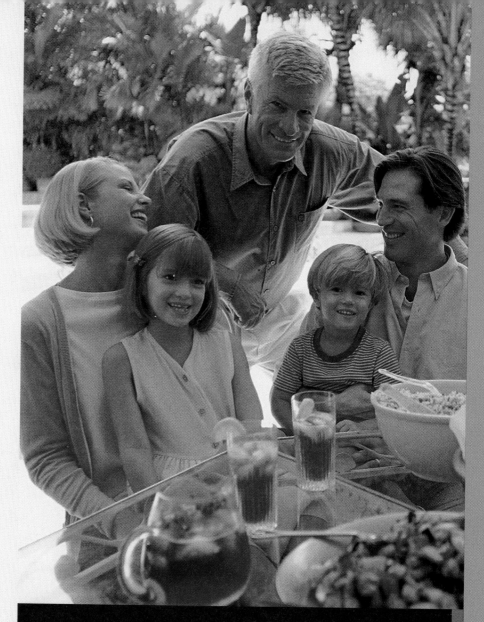

Lifespan and Wellness Concerns in Promoting Health and Managing Illness

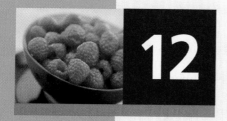

12 Maternal and Infant Nutrition in Health and Disease

OBJECTIVES

After completing this chapter, you should be able to:

- Identify nutritional needs during pregnancy, lactation, and infancy.
- Describe lactation management techniques.
- Describe infant feeding strategies.
- Identify women's health concerns.

TERMS TO IDENTIFY

Antidiuretic hormone
Bipolar disorder
Colostrum
Denver Developmental
  Screening Test
Diuresis
Embryo
Esophageal sphincter
Failure to thrive (FTT)
Fetal alcohol syndrome
Fetus
Fore milk
Gavage feeding
Gestational
Hind milk

Hyperemesis gravidarum
Immunoglobulin A (IgA)
Lactation
La Leche League
Let-down reflex
Milk anemia
Nursing-bottle mouth
Obstetrician
Otitis media
Oxytocin
Pediatrician
Physiologic anemia
Pica
Pincer grasp
Placenta

Postpartum blues
Postpartum psychosis
Preconception
Preeclampsia
Pregnancy-induced
  hypertension (PIH)
Premenstrual syndrome
  (PMS)
Prenatal
Preterm milk
Products of conception
Spina bifida
Toxemia
Weaning

INTRODUCTION

The human species is very resilient, having survived over the centuries with wide variation in nutritional intake. Many adults are healthy today, even though they were fed under less than ideal circumstances as infants. Only in this century have nutritional health, reproduction, and ways to raise healthier babies been readily understood. It is now widely accepted that nutrition plays a vital role in a healthy pregnancy and baby.

Growth of the **fetus** (the unborn baby; Box 12-1) may be affected by various maternal factors, for example, the ingestion, digestion, and absorption of nutrients from the mother's intestinal tract. The fetus is dependent on these processes and on maternal metabolism of the absorbed nutrients and transfer of nutrients through the **placenta** (an organ that allows the transfer of maternal nutrients to the fetus via the umbilical cord). An intact placenta of good size is critical for ideal growth of the fetus.

The impact of maternal nutrition does not stop at birth. Breast-feeding, preparation for a future successful pregnancy, and even the infant's feeding environment are all influenced by the mother's nutrition. A well-nourished mother is better able to cope with the demands of infant care, and a well-nourished infant displays a pleasant disposition, facilitating the return of the mother's strength and vitality. The relationship between maternal and infant nutrition is very much reciprocal.

HOW DOES NUTRITION INFLUENCE THE OUTCOME OF PREGNANCY?

The first trimester, during which the **embryo** (as the fetus is called in this period) develops, is the critical period of pregnancy (see Box 12-1). In this period all formation of organs occurs, such as that of the heart, brain, liver, and intestinal tract. Unfortunately, pregnancy is often not recognized until a significant amount of time in the first trimester has passed. It is for this reason that the **preconception** (before conception) nutritional status is now considered so important. This is especially true for women with diabetes, who need to have approximately normal blood sugar levels to help prevent birth defects that can occur in the first trimester (see later discussion on the management of diabetes during pregnancy). Maternal nutritional counseling should cover the preconception and postpartum periods and the more traditional **gestational** period (time of pregnancy).

Adequate nutrition without excess intake can help prevent some birth defects. For example, **spina bifida** (a neural tube birth defect in which the spine does not close) is associated with inadequate folate intake. Neural tube defects are among the most common and serious birth defects. Certain foods are now fortified with folate as a means to reduce the nation's incidence of these defects. Folate (also called folic acid) needs to be consumed within the first few weeks of pregnancy. Because pregnancy is usually not confirmed until later, it is advised

▌ BOX 12-1
▌ FETAL DEVELOPMENT

FIRST TRIMESTER (EMBRYO; CRITICAL STAGE)
Organs develop (4 to 12 weeks)
Central nervous system develops (4 to 12 weeks)
Skeletal structure hardens from cartilage to bone (4 weeks)

SECOND TRIMESTER (FETUS)
Growth and development continue (13 to 40 weeks)
Teeth calcify (20 weeks)
Fetus can survive outside womb (24 weeks)

THIRD TRIMESTER TO BIRTH
Growth and development continue
Storage of iron and other nutrients (36 to 40 weeks; premature babies often deficient in iron)
Development of necessary fat tissue (36 to 40 weeks)

that all women of childbearing age consume adequate folic acid either in food or in supplementation. Appropriate weight gain and **prenatal** (during pregnancy) avoidance of excess nutrients such as vitamin A are further associated with reduced morbidity and mortality.

WHAT NUTRITIONAL ADVICE IS RECOMMENDED DURING PREGNANCY?

Weight Gain

A major determinant of fetal outcome during pregnancy is maternal weight gain. Before 1960, pregnant women were encouraged to restrict their weight gain to less than 15 lbs. Current research shows that more liberal weight gain improves fetal growth. A woman who is underweight before pregnancy needs to gain more weight than is typically recommended to best promote growth of the **products of conception** (Figure 12-1). It is imperative that the placenta grow adequately because it transfers maternal nutrients to the fetus.

Ideal weight gain is now considered to be about 25 to 35 lbs for normal-weight women (that is, those who have a body mass index [BMI] of 20 to 26; see Appendix 12 for a nomogram for easy calculation), 28 to 40 lbs for an underweight (BMI <20) woman, and 15 to 25 lbs for an overweight (BMI >26) woman with an average weight gain of about 1 lb per week in the second and third trimesters of pregnancy. A grid can be used to plot weight gain throughout the pregnancy (Figure 12-2). Excess weight gain during pregnancy should be discouraged, but not if doing so would cause nutrient deficiencies.

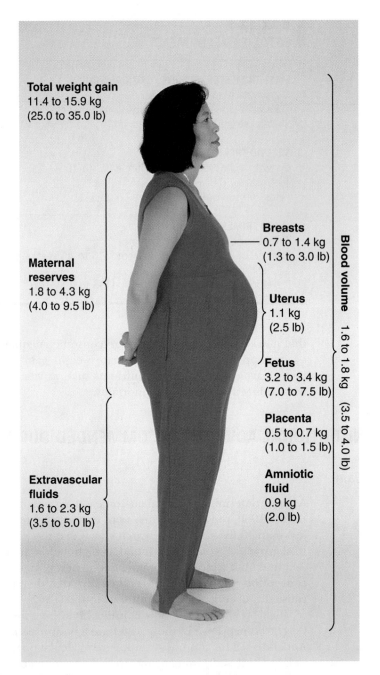

Total weight gain
11.4 to 15.9 kg
(25.0 to 35.0 lb)

Maternal reserves
1.8 to 4.3 kg
(4.0 to 9.5 lb)

Extravascular fluids
1.6 to 2.3 kg
(3.5 to 5.0 lb)

Breasts
0.7 to 1.4 kg
(1.3 to 3.0 lb)

Uterus
1.1 kg
(2.5 lb)

Fetus
3.2 to 3.4 kg
(7.0 to 7.5 lb)

Placenta
0.5 to 0.7 kg
(1.0 to 1.5 lb)

Amniotic fluid
0.9 kg
(2.0 lb)

Blood volume   1.6 to 1.8 kg   (3.5 to 4.0 lb)

FIGURE 12-1 Components of weight gain during pregnancy. (From Murray SS, McKinney ES, Gorrie TM: Foundations of maternal-newborn nursing, ed 3, Philadelphia, WB Saunders, 2002.)

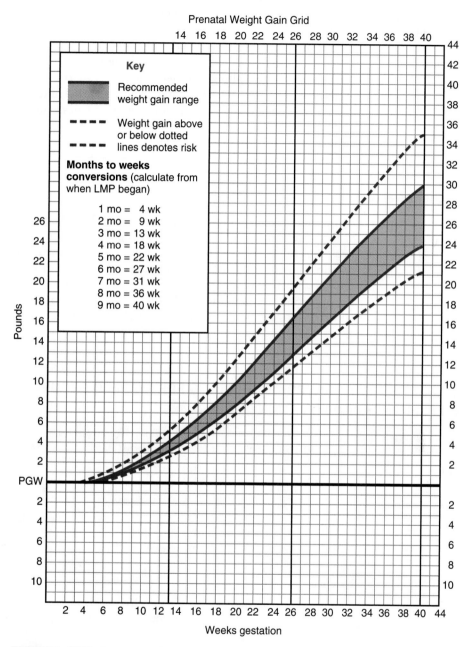

FIGURE 12-2 Recommended prenatal weight gain. Chart to monitor weight gain throughout pregnancy. KEY: PGW = pregestational weight (weight before conception). (From the New York State Health Department, WIC Program.)

Fallacy: Because a pregnant woman is "eating for two," she should eat twice as much.

Fact: It should be remembered that the second person is very small—about 7 lbs at birth. Although some nutrient requirements increase dramatically during pregnancy, the overall caloric need increases by only about 15%, amounting to about an extra 150 kcal a day during the first trimester and an additional 350 kcal per day for the remainder of the pregnancy. Thus it is important that a pregnant woman consume mainly nutrient-dense foods (foods that have a lot of nutrients for the number of kilocalories).

Nutrient Needs

To promote a healthy diet, a pregnant woman should be encouraged to consume at least the minimum number of servings recommended by the Food Guide Pyramid (Table 12-1), with a focus on the use of whole grains and unprocessed or minimally processed foods. Protein intake needs to be adequate; the minimum intake should be 60 g, which is met by the inclusion of the minimum number of servings listed in the Food Guide Pyramid. An intake of up to 100 g of protein daily has been advocated to ensure a healthy pregnancy. The kilocalories

TABLE 12-1
CHANGES IN FOODS FROM THE FOOD GUIDE PYRAMID GROUPS DURING PREGNANCY AND LACTATION

FOOD GUIDE PYRAMID GROUPS*	NONPREGNANT WOMEN	PREGNANT WOMEN (SECOND HALF OF PREGNANCY)	LACTATING WOMEN
Milk			
Adult	2 c or more	3 c or more	4 c or more
Adolescent	4 c or more	5 c or more	5 c or more
Vegetable and fruit			
Citrus and substitute	1 serving	2 servings	2-3 servings
Dark green, leafy or deep orange vegetable	1 serving at least every other day	1 serving daily	1-2 servings daily
Other fruits or vegetables, including potatoes	3-4 servings	2 servings	2 servings
Meat or alternate	2 servings or more	3 servings or more (6 oz cooked or more)	3 servings or more (6 oz cooked or more)
Cereal and bread whole grains	6 servings or more	6 servings or more	6 servings or more

If fortified milk is not used, obtain physician's instructions for vitamin D supplementation.
Use iodized salt.
Use water or other beverages—at least 6 to 8 c daily.
*Additional servings of these or any other food may be added as needed to provide the necessary calories and palatability.

needed to provide appropriate weight gain are supplied from additional carbohydrates and fat. A minimum of 30 g of fat is required to provide all of the essential fatty acids required for fetal growth and development. There is a wide range in the need for kilocalories during pregnancy and lactation because of variation in activity levels and possibly increased metabolic efficiency, among other factors. Specific recommendations for carbohydrate and fat intake during pregnancy and lactation are not possible for every woman (Catalano, 1999).

The type of fat in the diet has increasingly been examined in relation to neurologic development of the fetus. It has been advised that pregnant and lactating women include some food sources of omega-3 fatty acids that can affect fetal status (Koletzko et al., 2001). This type of fat is found in plentiful amounts in cold-water fish such as tuna and salmon. Small fish such as sardines are less likely to have high levels of mercury or other toxic substances harmful to a growing fetus. Vegetarians should be advised to consume walnuts, canola oil, or seaweed for alternative plant sources of omega-3 fatty acids. Reduced intake of trans fatty acids, as found in hydrogenated fats, during pregnancy can promote adequate levels of omega-3 fatty acids in infants at birth (Decsi et al., 2001). One study implicates saturated fat and associated oxidative damage with premature delivery (Scholl and Stein, 2001).

Fortunately, there are biologic mechanisms that allow for adequate nutrient availability to the fetus if the mother's diet is inadequate. For example, there is increased absorption in the intestinal tract of some nutrients during pregnancy. This has been found with calcium and zinc. Other nutrients, such as selenium, are maintained at a high level because of reduced excretion through the mother's kidneys (King, 2001).

Although a woman's ability to absorb minerals is enhanced during pregnancy, an adequate dietary intake is still best. Minerals such as zinc, copper, and magnesium are found in whole grains and legumes. Adequate consumption of dark green, leafy vegetables and deep orange vegetables and fruits should be encouraged for a source of beta-carotene (vitamin A). Vitamin C foods, such as citrus fruits and dark green, leafy vegetables, should be increased during pregnancy and lactation. A well-balanced diet will help the fetus grow well and allow the mother to stay healthy for future pregnancies. Table 12-2 shows a sample menu.

Vitamin supplements should be used only as added insurance, not as a replacement for nutrients found in foods. Supplements should not exceed the Dietary Reference Intakes (DRIs) (see inside back cover). Iron is the only nutrient specifically advised for supplementation during pregnancy. However, most obstetricians advocate the use of a prenatal vitamin and mineral supplement.

Pregnant women following a vegan diet need to ensure adequate intake of vitamin B_{12} through fortified foods or supplements. Vitamin D is also difficult to obtain in a vegan diet; the pregnant woman's diet should therefore be supplemented unless she receives adequate sun exposure of at least 15 minutes daily. Good nutritional intake should be maintained after delivery for healthy lactation and in preparation for a future pregnancy.

Women who have difficulty adhering to these guidelines or who have high-risk pregnancies are encouraged to consult a registered dietitian or qualified nutritionist.

TABLE 12-2
SAMPLE MEAL PLANS FOR PREGNANCY

	PREGNANT WOMAN	PREGNANT ADOLESCENT*
Breakfast	Orange juice, 1 c[†]	Orange juice, 1 c[†]
	Shredded wheat	Shredded wheat
	Scrambled egg	Scrambled egg
	Toast, 1 slice	Toast, 2 slices
	Milk, 1 c	Butter or margarine
	Decaffeinated coffee	Marmalade[†]
		Milk, 1 c
Lunch	Tuna sandwich	Tuna sandwich on whole wheat bread
	Carrot and green pepper sticks	Carrot and green pepper sticks
	Oatmeal cookies[†]	Cheese cubes
	Milk, 1 c	Oatmeal cookies[†]
		Fresh fruit
		Milk, 1 c
Midafternoon	Milk, 1 c	Chicken sandwich
		Milk, 1 c
Dinner	Broiled steak	Broiled steak
	Steamed broccoli	Steamed broccoli with melted cheese
	Baked potato	Baked potato with sour cream
	Tomato salad with French dressing	Vegetable salad with French dressing
	Apple slices	Apple with peanut butter
		Milk, 1 c
Bedtime	Hot milk or cocoa,[†] 1 c	Milk or cocoa,[†] 1 c

*Needs more kilocalories, protein, and calcium.
[†]For women with gestational diabetes, juice may be deemed inappropriate for control of blood glucose; oranges or other vitamin C-containing fruit may be advised later in the day rather than at breakfast and desserts should be restricted based on values obtained from the woman's self-monitoring of blood glucose levels (SMBG).

Fallacy: A few cups of coffee per day pose no risk during pregnancy.

Fact: There is conflicting evidence about how much caffeine is safe during pregnancy. Caffeine is known to cause blood vessels to constrict, potentially limiting blood flow through the placenta to the growing fetus. Until more is known, the prudent approach is to cut back on coffee and other caffeine sources gradually to no more than one cup (200 mg of caffeine) daily.

WHAT ARE SOME CLINICAL PROBLEMS DURING PREGNANCY?

Nausea

Nausea or morning sickness commonly occurs in the first trimester and for some women throughout the entire pregnancy. The cause of the nausea is not fully understood but is probably related to hormonal changes during pregnancy. Reduced motility throughout the gastrointestinal (GI) tract occurs, which is believed to allow for the increased absorption of nutrients. However, the reduced motility may also lead to feelings of fullness and nausea. Because high-fat foods further slow the movement of food through the GI tract, they should be avoided unless tolerated and allowable within weight gain goals.

Nausea may be related to low blood sugar levels because nausea seems to increase when a woman has not eaten for a time. Although there is no direct evidence indicating this, indirectly it is known that the need for insulin in those women who take it decreases during the first trimester. The resultant ketone formation and glucagon production that occurs with hypoglycemia or inadequate carbohydrate intake are known inducers of nausea and vomiting. Eating high-carbohydrate foods, such as dry toast or crackers, before rising may alleviate the problem. A gradual increase of food consumption during the late afternoon and evening can replace nutrients that were not consumed in the morning (a common time for nausea). Including carbohydrate snacks with a protein source may help to stabilize blood sugar levels during the night and help prevent morning sickness.

Hyperemesis Gravidarum

Hyperemesis gravidarum, commonly referred to as simply hyperemesis, is characterized by excessive and prolonged vomiting. It is probably more common than statistics show because treatment may be in a physician's office rather than in a hospital setting. One study found that over half of all pregnancies involve some nausea and almost 1 in 10 complain of severe or prolonged nausea with vomiting. About 2% of women with hyperemesis require hospitalization (Power et al., 2001).

Hyperemesis can cause serious dehydration and a weight loss of over 5% is considered indicative of this disorder. The effects of prolonged vomiting can be serious. Wernicke's encephalopathy (see Chapter 4) resulting from thiamin deficiency from hyperemesis has been noted (Tan and Ho, 2001). Charlotte Brontë, the famous writer, died of hyperemesis in 1855.

The cause of hyperemesis is generally unknown. It is interesting to note, however, that women with hyperemesis are more likely to deliver a female baby (Del Mar Melero-Montes and Jick, 2001). Hyperthyroidism is one possible cause of hyperemesis (Corssmit et al., 2001). One study found that infection with *Helicobacter pylori* is one of the important factors in the development of this disorder (Hayakawa et al., 2000). Intestinal obstruction during pregnancy can also be a contributing factor (Hardikar, 2000).

Hyperemesis has been noted to increase bitter-taste perception (Sipiora et al., 2000). It is partially for this reason that all foods that are tolerated are considered acceptable when severe nausea and vomiting are adversely affecting weight gain. Nutrient density becomes a minor issue when weight gain is paramount to combat the effects of hyperemesis. If a woman with hyperemesis can tolerate jelly beans or potato chips, they may be warranted as a source of carbohydrates and kilocalories. Once the hyperemesis is resolved, more nutrient-dense foods can be included.

Hospitalization with administration of intravenous fluids may ultimately be necessary, as may more aggressive medical management. Total parenteral nutrition (TPN) may be prescribed to resolve the nutrient deficiencies and help correct hyperemesis. This author helped initiate TPN for one woman with seemingly intractable hyperemesis that was then simply cured within 72 hours. An alternative option may be use of enteral nutrition with nasojejunal tube feeding (refer back to Chapter 5) if problems with aspiration are monitored and controlled.

Other causes of weight loss and vomiting need to be ruled out to develop the most effective management plan. Possibilities unrelated to the usual physiologic causes of hyperemesis include eating disorders such as anorexia nervosa and bulimia nervosa, which are related to miscarriage, low birth weight, and postpartum depression.

Fallacy: Hyperemesis is psychologic in origin.

Fact: There is little evidence that hyperemesis is caused by psychologic problems; rather, it is more likely that it causes psychologic distress itself. Stronger evidence indicates that hormonal or other physical issues are the basis of the development of hyperemesis. Smells, odors, and motion also often precipitate nausea and vomiting.

Anemia

Anemia from iron deficiency may occur during pregnancy when iron intake and stores do not meet the demand. This is preventable and treatable by daily supplements of 30 to 60 mg of ferrous salts.

Anemia from folate deficiency may occur if intake is inadequate. A daily supplement of 400 μg of folacin and improvement in eating habits will correct this condition. Anemia from folate deficiency is less likely to occur because the public health measure of fortifying food with this vitamin was instituted.

Physiologic anemia also results from expanded blood volume (plasma increases without a concomitant increase in red blood cells). There is controversy in the medical field over whether this form of anemia needs to be treated. However, until further research indicates otherwise, increased iron intake is advised.

Constipation

Constipation can be related to iron supplementation and to decreased intestinal motility, which is believed to be a normal physiologic process that assists in nutrient absorption during pregnancy. Increased production of the hormone *progesterone* is believed to be the physiologic basis for decreased peristalsis. Also, by the end of pregnancy, the associated pressure from the growing fetus contributes to constipation. Adequate fiber and fluid intake and appropriate exercise can help control constipation. A fiber intake of 20 to 35 g is generally advocated with a fluid intake of at least 2 L daily. Laxatives should only be used on the advice of an **obstetrician** (a physician specializing in pregnancy).

Heartburn

Heartburn in pregnancy is believed to be caused by the pressure of the growing fetus on the stomach, resulting in hydrochloric acid being forced into the esophagus. For this reason, pregnant women may find it helpful to eat smaller, more frequent meals and to avoid a reclining position after eating. Excess fat intake can contribute to heartburn by causing food to remain in the stomach for longer periods. Excess fat is also associated with relaxed muscle tone of the **esophageal sphincter** (the muscle connecting the stomach and esophagus), which further promotes the forcing of hydrochloric acid up into the esophagus. Pregnant women should not take over-the-counter medication for heartburn without consulting their obstetrician.

Pica

The practice of **pica** (eating nonfood items, especially clay or laundry starch) during pregnancy is a carryover from a tradition in Africa, where it is still practiced in some areas. The consumption of clay can provide a source of calcium, iron, and other minerals; however, it can also provide toxic contaminants. When clay is not available in this country, laundry starch is sometimes substituted. Consumption of these substances can interfere with absorption of adequate nutrients and should be discouraged.

The practice of pica is not often revealed, especially if the health care professional appears to have a judgmental attitude. The health care professional must demonstrate great sensitivity to elicit an accurate assessment of the practice of pica. Because pica is generally related to cultural heritage and beliefs, changing the practice may be difficult. Using objective measures, such as informing patients about the danger of anemia or lead poisoning, may help them understand the negative consequences of pica.

Closely Spaced Pregnancies

Although many parents plan to space their children close together so that the children can be playmates, it is healthier for the mother and the fetus for pregnancies to be at least 12 to 18 months apart. Longer spacing helps the mother reestablish good nutritional stores and recover from childbirth.

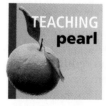

TEACHING pearl   Two effective assessment questions concerning nutritional preparation for subsequent pregnancies are: "Are you planning to have another child in the future?" and if so, "What have you heard is the ideal spacing between pregnancies?"

Obesity

Of women of childbearing age, it has been estimated that almost half are either overweight or obese (BMI ≥26); furthermore, one third of pregnant women gain more weight than is recommended (Cogswell et al., 2001). Excess weight gain during pregnancy increases the mother's body fat levels and is associated with pregnancy complications and delivery problems (Lederman, 2001). However, weight reduction should not be promoted during pregnancy because this may be detrimental to the health of the baby as well. Overweight women should observe the same principles of prenatal nutrition as do women of normal weight. The total weight gain, however, should be smaller, averaging about 15 to 20 lbs; thus limiting sugar and fat intake becomes important.

Fallacy: You can safely avoid gaining too much weight during pregnancy by taking calcium supplements instead of drinking milk.

Fact: Milk provides more nutrients than just calcium. A calcium supplement will not give you the extra 30 g of protein found in the recommended 4 c of milk. Riboflavin and other nutrients, such as potassium, magnesium, phosphorus, vitamins A and D, and other trace elements, are found in milk as well. Low-fat or skim milk can be used by weight-conscious women.

Pregnancy-Induced Hypertension

Pregnancy-induced hypertension (PIH), formerly known as **toxemia**, is a condition that may occur during the third trimester of pregnancy. Its cause is not known, but it is no longer felt to be a toxic condition; therefore the term *toxemia* is no longer used. It affects 10% of pregnancies in the United States and remains a leading cause of both maternal and fetal morbidity and mortality. Risks to the fetus include premature delivery, growth retardation, and death (Garovic, 2000). Pregnancy-induced hypertension is characterized by proteinuria, elevated blood pressure, and rapid weight gain. It is also an important risk factor for stroke (Lanska and Kryscio, 2000). Research is linking the insulin resistance syndrome with the development of hypertension in pregnancy (Innes et al., 2001).

Preeclampsia is associated with symptoms of PIH. *Eclampsia* (the most severe form of preeclampsia) is associated with convulsions and coma. Some symptoms that can indicate its development include a sudden rise in blood pressure, severe headache, blurred vision, and proteinuria (protein in the urine). The cause of eclampsia is not well understood. It is interesting to note, however, that postmenopausal women with a history of eclampsia and recurrent hypertension during pregnancy have a high rate of dyslipidemia (Hubel et al., 2000). This appears to be in line with the research mentioned earlier linking the insulin resistance syndrome with the development of hypertension and eclampsia.

The former practices of restricting kilocalories and sodium to reduce the risk of PIH complications are now considered obsolete. To the contrary, there is a greater incidence of PIH among underweight women who fail to gain weight normally during pregnancy. The evidence indicates that the total amount of weight gain per se is not the significant factor. Sodium restriction is no longer recommended and may actually be harmful because sodium requirements increase during pregnancy. However, avoiding excessive salt intake is recommended for pregnant women and for the general population. Found on food labels, the guidelines advocating 2400 mg of sodium for the general public are appropriate for women who are pregnant, with or without hypertension.

Diabetes

Type 1 diabetes was once considered an automatic cause for alarm if pregnancy occurred. Even with long-standing diabetes it is now felt that the outcome for mother and child is likely to be favorable if the various health concerns are managed well (Rosenn and Miodovnik, 2000). We now know that if a pregnant woman with this type of diabetes maintains near normal blood glucose levels before conception and throughout the pregnancy, she is just as likely as a woman without diabetes to bear a healthy, normal infant. It is paramount, however, that tight control over blood sugar levels be kept before conception to help prevent birth defects from developing during the critical first trimester. For women with preexisting Type 2 diabetes, the same precautions need to be taken.

An added concern of women who are taking insulin to manage their diabetes is nighttime hypoglycemia. One study found that over one third of pregnant women treated with insulin had nighttime hypoglycemia during the first trimester. Occurrence of hypoglycemia could be predicted in the majority of these women by measurements of blood glucose before bedtime (Hellmuth et al., 2000).

Gestational diabetes mellitus (GDM), a form of diabetes that occurs only during pregnancy, is not associated with birth defects because the elevated blood sugar does not develop until after the critical first trimester is over. The consequences of uncontrolled GDM are more problematic at the time of birth. A woman with GDM has an increased likelihood of delivering a large baby who is very susceptible to hypoglycemia in the first few hours after birth. Strict control of blood glucose during pregnancy will increase the chances of normal labor and delivery of a healthy baby without complications. Routine screening for GDM is now done between the twenty-fourth and twenty-eighth weeks of pregnancy. Women who have a family history of Type 2 diabetes, are of older age, or are overweight are all at increased risk of GDM and may benefit from earlier glucose screening.

Control of pregnancy with diabetes is best handled with a medical team approach, so that the most appropriate plan and means of control are developed, including aspects such as insulin, diet, and home glucose monitoring. Maternal blood sugar levels should range from 60 to 90 mg/dL fasting to 120 mg/dL postprandially (2 hours after eating, using a whole-blood glucose meter; 135 mg/dL is used with plasma meters as per the American Diabetes Association). High postprandial blood sugar levels may indicate a need for further carbohydrate restriction (particularly at breakfast), a need for insulin, or both. Morning urine ketone levels must also be monitored. Too little carbohydrate intake, too little insulin production, or weight loss of any amount can cause the mother's body fat to break down excessively. The resulting ketone buildup is potentially detrimental to the growing fetus and needs to be corrected with increased carbohydrates—especially at night—insulin, or both. On occasion, a middle-of-the-night carbohydrate snack may be necessary to stop the morning ketonuria, which is quite easy because it is most likely to occur in the third trimester when the mother is up in the night using the bathroom.

Restless Leg Syndrome

A cause of poor sleep during pregnancy is related to restless leg syndrome. One study found that 23% of women in their third trimester have this condition. It has been found to be associated with low ferritin and folate levels. Depression has been linked to this syndrome as well, probably stemming from inadequate deep sleep (Lee et al., 2001).

Phenylketonuria

Women who were born with the metabolic disorder phenylketonuria (PKU) may choose to conceive, but are at high risk of delivering a baby with growth retardation and birth defects. These abnormalities are proportional to the woman's serum phenylalanine levels. It has been found that with a strict low-phenylalanine diet that is followed before conception and throughout gestation, there is no greater risk of abnormalities than for a woman without PKU. The maternal blood phenylalanine levels must be maintained between 120 and 250 μmol/L and the tyrosine blood levels between 45 and 90 μmol/L. Weekly blood analyses are mandatory to ensure the safety of the growing baby (Matthieu et al., 2001). These women's diets must be monitored by a registered dietitian to ensure a nutritional intake sufficient to support a healthy pregnancy.

Alcohol Use

Fetal alcohol syndrome results from excessive alcohol intake by the mother during pregnancy. It is characterized by wide-set eyes and mental retardation or another dysfunction of the central nervous system. Because the safe limit of alcohol intake is not known, the best advice for the pregnant woman is to abstain from alcohol. Professional counseling may be necessary.

Drug Addiction

The use of illegal drugs (and legal drugs, such as alcohol and those found in tobacco) impairs fetal growth. Women who are addicted before conception often deny their dependence, presenting a challenge to the health care professional. Good nutrition is vital so that complications associated with drug use are not exacerbated.

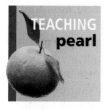

A description of the effect of tobacco use on the growing infant is to relate this to scuba diving. It can be explained to a patient that the fetus is essentially scuba diving in utero and is dependent on oxygen from the mother. Tobacco use decreases the amount of oxygen the fetus is able to receive, essentially suffocating it. Putting your hands around your neck and making gasping sounds definitely gets the patient's attention. She may, however, need assistance in smoking cessation.

Adolescent Pregnancy

Depending on the age of the mother and other factors, an adolescent pregnancy may be perfectly normal or extremely high risk. Younger teenagers and those who become pregnant near the time of menarche are at greatest risk. Pregnant teenagers may have dietary habits that include foods low in essential nutrients, resulting in an insufficient intake of nutrients especially important during pregnancy. A concern about body image may result in inadequate weight gain.

Programs for pregnant teenagers, common in most communities, offer social support, encouragement to seek good medical care, and assistance in completion of school. The Women, Infants, and Children (WIC) Supplemental Nutrition Program is generally available to all low-income pregnant teenagers and referral should be made by the health care professional (see Chapter 15). It provides the pregnant teenager with vouchers for purchasing specified foods that meet needs for calcium, vitamin C, and iron. Nutrition assessment and education is also provided by registered dietitians or nutritionists within the program.

Breast-feeding is possible for the motivated teenager, although other life concerns may take precedence. Nevertheless, breast-feeding should be recommended for all women unless specifically deemed unadvisable by a doctor. Even a few days or weeks of breast-feeding can be beneficial to the newborn infant.

Celiac Disease

Studies show that women with celiac disease are at increased risk of infertility, miscarriages, having children with low birth weight, and short duration of breast-feeding. Folic acid deficiency can occur because of poor intestinal absorption, which leads to neural tube defects and cleft palates. Minor symptoms may lead to misdiagnosis. Proper diagnosis of celiac disease followed by a gluten-free diet may improve fertility and pregnancy outcomes (Hozyasz, 2001). Refer back to Chapter 3 for more on celiac disease.

Postpartum Depression

Although it is common for women to experience the **postpartum blues** (a feeling of depression) within a few weeks after pregnancy, the more severe depression associated with **postpartum psychosis** (a condition following delivery that is attributed to hormonal changes in susceptible women) requires medical monitoring and intervention, including hospitalization. It has been estimated that 10% to 15% of women will develop syndromal depressions within the first 2 to 3 months postpartum, making this the most common serious medical complication following pregnancy. Postpartum psychosis is estimated to occur in approximately 1 to 2 deliveries per 1000 women. History of **bipolar disorder** (manic depression) increases the risk of postpartum psychosis to as much as 25%. Prior episodes further increase the risk to 50% to 75%. Causation has been attributed to low levels of total and free thyroxine concentrations during late pregnancy (Pedersen, 1999). It has been noted that persons with diabetes have a higher rate of bipolar disorder. This combination may result from excess levels of cortisol, a substance which induces diabetes and contributes to mania (Cassidy et al., 1999).

It may help to advocate the regular consumption of balanced meals to help prevent or treat postpartum depression. A highly insulin-resistant state develops by the end of pregnancy. The natural production of insulin increases in response to the opposing action of placental hormones. Once delivery occurs, the mother's insulin production may not lessen adequately. By including several meals and snacks over the course of the day, a postpartum woman's glucose levels are more likely to be stabilized. This can help prevent or manage depression, in part by reducing the production of cortisol.

HOW DOES DIET INFLUENCE THE NURSING COUPLE?

The affect of maternal diet on infant growth does not end at delivery. This is true even for nonnursing mothers, who need to maintain their nutritional status to cope best with the demands of a new baby. During **lactation** (production of milk for breast-feeding, also called *nursing*), adequate diet becomes more critical. Caloric intake can affect the quantity of milk produced; thus it is important for a breast-feeding woman to lose any excess weight slowly. (An initial rapid loss will result from fluid loss after delivery, which is unrelated to caloric intake.) Other nutrients vary in their effect on the quality of breast milk. In general, problems are limited to excessive intake of fat-soluble vitamins through the indiscriminate use of supplements in megadoses and insufficient intake of water-soluble vitamins. Mineral levels do not generally affect the quality of breast milk because development of maternal deficiency and toxicity states is uncommon.

Drinking milk is not a prerequisite for successful lactation, contrary to what is often believed. However, to help prevent maternal bone loss, other calcium-rich foods such as cheese, yogurt, pudding, or soybean products such as tofu (see Table 12-1 for recommended intakes during lactation) should be encouraged for the breast-feeding woman who cannot or will not drink milk. Women who avoid drinking milk and live in cloudy regions may have inadequate levels of vitamin D, which is reflected in breast milk. A vitamin D supplement may be advisable in such situations.

The omega-3 fatty acid docosahexaenoic acid (DHA) promotes visual development of infants. Lactating women's intake of DHA from fish affects the amount found in their breast milk. However, the optimal amount of DHA intake for lactating women is not known (Jorgensen et al., 2001).

As long as the mother's nutritional intake is adequate, breast milk provides all the necessary vitamins for the infant, with the possible exception of vitamin D. During both pregnancy and lactation, vegans may need vitamin D and vitamin B_{12} supplements and their infants may need some as well.

One known health benefit of breast milk for the infant is an increased immune response, resulting from the transferal of the mother's immune factors through **colostrum** (the substance that precedes breast milk) and breast milk. In these fluids, a substance called **immunoglobulin A (IgA)** helps guard against intestinal organisms and antigens, the latter of which are a cause of allergy development.

The improved learning ability of breast-fed infants may be caused by the high level of essential fatty acids naturally found in breast milk but not in cow's milk. These fats are likely involved in improving neurologic development of the growing infant. Another interesting aspect of breast-feeding has to do with exposure to food flavors. Breast milk will vary in flavor depending on the mother's diet. This may increase the infant's later acceptance of a variety of table foods (Mennella et al., 2001).

WHAT ARE LACTATION MANAGEMENT ISSUES?

Although many people believe that breast-feeding is both beneficial and natural, several important pieces of "how-to" information are not widely known. Nurses who see lactating mothers during the first weeks following delivery can play a vital role in the success (or failure) of breast-feeding. Positive verbal encouragement and support are of crucial importance.

Frequency of Feeding

A primary rule of thumb is that the more frequently a woman nurses, the more breast milk she will produce (Figure 12-3). This is referred to as *supply and demand.* Because the quantity of breast milk production is difficult to ascertain, other guidelines are used to determine adequacy. For the neonate and infants to 3 months of age, these guidelines are the following: weight gain by the infant of 1 to 2 lbs per month; 8 to 12 nursings per 24-hour period; and 6 or more wet diapers per 24-hour period (assuming the infant is not given any bottles of water).

Infant Weight Gain

Some breast-fed infants gain more than the recommended 2 lbs per month, but this is usually not a cause for concern because it is not possible to force-feed an infant who is fed only breast milk.

If the infant gains less than the recommended 1 to 2 lbs per month, great care must be taken not to discourage the lactating mother, but rather to assess possible causes and provide appropriate counseling in a highly sensitive manner. On average, breast-fed infants gain weight more slowly than formula-fed infants after the first 2 to 3 months. However, this slower weight gain should not be viewed as problematic as long as consumption of breast milk remains substantial and the infant is healthy.

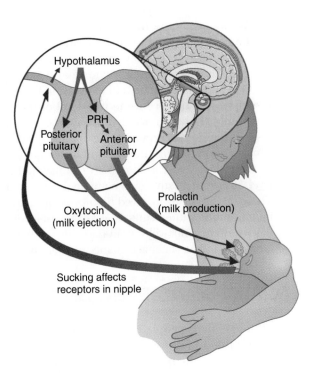

FIGURE 12-3 Milk release during breast-feeding.

Inverted Nipples

A simple exercise can determine whether a woman has inverted nipples (Figure 12-4). Either the Hoffman technique or a milk cup (not a soft rubber shield) can be used to alleviate the problem (Figure 12-5).

Poor Let-Down Reflex

Particularly for a first-time nursing mother, anxiety can be high and can inhibit the **let-down reflex**, which occurs when the milk descends from the upper parts of the breast (**hind milk**) comes down to the areola (the darker skin around the nipple). **Oxytocin** (a hormone) promotes this reflex. A lactating woman can usually identify when the let-down reflex is occurring because there is a momentary "pins-and-needles" feeling in the breast area.

The hind milk is richer and higher in fat content than milk from other parts of the breasts. Because of the high caloric value of fat found in the hind milk, the let-down reflex is crucial for the infant's adequate weight gain. Relaxation techniques are thus important for successful lactation. Humor is useful in helping the nursing mother relax; it should be encouraged by the nurse or other health care professional.

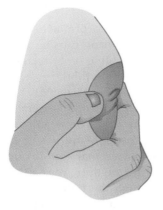

Inverted Nipple

An inverted nipple looks like a slit or a fold. A partially inverted nipple folds in on one side only.

A woman can tell if she has an inverted nipple by gently pinching the nipple at the base using the thumb and forefinger. If the nipple shrinks back, it is an "inverted" nipple.

Many women with inverted nipples have successfully breast-fed, but special preparation is very helpful. Using the Hoffman technique and wearing a hard plastic cup such as the Confi-Dry will encourage the nipples to stick out.

FIGURE 12-4 Inverted nipple. (From Health Education Associates, Sandwich, MA.)

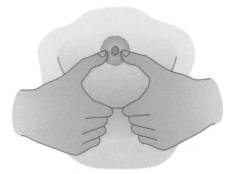

Hoffman Technique
For women with flat or inverted nipples

Place your thumbs opposite each other on either side of the nipple. Gently draw your thumbs away from the nipple. Then place your thumbs above and below the nipple and repeat.

Do this twice a day for a few minutes.

A

Milk Cup
For women with flat or inverted nipples

Begin by wearing the cup under the bra for short periods and gradually work up to 8 to 10 hours a day.

B

You can allow your skin to breathe by removing the cup for short periods or by wearing only the base part.

Wearing the cup is painless. It is not noticeable when worn in the bra unless the woman is wearing a tight-fitting jersey.

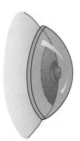

Milk cups/shells can be purchased from La Leche League International, 1400 N. Meacham Road, P.O. Box 4079, Schaumburg, IL 60168–4079 or call 1-800-LALECHE.

FIGURE 12-5 A, Hoffman technique. **B**, Milk cup. (From Health Education Associates, Sandwich, MA.)

Insufficient Feedings

If the let-down reflex does not seem to be a problem (the nurse can ask the mother if she feels a tingling sensation during nursing), the nurse should ask how often breast-feeding occurs. Women often try to maintain a feeding schedule and ignore the hunger cues of their baby, thinking, "the baby can't be hungry yet." Alternately, the infant may be a "sleepy baby," that is, one who does not indicate his own hunger. An appropriate schedule generally allows for feeding about every 2 to 3 hours, but for infants who gain weight slowly, more frequent feedings may be in order until the milk supply and weight gain increase.

During periods of growth spurts the baby may want to nurse more often than usual. Growth spurts often occur during the third week after delivery (just when the mother is likely to be going through the postpartum blues) and again at 6 weeks and 3 months. This does not mean formula needs to be added; rather, it is nature's way of increasing milk production to meet additional needs. Good advice is to encourage bed rest with continuous nursing (although strong family support is a prerequisite for this approach). After a couple of days of very frequent nursing, milk production will have increased, and the baby will go for longer periods between feedings.

Another helpful point concerning frequency of feeding is that the total number of feedings is more important than their spacing. For example, an infant who sleeps through the night, but feeds more frequently during the day and has the recommended 8 to 12 feedings will most likely gain weight just the same as the infant who wakes up regularly all night and day, but nurses the same number of times.

Breast Engorgement

Breast engorgement is a common occurrence in the first few days after delivery. Temporary measures to release excess milk include taking a warm shower or leaning with exposed breasts over a sink full of warm water. When engorgement is diminished, the infant will be better able to grasp the nipple, thereby allowing emptying of the breasts. Short, frequent nursings can help keep engorgement under control. The amount of milk produced by the new lactating mother will eventually even out to meet the infant's needs.

Sore or Cracked Nipples

Comfort measures for sore or cracked nipples include the following:

1. Relaxation techniques, such as deep breathing, at the beginning of each feeding and warm washcloths with gentle breast (not nipple) massage to encourage milk flow before the infant's suckling
2. Nursing on the less sore side first
3. Changing feeding positions, using the football hold (where the baby's feet point outward from the mother rather than inward toward her), the regular position, or even lying down with the baby's feet pointing up toward the

mother's head (awkward, but effective, in getting the baby's tongue off the sore spot on the mother's nipple)

4. Giving short, frequent nursings (the major portion of breast milk is removed within about 5 to 10 minutes; frequent nursings will prevent the baby from becoming overly hungry, thereby lessening excessive suckling)
5. Making sure the baby's mouth is well back on the areola and the tongue is underneath the nipple
6. Making sure that the baby is removed properly from the breast, breaking suction with the mother's finger inserted into the corner of the baby's mouth
7. Air-drying the nipples after each feeding
8. Using cold compresses or washcloths between nursings

Fallacy: A lactating woman who is experiencing sore nipples should be advised to wear a soft rubber nipple shield while breast-feeding.

Fact: Although this solution may provide relief in the short term, it can cause severe problems in the long term. Because tactile stimulation is necessary to continue producing milk, the physical barrier of the shield between the mother's nipple and the baby's jaw and tongue will inhibit milk production.

Twins

Many people believe that twins preclude the option of breast-feeding. However, because milk supply is most strongly influenced by frequency of feeding (remember supply and demand: the more the mother nurses, the more milk is produced), it is feasible to nurse twins. Babies can be positioned at each breast simultaneously with the infants' feet both facing the same direction or with each twin's feet facing outward from the mother. For multiple births, a combination of breast- and bottle-feeding may be the ideal solution. Any amount of breast-feeding still affords some immune system protection against illness and therefore should not be automatically precluded for women with multiple births.

Inappropriate Fluid Intake

Milk production necessitates increased fluid intake; however, the mother only needs to drink enough fluids to satisfy her thirst. A sudden excess in fluid intake may actually decrease milk yield because the release of **antidiuretic hormone** (a hormone that regulates water loss through the kidneys) is inhibited when fluid intake is in excess of need, resulting in **diuresis** (excess water loss through the kidneys).

The Premature Infant

Premature infants or those with cleft palate may be fed breast milk or commercial formula using bottles with special nipples. **Gavage feeding** (a form of force-feeding through a flexible tube or pump) may be required for those premature infants who do not have adequate suckling ability. Premature infants have special nutritional needs, primarily because of immature GI functioning. These infants now use either special formula or fortified breast milk. This breast milk ideally comes from the infant's own mother and is called **preterm milk**. In addition, commercial fortifiers are added to this breast milk to increase the amount of kilocalories and other nutrients.

The mother who is collecting milk for her premature infant probably will need extra support to maintain breast-feeding, particularly to relax in this tense situation. A picture of the baby that she can look at during the milk-collection process can help elicit positive feelings: "Oh, don't I have a beautiful baby!"—feelings that are difficult to experience while the baby lies in the intensive care unit hooked up to tubes and other medical paraphernalia. A relaxed nursing staff is of particular importance; again, the use of humor is a positive approach to help encourage the let-down reflex. It is difficult to achieve the same high level of tactile stimulation to the nipple by artificial means because no pumping machine fully mimics the action of the baby's tongue and jaw movements.

Women in the Workforce

Surveys suggest that one fourth of employed women with a child less than 1 year of age will be concurrently breast-feeding and working for at least 1 month (Zinn, 2000). The combination of working outside the home and breast-feeding can continue longer than this if there is adequate support such as refrigeration at the worksite for storage of the breast milk and time and space for women to pump their breast milk. Good family and daycare support is also required in such issues as avoiding the early introduction of solid foods. Once a woman's breast milk production is well established, the maintenance of breast-feeding, even with supplemental formula, can continue long term.

Weaning

The **La Leche League** (a breast-feeding support group) generally advocates baby-led **weaning** (accustoming the baby to nourishment other than breast milk). However, if the mother needs or wants to wean before the baby does, a variety of strategies may be used. The early-morning and late-night feedings are often the most difficult for the baby to give up. This can be the ideal situation for the working woman who wants to continue partial breast-feeding because she can continue to breast-feed her baby in the mornings before work. Then, when the mother is ready to stop the morning feeding, the baby is often old enough to sit in a high chair. When babies are fed cereal before the morning nursing, they often begin to wean themselves. Parents may need to try a variety of bottle nipples before the baby accepts one. Older infants (9 to 12 months of age and older) may be weaned directly to a cup.

WHAT ARE SOME BOTTLE-FEEDING CONCERNS?

Although it is preferable for infants to be breast-fed because of the nutritional benefits, commercial formulas that closely resemble breast milk have fortunately been developed for those women who cannot breast-feed because they are taking medications that contraindicate it or who have medical problems. The perfect food for human babies is clearly breast milk, but many successful adults were bottle-fed as infants.

Recently it has been shown that infants fed formulas devoid of the essential long-chain polyunsaturated fatty acids arachidonic acid and DHA (see Chapter 2) have poorer retinal and neurologic development than do babies who have been breast-fed. A significant increase in cognitive and motor skills was found among infants who were fed commercial formulas fortified with DHA and arachidonic acid compared with those fed formulas that were not fortified (Birch et al., 2000). Preterm infants are at the greatest risk for deficiency of these essential fats. The FDA has recently approved the addition of the omega-3 fatty acids to commercial infant formulas.

Although bottle-feeding may be the more practical method of feeding for the working mother, many working mothers find that a combination of bottle- and breast-feeding works well, particularly if their work is part-time. Expression of breast milk for use in a bottle can be an alternative, as shown in Figure 12-6.

It is helpful to tell a mother that if she expresses only 1 or 2 oz of breast milk initially, she is doing very well. Expressed milk cooled in the refrigerator can be added to previously frozen expressed milk to obtain full bottles (4-oz bottles are the handiest for collecting and storing expressed milk). Such bottles are visually

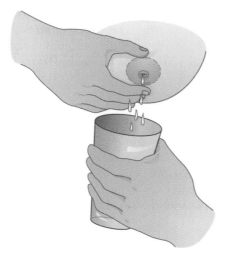

1. Do breast massage.

2. Place the thumb and index finger on the areola or darker skin around the nipple—about an inch back from the nipple. Press inward toward the chest wall and squeeze the thumb and finger together gently: push back and squeeze. Don't slide the thumb and finger. Don't pull the nipple out.

3. Keep the thumb and finger in that position and express until no more drops come out. Then move to another location around the nipple and repeat.

4. Lean over the sterile container and catch the milk. Switch to the other breast and again massage before beginning to express.

FIGURE 12-6 Instructions for hand expression of milk. (From Health Education Associates, Sandwich, MA.)

very interesting in that blue layers (composed of **fore milk**, the milk from the front of the breast) and thick white layers (composed of fat-rich hind milk) are formed. Women expressing milk should be relaxed and may find it easier after a warm shower. After a woman is comfortable with the technique and her ability, she can easily express milk any time, such as during her lunch break at work. The milk can then be stored in a portable ice chest or refrigerator (if available). Expressed milk can be kept for 1 to 2 days in sterile bottles at refrigerator temperature, for 1 to 2 weeks in a freezer, or for up to 6 months if the freezer maintains a constant temperature of 0° F (about −17.8° C) or lower.

Nursing-Bottle Mouth

Nursing-bottle mouth (also known as baby-bottle tooth decay; see Figure 13-2) is a condition in which the two front top teeth are severely decayed or completely eroded away in the older infant or child. This condition is caused by the infant's continuous suckling on a bottle that contains a source of carbohydrates. Sleeping with a bottle is particularly harmful because of decreased production of saliva that helps cleanse the teeth. As a general rule, juice should be given in a cup and only water bottles should be allowed at bedtime. It is also possible for a breast-fed infant who continually nurses throughout the night (i.e., an infant who sleeps with the mother) to develop similar tooth decay.

Milk Anemia

Milk anemia is caused when so much milk (not iron-fortified formula) is consumed that it replaces the consumption of food high in iron. Older children who use bottles may drink excess milk. A reduction in milk consumption to that recommended in the Food Guide Pyramid may be in order; water bottles can be substituted as necessary. When the young child begins to drink from a cup, milk intake will likely decrease to the recommended amount. Juice intake, when excessive, can also contribute to anemia by replacing foods high in iron.

Microwave Heating

The excess steam that results when bottles are heated in a microwave oven can cause bottles to explode in the infant's face. Also because hot spots in the liquid can develop, a seemingly safe temperature can actually cause the infant's mouth to be severely burned. The safest way to heat a bottle is to allow very warm water from a faucet to flow over it until the chill is gone.

Use of Inappropriate Liquids

The only appropriate liquids for regular use in a bottle are expressed breast milk, formula, and water. Although occasional use of juice is acceptable (such as in a car, when drinking from a cup is difficult), the regular use of juice in a bottle can cause nursing-bottle mouth (see earlier discussion). Other sweet liquids such as Kool-Aid or soft drinks should be avoided entirely. Formula replacements, such as nondairy creamer or milk products that are not specifically designed for infant use, should never be used. Formula should be mixed according to directions, not underdiluted or overdiluted unless specifically recommended by a **pediatrician** (a physician specializing in the care of infants, children, and adolescents) or a registered dietitian.

Types of Infant Formulas

Commercial Cow's Milk-Based Formulas

Made from cow's milk, these formulas closely approximate human milk. They are available in powder, liquid concentrated, and ready-to-feed form. Powdered forms are more economical, but require mixing and careful measuring. Liquid concentrated formulas require proper dilution with water (in a 1:1 ratio) before they are used. Commercial formulas are fortified to meet all known infant vitamin and mineral requirements. Formulas containing iron are available and are recommended by the American Academy of Pediatrics. Examples of infant commercial formulas are Enfamil and Similac.

Soybean-Based Formulas

If the infant shows signs of allergy to cow's milk, or if the parents are vegans, soybean-based formulas are generally used. Soybean-based formula is often the supplement of choice to breast-feeding because of the reduced likelihood of allergies. Commercially prepared formulas are fortified with vitamins and minerals. Bottle-fed infants who have an intolerance for lactose can use soy formulas. Examples of soybean-based formulas are ProSobee, Neo-Mull-Soy, and Isomil. Soy formulas have vitamin B_{12} added.

Special Formulas

Special formulas may be necessary for infants with digestive disturbances, allergies, or inborn metabolic errors. Examples are Portagen, Pregestimil, Lonalac, and Lofenalac. For infants with a strong family history of allergies, the elemental formulas may be the best choice if the mother cannot breast-feed.

WHAT ARE THE FEEDING GUIDELINES DURING THE FIRST YEAR?

Although it was once a common practice to wait until the infant reached 4 months of age to start introducing cereal and other solid foods, many parents today feel that is too long. Before 1920, solid foods were seldom offered to infants younger than 1 year. As time progressed, our knowledge of infant nutrition expanded, and women relied more on bottle-feeding. By the 1960s the age at which solid foods were commonly introduced had become a few months or even weeks. This trend, however, was a rational response to the nutritionally inadequate formulas used at that time (often evaporated milk mixed with water and corn syrup). A source of vitamin C such as orange juice and iron-fortified cereal were necessary then at an early age.

With the current return of breast-feeding and the development of highly nutritious commercial infant formulas, the risks associated with early introduction of solids (such as development of an allergy from orange juice and cereal) outweigh any benefits. The reasons to delay the introduction of solid foods until 4 to 6 months are:

1. The inability of the young infant to digest complex carbohydrates such as those found in cereal, vegetables, and fruits (thus infants can fill up their stomachs without getting the nutrients they need to grow)
2. The immature intestinal tract of the young infant that allows large, undigested food molecules to pass through the intestinal wall (which can activate an allergic reaction and may become a permanent condition)
3. Inadequate physiologic readiness of the infant to use tongue-thrust (it is felt that the human species may have developed this characteristic to prevent inappropriate ingestion of food)
4. The inability of the infant to indicate a desire for food by opening her mouth when a spoonful of food is presented or to indicate satiety by leaning back and turning away; it is felt that until an infant can respond in this manner (at about 5 months of age), feeding solid food may represent a type of force-feeding

Neither breast milk nor a milk formula will furnish adequate amounts of all nutrients required by the infant in later months. One important reason for introducing some solid foods into the infant's diet is to replenish the depleting stores of iron between 4 and 6 months of age. The general guidelines for the introduction of foods are as follows:

1. Introduce iron-fortified baby rice cereal at about 4 to 6 months of age.
2. Add pureed vegetables and fruits, one at a time, at about 6 to 8 months (starting with vegetables may help to increase acceptance by the infant not yet exposed to the sweet taste of fruits).
3. Add pureed meats at about 6 to 8 months.
4. Add juice when the infant is old enough to drink from a cup, at about 9 months.
5. Add foods with more texture and finger foods at about 9 months (chopped meats, crackers, and so on).
6. Add allergenic foods, such as egg whites (or whole eggs), whole milk, and orange juice, after 1 year (especially important for the infant with a family history of allergies or asthma).

Infants who are fed a vegan diet (no animal products) can receive adequate nutrition if they are breast-fed or receive soy milk formula. Breast-fed infants of vegan mothers may need a vitamin B_{12} supplement; older infants need a good source of vitamins D and B_{12} and the mineral zinc. Legumes may provide additional protein starting at about 7 to 8 months (Mangels and Messina, 2001).

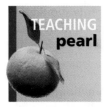

A good question to ask is, "Are you aware of what formula is made from?" followed by explaining that it is cow's milk with the excess protein removed and vitamins and minerals added to make it more nutritious, like breast milk. A further explanation can be provided by saying that so much protein is needed in cow's milk to help the baby cow grow that it causes GI irritation (stomach bleeding) in the human baby (using your hands to depict the size difference between a calf and a human baby can be very effective). This can support the continued use of formula versus changing to whole milk before the infant is physiologically ready to do so.

Fallacy: Cereal helps babies sleep through the night.

Fact: There is no scientific evidence to support this belief. Many experienced parents admit that their babies wake up regardless of how much food they have eaten. Parents should be strongly discouraged from giving an infant cereal before he or she is 4 to 6 months old, particularly when there is a family history of allergies.

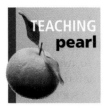

With regard to the introduction of solid foods, a good assessment question is, "Have you thought about when you are going to start solid foods such as cereal?" followed by, "What have you heard from other people about when to start?" This will help tailor the message to the beliefs the parents may hold.

At about the time the growing infant develops the **pincer grasp** (the ability to put the thumb and index finger together)—about 8 months—a sense of independence also begins to grow. This can be exasperating to a parent, particularly as the baby begins to spill food on the floor or decides to empty a full bowl of food on his own head. Because this is believed to be a normal part of development, parents are advised to cope with this behavior through positive strategies: an old shower curtain can be placed under the high chair to catch spills; a large bib can help prevent damage to the baby's clothes; small quantities of food can be given at one time to lessen waste; and bath time can be scheduled after meal time. If the infant is being allowed additional servings, he can receive an adequate intake while the parents enjoy a lowered frustration level. Bribing and coaxing the infant to eat and not to spill food can cause repetition of the negative behaviors as the infant learns he or she can control the parents' actions (as in thinking, "Let's see if I can get Mom and Dad to jump up and down if I drop this glass of juice."). Older infants prefer finger foods.

Inappropriate Foods

Aside from the special requirements for allergy-sensitive infants or for those who have metabolic disorders (a referral to a registered dietitian or a qualified nutritionist is in order in these cases), it should be stressed that parents should not give honey to babies because of the potential for botulism because honey contains botulism spores (in a quantity too low to cause adverse effects in older children and adults).

The high sodium content of some processed foods (such as canned vegetables or cured meats) can be detrimental to the immature renal functioning of infants. Steamed fresh vegetables, fruits, and other low-sodium foods may be safely used in preparing homemade baby foods. Special baby food grinders can be purchased for a reasonable price and allow the baby to eat the same foods as the family. It is important to avoid excess salt and sugar in baby food, whether store-bought or prepared at home.

To prevent choking, parents should avoid serving their infant any foods that have a hard texture (such as a raw apple or carrot) or are served in large pieces until the infant is old enough to chew adequately. Hot dogs should never be given to an infant and can also be problematic for an older child unless they are sliced into thin strips so they cannot cause choking if chewed inadequately.

HOW DOES AN INFANT GROW AND DEVELOP?

A well-nourished infant shows a steady gain in weight and height (with some fluctuations from week to week), is happy and vigorous, sleeps well, has firm muscles, has some tooth eruption at about 5 to 6 months (about six to twelve teeth will have erupted by 12 months), and has good elimination characteristic of the type of feeding—breast or formula. The nutrients found in milk, especially the protein, are essential in the development of the new tissues that accompany this growth.

Each infant has an individual rate of growth, but all grow faster in weight than in height. A steady weight gain is more important than a large amount gained. In interpreting growth with the National Center for Health Statistics growth charts (see Appendix 10), percentiles are used. A child at the fiftieth percentile for age is considered average. There is no concern with growth if the height and weight for age are above the tenth percentile and are consistent (i.e., not dropping in percentile). Weight for height should be between the twenty-fifth and ninetieth percentile without showing a significant change in percentile.

WHAT ARE SOME CLINICAL PROBLEMS IN INFANCY?

Babies born before they have had a chance to grow adequately are at nutritional risk. Babies less than 5 lbs at birth generally stay in the hospital after delivery until they have reached at least this weight. Lung function may be compromised. The ability to suckle may be impaired because of immature muscle development. Special feeding devices, including feeding tubes, may be required until the infant is strong enough to suck. Oral stimulation, such as use of a pacifier, is important for the infant who is tube-fed. Guidance on the introduction of solid foods needs to account for how early the premature infant was born. For example, cereal is usually started at 4 months. If the infant was born 3 months prematurely, the introduction of cereal should be delayed until the infant is 7 months old. This is especially true if there is a strong family history of allergies.

Failure to Thrive

The **failure to thrive (FTT)** syndrome was first observed in infants raised in institutional settings in which they did not receive adequate amounts of attention (physical touch and emotional warmth). As a result of this recognition, volunteers are now used to cuddle premature infants in hospital settings to help their chance of survival and growth.

Failure to thrive is a medical diagnosis that includes a weight and height of less than the third percentile for the infant's age (see Appendix 10) and less than normal ability in the **Denver Developmental Screening Test** (an observational test based on infant developmental progress). A total health care team approach may be in order.

WHAT ARE SOME OTHER NUTRITION ISSUES FOR WOMEN?

Premenstrual Syndrome

Premenstrual syndrome (PMS) occurs the first few days before the onset of the monthly menstrual cycle and disappears after menstruation. The majority of American women experience some degree of PMS; an estimated 10% to 15% experience severe or disabling symptoms, including symptoms of hypoglycemia such as increased appetite, anxiety, irritability, and headaches. However, eating does not always relieve these symptoms as would be expected in treating hypoglycemia. Nutrition has no known affect on PMS. However, eating balanced meals at regular times is a prudent approach.

Osteoporosis

This condition of brittle bones is more prevalent in women than in men. Women have less bone mass than do men and often have inadequate calcium intake. Women of Northern European and Asian heritage are especially at risk of osteoporosis. Thin women are at high risk as well. A new concern has been noted among adolescent girls who use Depo-Provera for contraception: it has been found that there is a significant decrease in bone mass density in normal adolescents up to the age of 21 who use this form of contraception (Kass-Wolff, 2001). Bone loss increases after menopause. Emphasizing milk or other calcium-rich foods in the diet helps maintain bone integrity. The equivalent of 3 to 4 c of milk daily is recommended to help prevent bone loss. Hormonal therapy with estrogen and weight-bearing exercise further help maintain bone integrity. For more information on osteoporosis, see Chapter 14.

Menopause

Women have symptoms of menopause for a number of years before complete onset. This period is referred to as *perimenopausal,* or the time around menopause. These symptoms consist of weight gain, mood swings, and hot flashes. The Chinese do not have a word for hot flash and it is felt this may be because of their lack of such symptoms. Consumption of soy products in large amounts, which are high in the estrogen-like substance called *estradiol,* may be the reason. Traditional medical approaches include the use of hormone replacement therapy (HRT) for estrogen and progesterone. For women who choose not to take HRT, a higher intake of calcium is recommended (1500 mg) to help prevent bone loss. An herb, black cohosh, has shown to be of use for menopausal symptoms (Hardy, 2000). However, as discussed in Chapter 4, there is little regulation over the supplement and herbal industry; caution must be exercised.

WHAT IS THE ROLE OF THE NURSE OR OTHER HEALTH PROFESSIONAL IN MATERNAL AND INFANT NUTRITION?

During Pregnancy

A nurse or other health care professional should be aware of potential biopsychosocial barriers to adequate nourishment during pregnancy. Examples are poor attitude (denial of pregnancy or desire to maintain slimness), misinformation (belief that salt restriction and low weight gain are desirable), or physical barriers to adequate nourishment (insufficient money for food, lack of adequate food preparation facilities, or hyperemesis). Once such a barrier is identified, referral to a registered dietitian or a qualified nutritionist, such as one associated with the WIC program, may be in order; immediate contact with the woman's obstetrician is also recommended.

It is especially important for health care professionals to recognize the strong need of pregnant teenagers (and in fact all adolescents) to rebel against authority figures. Rather than telling a pregnant teen what to do, the health care professional should inform her of alternative actions and their likely outcomes. Work as the teen's advocate and ask her in a positive manner how you can best assist her. Ask her what her perceived needs are and how she feels about your concerns. Encourage her involvement in other supportive programs in your community. Be a good listener and a supportive advocate for her.

After Pregnancy

After delivery, women should be encouraged to maintain good nutritional status to help provide themselves with adequate energy for infant care and to help restore nutritional stores for subsequent pregnancies. This is particularly true for the inclusion of folic acid. Counseling can be provided as needed to encourage adequate spacing between pregnancies and proper nutrient intake to prepare the body for a healthy future pregnancy.

New mothers should also be monitored for postpartum depression. A personal history of mood disorder (bipolarity or major depression) or PMS before pregnancy places a woman at high risk for postpartum mood disorders, which can lead to serious psychologic and social consequences and in some cases can even lead to suicide or infanticide. Psychologic intervention is warranted before pregnancy for women at high risk for mood disorders. The encouragement of eating well-balanced, frequent meals, which can allow blood glucose levels to remain stable, may help to ward off or treat postpartum depression.

During Lactation

The obstetric nurse plays an important role in promoting successful breast-feeding in the hospital setting. Of crucial importance is positive verbal encouragement and support. Flippant remarks can damage a woman's already sensitive emotions (related to hormonal changes associated with giving birth) and may impair her ability to breast-feed successfully.

The use of humor can help a tense new mother relax, which is important for a successful let-down reflex. All new breast-feeding women should be alerted to the following support and information services:

- A local La Leche League
- The WIC Supplemental Nutrition Program, which supports breast-feeding education
- The Cooperative Extension's Expanded Food and Nutrition Education Program (EFNEP), which may have breast-feeding support available through trained nutrition teaching assistants (see Chapter 15)
- The local hospital's obstetrics department, which will likely have nurses trained in lactation management; this can be especially helpful for problems that occur in the middle of the night

Breast-feeding buddy systems also exist in many communities. Volunteers experienced in breast-feeding are paired up with new mothers until breast-feeding is fully established. A nurse or other health professional can help set up such a system or make referrals to one already in existence.

For Bottle-Fed Infants

In the case of a bottle-fed infant, it is important for the nurse or other health care professional to be aware of the parents' philosophy and knowledge about feeding. Do they adhere to rigid feeding schedules that impair the infant's consumption of formula, or do they go solely by the infant's crying with the potential for either overfeeding or underfeeding? Are the parents receiving conflicting advice (which is likely) that undermines their confidence or that makes them adhere to inappropriate feeding practices? Do they believe that formula is made from "a bunch of chemicals" and that therefore whole milk is better? Do they realize that formula requires refrigeration after it has been prepared? Do they know how to properly prepare it? Is nursing-bottle mouth a potential problem? If so, recommend water bottles at bedtime (an older child may be given a choice: water bottle or no bottle).

Regarding the Introduction to Solid Food

Explaining why a grandmother or a mother-in-law may be giving one piece of advice while you are giving another can go a long way in building a new mother's trust in her own common sense. Because many new mothers are anxious and insecure in their first encounters with their infants, your efforts are best aimed at building confidence and strengthening decision-making skills.

CHAPTER STUDY QUESTIONS AND CLASSROOM ACTIVITIES

1. What benefits may the mother-to-be expect if she is well nourished?
2. Why should the pregnant teenager be sure she receives adequate kilocalories and sufficient amounts of all the other important nutrients?
3. How and why do the foods needed in the daily diet during pregnancy and lactation differ from those needed by nonpregnant women?
4. What can a nurse do to support breast-feeding in the hospital setting? What are the immediate and long-term concerns and their possible resolutions?
5. What guidelines would you give to a breast-feeding mother to help her determine whether breast-feeding is going well once she leaves the hospital?
6. Describe the likely effect of growth spurts on the nursing behavior of babies.
7. What are the advantages of breast-feeding? Why is breast milk so suitable for the infant?
8. What considerations for meal planning would be recommended for a pregnant or breast-feeding woman with diabetes (see Chapter 9 as needed)?
9. Have class members each provide at least one joke that can be compiled for later use with new lactating mothers to help promote the let-down reflex.

Case Study

CRITICAL THINKING

Andrea was plotting her weight on the pregnancy grid given to her by her obstetrician. She was 32 weeks pregnant. The doctor had advised that she gain up to 30 lbs, but she had already gained that amount. She could not understand how it had happened. There did not seem to be any history of weight problems from her family in Mexico. She had been avoiding fatty foods and ate very few sweets. She finished drinking her can of juice from lunch and headed back to the office for a long afternoon of sitting at her desk.

Critical Thinking Applications

1. What might be a source of excess kilocalories in Andrea's diet?
2. How might her work influence her weight gain?
3. What trimester of pregnancy is Andrea in?
4. What advice might you provide to Andrea regarding weight management?

REFERENCES   Birch EE, Garfield S, Hoffman DR, Uauy R, Birch DG: A randomized controlled trial of early dietary supply of long-chain polyunsaturated fatty acids and mental development in term infants. Dev Med Child Neurol. March 2000; 42(3):174-181.

Cassidy F, Ahearn E, Carroll BJ: Elevated frequency of diabetes mellitus in hospitalized manic-depressive patients. Am J Psychiatry. September 1999; 156(9):1417-1420.

Catalano PM: Pregnancy and lactation in relation to range of acceptable carbohydrate and fat intake. Eur J Clin Nutr. April 1999; 53:S124-S131.

Cogswell ME, Perry GS, Schieve LA, Dietz WH: Obesity in women of childbearing age: risks, prevention, and treatment. May 2001; 8(3):89-105.

Corssmit EP, Wiersinga WM, Boer K, Prummel MF: Pregnancy (conception) in hyper- or hypothyroidism. Ned Tijdschr Geneeskd. April 14, 2001; 145(15):727-731. [Article in Dutch.]

Decsi T, Burus I, Molnar S, Minda H, Veitl V: Inverse association between trans isomeric and long-chain polyunsaturated fatty acids in cord blood lipids of full-term infants. Am J Clin Nutr. September 2001; 74(3):364-368.

Del Mar Melero-Montes M, Jick H: Hyperemesis gravidarum and the sex of the offspring. Epidemiology. January 2001; 12(1):123-124.

Garovic VD: Hypertension in pregnancy: diagnosis and treatment. Mayo Clin Proc. October 2000; 75(10):1071-1076.

Hardikar JV: Malrotation of the gut manifested during pregnancy. J Postgrad Med. April 2000; 46(2):106-107.

Hardy ML: Herbs of special interest to women. J Am Pharm Assoc (Wash). March 2000; 40(2):234-242.

Hayakawa S, Nakajima N, Karasaki-Suzuki M, Yoshinaga H, Arakawa Y, Satoh K, Yamamoto T: Frequent presence of *Helicobacter pylori* genome in the saliva of patients with hyperemesis gravidarum. Am J Perinatol. 2000; 17(5):243-247.

Hellmuth E, Damm P, Molsted-Pedersen L, Bendtson I: Prevalence of nocturnal hypoglycemia in first trimester of pregnancy in patients with insulin-treated diabetes mellitus. Acta Obstet Gynecol Scand. November 2000; 79(11):958-962.

Hozyasz K: Celiac disease and problems associated with reproduction. Ginekol Pol. March 2001; 72(3):173-179. [Article in Polish.]

Hubel CA, Snaedal S, Ness RB, Weissfeld LA, Geirsson RT, Roberts JM, Arngrimsson R: Dyslipoproteinaemia in postmenopausal women with a history of eclampsia. Br J Obstet Gynaecol. June 2000; 107(6):776-784.

Innes KE, Wimsatt JH, McDuffie R: Relative glucose tolerance and subsequent development of hypertension in pregnancy. Obstet Gynecol. June 2001; 97(6):905-910.

Jorgensen MH, Hernell O, Hughes E, Michaelsen KF: Is there a relation between docosahexaenoic acid concentration in mothers' milk and visual development in term infants? J Pediatr Gastroenterol Nutr. March 2001; 32(3):293-296.

Kass-Wolff JH: Bone loss in adolescents using Depo-Provera. J Soc Pediatr Nurs. January-March 2001; 6(1):21-31.

King JC: Effect of reproduction on the bioavailability of calcium, zinc and selenium. J Nutr. April 2001; 131(4):1355S-1358S.

Koletzko B, Agostoni C, Carlson SE, Clandinin T, Hornstra G, Neuringer M, Uauy R, Yamashiro Y, Willatts P: Long-chain polyunsaturated fatty acids (LC-PUFA) and perinatal development. Acta Paediatr. April 2001; 90(4):460-464.

Lanska DJ, Kryscio RJ: Risk factors for peripartum and postpartum stroke and intracranial venous thrombosis. Stroke. June 2000; 31(6):1274-1282.

Lederman SA: Pregnancy weight gain and postpartum loss: avoiding obesity while optimizing the growth and development of the fetus. J Am Med Wom Assoc. Spring 2001; 56(2):53-58.

Lee KA, Zaffke ME, Baratte-Beebe K: Restless legs syndrome and sleep disturbance during pregnancy: the role of folate and iron. J Womens Health Gend Based Med. May 2001; 10(4):335-341.

Mangels AR, Messina V: Considerations in planning vegan diets: infants. J Am Diet Assoc. June 2001; 101(6):670-677.

Matthieu JM, Boulat O, Bianchi N: Maternal phenylketonuria. Rev Med Suisse Romande. April 2001; 121(4):297-300. [Article in French.]

Mennella JA, Jagnow CP, Beauchamp GK: Prenatal and postnatal flavor learning by human infants. Pediatrics. June 2001; 107(6):E88.

Pedersen CA: Postpartum mood and anxiety disorders: a guide for the nonpsychiatric clinician with an aside on thyroid associations with postpartum mood. Thyroid. July 1999; 9(7):691-697.

Power ML, Holzman GB, Schulkin J: A survey on the management of nausea and vomiting in pregnancy by obstetrician/gynecologists. Prim Care Update Ob Gyns. March 2001; 8(2):69-72.

Rosenn BM, Miodovnik M: Medical complications of diabetes mellitus in pregnancy. Clin Obstet Gynecol. March 2000; 43(1):17-31.

Scholl TO, Stein TP: Oxidant damage to DNA and pregnancy outcome. J Matern Fetal Med. June 2001; 10(3):182-185.

Sipiora ML, Murtaugh MA, Gregoire MB, Duffy VB: Bitter taste perception and severe vomiting in pregnancy. Physiol Behav. May 2000; 69(3):259-267.

Tan JH, Ho KH: Wernicke's encephalopathy in patients with hyperemesis gravidarum. Singapore Med J. March 2001; 42(3):124-125.

Zinn B: Supporting the employed breast-feeding mother. J Midwifery Womens Health. May 2000; 45(3):216-226.

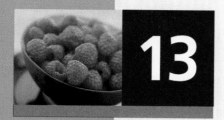

13 Growth and Development Issues in Promoting Good Health

OBJECTIVES

After completing this chapter, you should be able to:

- Describe nutritional needs during childhood and adolescence.
- Describe methods to promote good nutritional intake.
- Describe assessment and intervention strategies for psychologic eating disorders.
- Identify the factors related to dental health.
- Define developmental disability.
- Describe specific nutritional problems and conditions of the developmentally disabled.
- Apply knowledge of the nutrient needs to the meal environment.

TERMS TO IDENTIFY

Adenosine triphosphate (ATP)
Adipose tissue
Amenorrhea
Anorexia nervosa
Attention deficit
  hyperactivity disorder
  (ADHD)

Autism
Baby-bottle tooth decay
Bone growth
Bulimarexia
Bulimia
Carbohydrate loading
Cariogenic

Cerebral palsy
Creatine
Decalcification
Dental caries
Dental enamel
Dental erosion
Dental plaque

Continued

355

INTRODUCTION

Although the rapid growth that occurs prenatally and during infancy slows in childhood and only picks up in adolescence, developmental changes are rapid. From learning to walk to climbing trees, from uttering first words to chattering nonstop and monopolizing phone lines, and from being totally dependent to growing into independence, the changes that take place from early childhood to adolescence are truly remarkable.

Nutrition plays a key role in this process. Sources of food that provide good nutrition change throughout the period of childhood. Breast-feeding may continue for the first few years. Some children need to rely on bottle use beyond the first year, although this is generally discouraged because of concerns about dental health. The texture of foods also changes as children begin to eat more solid food as they develop the full ability to chew. Peer pressure becomes more of a factor in food choices as childhood advances (Table 13-1).

Eating disorders generally have their roots in childhood. This includes issues of eating for nonhunger reasons, which can lead to obesity. Anorexia nervosa is a psychologic problem leading to a strong fear of eating. Negative family functioning may be part of the cause of an eating disorder or may result from attempts to deal with food issues. Involving families in the assessment and planning stage promotes their support of the intervention plan. The school setting and the peer group also have an important impact on food choices.

WHAT IS MEANT BY GROWTH AND DEVELOPMENT?

Growth is the increase with age in weight and height, or size as it is popularly designated, that comes about as a result of the multiplication of cells and their differentiation for many different functions in the body. Growth is a continuous, but not uniform, process from conception to full maturity. During fetal life and infancy the rate of growth is very rapid. This period is followed by one of slower growth during early and middle childhood. Another period of very rapid growth occurs during adolescence, followed by a tapering off until the growth period ends.

TABLE 13-1
AGE-RELATED CHILDHOOD FOOD GUIDELINES

AGES (YEARS)	SUGGESTIONS
1 to 2	Provide plain, simple finger foods. Place small amounts on the plate (about 1 tbsp of each food for each year of child's age). Provide cups with handles that do not tip easily, large-handled silverware, and plates with edges (for pushing food against). Trust child's hunger cues, because appetite can vary from day to day.
2 to 3	Encourage the "one-taste" rule to expose children to new foods, but do not force child to eat. Make mealtimes pleasant and enjoyable. Offer structured food choices to allow for a growing sense of independence. Recognize that food jags (eating the same food day after day) are common at this age and beyond. Continue to increase the variety of foods offered.
3 to 5	Begin to include the child in food shopping (the young child can recognize numbers on food labels; give guidelines such as cereals with no more than 6 g of sugar per serving). Include the child in simple cooking techniques such as stirring and pouring. Avoid using food as a bribe or as a reward. Continue to increase the variety of foods offered.
5 to 10	Continue to provide breakfast, which is especially important for better school performance. Help the child categorize foods into groups of the Food Guide Pyramid. Be sensitive to the effects of food advertising; help the child understand that many foods advertised are high in fat and sugar.
10 to 18	Recognize that increased body fat often precedes puberty. Be sensitive to the influence of friends on food and beverage choices. Provide information on healthy food choices at fast-food restaurants and for snacks. Help the child find time to eat breakfast and to eat around sports and school events.

Development refers to the increasing ability of body parts to function. For example, being able to use a knife and fork successfully is a fine motor skill that is age dependent (see Table 13-1). Factors affecting the rate of growth and development include heredity, or inborn capacity to grow, and environment. An extremely important environmental factor is nutrition. Better diets, which accompany improved economic conditions, are credited for the taller stature of children and adults in the United States today. Adults were significantly smaller in past decades. In technologically advanced countries, the average height and weight of children of any given age have increased over the past 100 years, which is evidence that well-nourished children reach the potential set by their heredity, not only in physical growth, but also in mental development.

What Is the Importance of Nutrition to Healthy Growth and Development?

Without an adequate supply of nutrients, optimal growth and development to adulthood would not be possible. Nutrients supplied by food that the child consumes provide energy and the necessary building blocks for synthesis of new tissues. Foods for growth include those in the three lower levels of the Food Guide Pyramid.

Breast milk can continue to provide good nutrition for several years. Breast milk is a source of protein and calcium and other nutrients needed for good growth. With the ample food supply in the United States, the nutritional component of breast-feeding the older child is secondary to the emotional needs provided by close contact with the mother. All children will eventually become weaned (stop nursing or using the bottle) without assistance (see Chapter 12 for weaning guidelines).

Brain growth stops in early childhood, but other important organs continue to grow. Although the weight of the child (specifically **adipose tissue** [body fat]) is more affected by the total quantity of kilocalories consumed, **bone growth** (the growth that occurs in length and thickness of bones) and **lean tissue** (muscle) growth are affected by both the quantity and quality of the diet. Parents should strive for a high-quality diet and an adequate quantity of kilocalories.

Every child has different nutrient requirements based on factors such as chronologic age, individual growth rate, stage of maturation, level of physical activity, and the efficiency of absorption and utilization of nutrients. Guidelines, such as Dietary Reference Intakes (DRIs) and the Food Guide Pyramid give general indications of needed nutrients for growth. Growth charts are another important tool (see Appendix 10 and discussion below). If the child's growth is appropriate, it can be generally assumed that nutritional intake is adequate. Health problems can lead to poor growth even though an adequate diet is being consumed.

Because the human is a social being, appropriate interaction is important for growth and development. Food often serves as a social link, such as at mealtimes (see Figure 1-5). Children should eat as part of a family unit, ideally at the table. Eating with others can stimulate appetite and reinforce that eating is a pleasurable experience.

Research shows that children have inadequate intakes of zinc, folate, vitamin E, and vitamin D. This same research also found that children had the least variety of intake of vegetables with the least preference for them (Skinner et al., 1999). The importance of adequate intake of antioxidant vitamins such as vitamin E and magnesium, as found in vegetables and other plant-based foods, appears to lower the risk of asthma (Hijazi et al., 2000).

It is paramount that families and caretakers work to help make vegetables fun and appealing to eat. This might include making carrot curls using a vegetable peeler or melon balls using both cantaloupe and honeydew melons for good visual appeal. Spinach topped pizza flavored with pesto (an Italian sauce made with olive oil and basil which can easily be purchased commercially) is particularly appealing to young children when it is called "Popeye Pizza" and they sing the Popeye song:

> *I'm Popeye the sailor man,*
> *I'm Popeye the sailor man,*
> *I'm strong to the finish,*
> *'Cause I eat my spinach,*
> *I'm Popeye the sailor man,*
> *Toot, Toot!!*

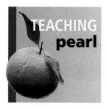

One woman captured the idea of positive values associated with vegetables. When someone commented on the wide variety of vegetables her children liked, her reply was, "Do you know how I did it? Whenever I offered a reward I would say, 'If you are good you can have a vegetable!'" Rewarding with food is not recommended, especially because candy is often the reward of choice. Rewarding with vegetables in this scenario, however, allowed the children to develop a strong appreciation for a healthy food group.

Why Were the Growth Charts Revised?

New childhood growth percentiles have been published recently by the Centers for Disease Control and Prevention. These new growth charts are designed to replace the widely used 1977 National Center for Heath Statistics percentiles (see Appendix 10). The new charts include updated percentile comparisons and the concept of the body mass index (BMI). As you may recall from Chapter 7, BMI is a mathematical equation of weight in kilograms divided by the square of the height in meters. There are various tables that allow BMI determination without doing the math such as with nomograms (an adult version of the nomogram is found in Appendix 12). The CDC Web site provides a multipaged chart to determine BMI for young children (see Appendix 1 for the Web site address).

Percentiles are used to compare a child's growth with other children of the same age and gender to reflect the changes in children's sizes. Percentiles are based on a given population. Because children are taller and consequently heavier than previous generations, the growth charts have been updated to reflect these standards. For example, a child who is on the fiftieth percentile means that there are as many children who are bigger as are smaller. The fiftieth percentile equates with the average size.

fact
FALLACY

Fallacy: All children should take a multivitamin and mineral supplement.

Fact: Although commercial vitamin and mineral supplements contain much of what is needed for good health, food contains even more such as protein and phytochemicals. A balanced diet consisting of a variety of foods is more likely than a vitamin preparation to supply all the necessary nutrients for growth and repair. In addition to being unnecessary most of the time (and therefore a waste of money), excess vitamin intake can be fatal. If a parent feels safer giving vitamins, he or she should make sure that the content does not exceed 100% of the Recommended Dietary Allowance (RDA).

WHY IS IRON-DEFICIENCY ANEMIA SO COMMON AMONG CHILDREN?

Young children and adolescents are particularly susceptible to iron-deficiency anemia because of the rapid use of iron during growth and the love of foods that

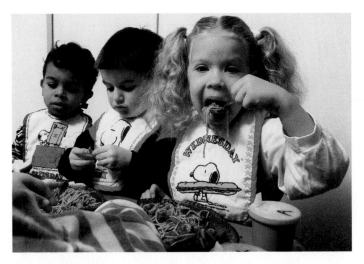

FIGURE 13-1 Pasta is a favorite dish of young children.

are generally low in iron (Figure 13-1). Other reasons include blood loss caused by parasites among young children who do not practice good hand washing. Teenaged girls are at an increased risk of anemia because of the start of menstruation, the rapid growth of adolescence, and insufficient iron in their diets.

With regard to diet, children often find eating meat difficult. This may be because the meat is too tough from being overcooked (meat cooked at low temperatures using moist methods, such as the meat cooked in stews, is more tender); because they have not acquired a taste for meat (such as with liver); or because the family avoids meat for economic, religious, moral, or other reasons.

Prevention of Iron-Deficiency Anemia

Aside from increased meat intake, other foods that are high in iron should be consumed freely. As noted in Chapter 4, the iron found in meat, referred to as heme iron, is well absorbed, whereas other food sources of iron (called nonheme iron) need to be eaten with a vitamin C food to enhance absorption. For example, iron-fortified cereal followed by a glass of orange juice or other food high in vitamin C will greatly enhance the absorption of iron (see Chapter 4 for other iron sources and Box 13-1 for suggested vitamin C foods that can be packed for school lunches).

Diagnosis and Treatment of Iron-Deficiency Anemia

Because iron-deficiency anemia continues to be a major health problem in the United States, there is widespread screening among children (particularly children from low-income families, who tend to have difficulty obtaining adequate amounts of iron in their diets). Programs such as the Well Child Clinic (operated

BOX 13-1
HOME-PACKED SCHOOL LUNCH IDEAS

Choose one food or a combination of foods from each group to meet one-third of the RDA:

VITAMIN A ($\frac{1}{2}$ CUP OR EQUIVALENT)
Apricot or apricot nectar
Broccoli (raw florets)*
Cantaloupe*
Carrot sticks or juice
Peaches
Spinach (raw for a salad)*
Sweet potato (as in pudding)
Tomato slices, juice, or soup*
Watermelon ($\frac{1}{2}$ slice)*

VITAMIN C ($\frac{1}{2}$ CUP OR EQUIVALENT)
Cabbage (for coleslaw)
Cauliflower (raw florets)
Grapefruit or juice
Orange or juice
Strawberries
Tangelo or juice
Tangerine or juice

PROTEIN (1 OZ OR $\frac{1}{4}$ CUP OR EQUIVALENT)
Any meat, chicken, or fish
Peanut butter (2 tbsp)
Egg (hard cooked or egg salad)
Cottage cheese
Hard cheese
(Meat and peanut butter are also high in iron and B vitamins)

CALCIUM (1 CUP OR EQUIVALENT)
Milk
Yogurt
Hard cheese ($1\frac{1}{2}$ oz)
Cream soup
(These foods are also high in protein and vitamins D and B_2)

Other foods are important, for example, whole-grain or enriched white flour products such as muffins, graham crackers, bread, noodles, rice, or pasta and other foods, for variety and to contribute other essential nutrients.
*Also contributes one-third of the RDA for vitamin C.

out of Public Health Departments) and the Women, Infants, and Children (WIC) Supplemental Nutrition Program commonly screen for iron-deficiency anemia using either the test for hemoglobin (the part of the blood that carries oxygen and is rich in iron) or the test for **hematocrit** (the amount of packed red blood cells) values.

Controversy exists regarding the blood levels that constitute iron-deficiency anemia. Generally, hemoglobin values greater than 12 g/dL and hematocrit values greater than 37% are considered normal. Hemoglobin readings of less than 11 g/dL and hematocrit readings of less than 33% should be evaluated further and complete blood counts will often show low transferrin saturation levels (transferrin is an important constituent of red blood cell formation). Hemoglobin values of less than 10 g/dL (which is roughly equivalent to a hematocrit value of less than 30%) are signs of iron-deficiency anemia and require immediate medical attention with iron supplementation. A test dose of iron may be used to help determine whether anemia is the result of iron deficiency. Increased focus on dietary intake of iron is also imperative to help resolve the anemia and prevent future episodes. It appears there is an increased need for folate (Kennedy et al., 2001).

Sickle Cell Anemia

In **sickle cell anemia** the red blood cells are a sickle shape. It is a genetic predisposition occurring mainly in persons with African or Mediterranean heritage. It is now believed that, historically, persons with the sickle cell trait were protected against malaria. This form of anemia is not caused by dietary deficiencies; however, diet has health implications. Because of the rapid turnover of blood cells, increased folic acid intake is beneficial.

WHAT CAUSES THE DEVELOPMENT AND PREVENTION OF DENTAL DECAY?

Dental caries, or tooth decay, begins with a genetic predisposition to a thin layer of **dental enamel** (the outer hard surface of the teeth) or from inadequate intake of calcium by the mother during pregnancy. Childhood dental caries develop from a complex process of demineralization of the tooth (**decalcification** [removal of calcium from the tooth structure]) and acid destruction.

Bacteria found in the mouth feed on carbohydrates—both sugars and starches—which results in the production of acid. Carbohydrates are **cariogenic** (able to induce dental caries or cavities). Saliva helps neutralize the normal acid production that occurs with the combination of oral bacteria and carbohydrate intake. Keeping the oral cavity clean from tooth brushing, flossing, and regular dental visits for professional removal of **dental plaque** (a buildup on dental surfaces that provides a medium for bacteria to grow) can significantly reduce the risk of dental caries.

Another source of acid destruction is related to erosion of the dental enamel. **Dental erosion** does not involve bacterial action, but happens in cases such as bulimia, in which constant purging of meals allows the acid contents of the stomach to severely erode the dental enamel. A new role for the dental profession in diagnosing bulimia has evolved as a consequence of this nation's obsession with weight. Excess intake of acidic beverages such as some soft drinks can lead to dental erosion. Chewable vitamin C tablets, also known as ascorbic acid, have also been found to be destructive to dental enamel.

Individuals with **Down syndrome** have a normal-sized tongue, but because of their facial structure, the oral cavity is frequently too small to accommodate the tongue, which may have deep fissures that can retain food particles. Consequently, tongue brushing should be part of daily oral hygiene. Autistic children may pouch their food rather than swallow it and prefer soft foods that require little chewing. This puts them at greater risk for dental caries. Suppressed immune function, drug therapy, oral motor dysfunction, and modified diets put the developmentally disabled child at high risk for oral infections. Caregivers are often so overwhelmed with medical, physical, psychologic, and feeding concerns that regular home dental care can be neglected.

Dental decay is difficult to control through food choices alone. Limiting the frequency of carbohydrate snacks can help. Snacks containing carbohydrate foods that tend to stick to the teeth should be limited. Including a protein source at snack time can also help. A snack that contains some fat, as found with protein foods, helps neutralize the acid production by the oral bacteria. Good dental hygiene with regular dental checkups and the use of topical fluoride are the most effective and appropriate preventive measures. The role of the dental professional should include the assessment of eating disorders (see section below) and between-meal snacking patterns.

The development of an immunization that inhibits growth of oral bacteria has shown success in reducing dental caries. This may, one day, become standard practice of immunization against dental caries.

What Steps Can Be Taken to Promote Good Dental Health Among Children and Adolescents?

Beginning in utero, pregnant women should be encouraged to consume adequate amounts of calcium via 3 to 4 c of milk or the equivalent minimum of 1000 mg of calcium to provide the building material for fetal development of strong dental enamel. Once born, young infants need a good source of calcium such as with breast milk or formula. Parents of infants should never replace these high-calcium sources with alternatives such as nondairy creamer.

Baby-bottle tooth decay (also referred to as nursing-bottle mouth) occurs in babies and young children who use a bottle excessively, especially at bedtime (Figure 13-2). Sweet liquids such as juice and other soft drinks are believed to be the primary culprits in baby-bottle tooth decay. Older babies and toddlers should not use a bottle, especially at nighttime. This not only helps prevent baby-bottle tooth decay, but also helps prevent choking, emesis, and aspiration. Use of a cup is recommended for older babies and children because the liquid does not continually bathe the teeth, unlike a bottle that is held in the mouth

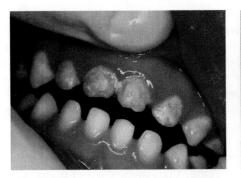 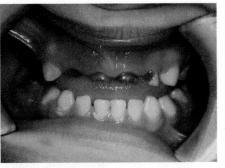

A   B

FIGURE 13-2 Examples of baby-bottle tooth decay. (Courtesy of Ferguson F, Department of Children's Dentistry, School of Dental Medicine, SUNY at Stony Brook, Stony Brook, NY 11733.)

for long periods. During sleep there is reduced production of saliva. For a child who cannot sleep without a bottle, a compromise of plain water in the bottle may be acceptable.

As soon as teeth first erupt, the older baby or toddler should have their teeth cleaned daily at home. This can be accomplished with the parents using a clean washcloth to wipe off the teeth or a child-size toothbrush may be used. The American Academy of Pediatric Dentistry recommends that infants be scheduled for an initial oral evaluation within six months of the eruption of the first primary tooth, but by no later than 12 months of age (Sanchez and Childers, 2000). This generally allows a positive first dental visit for a professional dental cleaning, which can help prevent future dental decay.

All children should be encouraged to thoroughly chew their foods. This helps in a lot of areas, but in the case of dental health, chewing promotes the production of saliva. Saliva helps to neutralize the acid formed in the mouth by bacteria feeding on carbohydrate and also helps to rinse the mouth of food debris. Saliva also contains a variety of minerals, such as calcium, that bathe the teeth, thereby encouraging the retention of dental enamel.

Older children can chew sugar-free gum after meals that further stimulates the flow of saliva and can help cleanse the teeth if using a toothbrush after meals is not possible. The use of chewing gum is not feasible for children with braces. For these children, at least a thorough rinsing of the mouth with water after meals is imperative to avoid dental caries. Other means to protect the enamel surface of the teeth include avoiding harsh abrasives on the teeth, not chewing ice (which can chip the teeth), not opening bottles with the teeth, and using pliable mouth guards in sports. **Fluoride**, a mineral that helps promote the formation of strong enamel in childhood, can be obtained through fluoridated drinking water or, for children under the age of 12, from fluoride drops or tablets. Once the adult teeth are fully formed, fluoride rinses continue to be an effective preventive treatment by promoting retention of the enamel surface. Fluoride is believed to actually promote remineralization of the dental surface.

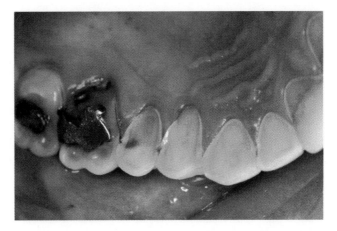

FIGURE 13-3 Bulimia-induced dental erosion. (From Neville BW, Damm DD, Allen CM, and Bouquot JE: Oral and maxillofacial pathology, ed 2, Philadelphia, WB Saunders, 2002.)

In addition to the use of fluoride, good dental hygiene and control of carbohydrate foods help control loss of dental enamel. All carbohydrate foods, especially sugar, contribute to acid production in the presence of oral bacteria. Eating sweet foods with a meal containing protein, fat, or both will further promote dental health. Eating carbohydrate foods with a thoroughly clean mouth will also be of great benefit. Acid production begins shortly after eating is begun, so brushing the teeth and flossing before eating may be as helpful as brushing after a meal. Limiting the time of exposure to acidic beverages is also important.

The supporting structure of the teeth, the gums or gingiva, requires a good nutritional status to remain strong and healthy. **Gingival** disease means disease of the gums. Irritants, such as plaque, can increase the risk of gingivitis. Brushing the teeth regularly and flossing daily, with at least annual dental visits for plaque removal, can help decrease the risk for **periodontal disease** (a painless gum disease that results in tooth loss in adulthood). One study found that gingival health was better maintained with a diet high in milk and fiber (Petti et al., 2000).

Adolescents who have bulimia nervosa (see section below), which includes **purging** (intentional vomiting) after eating, can develop irreversible enamel erosion by increasing the acid content of the mouth (Figure 13-3). **Xerostomia** (diminished or absent production of saliva) and irritation of the lining of the mouth can also occur in connection with frequent purging. Xerostomia can also be caused by certain medications such as antihistamines and from destruction of **salivary glands** (glands near the mouth that produce saliva) that may occur in radiation treatment of cancers near the throat. Dehydration and a resulting dry mouth are caused by other forms of purging such as laxative and diuretic abuse.

Persons with a dry mouth might suck on sugar-based candies, which further exacerbates dental decay. Use of sugar-free candies does not promote tooth decay, but adequate fluid intake is still important.

What Are Orthodontic Concerns?

Orthodontists often advise their patients to eat soft foods after orthodontic treatment to avoid pressure sensitivity. Any time there are food restrictions, there is an increased risk of nutritional deficiencies. This has potential to suppress the rate of growth and development among children who have braces or other orthodontal treatments. Thus it may be beneficial to provide nutritional guidance in choosing soft-food diets.

Fallacy: The development of baby-bottle tooth decay is not important because the baby teeth are going to be replaced with adult teeth.

Fact: The physical significance of baby-bottle tooth decay is that removal of the decayed teeth can cause jaw misalignment, preventing normal spacing for adult teeth as they erupt. The pain of dental decay is not pleasant for the infant or child and can cause excess crying and screaming—not pleasant for the child or the family. Further, a young child with dental decay experiences a frightening and painful first dental visit. It is best to prevent dental caries in infants and young children for the sake of the child, the family, and the dental professional.

WHAT ARE ISSUES OF CHILDHOOD OBESITY?

Among older children, obesity is an increasingly important predictor of adult obesity. There is an increasing rate of Type 2 diabetes in children, which is believed to be caused by increased obesity and decreased activity levels. Because there is a genetic predisposition to Type 2 diabetes, those children of high-risk ethnic populations with a strong family history of diabetes may benefit from diabetes screening and education to lessen the risk of diabetes development. Some adolescents have been shown to have cardiovascular risk factors, which are also correlates of the insulin resistance syndrome, including higher blood pressure levels, dyslipidemia, and obesity, all of which continue into young adulthood.

Great care needs to be taken to ensure that an overweight child's self-esteem is not damaged in attempting to control weight gain. It is important to use a positive approach with obese children, with an emphasis on good nutritional choices in a variety of social settings. Care needs to be taken to avoid labeling foods as good or bad. The causes of weight gain should be assessed, such as inactivity (for example, excessive television watching), eating for emotional reasons, drinking beverages high in sugar content, or physiologic reasons that can predispose some children for obesity even though they may be eating the same amounts of food as their friends. The health care professional needs to address the underlying causes of obesity appropriately rather than simply giving the child's parent or guardian a diet sheet for weight loss. Refer to Chapter 7 for guidance on long-term weight management.

WHAT IS THE AFFECT OF MALNUTRITION AND EATING DISORDERS ON GROWTH AND DEVELOPMENT?

Very severe malnutrition in infancy, if of long duration and followed by childhood undernutrition, can produce irreversible effects on neurologic development, which in turn can impair a child's ability to learn later in life. Children who do not get enough to eat and are malnourished tend to be smaller and are more likely than well-fed children to become ill because of decreased immunity. Such children may also be less able to learn. The extent to which malnutrition occurs in the United States means that many children will not be able to achieve their full potential. For developing nations worldwide, where children may constitute a large percentage of the population, malnutrition may limit the country's future social and economic development.

A prolonged lack of one or more nutrients retards physical development or causes specific clinical conditions to appear. For example, anemia, goiter, and rickets reflect a state of malnutrition. An adequate intake of iron and folate helps prevent anemia. Adequate iodine from fortified salt or sea fish can help prevent goiter. Rickets, which leads to bowing of the legs from soft bones occurs in young children as they start to walk. Rickets is most likely to occur among children of color with inadequate intake of calcium and vitamin D and with insufficient exposure to sunlight (Hartman, 2000).

Severe malnutrition, which is characterized by clinical manifestations, is of two basic types: kwashiorkor, a protein deficiency (Figure 13-4); and marasmus, an overall deficit of food, especially kilocalories (also known as protein energy malnutrition [PEM]) (Figure 13-5). Kwashiorkor generally occurs at or after weaning, when milk high in protein is replaced by a starchy staple food providing insufficient protein. A child with this type of malnutrition usually has stunted growth, edema, skin sores, and discoloration of dark hair to red or blond. Infantile marasmus is frequently the result of early cessation of breast-feeding, overdilution of formula, or gastrointestinal infection early in life, and it is accompanied by wasting of tissues and extreme growth retardation. See Chapter 2 for more discussion of kwashiorkor and marasmus.

Undernourished children are identified most often by biochemical and clinical signs, but the value of these signs is limited to identifying an extremely inadequate diet. Chronic long-term undernutrition generally results in stunted growth (Figure 13-6). Inadequate intake of calcium was noted among children with reduced bone mineral content (Hoppe et al., 2000). Adequate intake of vitamins and minerals found in fruits and vegetables, such as magnesium and potassium, are also associated with high bone-mass density important in later prevention of osteoporosis (New et al., 2000).

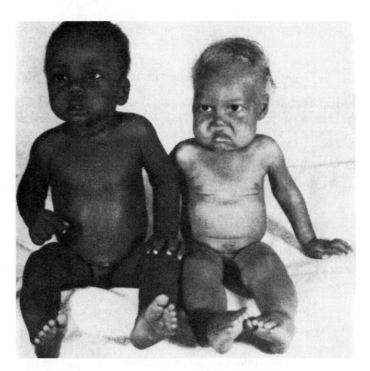

FIGURE 13-4 (*Right*) Infant with "sugar baby" kwashiorkor, attributed to a high-sugar, low-protein diet. The infant has stunted growth, edema of the feet and hands, fatty liver, moon face, and dyspigmentation of the skin and hair. (*Left*) Normal infant. (From Jellife DB: Hypochromotrichia and malnutrition in Jamaican infants. J Trop Pediatr. 1995;1:25; by permission of Oxford University Press.)

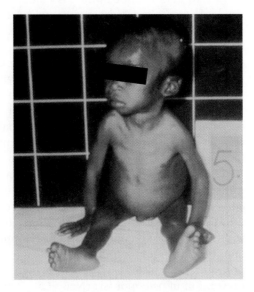

FIGURE 13-5 Marasmus. (From Zitelli: Atlas of Pediatric Physical Diagnosis, ed 3, London, Mosby-Wolfe, 1997.)

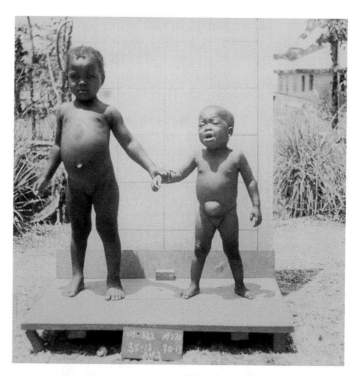

FIGURE 13-6 Stunting is shown with Nigerian children, born in the same month in the same village, who have genetically similar parents. (Photo courtesy of Michael Latham, Division of Nutritional Sciences, Cornell University, Ithaca, New York, and David Morley, Institute of Child Health, London, England.)

The degree of malnutrition is often proportional to the degree to which the child is subnormal in height or weight. Therefore anthropometric measurements (height, weight, and amount of body fat; see Chapter 5 for more on anthropometrics) are the most commonly used indices of undernutrition.

Types of moderate malnutrition include (1) those caused by chronic food reduction (manifested by growth retardation) and (2) those resulting from vitamin or mineral deficiency and accompanied by clinical symptoms such as rickets or pellagra. Malnutrition is most often associated with poverty resulting from a **food distribution system** (how food is allocated to the world's population) that is based on purchasing power. Exact determination of the effect on the individual is difficult because other factors influence human growth and behavioral development, including individual innate potential, health status, and environment.

Marasmus and kwashiorkor do occur in the United States, but are quite rare. Chronic undernutrition occurs more commonly. This can lead to iron deficiency and anemia, which is relatively common, especially in growing children. A child's growth record is a more accurate measure of whether he or she is receiving sufficient nutrients than are DRIs because the gross estimates of nutritional needs are not designed to assess an individual's nutritional status.

Malnutrition impairs the body's defense against disease. Therefore infection, which is rampant in underdeveloped regions of the world because of poor sanitary conditions, occurs more frequently in malnourished children.

What Are Some Psychologic Issues That May Lead to Eating Disorders?

Psychologic eating disorders are increasingly recognized in childhood. Anorexia nervosa and bulimia not only are problems of weight control, but also involve biologic, psychologic, and social factors. Obsessive dieting, refusal to eat, binge eating, gorging, purging, fasting, and laxative and diuretic abuse can lead to malnutrition, electrolyte imbalance, and cardiac arrhythmia, which can result in death. There are a variety of forms of eating disorders. The most common include **anorexia nervosa** (food restricting), **bulimia** (purging behavior), **bulimarexia** (food restricting with purging behavior), and binge eating disorder. There is evidence that a significant contributor to eating disorders is genetically based. The genetic factors include predisposition to anxiety disorders or traits, body weight, and possibly major depression (Klump et al., 2001). Any nonphysiologic reason to restrict or alter food intake might be termed an eating disorder when health is adversely affected.

Family relationships seem to contribute to the development of psychologic and behavioral traits for risk of some eating disorders. Other psychiatric problems, such as bipolar disorder (see Chapter 12) and schizophrenia, are associated with behavioral eating problems. Monitoring weight and diet is important in the management of psychiatric illness.

Anorexia Nervosa

Anorexia nervosa is characterized by a refusal to eat. This is often caused by a need to exert control. Such a child or teen can gain control in this area of his or her life, where he or she may not feel able to gain control in other realms. Initially there is no real loss of appetite. However, once severe weight loss has occurred, hormonal changes are believed to take place that alter perception. The syndrome occurs mainly in girls, after puberty. There is an increased risk of anorexia nervosa among high achievers and upper socioeconomic populations. Some common correlates of anorexia are as follows:

- An intense fear of becoming obese that does not lessen as weight loss progresses
- A disturbance of body image, such as claiming to feel fat even when emaciated
- Weight loss of at least 25% of original body weight
- Refusal to maintain body weight over a minimal healthy weight for age and height
- No known physical illness that would account for the weight loss
- Amenorrhea caused by altered hormonal states
- Bizarre eating habits such as cutting food into tiny pieces or limiting intake to only a few foods
- Underlying low self-esteem
- Compulsive exercise habits

Dietary Treatment. The goal of treatment should be to restore good nutritional status and resolve the underlying psychologic problems. Outpatient treatment is the preferred method and should involve the whole family. The person with anorexia nervosa who is 30% below normal weight and fails to gain weight and is in complete denial, or is suicidal should be hospitalized. All members of the health care team must be aware of the need to individualize the care plan. The nurse's role includes closely supervising and encouraging the patient to eat all of the food provided. A trusting relationship between patient and health care professional is absolutely essential. It should be recognized that treatment will require a long-term, family-based approach, and a considerable amount of time will be needed. Treatment is not always successful.

Bulimia

Bulimia is characterized by binge eating followed by purging through self-induced vomiting, abusive use of laxatives, or both. The person is afraid of becoming overweight and is aware that the eating pattern is abnormal. However, the bulimic patient loses control over eating and often eats large amounts of food rapidly. High-kilocalorie, easily ingested foods are chosen during binge episodes. Fasting then follows, often resulting in a weight fluctuation of as much as 10 lbs. Bulimarexia or bulimia nervosa is the term used to describe cycles of binge eating and purging (vomiting or laxative abuse) with undereating. Health care professionals need to be aware of the existence of bulimia and its detrimental effect on dental health. A health care team approach is advised for bulimia, but also for dental care in general.

Dietary Treatment. In the hospital, food intake should be normalized to appropriate mealtimes, with close supervision after eating to control vomiting. Psychologic assessment should take priority and plans should be made for long-term, outpatient, family-based counseling with a health care professional trained in eating disorders. A total health care team effort is essential to ensure effective treatment. Short-term mortality, as compared with anorexia nervosa, is significantly lower, but bulimia nervosa was found to become an entrenched pattern of eating in 20% of women studied (Keel and Mitchell, 1997). Outpatient dietary treatment of bulimia emphasizes regular mealtimes with appropriate food portions to satisfy hunger needs. Food is discouraged as a means of reward or comfort.

Autism

Autism includes a range of sensory deficits that lead to diminished social interaction. Autism is characterized by extreme withdrawal and an obsessive desire to maintain the present status; temper tantrums and language disturbances are also evident. It generally occurs in young children after a seemingly normal infancy. An increased incidence from 1 child in 10,000 to as many as 1 in 300 has occurred since 1978. There is some research that links genetically susceptible children with pertussis in the DPT vaccine. This is postulated to cause a retinoid receptor defect. Natural vitamin A may help reconnect the retinoid receptors needed for vision, sensory perception, language processing, and attention (Megson, 2000). This evidence is still very limited and controversial, however, increasing intake of vitamin A, such as in liver, cannot hurt, and may help. Because children with autism tend to eat a very limited number of foods, this goal may not be easy to accomplish. There is a tendency to accept dry foods such as bread and crackers and meat by children with autism. A family might have the local meat market grind liver into hamburger to increase the child's acceptance. Including liver in the usually very limited diet of an autistic child further increases intake of a vast array of trace minerals that are known to support growth and development. Although it is not likely for a child to be exposed to polar bear liver, as discussed in Chapter 4, the extremely high level of vitamin A in this type of liver can be fatal.

Attention Deficit Hyperactivy Disorder

Attention deficit hyperactivity disorder (ADHD) is the official term sanctioned by the American Psychiatric Association. The term attention deficit disorder (ADD) is an older, but still used, term. This disorder relates to a child's inability to pay attention and to sustain effort.

Many dietary theories have evolved over the years. It is widely believed that sugar and food additives cause hyperactivity among children, although research has shown this to be generally false. Part of the public's confusion with the belief that sugar causes hyperactivity is that the consumption of sweets often coincides with stimulating activities such as school recess, birthday parties, or holidays (at which time the activity or excitement, and not the sugar, causes excess activity).

Many families and teaching personnel may limit intake of sugar-based foods among children with ADHD in a belief that it is a causal factor. This may lead to negative dynamics between the child and adult caretakers or parents that leads to disordered eating by the child with ADHD. Families and caregivers of ADHD children may need to be reminded of the adage "cause no harm" when it comes to restricting foods from the child's diet. This is especially true with ADHD because there is no proven dietary treatment at this time.

What Are Other Causes of Underweight Children and How is the Condition Treated?

A child may weigh less than is desirable for many reasons. The child may be consuming the normal recommended amount of food and kilocalories, but have increased needs because of hypermetabolism. A hypermetabolic state occurs, for example, with fevers. A child who has chronic ear infections will have difficulty gaining adequate weight because of a reduced appetite in conjunction with an increased need for kilocalories. Children with intestinal parasites or chronic diarrhea will not grow to the optimal level. A child who is constantly on the go will have increased needs for kilocalories from the excessive activity level. If sudden or excessive weight loss occurs, serious organic illness, such as diabetes or psychologic problems, should be ruled out.

An increase of 500 kcal/day in excess of need should result in a weight gain of 1 lb/week, assuming adequate intestinal absorption. An additional intake of two slices of bread, 2 tbsp of peanut butter, or 2 oz of cheese, and an extra glass of whole milk provides 500 kcal. If there is an adequate nutritional intake (at least the minimum number of recommended servings according to the Food Guide Pyramid), the additional kilocalories can appropriately come from added fats and sugars. Adding gravy, butter, mayonnaise, or heavy cream to foods can increase the kilocalorie density of foods. Between-meal snacks, such as milkshakes, puddings, and ice cream, can also help promote weight gain. Treatment is aimed at developing appropriate food habits so that good nutritional status and weight gain can be maintained. Persons with a family history of heart disease or diabetes would benefit from increased amounts of unsaturated fats (liquid oils and mayonnaise) versus solid fats (butter and hydrogenated fats—see Chapters 8 and 9).

WHAT ARE IMPORTANT CONSIDERATIONS IN FEEDING THE TODDLER AND PRESCHOOL-AGED CHILD (1 TO 5 YEARS OLD)?

As children grow, their eating habits change. These changes are reflective of their stage in development. Among toddlers, simple foods that are fun to eat are favorites (see Box 13-2 and Figure 13-1). Mixed foods are generally unpopular with this age group. Differences in food textures interest children. Each meal might include something soft (such as macaroni and cheese), something chewy or crunchy (such as pineapple chunks and thinly cut carrot sticks), and something dry (such as peas). Small portions of a variety of foods at a meal can enhance satiety—the recognition of hunger being satisfied.

▌ BOX 13-2
▌ SUGGESTED SNACKS AND FINGER FOODS

FRUITS	VEGETABLES
Apple wedges	Cabbage wedges
Banana slices	Carrot sticks
Berries	Cauliflower florets
Dried apples	Celery sticks*
Dried apricots	Cherry tomatoes
Dried peaches	Cucumber slices
Dried pears	Green pepper sticks
Fresh peach wedges	Tomato wedges
Fresh pear wedges	Turnip sticks
Fresh pineapple sticks	Zucchini or summer squash strips
Grapefruit sections (seeded)	
Grapes	**MEATS AND MEAT SUBSTITUTES**
Melon cubes or balls	Cheese cube
Orange sections (seeded)	Cooked meat cubes
Pitted plums	Hard-cooked eggs
Pitted prunes	Small sandwiches (quartered)
Raisins	Toast fingers
Tangerine sections	Whole-grain crackers

From U.S. Department of Agriculture: A Planning Guide for Food Service in Child Care Centers, FNS-64. Food and Nutrition Service, Washington, DC.
*May be stuffed with cheese or peanut butter.

The child should be equipped with eating utensils and dishes that are easy to handle. The child should be offered only small amounts of food at a time. By eating at the table with the family, children are likely to develop an interest in food that mirrors that of their parents. By the age of 3 or 4 years, the child will be able to dish food onto a plate if smaller serving dishes and utensils are used. This further helps the child develop a sense of mastery over eating.

When compared with the infant, the preschool-aged child experiences a slowing rate of growth and development. A decrease in the consumption of food generally parallels this decrease in metabolic rate. A parent should not become alarmed if the following changes in eating behavior occur; rather, these changes are considered normal for the preschool child:

- Wanting foods plain, with no sauces and not mixed together
- Varying interest and lack of interest in food, with appetites that go up and down
- **Food jags**—eating only a few foods day after day or week after week until the next food jag starts

Keeping a record of food portions may help to allay parents' fears that their child is not eating enough. Being able to see the whole day or a whole week very often makes it apparent that the child is eating the recommended food servings of the Food Guide Pyramid. This knowledge, in addition to a comparison of the child's growth with a growth chart, can be very helpful in calming parents' fears of nutritional inadequacy. A healthy appearance and high levels of energy in children is further evidence of good nutritional status (Figure 13-7).

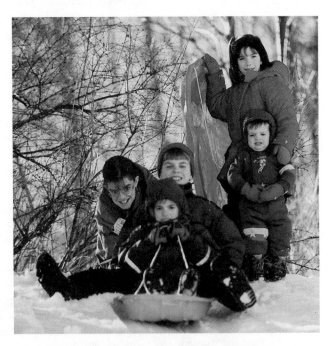

FIGURE 13-7 Healthy children love to play.

If the child's diet does appear to be lacking in a food group that is affecting growth, offering previously omitted foods at the times when the child is most hungry can help. Getting children to accept new foods may take time and patience. A child may need to be exposed to the food on several occasions before deciding that it is worth eating. Seeing the food in the grocery store or being prepared in the kitchen and a small portion served on the plate all help. The use of choice also helps.

Juice has increasingly become a staple beverage for toddlers. Because of excess kilocalories or replacement for milk, the amount of juice should be limited. A maximum of 12 oz/day of juice is recommended for children.

Snacks should be planned to enhance the nutritional value of the diet (see Box 13-2) while decreasing risk for dental caries (Box 13-3). Snacks should be served at least 1 hour before the meal to allow sufficient intake of food at mealtime. However, sometimes a compromise is needed if the child is very hungry. A premeal snack before dinner can be considered an appetizer. Good choices for snacks include a dish of peaches or yogurt, both nutritious for the young child.

Recommended amounts of foods for preschoolers can be found in Table 13-2. Good food habits developed at this time will help ensure an adequate diet throughout life.

Fallacy: Once a picky eater, always a picky eater!

Fact: It takes time for food likes to develop. Children do not like many foods when they first try them, but with repeated exposure in a positive environment, even the most finicky eaters can learn to appreciate a wide variety of foods. Children should be encouraged to have one taste of all foods served, but beyond that, forcing or begging a child to eat has no place in the development of long-term food preferences. It may be helpful for the anxious parent to follow the advice of Ellyn Satter, registered dietition, social worker, and author of "How to Get Your Kid to Eat . . . Not Too Much," who asserts that it is the parent's responsibility to offer nutritious foods in a positive meal setting, but that it is the child's responsibility to determine how much and what he or she eats. Children seem to eat better if they perceive they are eating because it makes them feel good and not simply to please their parents. It should be remembered, however, that it is common for a child to need at least 10 tries of a new food before it becomes a well-liked food.

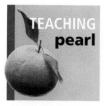

The self-fulfilling prophecy should be recalled when parents are encouraging their children to try new foods. The focus should be on the positive. For example, it is better to say, "Now that you are older, you may find you like spinach, and want more." Focusing on the negative discourages acceptance; that is, avoid saying, "If you don't like it, you don't have to eat it."

BOX 13-3
GOOD SNACK FOODS FOR DENTAL HEALTH

Carrot and celery sticks
Zucchini "matchsticks"
Radishes
Green and red pepper rings
Cucumber slices
Peanuts and other nuts (for children over 3 years, to avoid choking)
Cheese, regular in moderation or low-fat varieties
Hard-cooked egg, with or without the yolk (for cholesterol control)
Grain products (crackers, toast, bagels) with peanut butter or cheese
Apple wedges with peanut butter
Milk or yogurt

TABLE 13-2
PATTERN OF FEEDING FOR PRESCHOOL-AGED CHILDREN

MEAL	CHILDREN 1 TO 3 YEARS	CHILDREN 3 TO 6 YEARS
BREAKFAST		
Milk, fluid*	½ c	¾ c
Juice or fruit	¼ c	½ c
Cereal or bread, enriched or whole-grain[†]	¼ c[‡]	⅓ c[§]
cereal or bread	½ slice	½ slice
MIDMORNING OR MIDAFTERNOON SUPPLEMENT		
Milk, fluid,* or juice or fruit or vegetable	½ c	½ c
Bread or cereal, enriched or whole-grain[†]	½ slice	½ slice
bread or cereal	¼ c[‡]	⅓ c[§]
LUNCH OR SUPPER		
Milk, fluid*	½ c	¾ c
Meat or meat alternate[¶]		
Meat, poultry, or fish, cooked**	1 oz	1½ oz
Cheese	1 oz	1½ oz
Egg	1	1
Cooked dry beans and peas	⅛ c	¼ c
Peanut butter	1 tbsp	2 tbsp
Vegetables and fruits[††]	¼ c	½ c
Bread, enriched or whole-grain[†]	½ slice	½ slice

From U.S. Department of Agriculture: A Planning Guide for Food Service Child Care Centers, FNS-64. Food and Nutrition Service, Washington, DC, p. 5.
*Includes whole milk, low-fat milk, skim milk, cultured buttermilk, or flavored milk made from these types of fluid milk, which meet state and local standards.
[†]Or an equivalent serving of an acceptable bread product made of enriched or whole-grain meal or flour.
[‡]¼ c (volume) or ⅓ oz (weight), whichever is less.
[§]⅓ c (volume) or ½ oz (weight), whichever is less.
[¶]Or an equivalent quantity of any combination of foods listed under meat and meat alternates.
**Cooked lean meat without bone.
[††]Must include at least two kinds.

WHAT ARE SOME NUTRITION ISSUES IN THE PROCESS OF GROWTH AND DEVELOPMENT?

A Growing Sense of Independence among Preschoolers

A growing sense of independence occurs naturally in preschoolers. Parents will be well advised to offer the preschooler structured choices to allow for a sense of independence. This applies to food and to other daily activities (for example, "Are you going to put on your shoes or am I?"). Recognition of this facet of the growing child can foster positive parent-child interaction and healthy food selection. A structured food choice at the dinner table might be, "Would you like apple slices or a banana for dessert?" A structured food choice at the supermarket might be to allow the child a choice of cereals with less than 6 g (1.5 tsp) of sugar.

Promoting Sound Food Values

The manner in which food is offered is fundamental to the development of interest in a variety of nutritious foods. If you reflect for a moment on the types of holiday foods promoted, such as chocolate on Valentine's Day and candy at Halloween, you will quickly realize the value our society places on food. However, it is possible to promote nutritious foods. Kiwi fruit might be offered in Easter baskets and dried fruit offered at Halloween.

Parents and caregivers are the most effective nutrition educators of children. They teach by example and by attitude. Parents and daycare providers should be encouraged to promote positive food choices in an enjoyable manner.

Fallacy: Once a sweet tooth, always a sweet tooth.

Fact: Children whose diets are continually high in sugar can lose their ability to appreciate the natural taste of foods. As with salt and other substances, the taste for sweetness can be both learned and unlearned. Gradual reduction in quantities used is the easiest and surest way to overcome a sweet tooth.

Coping with Food Advertisements

Because many television or written advertisements promote foods that are not very nutritious (when was the last time you saw an ad for broccoli?), children need to be empowered to resist the negative messages. One approach is to divide food into two categories: foods that help you grow and those that do not, or foods that make you grow tall versus those that make you grow wide. This approach can help the child appreciate that the adult is being helpful by providing nutritious foods that are not advertised on television.

Working Parents

Two parents working or single mothers working can put added stress on mealtime. Finding time to prepare meals and to offer meals in a relaxed, positive manner can be difficult. Quick meal ideas for the working family may be helpful. Examples include a meal of scrambled eggs, whole-grain toast, mini carrots, and milk, or a meal might consist of bean and cheese burritos using either commercial or homemade refried beans rolled into flour tortillas and served with fresh fruit and beverage of choice.

WHAT ARE IMPORTANT CONSIDERATIONS IN FEEDING THE SCHOOL-AGED CHILD (5 TO 11 YEARS OLD)?

Meeting the nutritional requirements of the 5- to 11-year-old child takes larger amounts of the same foods needed by the preschool-aged child. Growth during prepuberty is slow and steady, with gradual increases in height and weight.

With the introduction of school into the child's daily routine, the child's meal pattern is likely to change. The child may have to eat breakfast earlier to allow sufficient time to get to school or plan on eating a school breakfast. Children who skip breakfast are less well fed because it is difficult to make up missed nutrients at other meals. If the family has good breakfast habits, the child will likely continue this practice. The child may be taught to prepare a simple, but nutritious, breakfast. Parents should eat breakfast with their children; even setting aside 5 minutes for eating a quick bowl of non–sugar-coated cereal is helpful. The importance of eating with the family continues with other meals. One study found beneficial effects on nutritional intake when children eat dinner with their families (Stockmyer, 2001).

At school the child is introduced to group feeding. Peers and teachers may influence eating behavior and the child may be more or less willing to try an unfamiliar food, depending on the eating behavior of others in the group. A child who has been exposed to a wide variety of foods at home is more likely to try new foods at school or at a friend's house.

Whether the child brings a lunch prepared at home or buys lunch from the National School Lunch Program, lunch should supply approximately one third of the DRI for all nutrients (see the table on the inside back cover). Nutrition education may occur at school through such means as cooking and identifying foods. Ideally, this food exposure at school should positively promote sound food choices without labeling foods as good or bad.

HOW DO THE CHANGES OF ADOLESCENCE AFFECT EATING PATTERNS AND NUTRITIONAL NEEDS?

Although children may be best friends and equals in elementary school, the onset of adolescence creates vast differences. Girls especially tend to increase their amount of body fat just before puberty and their growth spurt (the time of increased long-bone growth). Their male peers, who do not reach puberty as early and retain their boyish frames, may begin to question their masculinity. Eventually boys catch up to the girls with increased muscle mass and long-bone growth. All this is happening as the adolescent's face begins to look like a war zone covered with acne—or so it is perceived, even if there is only one pimple. All of these changes are hormonally related.

Intense concern with nutritional intake develops as a consequence of these changes, but too often in a negative way. Some teenagers try weight-control diets either to lose their baby fat or to regain a sense of control over their rapidly changing bodies. This can result in conditions such as anorexia and bulimia. Others ignore sound nutritional practices (for example, by eating potato chips in place of fruits or by drinking soft drinks in place of milk) to feel accepted among their peers. The need for a sense of self-worth and of identity can take priority over good nutritional practices.

Other barriers to good nutritional intake that adolescents encounter include the following:

1. *Society's emphasis on slimness.* There are clothes sold today that are actually size 0. Young women still aspire to the 19-inch waists once common among nineteenth-century women, who achieved their hourglass figures by wearing tight-laced corsets and commonly fainted from the inability to breathe with these corsets. We tend to forget that we are twenty-first-century women who are taller and proportionally larger than our earlier counterparts. Good nutrition can suffer, particularly among adolescent girls, in the attempt to achieve this unrealistic image.
2. *Access to jobs and spending money.* This allows the adolescent greater freedom in purchasing food and restricting the time to eat because teenagers often dash to part-time work directly from school. Fast-food outlets are a common lure for this population. Adolescents' sense of immortality can overshadow their knowledge of the importance of good nutrition, which can result in an increased intake of fat and sugar. If this type of eating habit becomes entrenched, it can be difficult to alter eating habits as an older adult, when the need becomes more apparent.
3. *Athletic sports.* After-school sports, although a positive influence on teen's physical and mental health, can make it difficult for the student to eat appropriately. Dinnertime with family is often usurped by practice or game times. Limited mealtime promotes reliance on processed foods, which often are high in fat and sugar. Safe portable foods can be packed by the teen, such as a peanut butter sandwich and banana or dried apricots and nuts with bottled water or juice as a beverage. Milk intake can be promoted at other meals and as a bedtime snack in the form of yogurt or a bowl of cereal with milk. A new carbonated milk called e.moo is being sold in some parts of the country, which is hoped to compete with soft drinks. Other adverse associations with athletics on nutritional status can also occur such as dieting to meet weight goals for wrestling.
4. *More time spent away from home.* Adolescents are increasingly in a position to determine what or if they eat. This freedom, coupled with adolescent rebel-

lion, can result in their consuming the opposite of what they know they should. If this is a problem for the adolescent's health needs, problem-solving with the teen should be emphasized. Just as young children better accept and practice desired behaviors when they are given choices, so do persons of all ages.

5. *Alcohol as a rite of passage.* Alcohol increasingly becomes an issue for teenagers. Television advertising can lure them into thinking that alcohol, such as beer, brings with it fun and glamour. Alcohol use can make teenagers feel more adult and independent. Many teenagers regularly drink beer and wine and alcoholism can occur. Alcohol can seriously impair the final stages of growth and development by replacing foods or more nutritious beverages such as milk and juice. The sense of immortality in adolescence can contribute to drunk driving accidents and alcohol poisoning from excess intake.

What Are the Nutritional Requirements of the Adolescent (12 to 18 Years Old)?

During the rapid growth period of adolescence, kilocalorie and nutrient needs are higher to provide for increases in bone density, muscle mass, blood volume, and for the developing endocrine system. There is an increased need for kilocalories, calcium, iron, and iodine (see the table on the inside back cover). Unfortunately, this message has not been adequately heard by teens with inadequate nutrient intake. There is increasing evidence that calcium intake up to the threshold amount, about 1500 mg, increases bone mass during growth. Nutrient needs can be met by increasing the serving size or number of dairy servings to four per day with the addition of other calcium foods such as legumes and certain leafy, green vegetables (see Chapter 4). A minimum of 3 c of milk equivalent (or about 1000 mg of calcium) needs to be recommended to all teens. A vegan or macrobiotic diet (no animal products including milk) can result in decreased bone mass in adolescents, which may increase the risk of fracture in later life.

WHAT ARE NUTRITION CONCERNS FOR CHILDREN AND ADOLESCENTS INVOLVED IN SPORTS OR OTHER PHYSICAL ACTIVITIES?

Maintaining a good level of physical activity is important for the health of growing children and adolescents. Aerobic exercise such as walking, running, and biking helps to increase the intake of oxygen, which promotes metabolic processes. Simply supporting the weight of the body through various forms of physical activity promotes the development of strong bones. Exercise promotes good emotional health and a sense of well-being. Physical activity accompanied by an adequate diet best allows for optimal growth and development. For example, a combination of adequate calcium intake with vitamins C, D, and K with weight-bearing exercise in adolescence is important for optimal bone growth (Branca and Vatuena, 2001).

The nutrient needs for children and adolescents who are involved with endurance levels of physical activity have increased needs for kilocalories, protein, and fluids.

Energy Requirements

Specific energy needs depend on one's age, gender, type of exercise, and degree of exertion. Adolescent male athletes may require as many as 5000 kcal to maintain weight. With a few exceptions, an adolescent male athlete should eat no fewer than 2000 kcal per day and a female athlete should eat at least 1700 to 1800 kcal per day.

Calculation of Kilocalorie Needs

A simple formula can also be used to calculate approximate kilocalorie needs as follows:

20 to 25 kcal per kilogram of body weight for low to moderate activity (10 to 12 kcal per pound of body weight)
30 kcal/kg body weight for high activity (15 kcal/lb body weight)
38 kcal/kg body weight for active adolescent females
45 kcal/kg body weight for active adolescent males
80 kcal/kg body weight for prepubescent children

Carbohydrate Needs

Most of the energy that is used during exercise comes from carbohydrates, especially for nonathletes, for long-distance or marathon athletes, and those involved in other endurance sports. Carbohydrate is the nutrient that is most readily digested, stored, and metabolized. It is found in the form of glucose in the blood and the storage form, glycogen, is found in both the liver and muscle.

Carbohydrate loading is a means of manipulating diet and exercise in an effort to maximize glycogen stores during an endurance competition. It is most often practiced by long-distance runners, cyclists, and swimmers. Athletes practicing carbohydrate loading may eat large quantities of pasta, bagels, fruits, and other carbohydrate foods for a few days before an athletic event. Exhaustion is delayed simply by increasing muscle glycogen stores. Gender differences exist in the practice of carbohydrate loading. Females metabolize more body fat and less carbohydrate during endurance exercise. In addition, the ability to build glycogen stores is more difficult for females. In order for females to carbohydrate load, they may need to consume greater than 8 g of carbohydrates per kilogram of body weight (Tarnopolsky, 2000). Children and adolescents are well adapted to prolonged exercise of moderate intensity because they have a greater reliance on fat metabolism than on carbohydrate metabolism (Boisseau and Delamarche, 2000).

Glycogen is readily available during exercise, assuming the glycogen stores are not depleted. For endurance events, carbohydrate intake at regular intervals should be emphasized to maintain blood glucose levels and to help prevent the depletion of the glycogen stores. The recommended amount of carbohydrate intake during exercise is 30 to 60 g/hour (Paquot, 2001). Glycogen is the limiting factor in the length of time exercise can be sustained.

Fallacy: Candy bars are a good source of quick energy before a sports event.

Fact: The fat in the candy bars slows the rate of digestion and the sugar that is quickly absorbed causes an increase in insulin production, which can lead to hypoglycemia, premature fatigue, and decreased performance.

Role of Protein for Physical Fitness

The major role of protein is to build and repair body tissues. Recent evidence suggests that the RDA of 0.8 g of protein per kilogram of body weight is too low for an athlete. The daily suggested protein requirement is now set at 1 to 1.5 g/kg body weight. This protein level is easily met by a diet containing 1800 to 2000 kcal per day. With such a diet, protein supplements are not necessary and are potentially detrimental to health and athletic performance. Dehydration and renal complications may result, for example. Also, a high-protein diet is often high in fat and kilocalories and can increase the risk for cardiovascular disease and obesity. Recreational sporting activities do not require an increased intake of protein.

Fallacy: Protein supplements are needed to enhance athletic performance.

Fact: It is easy to get enough protein from foods. An athlete weighing 180 lbs requires between 80 to 120 g of protein. The maximum number of servings in the Food Guide Pyramid provides this amount of protein.

Physical Fitness and Body Fat

For a well-trained athlete, body fat is a major source of fuel during endurance activity. This spares glycogen stores and helps prevent exhaustion. For children who are not physically fit, exercise is best done at a slow, steady pace until the body is better conditioned. Extremely lean athletes or anorexic athletes who have very low body fat stores may have better endurance levels if the body fat level is increased to more normal amounts. An increased intake of carbohydrates with an increased fat intake is the ideal fuel mix to promote weight gain as needed.

The Role of Vitamin and Mineral Supplementation in Sports Nutrition

Calcium
No supplementation is necessary for girls and women with normal menstrual cycles who have a balanced diet, including the recommended calcium intake of at least 1300 mg, and who perform weight-bearing exercises that promote bone resorption of calcium. However, calcium intake is frequently deficient among ado-

lescent female athletes. Additionally, **amenorrhea** (no menstrual period) is present in up to 20% of vigorously exercising women which increases the risk of early osteoporosis.

The term **female athlete triad** has been coined to describe the combination of menstrual irregularity, disordered eating, and premature osteoporosis seen in the female athlete. The risk of stress fractures is further increased among Caucasians who have low bone-mineral density, prior history of stress fractures, or both conditions. The best course of action is prevention that involves developing optimal bone-mass density through adequate calcium and caloric intake and ensuring optimal hormonal balance with weight-bearing exercise (Nattiv, 2000). There is no simple approach to managing the female athlete triad. Improved nutritional intake, however, is paramount. Adequate intake of calcium and other nutrients needed to prevent osteoporosis is essential. This includes an adequate intake of protein and kilocalories with vitamin D, magnesium, and potassium at a minimum. Calcium supplementation and hormone replacement therapy may be needed in adolescent girls with amenorrhea and low levels of estrogen production to help prevent the early onset of osteoporosis.

Iron

Adequate iron intake is essential from foods or supplements and is readily obtained from iron-fortified cereals, meats, legumes, and whole grains. To avoid excess intake, iron status should be evaluated in athletes before a supplement is prescribed. A common form of anemia is found in athletes that is not related to iron. **Sports anemia** is related to an increase in plasma volume (causing a dilution of the amount of iron in the blood) that is associated with the initiation of training. Sports anemia is not a clinical iron-deficiency anemia and should not be treated with iron supplementation.

Other Vitamins and Minerals

There is evidence of oxidative damage in athletes. Encouraging athletes to eat a variety of plant-based foods that increase intake of antioxidant vitamins is warranted. However, it has not been proven that additional supplements are needed (Clarkson and Thompson, 2000). The use of a good quality multivitamin supplement may be appropriate, but should not take the place of a good diet.

Ergogenic Aids

The use of some form of **ergogenic** aid (substance that enhances physical energy) is rampant among athletes, including adolescent athletes. Claims made by the manufacturers of such aids are not always based on actual data and may not be safe even though they are sold to the general public. Because of the misguided trust in the safety of these products, the use of ergogenic aids has become widespread. It has been estimated that one to three million athletes in the United States used anabolic steroids (Silver, 2001).

One ergogenic aid is **creatine**, a naturally occurring nitrogen compound found primarily in skeletal muscle. Increasing creatine levels may prolong skeletal muscle activity, enhancing work output. Using supplemental creatine is recognized to prevent the depletion of **adenosine triphosphate (ATP),** which is the substance that provides energy in our body cells. Evidence shows that supplementation can increase muscular force and power, reduce fatigue in repeated exertions or activities, and increase muscle mass. Creatine has also been used in various neuromuscular disorders (Persky and Brazeau, 2001).

Although there has been some benefit shown in a laboratory setting, the effect on athletic performance has not been proven. There is some question regarding the supplemental creatine's effect on the kidneys. With the concern for prevention of kidney damage and the fact that there is no research on its effectiveness with children and adolescents, this population, in particular, should be discouraged from using supplemental creatine (Pecci and Lombardo, 2000). This recommendation may be in contrast with current practice. One study on the prevalence of creatine supplementation found that among high school athletes, over 15% used creatine. Adverse effects were reported by 26% of these students (Ray et al., 2001). Among Division I collegiate athletes there was an even higher percentage of use with over 40% reporting the use of creatine. Its use was more prevalent among men than women and negative effects included cramping and gastrointestinal distress (Greenwood et al., 2000).

It has been noted that not all individuals benefit from creatine supplementation and that those who insist on taking it can gain the same benefit with 3 g/day rather than the research lab use of 20 g. Creatine supplementation leads to weight gain within the first few days of its use, likely caused by water retention in the muscle (Terjung et al., 2000).

One reason to limit the use of supplemental creatine is related to the quality of the creatine product. The more creatine ingested the greater the amount of possible contaminants consumed from the supplement. The French authorities have forbidden the sale of products containing creatine because of the possibility of contamination with mad-cow disease because bovine tissue may be used in the manufacture of creatine. Cyanamide is also used in the manufacturing process (Benzi and Ceci, 2001).

The Role of Water and Electrolytes in Sports Activities

Water is probably one of the most critical nutrients for athletic performance, yet it is the nutrient that so many active individuals tend to forget about or ignore. Approximately 50% to 75% of the human body is composed of water; water is essential for circulation, urine production, and temperature control. As the athlete exercises, heat is produced by the muscles. This heat needs to escape for a safe internal body temperature to be maintained. When sweat evaporates, heat is released from the blood circulating near the skin and the body is cooled. This water-cooling mechanism is extremely effective in maintaining the necessary body temperature.

Dehydration reduces aerobic endurance performance and results in increased body temperature, heart rate, and possibly increased reliance on carbohydrates as a fuel source. Less than 2% dehydration can affect performance, especially when the exercise is performed in the heat (Barr, 1999). Athletes should drink fluids before, during, and after exercise. In prolonged continuous exercise both fluid and carbohydrate intake has been shown to improve performance. For prolonged exercise, fluid intake should contain both carbohydrates and electrolytes and equal the fluid loss from sweating during exercise (Galloway, 1999). Prolonged exercise is generally of 1 hour or more duration, especially if the weather conditions promote excessive sweating. Two cups of water equates to 1 lb of water loss from sweating. Sports drinks are designed to include some carbohydrates and have added electrolytes. A homemade version is diluted orange juice or lemonade with some added salt; the palatability may not be as acceptable, however, as compared with commercial sports drinks.

For shorter bouts of exercise, cool or cold water is the ideal fluid, because it empties from the stomach most quickly. Other fluids, such as juices and soda pop, have a high sugar concentration, resulting in a slower gastric emptying time. Athletes should experiment before competition to find out what works best for them. Beverages containing caffeine or alcohol cause increased urine production and should not be considered as fluid replacement.

If adequate hydration is not maintained, sweating will diminish or cease entirely. Body heat cannot escape fast enough unless sweat is produced. As a result, body temperature quickly rises and heat exhaustion, heat stroke, or even death may result. General signs of thirst should not be relied on to determine when fluids should be consumed during athletic events. The warning signals that occur during severe dehydration are the following:

- Pronounced thirst
- Loss of coordination
- Mental confusion with irritability
- Dry skin
- Decreased urine output

Fallacy: Salt tablets should be taken by the athlete.

Fact: Although adequate sodium intake is essential when there is a high intake of water, salt tablets are not recommended. Salt tablets can remain whole in the stomach and cause irritation to the stomach lining. Excess salt also draws fluid away from the body cells where it is needed. Thus salt tablets are not necessary and are potentially harmful. Including sports drinks or canned broths as fluid sources or adding some table salt to foods will naturally replace the amount of sodium lost in sweat from exercise.

The Postevent Sports Meal

The athlete should consume carbohydrate foods or drinks as soon as possible after an endurance event. The first several hours after the exercise are most conducive to restoration of glycogen stores. Because there is the equivalent of $\frac{1}{2}$ lb of sugar stored in the liver as glycogen, at least 200 g of carbohydrates are required to replenish glycogen stores. Additional carbohydrates beyond this amount are needed to replenish blood glucose levels and muscle glycogen stores. Fruit juice can be easily consumed and provides the needed carbohydrates as well as being a fluid and electrolyte source. Drinking 1 c of juice every 15 minutes for about 4 or 5 hours after the sports event may be required. When the appetite returns to normal, sandwiches, fruit, and milk—which all contribute carbohydrates—may be appealing to the hungry athlete.

WHAT IS MEANT BY A DEVELOPMENTAL DISABILITY?

The term **developmental disability**, according to the Developmental Disabilities Assistance and Bill of Rights Act, refers to a severe, chronic disability that

1. is attributable to a mental or physical impairment or a combination of mental and physical impairments;
2. is manifested before the person reaches the age of 22 years;
3. is likely to continue indefinitely;
4. results in substantial functional limitations in three or more of the following areas of major life activity: self-care, receptive and expressive language, learning, mobility, self-direction, capacity for independent living, and economic self-sufficiency; and
5. reflects the person's need for a combination and sequence of special interdisciplinary or generic care, treatment, or other services that are lifelong or of extended duration and individually planned and coordinated.

The subcategories of developmental disabilities include the following: autism; **mental retardation**, a general term for a wide range of conditions resulting from many different causes, some of which are directly related to various diseases; **cerebral palsy**, characterized by a persistent qualitative motor disorder caused by nonprogressive damage to the brain; conditions that may involve sensory deficits and mental retardation; conditions that exhibit varying levels of **spasticity** (movements of the body); **epilepsy**, a group of symptoms or conditions that overstimulate nerve cells of the brain, resulting in seizures; and **neurologic impairment** that involves sensory, mentation, and consciousness functions (Table 13-3).

WHAT ARE THE NUTRITION-RELATED PROBLEMS AND CONCERNS OF THE DEVELOPMENTALLY DISABLED?

Eating problems may result from neuromuscular dysfunction such as hyperactive gag reflex, tongue thrust, poor lip closure, and inability to chew. *Neuromuscular dysfunction* refers to abnormal sensory input and muscle tone and is manifested in sucking, swallowing, and chewing movements that are hampered when oral muscles do not function properly. When chewing reflexes are lacking, ways must be found to stimulate them. For example, sweet and cold foods are found to be effective. The act of chewing also stimulates saliva production and facilitates swallowing. Neuromuscular dysfunction is common in cerebral palsy, Down syndrome, and the Prader-Willi syndrome (PWS). *Anatomic defects* and *malformations,* such as cleft palate, may cause food to pass into the nasal passages. Choking is a

TABLE 13-3
DESCRIPTION AND NUTRITIONAL IMPLICATIONS OF SOME CONDITIONS

COMMON CHARACTERISTICS	NUTRITIONAL IMPLICATION
DOWN SYNDROME (CAUSED BY CHROMOSOMAL ABNORMALITIES)	
Reduced muscle tone in varying degrees	Effects on chewing, swallowing, sucking, and tongue control
	Effects on appetite and behavior at mealtime
Growth retardation	Weight control
Small flattened skull	
Narrow nasal passage	
Delayed tooth development	Dental caries
Narrow palate	Problems with eating
CEREBRAL PALSY	
Neuromuscular impairment	Weight control
Motor disability	
Poor occlusion	Difficulties in chewing, swallowing, tongue control, and drooling
Types	
Spastic: disharmony of muscle movements	Overweight condition possible because of limited movement
Athetoid: involuntary movements of extremities	Underweight condition possible
Ataxic: inability or awkwardness in maintaining balance	
Hypotonic: muscles fail to respond to stimulation	
Hypersensitivity	Sensitivity to taste temperatures and consistency of food
PRADER-WILLI SYNDROME (ENDOCRINE, HYPOTHALAMIC DISORDER)	
Hyperphagia	
Obesity	Weight control
Short stature	Feeding difficulties in infancy
Small hands and feet	Dental caries
Hypogenitalism	
Mild mental retardation	
Bizarre eating behaviors (gorging, food stealing, eating inappropriate foods such as pet food)	
Poor sucking ability and failure to thrive in infancy	
Rapid weight gain after 1 year of age	
Slow motor development	
Obesity-related diabetes in later childhood	
Frequent lack of emotional control	

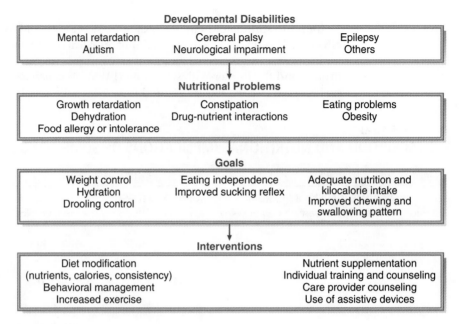

FIGURE 13-8 Flowchart for attaining nutritional goals for the developmentally disabled population.

major concern in such a condition. Poor lip closure and tongue control, a strong bite reflex, tongue thrust, excessive drooling, choking, and delayed hand-to-mouth coordination are likely to cause inadequate nutrient intake. **Tongue thrust** is a term used to describe the condition in which the teeth are not brought together to initiate swallowing, the tongue pushes out saliva, and drooling occurs. It should be noted that special feeders are available for babies with anatomic defects and that surgery can largely correct cleft palate (Figure 13-8).

Just as a period of anxiety can cause gastric distress in the normally functioning population, *behavioral problems* such as tantrums, agitation, rocking, and flailing of arms (forms of self-stimulation) can result in esophagitis, aspiration of food, dehydration, and malnutrition in the developmentally disabled. *Pica behavior* (the ingestion of nonfood items) may cause malabsorption of certain nutrients or even intestinal blockage. Food stealing is another behavioral problem that often occurs in conditions such as PWS.

Persons with Down syndrome and the **Prader-Willi syndrome (PWS)** (a genetic condition of unknown etiology) are frequently identified as being obese. Obesity is likely to occur whenever there is limited mobility, poor muscle tone, altered growth, lack of nutritional knowledge, hyperphagia, and feeding and eating problems, unless a preventive approach is taken by caregivers and parents. Unfortunately, some well-meaning people believe that food is the only source of enjoyment for those who are physically and mentally disabled. Such an attitude will only lead to more health problems. Estimation of kilocalorie needs for children with developmental disabilities is based on length in centimeters (Table 13-4).

TABLE 13-4
ENERGY REQUIREMENT CHART FOR INDIVIDUALS
WITH DISABILITIES

DIAGNOSIS	ENERGY REQUIREMENT
Cerebral palsy (mild spasticity), 5-11 years old	13.9 kcal/cm
Cerebral palsy (severe spasticity), 5-11 years old	11.1 kcal/cm
Down syndrome, boys	16.1 kcal/cm
Down syndrome, girls	14.3 kcal/cm

From Rhudy NT, Kristopher L, Miller A, Murphy P: Calculating Nutritional Requirements for Individuals with Disabilities. Morgantown, WV, Nutrition and Dietary Services, University Affiliated Center for Developmental Disabilities (UACDD).

Children with PWS need fewer kilocalories than are normally required to maintain weight. However, **hyperphagia** (excess hunger) is often present. Increased energy expenditure is helpful to control weight gain such as with walks or dancing to music. Kilocalorie needs are increased with **hyperkinesis** (excessive movement) and seizure activity. Persons with cerebral palsy often have very rigid muscles, which can increase kilocalorie needs (hypertonia). The hypotonic form of cerebral palsy will require reduced kilocalories to allow for appropriate weight.

Children with epilepsy have intermittent or chronic seizure activity. Grand mal seizures are those in which seizure activity is very pronounced and the person may be harmed through the extreme physical movements. Petit mal seizures may go unnoticed and last for only seconds at a time. An underweight child who has intermittent periods of "staring" may be having chronic seizure activity that increases the need for kilocalories, but diminishes the ability to consume adequate amounts of food.

The ketogenic diet was originally introduced in the 1920s and is once again increasingly being used to control seizure activity. This is a very rigid diet that limits carbohydrate intake to less than 5% of kilocalories, protein to 10% and the balance of kilocalories from fat. Medical oversight is critical before placing a child on a ketogenic diet.

What Are Conditions of Inborn Errors of Metabolism?

The term **inborn errors of metabolism** refers to a group of diseases that affect a wide variety of metabolic processes. Certain enzymes are lacking because of a genetic defect, requiring the diet to be modified to prevent toxicity from the excessive accumulation of by-products such as with phenylketonuria (PKU) (discussed below). Failure to detect inborn errors of metabolism at an early age results in a variety of severe problems, such as damage to the central nervous system and many body organs if an effective treatment is not started soon after birth. Many inborn errors of metabolism require specific diets for treatment. A specific diet order from the physician should be obtained and the dietitian should provide a list of acceptable foods for various special occasions.

Galactosemia

Features that characterize galactosemia include a lack of transferase (a liver enzyme that converts galactose to glucose), toxic levels of galactose in the blood, diarrhea, drowsiness, edema, liver failure, hemorrhage, and mental retardation.

The lack of the enzyme transferase requires elimination of all milk products or other milk ingredients including lactose, nonfat dry milk solids, casein, whey, and whey solids. Acceptable infant formulas are Isomil, Neo-Mull-Soy, ProSobee, Soylac, meat-based formulas, Nutramigen, and Pregestimil. Additional nutrients are provided according to the DRI.

It is very important that all ingredient labels for processed and packaged foods be read carefully. Any foods containing milk, lactose, nonfat dry milk solids, casein, whey, or whey solids cannot be tolerated by individuals with galactosemia. Lactate, lactic acid, and lactalbumin are acceptable. The complete list of ingredients may not be found on some foods, such as bread and imitation milk. Therefore frequent monitoring of red blood cell levels of galactose and galactose-1-phosphate is recommended to assure adherence to the diet.

Phenylketonuria

Phenylketonuria (PKU) is an autosomal recessive disorder characterized by a lack of the enzyme necessary to metabolize phenylalanine, one of the essential amino acids. Because phenylalanine is not metabolized, high levels accumulate and there is a characteristic excretion of phenylketones in the urine. Infants are usually blond, blue-eyed, and fair and often have eczema. All infants are now tested at birth for PKU. When untreated, the infants are hyperactive and irritable with an unpleasant personality and a musty or gamey odor. Severe retardation results if treatment is delayed. However, some studies have shown improvement in behavior in untreated individuals later in life even when the diet was not started at birth.

Bottle-fed infants with PKU require special infant formulas that prevent buildup of toxic levels of phenylalanine. Lofenalac, Phenyl-Free, and PKU-Aid are acceptable. A 10% to 30% increase of protein over the DRI is necessary to ensure adequate utilization of amino acids. Kilocalories need to be adjusted for the age, appetite, and growth pattern of the child. Special tables showing the phenylalanine content of various foods are available. Many products on the market contain aspartame, which is a source of phenylalanine and can be a problem for individuals with PKU.

Homocystinuria

This disease is characterized by a lack of the enzyme necessary for sulfur amino acid metabolism. The purpose of the diet for homocystinuria is to lower blood methionine and homocystine levels. Adequate L-cystine must be supplied; it is used to prevent the buildup of methionine and homocystine in the plasma and homocystine in the urine. Typically, the untreated child is retarded, has a fair complexion, and has detached retinas. Death usually occurs from spontaneous thrombosis.

Tyrosinosis

This disorder is a result of an error in tyrosine metabolism. The purpose of the diet for tyrosinosis is to reduce plasma tyrosine and phenylalanine levels and to prevent liver and kidney damage. It may prevent mental deterioration if started early in life.

Maple Syrup Urine Disease

In maple syrup urine disease (MSUD) there is an inability to utilize branched-chain amino acids. The purpose of the diet for this disease is to reduce leucine, isoleucine, and valine plasma levels to normal. The diet is used to prevent neurologic damage and rapid death by reducing these branched-chain amino acids in the diet.

Histidinemia

This condition is caused by a lack of the enzyme for histidine metabolism. The purpose of the diet is to lower the plasma histidine level and to treat the symptoms of histidinemia, which results in speech disorders and mental retardation. Special formulas are available for homocystinuria, tyrosinosis, MSUD, and histidinemia.

WHAT IS THE ROLE OF THE NURSE OR OTHER HEALTH CARE PROFESSIONAL IN PROMOTING GOOD NUTRITION DURING CHILDHOOD?

For Children

The terminology used with children needs to be concrete and nonscientific. Children cannot understand abstract concepts, such as the role of nutrients in foods, even though a young child can pronounce the words. Therefore it is more appropriate to focus on promoting positive attitudes toward eating nutritious foods. Children can appreciate the concept that eating is fun and this concept should be applied to nutritious foods. One method that strongly appeals to children (and even to the parents who may be present) is the use of puppet shows. Stick puppets are made easily with food pictures and with the addition of paper eyes and mouths they "come alive." Children's books such as *Green Eggs and Ham* or *Stone Soup* can also favorably influence a child's willingness to try new foods.

The importance of good dental care spans all ages, from infants to the very old. Emphasizing good oral hygiene with regular dental checkups for plaque removal is in order. Infants can have their teeth cleaned with a wet washcloth. Young children can be taught to brush their teeth or have their parents do it for them. The use of fluoride tablets should be promoted for children under 12 years of age if it is not in the local water supply. Assessment of dietary practices is important, especially that of between-meal snacking habits. Sugar is a known cariogenic food. If sweetened foods are eaten at mealtimes, they are less cariogenic. Cheese as part of a snack can help prevent dental decay, possibly because of the calcium and phosphate content, but certainly because of the protein and fat content. However, in the attempt to prevent dental caries we do not want to promote heart disease. To avoid excess intake of fat, food models might be used to show what 1 oz of cheese looks like. Local educational programs on dental health are usually offered by the health department or the WIC program (see Chapter 15). These programs generally focus on children's dental health. The health care professional should be aware of local programs to make referrals.

For Teenagers

A sensitive approach to teenagers' needs, recognizing their need for autonomy and acceptance by their peers, should be used in counseling or educational settings. The use of appropriate humor can help the teenager recognize that the health care professional is a caring human being, not merely an authority figure. Comments should be positive ones that help promote positive self-worth and do not undermine a teenager's already fragile self-image. Teenagers should be told about realistic body perceptions and eating patterns such as those represented in growth charts and the Food Guide Pyramid.

Nutrition counseling is especially important for the teenager who has failed to develop good food habits up to this point and for the teenager who has strayed from previously good habits. Information should be presented in an interesting and motivating manner. Because teenagers are very interested in their physical appearance, it should be emphasized that adequate nutrients allow for optimal growth and development of their bodies. A teenaged girl who believes that she is overweight and starts to lose weight too rapidly can use a growth chart to gain a better sense of normalcy. This tool can be particularly helpful to a teenager with anorexia or bulimia when she can visualize her growth fall from the normal curve (Figure 13-9). Although it is relatively rare, boys are also known to experience anorexia and bulimia. Health care professionals need to be aware of the existence of bulimia and its detrimental effect on dental health. A health care team approach is advised for bulimia.

It is important that the counselor respect the teenager's independence. Presenting the adolescent with flexible eating styles instead of a rigid eating pattern will increase the effectiveness of counseling. Special problems of teenagers, such as obesity, alcoholism, anorexia nervosa, and pregnancy, should be an important focus of nutrition counseling. Sports nutrition and appropriate use of supplements are issues increasingly facing American teens. Prevention of heart disease, cancer, diabetes, osteoporosis, and other diseases that may occur later in life need to be addressed with this population.

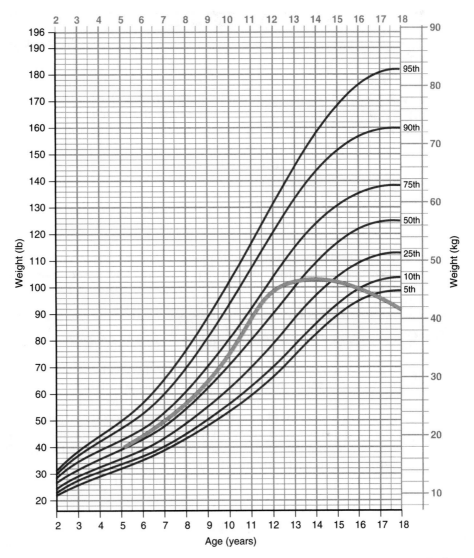

FIGURE 13-9 Sample growth fall from normal curve as assessed using the weight-for-age chart for girls 2 to 18 years of age.

**CHAPTER
STUDY
QUESTIONS
AND
CLASSROOM
ACTIVITIES**

1. How would you explain the terms *growth* and *development?*
2. What effects might be expected later in life from foods inadequate in quantity and quality during the growing period?
3. Why is it important to prevent baby-bottle tooth decay?
4. What would you advise parents who insist their toddler needs a bedtime bottle?
5. Why is it particularly important for an adolescent girl to have a nutritious diet?
6. What are the characteristics of anorexia nervosa and bulimia?
7. Why are persons with bulimia at high risk of dental erosion? What steps should be taken by one's dental hygienist if bulimia-induced dental caries are suspected?
8. What are some strategies to make snacking less harmful to dental health?
9. What advice would you provide to a high school sports team?

Case Study

**CRITICAL
THINKING**

Shannon was sitting in class and feeling very hungry. Her orthodontist had given her a whole list of foods she could not eat with her new braces. She could not eat raw fruits and vegetables. She needed to stay away from starches that would stick to her teeth, like pretzels and bread, unless she brushed her teeth afterwards. She could eat a sandwich from home, but did not like the thought of having to brush her teeth in the school bathroom. She used to eat an apple and a big tossed salad with cheese, kidney beans and croutons for lunch. Today she had eaten a yogurt, but it was not enough food. She had a soccer game after school and debated over what she could eat.

Critical Thinking Applications

1. List some foods that Shannon could eat to give her enough protein and kilocalories.
2. List foods from each group of the Food Guide Pyramid that Shannon could eat.
3. What unique needs might Shannon have as a soccer player?
4. If Shannon was to lose 3 lbs after a soccer game, how much water does she need to drink? If her weight is 140 lbs, what percentage of weight loss is this? What might you suggest to her for future soccer games?

REFERENCES

Barr SI: Effects of dehydration on exercise performance. Can J Appl Physiol. April 1999; 24(2):164-172.

Benzi G, Ceci A: Creatine as nutritional supplementation and medicinal product. J Sports Med Phys Fitness. March 2001; 41(1):1-10.

Boisseau N, Delamarche P: Metabolic and hormonal responses to exercise in children and adolescents. Sports Med. December 2000; 30(6):405-422.

Branca F, Vatuena S: Calcium, physical activity and bone health—building bones for a stronger future. Public Health Nutr. February 2001; 4(1A):117-123.

Clarkson PM, Thompson HS: Antioxidants: what role do they play in physical activity and health? Am J Clin Nutr. August 2000; 72(2 Suppl):637S-646S.

Galloway SD: Dehydration, rehydration, and exercise in the heat: rehydration strategies for athletic competition. Can J Appl Physiol. April 1999; 24(2):188-200.

Greenwood M, Farris J, Kreider R, Greenwood L, Byars A: Creatine supplementation patterns and perceived effects in select division I collegiate athletes. Clin J Sport Med. July 2000 ; 10(3):191-194.

Hartman JJ: Vitamin D deficiency rickets in children: prevalence and need for community education. Orthop Nurs. January-February 2000; 19(1):63-67.

Hijazi N, Abalkhail B, Seaton A: Diet and childhood asthma in a society in transition: a study in urban and rural Saudi Arabia. Thorax. September 2000; 55(9):775-779.

Hoppe C, Molgaard C, Michaelsen KF: Bone size and bone mass in 10-year-old Danish children: effect of current diet. Osteoporos Int. 2000; 11(12):1024-1030.

Keel PK, Mitchell JE: Outcome in bulimia nervosa. Am J Psychiatry. March 1997; 154(3):313-321.

Kennedy TS, Fung EB, Kawchak DA, Zemel BS, Ohene-Frempong K, Stallings VA: Red blood cell folate and serum vitamin B_{12} status in children with sickle cell disease. J Pediatr Hematol Oncol. March-April 2001; 23(3):165-169.

Klump KL, Kaye WH, Strober M: The evolving genetic foundations of eating disorders. Psychiatr Clin North Am. June 2001; 24(2):215-225.

Megson MN: Is autism a G-alpha protein defect reversible with natural vitamin A? Med Hypotheses. June 2000; 54(6):979-983.

Nattiv A: Stress fractures and bone health in track and field athletes. J Sci Med Sport. September 2000; 3(3):268-279.

New SA, Robins SP, Campbell MK, Martin JC, Garton MJ, Bolton-Smith C, Grubb DA, Lee SJ, Reid DM: Dietary influences on bone mass and bone metabolism: further evidence of a positive link between fruit and vegetable consumption and bone health? Am J Clin Nutr. January 2000; 71(1):142-151.

Paquot N: Sports nutrition. Rev Med Liege. April 2001; 56(4):200-203. [Article in French.]

Pecci MA, Lombardo JA: Performance-enhancing supplements. Phys Med Rehabil Clin N Am. November 2000; 11(4):949-960.

Persky AM, Brazeau GA: Clinical pharmacology of the dietary supplement creatine monohydrate. Pharmacol Rev. June 2001; 53(2):161-176.

Petti S, Cairella G, Tarsitani G: Nutritional variables related to gingival health in adolescent girls. Community Dent Oral Epidemiol. December 2000; 28(6):407-413.

Ray TR, Eck JC, Covington LA, Murphy RB, Williams R, Knudtson J: Use of oral creatine as an ergogenic aid for increased sports performance: perceptions of adolescent athletes. South Med J. June 2001; 94(6):608-612.

Sanchez OM, Childers NK: Anticipatory guidance in infant oral health: rationale and recommendations. Am Fam Phys. January 1, 2000; 61(1):115-120, 123-124.

Silver MD: Use of ergogenic aids by athletes. J Am Acad Orthop Surg. January 2001; 9(1):61-70.

Skinner JD, Carruth BR, Houck KS, Bounds W, Morris M, Cox DR, Moran J III, Coletta F: Longitudinal study of nutrient and food intakes of white preschool children aged 24 to 60 months. J Am Diet Assoc. December 1999; 99(12):1514-1521.

Stockmyer C: Remember when mom wanted you home for dinner? Nutr Rev. February 2001; 59(2):57-60.

Tarnopolsky MA: Gender differences in metabolism; nutrition and supplements. J Sci Med Sport. September 2000; 3(3):287-298.

Terjung RL, Clarkson P, Eichner ER, Greenhaff PL, Hespel PJ, Israel RG, Kraemer WJ, Meyer RA, Spriet LL, Tarnopolsky MA, Wagenmakers AJ, Williams MH: American College of Sports Medicine roundtable. The physiological and health effects of oral creatine supplementation. Med Sci Sports Exerc. March 2000; 32(3):706-717.

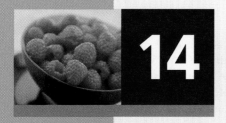

14 Nutrition Over the Adult Lifespan

OBJECTIVES

After completing this chapter, you should be able to:

- Explain how physiologic, economic, and social changes affect nutritional status.
- Discuss how nutrient needs are modified in the aging process.
- Explain how nutritional needs are identified in the elderly population.
- Name and describe nutrition programs for the elderly.
- Name some meal services and food safety considerations for older adults.

TERMS TO IDENTIFY

Aging
Alzheimer's disease
Arthritis
Dementia
DETERMINE Checklist
Geriatrics
Gerontology
Hyponatremia

Kyphosis
Macular degeneration
Meals on Wheels
Nutrition Screening
  Initiative
Older Americans Act
Osteoporosis

Over-the-counter
  medications
Parathyroid glands
Parkinson's disease
Pernicious anemia
Polypharmacy
Pouching

INTRODUCTION

The transition from childhood to young adulthood brings its own set of challenges. Learning how to cook, eating within the workplace, or having late-night snacks in college dorms (Figure 14-1) can have lasting health implications for the later years. Many chronic health problems have their roots in the habits of childhood and young adulthood. The promotion of good nutrition is an ongoing process.

The causes of mortality have changed since the beginning of the twentieth century. Additionally, about 30 years have been added to the average life expectancy, which was then only 47 years. This extension of life expectancy has had and will continue to have a profound effect on society and the health care system. Historically, infectious diseases were the most common cause of mortality. Currently, chronic health problems from years of poor-quality diets and lack of activity lead to most causes of morbidity and mortality. Furthermore, the process of **aging** diminishes the ability to ingest, digest, absorb, and metabolize nutrients in food. Thus inadequate food choices are of particular concern in the elderly population. **Gerontology** is the study of **geriatrics**, or the health concerns of older people.

Today's older adult is very different from those of past generations. There is more free time with early retirement. Many older adults choose to stay physically active even into their 90s. The age at which persons are physically active and involved with sports such as golf, swimming, and tennis will likely only continue upward.

Food and meal choices can stem from earlier life experiences. Older adults who grew up during the Great Depression often have a difficult time wasting food. This can lead to food poisoning from eating food that has been in the refrigerator too long or to obesity from trying to clean the plate, especially with the

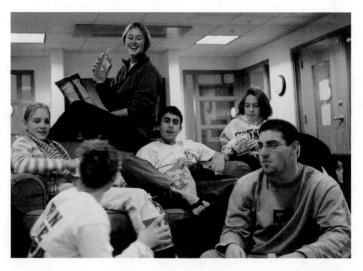

FIGURE 14-1 Late-night snacking is a common social experience in college dorms.

large portions now served in restaurants. Older adults might be very willing to eat sardines because it was a food commonly consumed throughout life and a younger adult would not dream of eating fish at all. Some adults still refuse to eat vegetables because they were forced to do so as children. The complexity of cultural food values and diversity of health requirements makes working with adults both challenging and rewarding in helping them to meet their nutritional needs.

By ensuring the good nutritional status of older adults, we can help them maintain their health and independence, thereby improving their quality of life and lessening the demands on institutional care. It has been noted that avoiding excess caloric intake while maintaining a good-quality diet and staying physically and mentally active may reduce both the incidence and severity of neurodegenerative disorders in humans (Mattson, 2000). The importance of good nutritional status in maintaining independence among the elderly cannot be overstated. Growing old need not be a burden on society, but increased attention to health is necessary, beginning in the younger years.

Fallacy: Amino acid supplements will promote longevity.

Fact: The older adult's protein requirement is essentially the same as that of a younger person, and there is no truth to the notion that amino acid supplements have any effect on the aging process. A wide variety of good protein sources are available, even for individuals who have poor dentition and sore gums. Eggs or egg whites, tuna, cottage cheese, peanut butter, and dried beans and peas are good substitutes for meat if chewing is difficult.

HOW DOES AGING AFFECT NUTRITIONAL STATUS?

Physical Changes

Once adolescence is past, the need for kilocalories decreases as the growth process ceases. This may result in weight gain if similar quantities of food are consumed. This is particularly true for previously athletic adolescents who find themselves sitting behind a work desk or studying for college exams. The additional challenge of changing food habits because of lifestyle factors can cause havoc with weight and long-term health.

During the aging process, the basal metabolic rate slows and the amount of lean body mass (muscle tissue) is reduced. Elderly persons have been found to have as much as 50% reduced muscular oxidation because of reduced numbers and functioning of mitochondria (the furnaces of the body cells) with age (Conley et al., 2000). With aging comes a reduced ability to use fat as a fuel source. This may help explain the age-related increase in body fat levels and insulin resistance with the resulting obesity, Type 2 diabetes mellitus, and cardiovascular

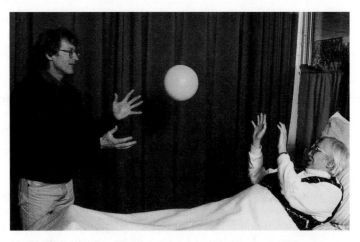

FIGURE 14-2 Exercise is possible even for bedridden adults.

disease (Blaak, 2000). Exercise needs to be part of daily activities. Even bedridden older adults can exercise (Figure 14-2).

Perceptual changes may affect eating behavior. Taste may be altered because of a decrease in the number of taste buds that occurs either as part of the aging process or as an effect of disease states, nutritional deficiencies, or medications. A reduced ability to detect odors and impaired hearing and sight may reduce the enjoyment of the social aspects of eating. All these perceptual changes may contribute to reduced food consumption.

Loss of teeth, common in the adult and elderly population, may lead to altered food choices that decrease the nutritive value of the diet.

If refined foodstuffs are eaten instead of raw fruits and vegetables, constipation may become a problem because aging is accompanied by a decrease in the body's ability to move waste products through the gastrointestinal tract. Increasing the fiber content of the diet and maintaining an adequate fluid intake and exercise will help control constipation.

The kidneys may not function in older individuals as they do in younger ones, especially if they have a chronic illness such as diabetes. Nutrient loss can occur because the kidneys are not able to conserve and reabsorb some nutrients. The buildup of toxins can also occur when the kidneys lose their ability to filter harmful substances. Because the sense of thirst diminishes with age, it is especially important to be aware of the need for fluids to promote the removal of wastes through the gastrointestinal tract and kidneys.

Decreases in body secretions also occur with aging. For example, swallowing may become more difficult because of decreased saliva production, and protein digestion is less efficient because of decreased hydrochloric acid secretion. The body's production of digestive enzymes decreases with aging as well. Table 14-1 summarizes the effect of the physiologic changes.

TABLE 14-1
PHYSIOLOGIC CHANGES IN THE OLDER ADULT

COMPONENT	FUNCTIONAL CHANGE	OUTCOME
Body composition	↓ Muscle mass	↑ Fat tissue in muscle size and strength
	↓ Basal metabolic rate	↓ Caloric requirements
	↓ Bone density	↑ Risk of osteoporosis
Perceptions	↓ Hearing	Feeling of isolation
		Reluctance to eat in public places or at large social affairs
	Slowing of adaptation to darkness	Need for brighter light to perform tasks
	↓ Number of taste buds	↓ Ability to taste salt, sweet
		↑ Ability to taste bitter and sour
	↓ Smell	↑ Threshold for odors
Gastrointestinal tract	↓ Motility	Constipation
	↓ Hydrochloric acid	↓ Efficiency of protein digestion
		More prone to food poisoning
	↓ Saliva production	Difficulty swallowing
Heart	↑ Blood pressure	↓ Ability to handle physical work and stress
	↓ Ability to use oxygen	
Lungs	↓ Capacity to oxygenate blood	↑ Fatigue
		↓ Capacity for exercise
Endocrine	↓ Number of secretory cells	↓ Blood hormone levels
	↓ Insulin production	↑ Blood sugar level
Kidney	↓ Renal blood flow	↓ Capacity for filtration and absorption

Even though little is known about an elderly person's nutritional needs, meals should be planned according to the five-food group system of the Food Guide Pyramid as discussed in Chapter 1. Six small meals a day are often more appropriate than three full-sized meals for someone with a small appetite. Eating smaller, more frequent meals can also help with weight stabilization for the younger adult. Caffeine- and alcohol-free beverages can be counted as fluids and should be included with each meal and snack to ensure adequate hydration.

Economic Changes

A young adult, often earning low wages, may find it difficult to purchase nutritious foods. Learning how to budget to include the essentials is an important step in maintaining health throughout life. With advancing age brings retirement from work. This usually results in a decrease in income at a time when an increased amount of money is being spent on medical care. As a result, less money may be available for food. High-protein foods may be consumed in lesser amounts because they are expensive, require preparation, and are difficult to chew and swallow. Young and old alike may consume excessive amounts of high-carbohydrate foods, which are inexpensive, easily stored without refrigeration, and simple to prepare.

Social Changes

Younger adults often see changes in eating habits once their children are born. Mealtimes may be rushed to take care of the needs of a newborn infant or because of older children's after-school activities. Older adults may stop cooking once children are grown, especially if living alone as a result of divorce or death of a spouse. Other older adults who are cared for by an adult son or daughter may have to eat what is offered them. Loss of mobility to shop for food occurs when physical impairments make driving a car or using public transportation difficult. Isolation from others will result unless there are friends or family on whom the elderly person can rely. Entering a nursing home profoundly changes eating habits. The loss of independence that often accompanies these changes in social structure may reduce elderly persons' self-esteem, possibly causing them to consume either more or less if they become depressed.

Grocery shopping may become more difficult for the older adult for two reasons. Food labels and prices can become hard to read because of visual impairment, and large supermarkets, which are a growing trend, require good mobility and physical stamina.

WHAT ARE THE NUTRIENT NEEDS OF THE ADULT?

Energy

Younger adults typically require 2000 to 2500 kcal daily. For this reason, the Daily Values found on food labels list the amounts of fat, carbohydrate, and protein based on these levels (see Figure 1-2). There is, however, a wide range in caloric needs for individuals, based on body composition, level of physical activity, age, and metabolism. For any adult, a minimum of 1200 to 1500 kcal is required to have an adequate nutritional intake and most young adults will even lose weight at these levels.

We know that energy needs are lower for the older adult because basal metabolism decreases gradually with aging, which in turn is caused by a decrease in lean body tissue. Older adults have the same minimum needs for food and kilocalories as younger adults, which equates to the minimum number of servings of the Food Guide Pyramid. This minimum number of kilocalories may be associated with weight stabilization for the older adult. Older adults should focus on nutrient-dense foods because the body's ability to conserve nutrients from renal loss (and metabolism in general) is less efficient than that of a younger adult.

Protein

Protein requirements do not decrease with age. It is now generally believed that a slightly higher need for protein exists for the elderly at 1.0 g/kg of body weight—versus 0.8 g/kg for the younger adult—because of the diminishing efficiency of protein utilization in the elderly. Athletic adults need a higher protein intake of up to 1.5 g/kg of body weight. Factors such as renal health and serum albumin levels can help determine individual protein needs. Also, with any age, protein requirements increase in response to certain types of physiologic stress, such as infection, bone fractures, surgery, and burns. The minimum number of servings of the Food Guide Pyramid easily meets the basic protein needs of most adults. Exceptions consist mainly of pregnant women, athletes, and those who have more immediate needs such as healing from trauma situations.

Vitamins and Minerals

The Dietary Reference Intakes (DRIs) for vitamins and minerals are for the older adult similar to those of the younger adult. However, the precise nutrient needs of the older adult are generally not well known.

Iron is one mineral known to be needed in smaller amounts in the elderly. For younger women, the higher amount of iron needed results from menstrual blood loss. In fact, women who experience very heavy menstrual periods can develop iron-deficiency anemia. Iron needs for older women and men are lower because of lack of regular blood loss. This difference is reflected in the lower amounts of iron found in multivitamin and mineral supplements designed for the older adult, such as Centrum Silver™ or men's preparations.

At least 1200 mg per day of calcium is required for most women; levels greater than 2500 mg are not recommended. To ensure adequate calcium absorption, a daily intake of 400 to 600 IU of vitamin D is recommended, either through adequate sun exposure or through diet or supplementation (North American Menopause Society, 2001).

Drinking vitamin D-fortified milk is a good way to ensure adequate intake of vitamin D and calcium in older persons who may be lacking appropriate sun exposure or who have lost the ability to manufacture vitamin D in the skin. This inability puts all elderly individuals at risk for vitamin D deficiency, particularly African Americans who live in northern climates (especially in winter when the sunlight is very weak) (Harris et al., 2000). Lactose-free milk products are available and may be necessary because the digestive enzyme lactase is less present among some population groups and with advancing age.

The elderly do not appear to be at risk for vitamin-mineral toxicity when taking supplements at the DRI level, but may be at increased risk when taking large doses because of decreased lean body mass and reduced kidney function. One study noted an elderly woman was documented to have vitamin A toxicity. Age, weight, and renal insufficiency increase the risk of vitamin A toxicity (Beijer and Planken, 2001).

A review of the older adult's vitamin and mineral use by the health care professional can help identify potentially toxic amounts of supplements. The general guidelines for all persons also apply to the older population. Use of a vitamin-mineral supplement may be appropriate and safe, but should be within the DRI range until safety guidelines establish otherwise. Increased intake of vitamins and minerals is still best achieved via food, in part because of other nutritional requirements such as protein, kilocalories, and phytochemicals.

It should be mentioned that excess nutrients can come from the use of forti-fied foods, including fortified cereals. One analysis of iron and folic acid content in breakfast cereals found amounts higher than listed. It is not uncommon for adults to eat greater than the labeled serving size of cereal. Consuming a large amount of cereal with a high level of fortification may contribute to excessive in-take of iron and folate (Whittaker et al., 2001).

Fluids

Adequate fluid intake is important throughout life. For athletic adults, increased attention to fluid intake is important, especially if they are engaged in high-endurance activities. There are two main circumstances when the sense of thirst is not an adequate indicator of fluid needs: during athletic events and for the el-derly population at any time. As adults age, the sense of thirst diminishes. Thus even young adults should develop the habit of drinking water regularly because it will make the habit easier to maintain into the elderly years.

Adults require an intake of 1 ml/kcal or 30 ml/kg of body weight. This equates to 2 L or 8 c of fluids daily for most adults. It is particularly important for the elderly to meet their fluid needs to help prevent dehydration, which may result in constipation, increased body temperature, low blood pressure, loss of balance resulting in falls, mental confusion, and dental decay.

There may also be a problem with overhydration. One study found that among hikers, about 15% had **hyponatremia**, or low levels of sodium in the blood. This was felt to result from excess water intake without concomitant in-crease in sodium. Symptoms included nausea, vomiting, headache, and dizzi-ness. With altered mental status or seizures during prolonged exercise in the heat, hyponatremia should be suspected (Backer et al., 1999).

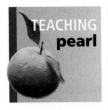

TEACHING **pearl**

A graphic description of the color of normal urine can help older adults recognize de-hydration, even though they may not feel thirsty. Urine that is dark yellow or amber gen-erally reflects dehydration. An adult who is trying too aggressively to increase fluid in-take will find a lightening in color of urine, sometimes until it is almost clear. Normal urine color is pale yellow. Comparing amount of fluid intake to the color of urine ex-creted can help to recognize a need for greater or lesser intake.

Fiber

Fiber is also important throughout life. It serves as a marker at any age for intake of a variety of trace minerals. Minerals are essential for the numerous metabolic activities that occur within the body cells.

In older adults, low fiber intake is related to chronic disorders such as diver-ticulosis and constipation. The recommended amount is about 25 g per day, which is reflected in the USDA Food Guide Pyramid's minimum number of serv-ings of fruits, vegetables, and whole grains. It is particularly easy to meet the fiber and mineral goals through the consumption of legumes, which on average contain 3 to 4 times the fiber content of any other plant-based food.

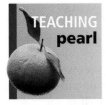

The correlation of fiber and mineral content of food can be related through the description of plant growth. Minerals are microscopic rocks (refer back to Chapter 4) that are drawn from the soil by the roots of various plants (whole grains, vegetables, fruits, etc.). The minerals are tied up with the fiber in plant-based foods.

WHAT MEDICAL CONDITIONS ARE COMMON IN THE OLDER ADULT?

Headaches

Headaches are a common malady often beginning in childhood. They are a frequent cause of physician visits and absences from work. Some headaches are now recognized to be related to the production of *histamine*. Histamine is a known gastrointestinal irritant, but newer evidence shows that it causes the release of nitric oxide from the vascular system, causing spontaneous headache pain (Thomsen and Olesen, 2001). Histamine may be released during periods of hypoglycemia (see Chapter 9). Thus small, frequent meals may be helpful in reducing the incidence of some forms of headaches. Red wine, chocolate, and aged cheese are common headache inducers; excess alcohol, dehydration, lack of sleep, and sudden withdrawal from caffeine can also trigger them.

Gastroesophageal Reflux Disorder

Gastroesophageal reflux disorder (GERD) is common among older adults. Treatment may involve weight loss for reduced pressure on the stomach from excess abdominal adipose tissue. The use of small, frequent meals further helps. Avoiding fatty meals, especially before bedtime, allows for quicker digestion. When the stomach is empty there is less likelihood of reflux to occur. Avoidance of fatty foods, alcohol, caffeine, and nicotine from smoking cigarettes helps the esophageal sphincter to function better, thereby helping to prevent reflux. Another common condition among older adults is hiatal hernia (see Figure 3-7), which may have symptoms and problems similar to those of GERD.

Diminished Immunity

It is well known that the elderly are at increased risk for infectious diseases such as pneumonia. Decreased immunity occurs with uncontrolled diabetes. There is also evidence that low zinc levels lead to diminished immunity (Fraker et al., 2000). The relationship of zinc deficiency to impaired immunity is highlighted by research that shows inadequate zinc intake among the elderly (Ma and Betts, 2000).

Arthritis

There are two major forms of **arthritis**: osteoarthritis and rheumatoid arthritis. Many misconceptions exist concerning the role of nutrition in preventing and managing arthritis. Nutrition is generally felt to play a minor role in prevention and management, except in regard to weight control, which helps decrease strain on joints affected by osteoarthritis.

Control of blood sugar levels may have an effect because low blood sugar levels—or the rise and fall in blood sugar levels after eating sweets—can trigger histamine production in some individuals. Although histamine production is related to allergies, there is no conclusive evidence that avoiding sugar will help control rheumatoid arthritis. Eating fewer sweets certainly will not cause any physical harm, however, and it helps to manage weight.

There is some belief that omega-3 fatty acids may help control rheumatoid arthritis by reducing inflammation, but there is no strong evidence to support it. However, including fatty fish such as salmon, sardines, or herring in the diet carries with it other benefits in addition to its possible role in managing rheumatoid arthritis.

Gout

Gout resembles arthritis and is characterized by pain in a single joint (often starting with the large toe) followed by complete remission. As the disease progresses, the attacks become more prolonged and more frequent. Eventually degenerative joint changes and deformity take place.

Gout is now recognized as a strong correlate of the insulin resistance syndrome (see Chapter 6). As research continues, our understanding of how to prevent and manage gout will be enhanced. For example, a low-purine diet, which limits the consumption of legumes, is sometimes advocated. Legumes, however, which are an example of a food high in complex carbohydrates that also contains soluble fiber and trace minerals such as zinc, potassium, and magnesium, may play a positive role in managing gout by controlling insulin resistance.

Alcohol and excess fatty foods are to be avoided with gout because they may inhibit excretion of urate and hinder weight control. Maintaining sufficient fluid intake and ideal body weight is important. Rapid weight loss should be avoided.

It should be noted that drugs are usually more effective in lowering blood uric acid than are dietary modifications. Thus dietary restrictions are usually no longer imposed.

Osteoporosis

Osteoporosis (porous bones) is a major health concern for the older adult; an estimated 20 million Americans are affected. Osteoporosis develops gradually over a lifetime, but age-related bone loss begins around the age of 35 to 40 years in both men and women. Current approaches increasingly focus on prevention, but for many older adults, osteoporosis has already been diagnosed. With the diagnosis of osteoporosis comes increased risk of bone fractures that can be caused simply by activities of daily living.

Including adequate amounts of calcium and vitamin D during adolescence and young adulthood decreases the risk of osteoporosis. If the bone is able to absorb adequate amounts of calcium at this time of life, osteoporosis will be less likely to occur. Beneficial effects of omega-3 fatty acids on bone metabolism and bone and joint diseases have also been noted (Watkins et al., 2001).

Aside from inadequate calcium and vitamin D intake, reduced levels of weight-bearing physical activity increase the risk of osteoporosis. Other risk factors include excess alcohol intake. However, there is some concern that even moderate drinking may have detrimental effects on bone (Turner et al., 2001). Cigarette smoking hinders the oxygenation process, thereby damaging all body cells, including bone.

Estrogen deficiency is a major cause of bone loss in postmenopausal women. Newer evidence has found that lower doses of estrogen in women may still prevent bone loss while minimizing the side effects seen with higher doses. Additionally, when adequate calcium, vitamin D, and weight-bearing exercise are used in combination with estrogen, bone density increases (Gallagher, 2001).

Medications known to adversely affect bone density include steroids, thyroid hormones, and chronic heparin therapy (South-Paul, 2001). Steroid medications cause rapid bone loss within weeks of their start, but bone loss continues for years with chronic use. About one third of patients using steroid medications will develop fractures. Postmenopausal women with low initial bone densities are at the highest risk when also using steroids. A skeletal assessment should be undertaken and bone density can be increased by use of hormone replacement (androgens for men and estrogen for women who have lowered levels of these hormones) or a *bisphosphonate* medication such as *etidronate, alendronate,* or *risedronate* (Reid, 2000).

Rheumatoid arthritis is also associated with bone loss. The use of steroid medications to treat the inflammation of rheumatoid arthritis further increases the risk of osteoporosis (Bijlsma and Jacobs, 2000).

Other associated causes of osteoporosis include resection of the ileum and malabsorption (see Chapter 3) and other inflammatory conditions such as Crohn's disease. Some of the risk of osteoporosis related to Crohn's disease is related to the use of steroids (Chinea et al., 2000).

In 1997 the Food and Nutrition Board of the National Academy of Science released the new DRIs for calcium. Recommendations were set at levels associated with retention of body calcium. The recommended intake for adults is 1000 to 1200 mg per day. The upper tolerable limit for calcium was set at 2500 mg (Bryant et al., 1999). A calcium intake in the range of 1300 to 1700 mg stops age-related bone loss and reduces fracture risk in individuals 65 and older. Intakes of 2400 mg daily restore the functioning of the **parathyroid glands** (glands integral in maintaining serum calcium levels) to young adult values. Milk is probably the most nutritionally and cost-effective means of meeting the calcium need in the elderly (Heaney, 2001).

For patients of older ages, treatment of osteoporsis may be altered. Hormone replacement therapy is rarely used after 70 years of age, whereas calcium and vitamin D are widely used with bisphosphonate medications. After 80 years, the calcium-vitamin D combination alone is useful. Renal function should be assessed annually in patients taking bisphosphonates (Daragon and Vittecoq, 2001).

Fallacy: Calcium-based antacid tablets will prevent osteoporosis.

Fact: Although this message may be advertised as an appropriate strategy to prevent osteoporosis, it is oversimplified and potentially harmful. Individuals who have consumed adequate quantities of milk and milk products throughout their lives are less prone to the development of osteoporosis in their later years. However, it is still not clear whether the calcium in milk or other combinations of nutrients (such as magnesium) in the milk are of the most benefit. The best approach is to eat or drink foods that are naturally rich in calcium and vitamin D, such as fortified milk. Moderate sun exposure will also help. Weight-bearing exercise, avoidance of excess alcohol, and consuming a well-balanced diet containing a variety of vitamins and minerals are all important in maintaining bone health and strength.

Pernicious Anemia

Individuals with **pernicious anemia** lack intrinsic factor and therefore cannot absorb dietary vitamin B_{12}; it must then be given by injection. This condition increases in prevalence among the elderly, but also can occur at any age when diseases of the gastrointestinal tract are involved.

Mood Disorders

Mood disorders such as depression can occur in childhood, but are more common in adulthood. A variety of dietary changes may help. Slow weight reduction can help to elevate mood. Eating breakfast regularly leads to improved mood, better memory, more energy, and feelings of calmness (Lombard, 2000). Diminished omega-3 fatty acid concentrations are associated with mood disorders. Evidence suggests a role for omega-3 fatty acids in managing schizophrenia (Freeman, 2000).

Alzheimer's Disease and Dementia

Alzheimer's disease and **dementia** are diseases that progress in frequency and severity with age. An increased risk of cognitive decline is related to low levels of the antioxidant selenium (Berr et al., 2000). There is evidence that omega-3 fatty acids reduce the risk of dementia (Freeman, 2000). Memory can be improved by increasing circulating glucose availability (Newcomer et al., 1999).

Several problems occur with these conditions, including forgetfulness and disorientation, pacing, inability to eat independently, weight gain or loss, dysphagia, food behavioral problems, and constipation usually from inadequate intake of fluids. Because of disorientation, a person with dementia needs to be reminded to chew, swallow, and drink water. All these problems may affect nutritional status. Responses might include increasing caloric intake to prevent weight loss, increasing fluid intake for constipation, or offering finger foods to encourage feeding independence.

Pouching (retaining bits of food between the cheeks and gums) is sometimes observed, especially in nursing home patients or those with developmental delays (see Chapter 13). If the food retained in the mouth contains fermentable carbohydrates (such as in fruit, candy, bread), acid production and plaque will occur, resulting in dental decay. Acidic foods, such as oranges, may cause erosion of tooth enamel if the food is pouched. Caregivers should inspect the mouth of persons known to pouch.

Parkinson's Disease

Parkinson's disease is a common neurodegenerative disorder with risk increasing with age. There is some evidence that neurodegenerative disorders occur from oxidative damage at the cell level. There is promise that a diet rich in antioxidant vitamins may help prevent the onset or progression of neurodegeneration.

Loss of Vision

Loss of vision occurs with uncontrolled diabetes (see Chapter 9). Another form is related to degenerative diseases of the retina. Many forms of retinal degeneration can be treated with vitamin A or other dietary changes. One common form of retinal degeneration is **macular degeneration**. The macula is found in the retinal area on the back of the eye. Degeneration of the macular disk results in slow or sudden, but painless, loss of central vision or visual distortion. A significant decrease in risk for macular degeneration occurs among those who consume a large amount of spinach, collard greens, and other dark green, leafy vegetables such as kale and broccoli. It is believed that the high carotene and lutein content of these vegetables is involved in the prevention of macular degeneration. However, prevention may also involve other substances such as vitamins C and E and the mineral zinc and further research is underway (Berson, 2000).

WHAT ARE SOME CONCERNS RELATED TO FOOD-DRUG INTERACTIONS?

A significant portion of all prescribed and **over-the-counter medications** (those not prescribed) are used by persons over 65 years of age. Older persons may often take three to seven separate drugs at any given time. Organ deterioration, underlying chronic diseases, dietary regimens, an unstable nutritional status, and other factors make the elderly particularly vulnerable to food and drug interactions. Quality of life and health may be affected as a result.

Polypharmacy, the excessive use of prescription and over-the-counter medications, increases risk for adverse drug reactions and drug-drug interactions. Medical nutrition therapy can help individuals avoid, reduce, or discontinue some medications.

HOW IS THE OLDER ADULT'S NUTRITIONAL STATUS ASSESSED?

The nutrition assessment process is discussed in detail in Chapter 5, but a few important aspects about the older adult need to be mentioned. The nurse is often the first person to discover nutritional problems. In taking a diet history, it is important for the nurse to note any type of food restrictions, ethnic or religious preferences, food aversions, and allergies. Certain signs of malnutrition may be noted during the physical examination; for example, low serum albumin is related to edema.

Factors such as bone loss and a shortening of the spinal column during later years indicate the need for current height measurement rather than relying on reported measurements from younger years. Height is frequently difficult to determine because of **kyphosis** (hunched shoulders), although knee height can be used to estimate true height (see Appendix 13).

A calibrated balance-beam scale is recommended for weighing ambulatory adults. A calibrated chair or bed scale may be used for those who are in wheelchairs or are bedridden. Weight should be monitored weekly in the hospital and monthly in other health facilities and the caregiver should keep in mind that fluid retention and dehydration can affect weight status.

What Is the Nutrition Screening Initiative and Its Role in Preventing Malnutrition in Older Adults?

The vast majority of the elderly suffer from chronic diseases that could benefit from changes in diet. Unfortunately, the warning signs of poor nutritional health are often overlooked.

The **Nutrition Screening Initiative** began in 1990 as a 5-year, multifaceted effort to promote nutrition screening and better nutritional care of older adults. This effort is a project of the American Academy of Family Physicians, the American Dietetic Association, and the National Council on Aging. Many related organizations and health professionals continue to help guide the initiative.

The Level I Screen of the Nutrition Screening Initiative is designed for social service and health professionals to identify older Americans who may need medical or nutritional attention. The Level II Screen provides more specific diagnostic information on nutritional status and is designed for use by health and medical professionals. A public awareness tool that older adults can use to assess their own nutritional risk is called the **DETERMINE Checklist** (Box 14-1).

Many circumstances can negatively affect an elderly person's nutritional status regardless of income. Warning signals include bereavement, physical or mental disabilities, and poor nutrition knowledge. Care providers can be taught to

BOX 14-1
■ **DETERMINE CHECKLIST**

Disease

Any disease, illness, or chronic condition that causes changes in eating habits or makes eating difficult increases nutritional risk. Four of every five adults have chronic diseases that are affected by diet. Confusion or memory loss that keeps getting worse is estimated to affect one or more of five older adults. This can make it hard to remember what, when, or if food has been eaten. Feeling sad or depressed, which happens to about one of eight older adults, can cause big changes in appetite, digestion, energy level, weight, and well-being.

Eating Poorly

Eating too little or too much leads to poor health. Eating the same foods day after day or not eating fruit, vegetables, and milk products daily will also cause poor nutritional health. One in five adults skips meals daily. Only 13% of adults eat the minimum amount of fruit and vegetables needed. One in four adults drinks too much alcohol. Many health problems become worse if more than one or two alcoholic beverages are consumed daily.

Tooth Loss or Mouth Pain

A healthy mouth, teeth, and gums are needed to eat. Missing, loose, or rotten teeth or dentures that do not fit well or cause mouth sores make it hard to eat.

Economic Hardship

As many as 40% of older Americans have incomes of less than $6000 per year. Having less—or choosing to spend less—than $25 to $30 per week for food makes it very hard to procure adequate foods to stay healthy.

Reduced Social Contact

One third of all older people live alone. Being with people daily has a positive effect on morale, well-being, and eating habits.

Multiple Medicines

Many older Americans must take medicines for health problems. Almost half of all older Americans take multiple medicines daily. Growing old may change the way we respond to drugs. The more medicines used, the greater the chance for side effects, such as increased or decreased appetite, change in taste, constipation, weakness, drowsiness, diarrhea, and nausea. When taken in large doses, vitamins and minerals act like drugs and can cause harm. Doctors need to be alerted to all medications taken.

Involuntary Weight Loss or Gain

Losing or gaining a lot of weight when not trying to do so is an important sign that must not be ignored. Being overweight or underweight also increases the chance of poor health.

Needs Assistance in Self-Care

Although most older people are able to eat, one in five has trouble walking, shopping, and buying and cooking food.

Elder Years Above Age 80

Most older persons lead full and productive lives. But as age increases, risk of frailty and health problems increase. Older persons should check their nutritional health regularly.

Modified with permission by the Nutrition Screening Initiative, Washington, DC, a project of the American Academy of Family Physicians, the American Dietetic Association and the National Council on the Aging, Inc., and funded in part by a grant from Ross Products, a division of Abbott Laboratories.

make observations in the home and then take appropriate steps to prevent the onset of a nutritional crisis. Practical actions can be simple, informal, and inexpensive. For example, the care provider might arrange for transportation to social activities and assist the older adult in grocery shopping and the preparation of food. However, independence should be encouraged as much as possible in all activities, including eating.

WHAT NUTRITION PROGRAMS ARE AVAILABLE FOR THE OLDER ADULT?

The federal **Older Americans Act** provides the states with money to conduct nutrition programs for the elderly. Under this Title III legislation, a hot noon meal is served to elderly persons 5 days a week in senior centers. This funding also provides transportation for individuals who are otherwise unable to get to the center. Nutrition education, health services, and recreational activities are planned around meals. For homebound elderly persons, up to a week's worth of meals are prepared at the center and delivered. Each of the one or two daily meals provides one third of the RDA of nutrients. The Title IIIc program is commonly called the Nutrition Program for the Elderly.

Meals on Wheels is a community-sponsored program that provides hot noon meals and cold evening meals to homebound elderly persons. The amount the elderly person is charged for the meals is based on the ability to pay. This program is often operated by local hospitals.

The Food Stamp Program is available to low-income individuals. In some states, food stamps can be used to pay for food provided by the Nutrition Program for the Elderly. Some older adults need to be persuaded that it is acceptable and appropriate for them to use food stamps because of the negative media coverage over the past decade about them.

These nutrition programs have helped to improve the nutritional status of the elderly population. Participation in these programs is enhanced by social work agencies that can direct the elderly population to the appropriate programs.

WHAT ARE SOME INSTITUTIONAL MEAL SERVICE CONSIDERATIONS?

Although most elderly persons remain in their own or their children's home, a significant number will eventually reside in nursing homes. The most common nutritional problems facing nursing home residents are weight loss and protein energy malnutrition. Mealtimes should be pleasant to promote adequate consumption. Prompt and courteous service is a must. Elderly persons are likely to eat better and enjoy meals more when dining with others and this habit should be encouraged whenever possible.

Food will be more appealing if it is served at the proper temperature and as soon as possible after preparation to maintain palatability. It may be necessary to cut meat into bite-sized pieces, butter bread, and open containers if the individual is unable to perform those tasks independently because of weakness or pain from arthritis, for example. Certain adaptive equipment may be needed to help maintain independence in eating. Plates and bowls can be stabilized with rubber pads (dycem mats) and suction cups. Soup can be more easily managed if poured into a cup. Foam-covered spoon and fork handles are useful for individuals who have lost some ability to handle silverware easily. See Chapter 5 for a description of various assistive eating devices.

Respect and dignity are important to the elderly. When serving a meal, the health care provider should address the person by the last name preceded by Mr., Miss, or Mrs., unless requested to do otherwise. Napkins and a damp cloth should be close at hand for wiping any spilled food from face or clothing. A vision- or hearing-impaired individual will appreciate patience and understanding. Food items and their location on the plate and at the place setting should be identified for a visually impaired person. For the visually impaired person who needs to be fed, it is vital that each bite of food be explained in advance to promote trust in the caregiver and to help the person distinguish among the foods being eaten.

WHAT ARE SOME FOOD SAFETY ISSUES FOR OLDER ADULTS?

Food preparation, shopping, and storage can be very demanding jobs for many elderly persons living alone. The elderly are highly susceptible to food poisoning because of their declining immune systems. Tight budgets and ingrained feelings about waste cause many elderly people to store food longer than is safe. With declining vision and sense of taste, food spoilage may go undetected. Food preparation leads to safety concerns. For instance, an older adult may forget that the stove is turned on. Microwave ovens can be helpful in this regard. The health professional must be alert in identifying problems in household management.

WHAT IS THE ROLE OF THE NURSE OR OTHER HEALTH CARE PROFESSIONAL IN PROMOTING THE NUTRITIONAL HEALTH OF THE OLDER ADULT?

Screening and identification of adults who are at nutritional risk, with referral to appropriate services, is an important role for all health care professionals. Use of the tools developed by the Nutrition Screening Initiative is appropriate for the elderly. Some practical actions, such as promoting a variety of foods from the Food Guide Pyramid; recommending seasonings such as herbs, spices, and lemon juice as alternative methods of flavoring to reduce salt and sugar intake; and advising on the importance of food safety to help prevent food poisoning are appropriate approaches for all health care professionals.

Because caloric needs are generally lower though nutrient needs remain high, using skim or low-fat milk and lean meats and limiting sauces, gravies, fats, and high-calorie desserts can be recommended for those individuals who are overweight. Low-calorie desserts can be encouraged because they enhance the nutritional value of the diet (e.g., canned fruits packed in their own juice, puddings and custard made with skim or low-fat milk, or low-fat cookies such as fig bars or ginger snaps).

Moderate consumption of alcohol is advisable at all stages of adulthood. The younger adult is at risk for overindulgence at social gatherings often based at bars or other venues, such as college fraternity parties. The older adult is at risk because of a diminished ability to tolerate alcohol as a result of physiologic changes.

If chewing is a problem for the adult lacking teeth, an acceptable nutritional solution may be in the form of tender, ground, or pureed meats; meat or fish loaves; or eggs. Stewed or canned fruits may be better tolerated than fresh ones. Regular foods can be chopped, ground, or even blended, providing a more appealing texture than baby foods. Adding meat to soups will also enhance the protein value of the diet. Breakfast-type foods are generally well accepted because they are easy to chew and swallow. When necessary, these breakfast-type meals can also be eaten for lunch and dinner, but they should include at least three of the food groups from the Food Guide Pyramid—for example, French toast with peach slices or scrambled eggs made mostly with egg whites and served with lightly toasted whole-grain bread and a side dish of fruit.

CHAPTER STUDY QUESTIONS AND CLASSROOM ACTIVITIES

1. Why is it necessary to understand the physiologic changes that occur with aging?
2. Why are young adults and the elderly vulnerable to nutritional deficiencies?
3. How have the nutrition programs for the elderly helped to improve their nutritional status?
4. Observe meal service at a local nursing home. How have the meals been modified to meet individual needs?
5. Take turns feeding a blindfolded classmate and, based on that experience, explain how a visually impaired adult would react to being fed. Pureed foods might also be tasted for additional perspective.
6. What dietary advice would be appropriate for an overweight widower who has hypertension, an elevated cholesterol level, and relies on convenience foods?

Case Study

CRITICAL THINKING

Sean was reading the menu at the restaurant. He and Rita were eating dinner together. He was considering ordering an appetizer instead of an entree because he knew the portions were too large. He would suffer later if he ate too large of a meal. Because he was taught as a young child that it is a sin to waste food, he had a difficult time when eating out. He decided he would just have to get a doggy bag if the portion was too large.

Critical Thinking Applications

1. What health conditions might Sean be dealing with?
2. What may occur with the use of a doggy bag?
3. What other alternatives might Sean use to limit his food portions?
4. What era helps to explain Sean's view that wasting food is a sin?

REFERENCES

Backer HD, Shopes E, Collins SL, Barkan H: Exertional heat illness and hyponatremia in hikers. Am J Emerg Med. October 1999; 17(6):532-539.

Beijer C, Planken EV: Hypercalcemia due to chronic vitamin A use by an elderly patient with renal insufficiency. Ned Tijdschr Geneeskd. January 13, 2001; 145(2):90-93. [Article in Dutch.]

Berr C, Balansard B, Arnaud J, Roussel AM, Alperovitch A: Cognitive decline is associated with systemic oxidative stress: the EVA study. Etude du Vieillissement Arteriel. J Am Geriatr Soc. October 2000; 48(10):1285-1291.

Berson EL: Nutrition and retinal degenerations. Int Ophthalmol Clin. Fall 2000; 40(4):93-111.

Bijlsma JW, Jacobs JW: Hormonal preservation of bone in rheumatoid arthritis. Rheum Dis Clin North Am. November 2000; 26(4):897-910.

Blaak EE: Adrenergically stimulated fat utilization and aging. Ann Med. September 2000; 32(6):380-382.

Bryant RJ, Cadogan J, Weaver CM: The new dietary reference intakes for calcium: implications for osteoporosis. J Am Coll Nutr. October 1999; 18(5Suppl):406S-412S.

Chinea B, Rosa A, Oharriz JJ, Ramirez M, Haddock L, Perez C, Torres EA: Osteopenia in Puerto Ricans with Crohn's disease. P R Health Sci J. December 2000; 19(4):329-333.

Conley KE, Jubrias SA, Esselman PC: Oxidative capacity and aging in human muscle. J Physiol. July 1, 2000; 526 Pt 1:203-210.

Daragon A, Vittecoq O: Osteoporosis in the elderly. Practical prevention and treatment. Presse Med. February 24, 2001; 30(7):317-320. [Article in French.]

Fraker PJ, King LE, Laakko T, Vollmer TL: The dynamic link between the integrity of the immune system and zinc status. J Nutr. May 2000; 130(5 Suppl):1399S-1406S.

Freeman MP: Omega-3 fatty acids in psychiatry: a review. Ann Clin Psychiatry. September 2000; 12(3):159-165.

Gallagher JC: Role of estrogens in the management of postmenopausal bone loss. Rheum Dis Clin North Am. February 2001; 27(1):143-162.

Harris SS, Soteriades E, Coolidge JA, Mudgal S, Dawson-Hughes B: Vitamin D insufficiency and hyperparathyroidism in a low income, multiracial elderly population. J Clin Endocrinol Metab. November 2000; 85(11):4125-4130.

Heaney RP: Calcium needs of the elderly to reduce fracture risk. J Am Coll Nutr. April 2001; 20(2 Suppl):192S-197S.

Lombard CB: What is the role of food in preventing depression and improving mood, performance and cognitive function? Med J Aust. November 6, 2000; 173 (Suppl):S104-S105.

Ma J, Betts NM: Zinc and copper intakes and their major food sources for older adults in the 1994-96 continuing survey of food intakes by individuals (CSFII). J Nutr. November 2000; 130(11):2838-2843.

Mattson MP: Neuroprotective signaling and the aging brain: take away my food and let me run. Brain Res. December 15, 2000; 886(1-2):47-53.

Newcomer JW, Craft S, Fucetola R, Moldin SO, Selke G, Paras L, Miller R: Glucose-induced increase in memory performance in patients with schizophrenia. Schizophr Bull. 1999; 25(2):321-335.

North American Menopause Society. The role of calcium in peri- and postmenopausal women: consensus opinion of the North American Menopause Society. Menopause. Summer 2001; 8(2):84-95.

Reid IR: Preventing glucocorticoid-induced osteoporosis. Z Rheumatol. 2000; 59 (Suppl 2):97-102.

South-Paul JE: Osteoporosis: part II. Nonpharmacologic and pharmacologic treatment. Am Fam Physician. March 15, 2001; 63(6):1121-1128.

Thomsen LL, Olesen J: Nitric oxide in primary headaches. Curr Opin Neurol. June 2001; 14(3):315-321.

Turner RT, Kidder LS, Kennedy A, Evans GL, Sibonga JD: Moderate alcohol consumption suppresses bone turnover in adult female rats. J Bone Miner Res. March 2001; 16(3):589-594.

Watkins BA, Li Y, Lippman HE, Seifert MF: Omega-3 polyunsaturated fatty acids and skeletal health. Exp Biol Med (Maywood). June 2001; 226(6):485-497.

Whittaker P, Tufaro PR, Rader JI: Iron and folate in fortified cereals. J Am Coll Nutr. June 2001; 20(3):247-254.

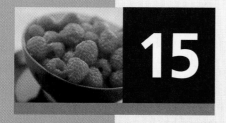

15 Public Health Issues in National and International Nutrition

OBJECTIVES

After completing this chapter, you should be able to:

- Identify the basic focus of the various federal community nutrition programs for referral purposes.
- Discuss the importance of controlling food quackery.
- Identify appropriate uses of food additives.
- Describe the principles of home-based food sanitation.
- Explain why public health professionals need to be advocates for consumer nutritional and health needs.

TERMS TO IDENTIFY

Ambulatory care
Clostridium botulinum
Clostridium perfringens
Communicable disease
Escherichia coli
Food additives
Food fads
Food insufficiency
Food irradiation

Food quack
Food resource management
Generally recognized as
    safe (GRAS) list
Genetically modified foods
Holistic
Hospices
Hyperparathyroidism
Listeria

Medicare
Organic foods
Palliative care
Paraprofessionals
Poverty
Salmonella
Staphylococcus aureus
Thrifty Food Plan

INTRODUCTION

Public health initiatives change as needs change. At the beginning of the twentieth century the average life expectancy was 47 years. Women routinely died from childbirth and approximately 1 in 10 infants died in the first year of life. Infectious respiratory diseases accounted for nearly a quarter of all deaths. Public health measures routinely focused on sanitation. The advent of immunizations and antibiotics helped to drastically reduce mortality from infections. Over the past century the percentage of child deaths caused by infectious diseases declined from over 60% to 2% (Guyer et al., 2000).

Currently the vast majority of deaths in the United States are from chronic illnesses such as heart disease and cancer. Obesity is becoming an issue worldwide and is contributing to morbidity and mortality of chronic illnesses such as diabetes and renal disease. The challenge for the twenty-first century is how to continue the fight against infectious diseases while helping to prevent chronic illnesses and providing for the health needs of an aging population.

The attacks on the World Trade Center and the Pentagon on September 11, 2001 and the subsequent deaths from anthrax delivered through the postal service began a new era of defense against terrorism. This included the temporary cessation of aerial spraying of crops out of concern for possible biologic contamination and germ warfare. Our nation's water supply will also undergo closer scrutiny to ensure the maintenance of public well-being.

Public health emphasizes an approach for community rather than individual needs. This approach includes public health initiatives such as the policy that restaurant workers must wash their hands after using lavatory facilities and use gloves in food handling to prevent widespread food poisoning. Public health departments are found in all locales and they regularly inspect restaurants for the safe storage, preparation, holding, and service of foods. Restaurants can be shut down by the agencies when they are deemed to be risking the health of the patrons they serve.

Public health messages are aimed at particular high-risk groups, such as children or the elderly, or else they concern themselves with specific conditions, such as hypertension or diabetes. National initiatives include the Food Guide Pyramid and food label guidelines, which help to improve food selection and thereby reduce obesity and heart disease. Iodized salt, vitamin D-fortified milk, and folic acid fortification of certain grain products are all designed to improve the health of large segments of the American population.

Public health programs may provide education, but they may also allow individuals to obtain nourishing food, such as in the Food Stamp Program and the Nutrition Program for the Elderly (see section later in the chapter). The Women, Infants, and Children (WIC) Supplemental Nutrition Program (see section later in the chapter) was developed in response to high rates of childhood anemia among low-income families. It provides both education and food vouchers for iron-fortified cereals to lower the rate of childhood anemia.

Public health messages are effective at getting simple information to large numbers of individuals. All health care professionals should promote public health messages such as the importance of eating less saturated fat and more high-fiber foods. More precise guidance and medical nutrition therapy provided by a registered dietitian (RD) are often needed at the individual level for the management of disease states.

WHAT IS OUR NATION'S NUTRITIONAL STATUS?

Approximately 10.2 million persons in the United States sometimes or often do not have enough food to eat, a condition known as **food insufficiency** (Dixon et al., 2001). The Continuing Survey of Food Intakes by Individuals (CSFII), 1994 to 1996, found that 7.5% of low-income families with children experienced food insufficiency. These children consumed fewer calories and total carbohydrates with less fruit than did children of higher-income families. Additionally, they had a higher cholesterol intake, were more overweight, and spent more time watching television (Casey et al., 2001). These data reinforce the belief that children from low-income families may benefit from public measures that increase their fruit consumption and provide a means for increased physical activity, such as after-school sports.

Data from the CSFII further show that the prevalence of overweight is high among women who experience food insufficiency. It has been noted that as food insufficiency increased, overweight increased proportionally. The percentage of overweight women in the CSFII study went from just under 35% with no food insufficiency to over 40% experiencing mild food insufficiency and over half of the women who were moderately food insufficient (Townsend et al., 2001). Furthermore, health care costs are higher for persons who are overweight, especially those with BMIs of at least 30 (Thompson et al., 2001). This evidence shows that a sounder national policy to eliminate food insufficiency may help lessen other national costs related to health care. However, nutrition education is important for all persons, whether coping with limited food resources or not.

Data from the Third National Health and Nutrition Examination Survey (NHANES III) found that families experiencing food insufficiency had a lower calcium intake and were more likely to have calcium and vitamin E intakes below half the recommended amounts. Fruits and vegetables were also consumed in lesser amounts, which was reflected in lower serum levels of vitamin A and carotenoids such as lutein. Older adults experiencing food insufficiency had lower intakes of kilocalories, vitamin B_6, magnesium, iron, and zinc and were more likely to have iron and zinc intakes below half the recommended amount. Both younger and older adults experiencing food insufficiency were more likely to have very low serum albumin—less than 3.5 mg/dL (Dixon et al., 2001).

The lower calcium intake among families experiencing food insufficiency is reflected in the outcomes of the Boston Low-Income Elderly Osteoporosis Study. This study found hyperparathyroidism (a condition related to excess activity of the parathyroid gland) to be significantly associated with reduced heel bone mineral density in African Americans. Higher calcium and vitamin D intakes are beneficial to this population group (Harris et al., 2001).

Hunger and Food Insufficiency in America

Hunger has always been and will always be with us, but the attempts to control its ravages have changed over the course of history. In the twentieth century, the Great Depression of the 1930s led to the establishment of soup kitchens and the Food Stamp Program. During the draft of World War II, poor nutritional status kept many young men from being admitted to the military service. In response to the observations made at that time, the School Lunch Program was expanded. During the 1960s the issue of domestic hunger received major attention from the Kennedy and Johnson administrations, which resulted in the expansion of food programs.

Beginning in the 1980s and continuing into the twenty-first century, underconsumption has again become an acute problem for many Americans. Starting in the Reagan administration, benefits were cut back or eliminated. Welfare reform enacted in the Clinton administration will likely lead to further food insuffiency for many Americans. Of the number of persons living in **poverty** (the condition of lacking the means to meet basic needs, such as housing and food), many are children, the innocent victims of some of our social policies.

Hunger, a side effect of poverty, continues not only in the United States, but also in other industrialized countries. Demand for food assistance in Canada has grown since the 1990s. Lower-income Canadian women were found to consume fewer servings of vegetables and fruit than the recommended minimum. One suggestion to enhance the nutritional status of the poor is through education and provision of foods that meet the goals of healthy eating by food banks (Jacobs Starkey and Kuhnlein, 2000).

Hunger can often be related to food availability issues as well. A person living in a rural area is relatively dependent on what the local grocery store carries, whether in rural Montana or on a Native American reservation. In more metropolitan areas, large grocery stores exist with foods from around the world, but these stores are often inaccessible to many because of transportation difficulties.

WHAT NATIONAL AGENCIES HELP IMPROVE NUTRITION?

Several federal programs give people access to food, and there are also local soup kitchens, food banks, and food pantries. These volunteer organizations depend on contributions and local, state, and federal grants. They help feed the homeless, unemployed, working poor, and developmentally disabled in many states. Other nutrition programs are discussed in the following paragraphs.

The Child and Adult Care Feeding Program (CACFP)

This program promotes good nutrition through financial reimbursement. Those who qualify are licensed home day care providers and day care centers that serve nutritious meals.

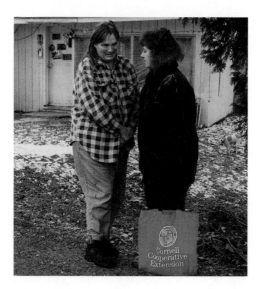

FIGURE 15-1 A nutrition teaching assistant with EFNEP visits the home of a low-income family.

The Expanded Food and Nutrition Education Program (EFNEP)

This program is offered by Cooperative Extension associations and is aimed primarily at the nutritional needs of low-income families. Local **paraprofessionals** (people who are trained by professionals) are trained in nutrition to provide free nutrition education at the homes of low-income families (Figure 15-1). They focus on **food resource management** (strategies to control food costs) and other areas relevant to nutrition, such as breast-feeding support for low-income mothers.

The Food Stamp Program

The Food Stamp Program provides stamps that can be used to purchase food or seeds to grow food. The allotment is based on the **Thrifty Food Plan**, a meal plan designed to meet the lowest possible cost for nutritional adequacy. The Thrifty Food Plan, although beneficial, was not intended to serve long-term nutritional needs. Thus relying on food stamps solely to meet food and nutritional needs is an extreme challenge for even the best-educated person.

Aid to Families with Dependent Children (AFDC)

This program is also referred to as the welfare program and was started in the Roosevelt administration during the Great Depression. Today there is still evidence that both AFDC and the Food Stamp Program have a positive effect on children's nutritional status. These programs are partly responsible for increased growth of children. However, the programs have their limitations. It has been found that the foods consumed by children in families receiving welfare benefits were of significantly lower nutritional value than foods consumed by other children, in part because of the limited funding a family can receive (Johnson et al., 1999). It is cheaper to buy white bread than it is to purchase whole grains, vegetables, and fruits. To get enough food and kilocalories, the nutritional quality of food choices can suffer when there is limited money to spend. Still, these programs are better than nothing: results suggest that participation in the Food Stamp Program is associated with food sufficiency and preschoolers' micronutrient intake. Above-average intakes of kilocalories, vitamin B_6, folate, and iron have been noted as well (Perez-Escamilla et al., 2000).

Commodity Supplemental Food Program (CSFP)

This program is offered to lower-income women and their children up to age six who are eligible for other public assistance. It is also available for seniors over 60 with income less than 130% of the Federal Poverty Level. Food or cash benefits may be provided. Seniors can receive direct deposit of funds after a home or telephone interview by their local Social Welfare office. The program targets population groups most at risk for malnutrition and helps farmers financially.

The Nutrition Program for the Elderly

The Nutrition Program for the Elderly provides nutritious meals through congregate meal settings and home-delivered meals for homebound elderly individuals. The meals provide at least $\frac{1}{3}$ of the DRIs for calcium, vitamin A, vitamin C, protein, and kilocalories. Nutrition education and counseling on social service needs are provided. Meals on Wheels, a similar program often run out of hospitals, is often used on a temporary basis during convalescence or as the need arises. It can also provide meals to a spouse while supporting the physical needs of a recuperating person.

Project Head Start

Head Start is aimed at children 3 to 5 years old whose parents' income is below the poverty line. The program combines nutrition, social services, parent involvement, and health services within an educational setting. Nutritious meals and snacks are provided. Family-style eating is promoted in that the classroom teachers eat the same foods as the children to serve as role models and promote a positive meal environment. Food is served family-style in common dishes and passed around the table so children can take their own portions. This helps build social and fine-motor skills and gives children a feeling of control over food choices.

The School Lunch and Breakfast Program

The School Lunch and Breakfast Program provides nutritious foods at reduced cost for children whose families fall within 185% of the poverty line. It further

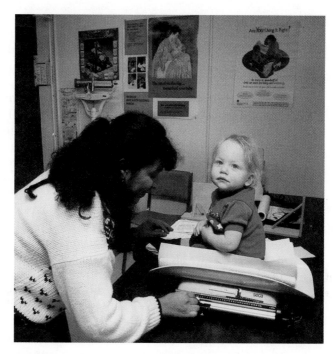

FIGURE 15-2 Monitoring growth of an infant in the WIC program.

provides free meals for those below the poverty line. Government guidelines for school lunch patterns are provided in Appendix 14.

Women, Infants, and Children (WIC) Supplemental Nutrition Program

This program provides nutrition education and vouchers for prescribed supplemental foods and is aimed at promoting the growth of the young child (Figure 15-2). Women who are pregnant or breast-feeding, infants, and children up to the age of five are eligible if the family income is within 185% of the poverty line. Nutritional risk criteria, such as low hematocrit, poor growth, frequent illness, or other qualifying medical conditions, are specified for eligibility for enrollment in the WIC program. To further promote child welfare, single fathers, foster parents, or other guardians of children can receive WIC benefits for their children.

WHAT ARE AMBULATORY CARE PROGRAMS?

Ambulatory care (health care in a noninstitutional setting) is increasing as the costs of hospital-based care continue to rise. For adequate health care services, insurance coverage is necessary. It is felt that the lack of universal health insurance contributes to the disparity between the health statuses of whites and

African Americans. African Americans have a higher prevalence of cardiovascular disease, cancer, hypertension, diabetes, obesity, and sexually transmitted infections. A variety of national, community, and individual efforts will be required to lower the health disparities in this population group (Dreeben, 2001).

Another reason for the disparity in health status of African Americans is their genetic predisposition to the insulin resistance syndrome. The same can be said of other population groups as well (see Chapter 6). As discussed throughout Section Two of this text, genetic predisposition to insulin resistance can be managed with lifestyle changes. Education regarding the physiology of insulin resistance, including its genetic basis and management, needs to be addressed through all national or other private ambulatory health programs and services to prevent later health problems.

During the last year of life, about one quarter of **Medicare** (a health plan primarily for older adults) expenditures for all adults occur, in part because of the cost of nursing home care. This statistic is unchanged from 20 years ago (Hogan et al., 2001). The Medicare program is increasingly recognizing prevention as a means to control spiraling health care costs. This focus allowed the addition of RDs as recognized providers for diabetes and predialysis renal disease in 2002. The American Dietetic Association continues to develop research documenting improved quality of life with less costly medical actions required through Medical Nutrition Therapy. As this evidence continues to be documented, Medicare will likely begin to cover other issues such as cardiovascular disease with RDs in the future.

Home Health Agencies

Home health agencies are private programs that have nurses and sometimes dietitians on staff to go to patients' homes. The attending nurse often provides the patient with nutritional care. Dietitians generally have limited roles in home health agencies because insurance policies often do not cover the cost of their services.

Hospices

Hospices are programs that offer supportive services for terminally ill patients and their families. **Palliative care** (noncurative care) and support are the general goals of hospices. The services may be provided in an institutional setting or based at home. The hospice movement is probably the best example of the change in attitude toward the **holistic** approach (one that takes into account all aspects of a person's health, such as emotional and spiritual needs, in addition to medical and nutritional needs).

In their services for terminally ill patients, emphasizing quality and not quantity of life, hospices have embraced the view espoused by Dr. Elisabeth Kübler-Ross that death is an integral part of life. Kübler-Ross was a pioneer in recognizing that terminally ill patients and their families go through stages of grief, which include denial, anger, depression, and acceptance. Nutritional goals promote palliative care of the patient as opposed to a curative approach. Therapeutic dietary restrictions may become more lenient. Goals become more short-term, such as preventing dehydration or controlling constipation. If a family member is in denial of the impending death, modifications to the patient's usual diet may not be accepted.

Appropriateness of Nutritional Support for the Terminally Ill

Nutritional support and other life-support measures for terminally ill patients can be viewed as either prolonging life or postponing death. Nutritional support for the person who is terminally ill generally focuses on oral feedings, but total parenteral nutrition (TPN) (see Chapter 5) or tube feedings cannot be ruled out. Each patient's case is unique and must be handled individually. The institution should have written guidelines for feeding the terminally ill patient. An RD can assist with deciding on an appropriate nutritional plan, based on objective criteria.

WHAT ARE SOME PUBLIC HEALTH CONCERNS THAT HAVE A BEARING ON NUTRITIONAL STATUS?

Food Irradiation

The use of radioactivity on foods to eliminate infectious pathogens is called **food irradiation**. Its use may have important positive health implications, such as the reduction of instances of *Escherichia coli* poisoning (see later section). However, there is still public concern about adverse effects of food irradiation. One study found that toxic by-products occur with light-based irradiation to vitamin B_6 (Maeda et al., 2000). Concerns such as this cause much of the public to be fearful of food irradiation. However, as a nation we need to keep the total perspective in mind. Irradiation may be appropriate when viewed as a means to prevent fatal infections from *E. coli* or *Salmonella* food poisoning outbreaks. Further research is justified to ensure that the benefits of irradiation outweigh the risks.

Organic Foods

The debate on the benefits of **organic foods** continues. Recent labeling regulations have gone into effect to ensure that consumers are actually purchasing organic foods, if they desire. *Organic* means the foods were grown without the use of commercial fertilizers and pesticides. Generally speaking, persons purchasing organic foods are concerned for the environment. For example, they favor less reliance on chemical pesticides that may be endangering health through contamination of the water supply. There is limited research on the nutritional advantages of organic foods. One study, however, found that vine-ripened tomatoes had significantly more lycopene and beta-carotene (Arias et al., 2000).

As the organic food movement continues, we will likely continue to learn more about the benefits of this approach. One lesson learned is that many consumers are willing to pay more for organic foods. Although this is positive in the sense that it encourages more farms to be less reliant on pesticides, the consumer can be paying excessively for the benefits provided.

Genetically Modified Foods

Genetically modified foods include traditional hybrid versions of plants and the more sophisticated genetically altered foods. Much of what we eat today was altered centuries ago through *hybridization*, otherwise called cross-pollination. Cross-pollination of plants occurs when the pollen from one plant is transferred to another. It can either be encouraged or discouraged, resulting in different varieties of the same plant. The cruciferous vegetables, for example, originated from one plant. Broccoli is biologically much like cauliflower except that it is green and, consequently, higher in beta-carotene and vitamin C.

Current genetic manipulation of plants has become more sophisticated thanks to the advances in the science of genetics. Through molecular biology, plants are now able to have a gene physically extracted or added to change the characteristics of new generations of plants. One positive use of genetic manipulation of plants is the ability to insert plant genes that are naturally resistant to insects. This can reduce our reliance on chemical pesticides while still feeding the world's population. Research generally shows genetically modified foods to be safe, but many want further research before widespread use of genetically modified foods are routinely developed.

Nutrition Misinformation

Food fads (a short-term, "quick-fix" diet or supplement) and nutritional quackery have multiplied as the science of nutrition has grown. A trained person can easily differentiate between accurate and unsound information, but unfortunately, the layperson often cannot. The dramatic manner in which fads and fallacies are presented covers the falseness. Anything that is out of line with current scientific evidence can be considered misinformation.

The **food quack** of today has been likened to the patent medicine man of the past. Food quacks use scientific jargon to sell the product, be it a special food or dietary supplement, special diet, regimen, book, magazine, or weight-reducing gadget. It is wise to be suspicious of any writer, lecturer, or television speaker who makes claims contrary to accepted information. Be wary of those who claim that wholesome food is harmful or undesirable in some way; use a scare technique in regard to health or claim to be a scientist or authority; or claim association with an unheard of organization or attack the Food and Drug Administration (FDA) or medical, public health, or nutrition authorities. One should always be suspicious of any material that comes from an anonymous source. The Internet is one example where sound nutritional advice and false and misleading information can be found. See Appendix 1 for Web site addresses of reputable health and nutrition organizations.

Individuals seeking health and nutrition information should make sure it is reliable and unbiased. As the expression states, "Question authority." The proposed authority on a given subject may not be a qualified authority at all. Registered dietitians are authorities that can be trusted to give sound, scientific advice on a variety of nutritional issues. Look for the credentials RD, licensed dietitian (LD), or certified dietitian-nutritionist (CDN) when looking for guidance on nutritional issues.

The FDA has long been concerned about the promotion of food supplements as cure-alls for conditions requiring medical attention. Misleading promotion of food supplements violates federal law, but nevertheless continues in the following ways:

1. Health food lecturers who claim, directly or indirectly, that the products they are promoting are of value in preventing and curing disease when in fact they are not.
2. Door-to-door sales agents who pose as experts on nutrition.
3. Pseudoscientific books and journals (written by persons with little nutritional background or training) that frequently recommend some particular food or food combination and that may include advertisements for various products in which the publisher has a commercial interest.

Nutrition authorities agree that the best way to buy vitamins and minerals is in the packages provided by nature: whole-grain breads and cereals, vegetables and legumes, fruits, milk, eggs, meat, and fish. The normal American diet now includes such a variety of foods that most persons can hardly fail to have an ample supply of the essential food constituents if they choose foods wisely. The public should distrust any suggestion of self-medication with vitamins and minerals to cure diseases of the nerves, bones, blood, liver, kidneys, heart, or digestive system.

Food Additives

The 1958 Food Additives Amendment was designed to protect the consumer. Because of this legislation, **food additives** (substances added to foods, generally to make them safer to eat) used in processed food must be proved safe by industry before they can be incorporated into any food product. The **generally recognized as safe (GRAS) list** is another approach used to control the safety of substances used in foods. Additives must meet strict guidelines for inclusion in the GRAS list. Examples of food additives include the use of nitrites to prevent botulism in cured meat products. Ascorbates and other ingredients are added to maintain quality in meat products. Only minute quantities of these additives are used, usually in amounts lower than might exist naturally in many food products. The U.S. Department of Agriculture requires that additives meet the following requirements:

1. They must be approved by the FDA and are limited to specific amounts.
2. They must meet a specific, justifiable need in the product.
3. They must not promote deception as to product freshness, quality, or weight.
4. They must be truthfully and properly listed on the product label.

Table 15-1 lists typical food additives. Table 15-2 lists food and nutrition-related responsibilities of federal agencies.

TABLE 15-1
TYPICAL FOOD ADDITIVES, WHY AND WHERE USED

REASONS FOR USE	SUBSTANCE USED	FOODS
TO IMPART AND MAINTAIN DESIRED CONSISTENCY Emulsifiers distribute tiny particles of one liquid in another to improve texture consistency, homogeneity, and quality; stabilizers and thickeners give smooth uniform texture, flavor, and desired consistency	Alginates, lecithin, mono and diglycerides, agar, methyl cellulose, sodium phosphates, carrageenan	Baked goods, cake mixes, salad dressings, frozen desserts, ice cream, chocolate milk, processed cheese
TO IMPROVE NUTRITIVE VALUE Medical and public health authorities endorse this use to eliminate and prevent certain diseases involving malnutrition: iodized salt has eliminated simple goiter; vitamin D in dairy products and infant foods has virtually eliminated rickets; and niacin in bread, cornmeal, and cereals has eliminated pellagra in the southern states	Vitamin A, thiamin, niacin, riboflavin, ascorbic acid, vitamin D, iron, potassium iodide products, margarine, milk, iodized salt	Wheat flour, bread and biscuits, breakfast cereals, cornmeal, macaroni, and noodles
TO ENHANCE FLAVOR Many spices and natural and synthetic flavors give us a desired variety of flavorful foods such as spice cake, gingerbread, and sausage	Cloves, ginger, citrus oils, amyl acetate, benzaldehyde	Ice cream, candy, gingerbread, spice cake, soft drinks, fruit-flavored gelatins, fruit-flavored toppings, sausage
TO PROVIDE DESIRED TEXTURE Leavening agents are used in the baking industry in cakes, biscuits, waffles, muffins, and other baked goods	Sodium bicarbonate, phosphates	Cakes, cookies, crackers
TO IMPART TARTNESS TO BEVERAGES	Citric acid, lactic acid, phosphates, phosphoric acid	Soft drinks
TO MAINTAIN APPEARANCE, PALATABILITY, AND WHOLESOMENESS Deterioration caused by microbial growth or oxidation is delayed and food spoilage caused by mold, bacteria, and yeast is prevented or slowed by certain additives; antioxidants keep fats from turning rancid and certain fresh fruits from darkening during processing when cut and exposed to air	Propionic acid, sodium and calcium salts of propionic acid, ascorbic acid, butylated hydroxyanisole, butylated hydroxytoluene, benzoates	Bread, cheese, syrup, pie fillings, crackers, frozen and dried fruits, fruit juices, margarine, lard, shortening, potato chips, cake mixes

From Chemical Manufacturers Association: Food Additives . . . Who Needs Them? Washington, DC, p. 11.

TABLE 15-1
TYPICAL FOOD ADDITIVES, WHY AND WHERE USED—cont'd

REASONS FOR USE	SUBSTANCE USED	FOODS
TO GIVE DESIRED AND CHARACTERISTIC COLOR		
Acceptability and attractiveness are increased by the correction of objectionable natural variations	FDA-approved colors, such as annatto, carotene, cochineal, chlorophyll	Confections, bakery goods, soft drinks, cheeses, ice cream, jams, and jellies
OTHER FUNCTIONS		
Humectants retain moisture in some foods and keep others, including salts and powders, free-flowing	Glycerine, magnesium carbonate	Coconut, table salt

TABLE 15-2
FOOD AND NUTRITION-RELATED RESPONSIBILITIES OF FEDERAL AGENCIES

AGENCY	FUNCTION
Bureau of Alcohol, Tobacco and Firearms (BATF)	Regulation of alcoholic beverages
Consumer Product Safety Commission (CPSC)	Safety of food-handling equipment
Department of Agriculture (USDA):	
Economics Research Service (ERS)	Analysis and reporting of food situation and outlook
Food and Nutrition Service (FNS)	Administration of the following programs: Food Stamps; School Lunch; Women, Infants, and Children; and Donated Food
Food Safety and Inspection Service (FSIS)	Inspection and labeling of meat, poultry, and eggs; grading of all foods; controlling nitrite in cured meats and poultry
Human Nutrition Information Service (HNIS)	Food consumption standard tables for nutritive value of food, educational materials
Science and Education Administration (SEA)	Extension Service, Agricultural Research Service Cooperative State Research Service, National Agricultural Library
Department of Health and Human Services (HHS):	
Centers for Disease Control (CDC)	Analysis and reporting of incidence of foodborne diseases
Food and Drug Administration (FDA)	Food labeling, safety of food and food additives, inspection of food processing plants, control of food contaminants, food standards
National Institutes of Health (NIH)	Research related to diet and health
Environmental Protection Agency (EPA)	Standards for drinking water, water pollution, and use of pesticides on food crops
Federal Trade Commission (FTC)	Food advertising, competition in food industry
National Marine Fisheries Service (NMFS)	Inspection, standards, and quality of seafood
Occupational Safety and Health Administration (OSHA)	Employee safety in food-processing plants

WHAT IS THE IMPORTANCE OF FOOD POISONING AND HOW CAN IT BE PREVENTED?

Food sanitation, although it appears at times unimportant to the general population, can be a matter of life and death, especially for the debilitated or acutely ill patient or young child. Eating can be hazardous to health unless three general principles are followed: (1) conditions when preparing and consuming food should be *clean;* (2) when in doubt, throw it out; and (3) keep hot foods hot and cold foods cold (above 140° or below 40° F; see Figure 15-3).

The health of a community depends on safe food and water supplies. Many agencies promote good sanitation practices to prevent and control **communicable disease** (disease that can spread from person to person, often through water and food). These agencies are concerned with all aspects of food quality, including food preservation and food additives, prevention of both natural and bacterial food poisoning, waterborne diseases, and the dangerous effects of pesticides and other toxic chemicals, such as the heavy metals lead and mercury. The U.S. Public Health Service, which is the principal health agency of the federal government, concerns itself with all factors affecting public health, including nutrition. FIGHT BAC is a national effort to educate the public on the importance of preventing foodborne illness and strategies to accomplish this.

Lack of sanitation, insufficient cooking, and improper storage can allow bacteria in food to increase to dangerous levels. Most foodborne illness results from bacterial growth in food held at an improper temperature and poor personal hygiene of food handlers. Some bacteria produce poisonous substances called toxins that cause illness when contaminated food is eaten. The following are some guidelines to preventing food poisoning:

- Serve food soon after cooking or refrigerate promptly. Hot foods may be refrigerated if they do not raise the temperature of the refrigerator to greater than 45° F (7° C).
- Keep food in the refrigerator until served or reheated.
- Speed the cooling of leftovers by refrigerating them in shallow containers.
- Keep hot foods *hot* (at temperatures greater than 140° F or 60° C) and cold foods *cold* (less than 40° F or 4° C). Food may not be safe to eat if held more than 2 or 3 hours at temperatures between 60° F (15° C) and 125° F (52° C), the zone in which bacteria grow rapidly. Remember to count time spent in preparation, storage, and serving.
- Thoroughly clean all dishes, utensils, and work surfaces with soap and water after each use. It is especially important to thoroughly clean equipment and work surfaces that have been used for raw food before using them for cooked food. This prevents the cooked food from becoming contaminated with bacteria that may have been present in the raw food. Bacteria can be destroyed by rinsing utensils and work surfaces with chlorine laundry bleach in the proportion recommended on the package. Cutting boards, meat grinders, blenders, and can openers particularly need this protection.
- Always wipe up spills with paper towels or other disposable material.

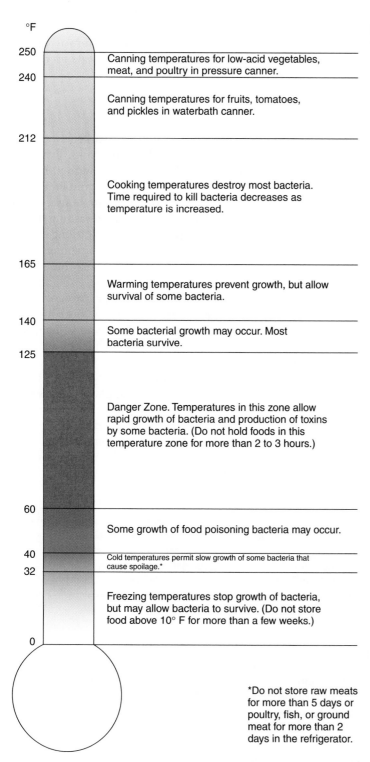

FIGURE 15-3 Temperature of food for control of bacteria.

°F

250

240 — Canning temperatures for low-acid vegetables, meat, and poultry in pressure canner.

Canning temperatures for fruits, tomatoes, and pickles in waterbath canner.

212

Cooking temperatures destroy most bacteria. Time required to kill bacteria decreases as temperature is increased.

165

Warming temperatures prevent growth, but allow survival of some bacteria.

140

Some bacterial growth may occur. Most bacteria survive.

125

Danger Zone. Temperatures in this zone allow rapid growth of bacteria and production of toxins by some bacteria. (Do not hold foods in this temperature zone for more than 2 to 3 hours.)

60

Some growth of food poisoning bacteria may occur.

40

Cold temperatures permit slow growth of some bacteria that cause spoilage.*

32

Freezing temperatures stop growth of bacteria, but may allow bacteria to survive. (Do not store food above 10° F for more than a few weeks.)

0

*Do not store raw meats for more than 5 days or poultry, fish, or ground meat for more than 2 days in the refrigerator.

- Thoroughly cook meat to avoid *E. coli* contamination.
- *If the odor or color of any food is poor or questionable, do not taste it. Throw it out. The food may be dangerous.* However, remember that there is not always an indication of food spoilage. *When in doubt, throw it out.*

How Does Personal Hygiene Affect Food Safety?

Infection of food with bacteria can begin in the farm fields by workers who have not engaged in good personal hygiene picking vegetables and fruits. Primarily for this reason, purchased raw fruits and vegetables need to be washed before consumption, but they should also be washed to reduce possible contamination from larvae left behind from insect exposure. Once food is in the house, it can be cross-contaminated from other foods, such as raw meat. Handwashing is crucial in preventing cross-contamination. Studies recommended washing hands frequently, using an antibacterial soap on areas that have been in contact with raw meat, poultry, seafood, eggs, vegetables, and other foods that may have been contaminated with an infectious agent (Toshima et al., 2001).

Anyone who has an infectious disease should not handle, prepare, or serve food. The bacteria in infected cuts or other skin infections may be the source of foodborne illness. Food handlers must always work with clean hands, hair, fingernails, and clothing. Hands must be washed after using the toilet or assisting anyone using the toilet; after cigarette smoking or blowing the nose; after touching raw meat, poultry, or eggs; and before working with other food. Food should be mixed using clean utensils rather than by hand; however, plastic gloves may be worn if it is easier to use the hands. Hands should be kept away from the mouth, nose, and hair. It is important to cover coughs and sneezes with disposable tissues and to wash hands afterward. The same spoon should not be used more than once for tasting food while preparing, cooking, or serving, unless the two-spoon method is used (see Teaching Pearl).

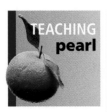

TEACHING pearl

The two-spoon method should be promoted for repeated tasting of food while cooking. One spoon is used to obtain a sample for tasting of the food item. This spoon is then used to transfer the portion for tasting onto the second spoon without having the spoons touch. This way there is no likelihood of personal contamination of food to be served to others. This method will also prolong the safety of remaining leftovers by preventing bacteria in saliva from growing and multiplying in them.

What Are Some Types of Food Poisoning?

To understand the importance of food poisoning prevention, the various types of foodborne illnesses must be recognized. The more common of these are caused by the following bacteria:

- *Salmonella*
- *Staphylococcus aureus;* causes staph poisoning

- *Clostridium botulinum;* causes botulism
- *Clostridium perfringens*
- *Escherichia coli*
- *Listeria*—a newly emerged pathogen that causes fever and possible death and is carried by raw and unprocessed foods such as soft cheeses, deli meats, and some vegetable products (Schlech, 2000).

Specific information on the causes, symptoms, and prevention of these bacterial foodborne illnesses is found in Table 15-3.

Fallacy: Adding an egg to a milkshake or making eggnog is a good idea for someone who is too ill to eat.

Fact: Raw eggs can contain *Salmonella,* a type of bacteria that can be deadly (especially when cracked or soiled) for a person with an already weakened immune system. Eggs should be used only in foods that are to be thoroughly cooked, such as baked goods or casseroles. Proper handling of foods containing cooked eggs is also important. Set custards and puddings in ice water to cool quickly after their preparation; then refrigerate promptly until serving. Pasteurized egg products are generally safe.

WHAT ARE SOME WORLD PROBLEMS IN NUTRITION AND WHAT ARE THE INTERESTED AGENCIES?

In less developed countries, a large number of individuals are undernourished, malnourished, and hungry. People in developing countries are hungry primarily because they are too poor to purchase the food that is available, although availability may also be limited by inadequate transportation or civil war.

Micronutrient deficiencies affect nearly half the world population, impairing child development, reducing work productivity, and increasing mortality and morbidity rates by affecting both infectious and chronic diseases. One micronutrient that may be deficient is selenium, which at high intake levels can reduce cancer risks (Combs, 2000). The micronutrient deficiencies of greatest public health significance include those of iron, vitamin A, and iodine (Chakravarty and Ghosh, 2000).

The problem of malnutrition is greatest among women and growing children. Millions of children in impoverished countries show signs of moderate vitamin A deficiency and are therefore more vulnerable to infection and scarring of the cornea, which can lead to blindness. The prevention of blindness in children is a priority within the World Health Organization's VISION 2020 program (Gilbert and Foster, 2001).

The four basic ways of dealing with the international hunger problem are through (1) donation of food; (2) international efforts that direct the food to vulnerable groups, such as women and children; (3) promotion of agricultural production, food technology, and better use of a given country's own food resources; and (4) economic assistance.

TABLE 15-3
BACTERIAL FOODBORNE ILLNESS: CAUSES, SYMPTOMS, AND PREVENTION

FOODS INVOLVED	SYMPTOMS	CHARACTERISTICS OF ILLNESS	PREVENTIVE MEASURES
SALMONELLOSIS: *SALMONELLA*			

Bacteria widespread in nature that live and grow in intestinal tracts of human beings and animals
Foods involved:
  Poultry
  Red meats
  Eggs
  Dried foods
  Dairy products
	Severe headache, followed by vomiting, diarrhea, abdominal cramps, and fever. Infants, the elderly, and persons with lower resistance are most susceptible; severe infections cause high fever and may even cause death	Transmitted by eating contaminated food or by contact with infected persons or carriers of the infection; also transmitted by insects, rodents, and pets
		Onset: Usually within 12 to 36 hours
		Duration: 2 to 7 days
			Salmonellae are destroyed by heating the food to 140° F and holding for 10 minutes, or to higher temperature for less time (e.g., 155° F for a few seconds)
			Refrigeration at 40° F inhibits the multiplication of Salmonellae, but they remain alive in foods in the refrigerator or freezer and even in dried food

PERFRINGENS POISONING: *Clostridium perfringens*			
Spore-forming bacteria that grow in the absence of oxygen; temperatures reached in thorough cooking of most foods are sufficient to destroy vegetative cells, but heat resistant spores can survive Foods involved: Stews, soups, or gravies made from poultry or red meat	Nausea without vomiting, diarrhea, acute inflammation of stomach and intestines	Transmitted by eating food contaminated with abnormally large numbers of bacteria *Onset:* Usually within 8 to 20 hours *Duration:* May persist for 24 hours	To prevent growth of surviving bacteria in cooked meats, gravies, and meat casseroles that are to be eaten later, cool foods rapidly and refrigerate promptly at 40° F or below, or hold them above 140° F
STAPHYLOCOCCAL POISONING: *Staphylococcus aureus*			

Bacteria fairly resistant to heat; growing in food, they produce a toxin that is extremely resistant to heat
Foods involved:
  Custards
  Egg salad
  Potato salad
  Chicken salad
  Macaroni salad
  Ham salad
  Salami
  Cheese
	Vomiting, diarrhea, prostration, abdominal cramps; generally mild and often attributed to other causes	Transmitted by food handlers who carry the bacteria and by eating food containing the toxin
		Onset: Usually within 3 to 8 hours
		Duration: 1 to 2 days
			Growth of bacteria that produce toxin is inhibited by keeping hot foods above 140° F and cold foods at or above 40° F.
			Toxin is destroyed by boiling for several hours or heating the food in a pressure cooker at 240° F for 30 minutes

From U.S. Department of Agriculture: Keeping Food Safe to Eat—A Guide for Homemakers. Home and Garden Bulletin No. 162, Washington, DC, and CDC Web site.

FOODS INVOLVED	SYMPTOMS	CHARACTERISTICS OF ILLNESS	PREVENTIVE MEASURES
BOTULISM: *Clostridium botulinum*			
Spore-forming organisms that grow and produce toxin in the absence of oxygen, such as in a sealed container Foods involved: Canned low-acid foods Smoked fish	Double vision, inability to swallow, speech difficulty, progressive respiratory paralysis. Fatality rate is high, in the United States about 65%	Transmitted by eating food containing the toxin *Onset:* Usually within 12 to 36 hours or longer *Duration:* 3 to 6 days	Bacterial spores in food are destroyed by high temperatures obtained only in the pressure canner.* More than 6 hours is needed to kill the spores at boiling temperature (212° F). The toxin is destroyed by boiling for 10 to 20 minutes; time required depends on type of food.
***Escherichia coli* (*E. coli* 0157:H7)**			
Organism that lives in the intestinal tract Foods involved: Beef Raw milk Lettuce Alfalfa sprouts Salami	Abdominal cramping Bloody diarrhea[†]	73,000 cases of infection and 61 deaths annually per CDC Kidney failure occurs in 2% to 7% of cases Illness usually resolves in 5 to 10 days	Thoroughly cook meat; do not eat burgers that are pink in the middle; handle food safely. Wash vegetables and fruits, especially if they will be served raw.
LISTERIA			
Bacteria found in soil, plants, and animals Foods involved: Soft and unpasteurized cheese Raw meat and poultry Raw and smoked seafood Raw milk	Fever Headache Nausea Vomiting Pregnant women can get flu-like symptoms of chills and fever meningitis	Symptoms occur from 2 days to 6 weeks Dangerous to unborn babies and persons with compromised immune systems Infections treated with antibiotics	Use pasteurized milk and milk products; use cottage cheese and cheese aged >60 days; pregnant women should reheat cold cuts. Wash fruits and vegetables; thoroughly cook meat; follow good food safety precautions. Do not use bulging canned goods.

*For processing times in home canning, see Home and Garden Bulletin No. 8, Home Canning of Fruits and Vegetables, and No. 106, Home Canning of Meat and Poultry. U.S. Department of Agriculture, Washington, DC.
[†]All persons with bloody diarrhea should have their stools tested for *E. coli* 0157:H7.

Food donations must reflect the health needs of the population. Lactose intolerance is commonly found worldwide; thus simply providing milk or milk powder may actually induce diarrhea and further impair nutritional status. Low-lactose milk powder was found to be well tolerated among nursing home residents in Hong Kong. This was a good alternative to other oral supplements and yogurt, which had unfamiliar tastes and were unpopular among the older Chinese. The milk supplementation increased intakes of calcium, vitamin D, vitamin A, riboflavin, and potassium among these malnourished nursing home residents (Kwok et al., 2001).

Policies designed to increase money available for food purchase can help lessen malnutrition. It was estimated in Bangladesh that if the money spent on tobacco were spent on food instead, at least an additional 500 kilocalories could be added to the diet of one or two children per person (Efroymson et al., 2001).

The United States has developed various programs and campaigns that assist developing countries in combating undernutrition. The U.S. Foreign Aid and Food for Peace programs and the activities of the Agency for International Development are coordinated with United Nations agencies. The governments of many nations contribute to the organizations that distribute food or money for the purpose of improving nutritional standards. Some of these agencies are listed in Table 15-4.

Countries in transition to Westernized lifestyles and foods may be at increased risk for inadequate micronutrient intake and for excess caloric intake from fats and sugars, which leads to obesity. The city of São Paulo, Brazil, found a decreased expenditure on nonprocessed foods by 35% in the last decade (Barretto and Cyrillo, 2001). Processed foods are typically lower in content of

TABLE 15-4
WORLD ORGANIZATIONS FOR BETTER NUTRITION

ORGANIZATION	PURPOSES
United Nations Food and Agriculture Organization (FAO)	Studying aspects of world food problems Raising nutrition standards by improving growth, distribution, and storage of food
World Health Organization (WHO)	Focusing on worldwide health problems, including nutrition
United National Education, Scientific and Cultural Organization (UNESCO)	Improving the standard of living through science education and elimination of illiteracy
United Nations International Children's Emergency Fund (UNICEF)	Directing the distribution of milk to children worldwide through emergency relief, school feeding, and maternal-child health care centers
Oxford Famine Society (OXFAM-UK)	Donating money and services for agricultural development
CARE	Receiving food from the Food for Peace Program for relief activities
World Bank	Sponsoring international projects through its agricultural and nutritional divisions

trace minerals such as zinc. Chile and the Latin American region are also experiencing a rapid change from underweight and stunting to obesity with the associated chronic illnesses of cancer, cardiovascular disease, and Type 2 diabetes (Albala et al., 2001). The worldwide increase in obesity will have an important effect on the global incidence of chronic illnesses such as Type 2 diabetes and cardiovascular disease. Obesity prevention programs should be high on the scientific and political agenda in both industrialized and industrializing countries (Visscher and Seidell, 2001).

WHAT IS THE ROLE OF THE NURSE OR OTHER HEALTH CARE PROFESSIONAL IN NATIONAL AND INTERNATIONAL NUTRITION PROGRAMS?

National Nutrition

Providing information related to the Food Guide Pyramid food groups such as portion sizes and low-sodium, low-saturated fat, or low-sugar alternatives is appropriate. Providing the patient with a reason for making dietary changes in line with physiologic needs particularly suits the nurse's skill level. Providing advice on low-cost food shopping is also appropriate (Box 15-1). Consultation should be made with an RD and physician regarding individual dietary needs that go beyond basic nutrition.

A health care team approach can help promote good nutritional status. The nurse or other health professional can help combat potentially dangerous nu-

---

■ BOX 15-1
■ MONEY-SAVING FOOD-SHOPPING SKILLS

- Use less tender cuts of meat, which are less expensive. To tenderize, cook slowly with moisture (such as in stews) or grind, cube, or pound the meat. Marinating in an acid such as lemon or tomato juice also helps to tenderize meat.
- Extend meat, poultry, and fish by making casseroles using legumes (dried beans), pasta, rice, or potatoes.
- Include meatless meals once or twice a week using legumes, eggs, cheese, or peanut butter in the place of meat for protein.
- Buy in bulk whenever possible and freeze as needed.
- Study unit pricing to determine the best buy per pound or ounce.
- Take advantage of specials and use coupons.
- Try lower-priced generic store brands, which are often similar in quality to more expensive brands.
- Plan meals to include leftovers.
- Shop for low-cost foods within each food group.
- Use food labels to compare nutritional value for cost to get your money's worth.

trition myths and fads by providing correct information and assisting the public in recognizing false nutritional health claims. On a larger scale, the health care professional can help raise societal health consciousness by documenting the health needs of those who have a low income or are homeless. This documentation is necessary to justify equitable allocation of resources to legislators and other policy makers.

It is important for the nurse or other health care professional to be aware of programs for referral purposes and direct care. Ambulatory care in particular is a growing type of health care, where the nurse is often called on to help patients cope with therapeutic diets and to help prevent the effects of poor food sanitation on the debilitated patient.

International Nutrition

Solving international nutrition concerns is more complex. The health care professional should be aware of programs that can be effectively promoted, such as recommending vitamin A tablets or foods to prevent blindness. Food programs meant to help should be closely examined. Attempts to end world hunger must be undertaken in a way that encourages independence. Individuals can have an effect on world hunger by contacting political leaders to express concern. Efforts by credible international agencies, such as the Agency for International Development and the United Nations (see Table 15-4), can be supported. For Americans, eating less meat contributes, if only in a small way: it takes about 4 lbs of grain to produce 1 lb of meat; grain grown to feed cattle could be redirected to feed the world's hungry population.

CHAPTER STUDY QUESTIONS AND CLASSROOM ACTIVITIES

1. What community programs might help a low-income family?
2. How has legislation affected public health in relation to food and nutrition issues?
3. What existing programs promote good nutrition?
4. What are the signs of a food faddist?
5. Visit or call your local health department. Learn about any nutrition activities that are conducted under the auspices of the department.
6. Identify other organizations in your area that focus on the promotion of nutrition. Describe who they are and what their programs cover.
7. Contact a federal or state legislator through a letter or a phone call to express your support for legislation on a particular public health issue.
8. A student volunteer will be assigned to swab the inside of a home refrigerator using a cotton-tipped swab. Students in the class can then rub the swab on a Petri dish and observe bacterial growth.
9. How might you assist a low-income individual who has hypertension and needs to rely on donated canned foods?

Case Study

Maria was trying to convince her mother-in-law that she needed to receive home-delivered meals, at least for now. Rita had undergone a hip replacement and could not prepare meals for herself. Because both Maria and Tony had to go to work, Joey had moved back east, Anna had her hands full with a toddler and a new baby, and A.J. was too young to help, it was the best way to ensure Rita could heal in a timely fashion from her operation. Rita, however, held the old-school belief that you did not take handouts. Maria was trying to convince her that she would heal more quickly and get back on her feet if she had a nourishing meal at noon.

Critical Thinking Applications

1. What nutrients are found in the Nutrition Program for the Elderly that would help Rita heal from her surgery?
2. What are some lunch alternatives that Rita could have that would allow healing, would not require preparation, and would stay safe to eat at room temperature?
3. If Rita did not have a family to help take care of her, what options would she have? What programs could help with health care needs and costs?

REFERENCES   Albala C, Vio F, Kain J, Uauy R: Nutrition transition in Latin America: the case of Chile. Nutr Rev. June 2001; 59(6):170-176.

Arias R, Lee TC, Specca D, Janes H: Quality comparison of hydroponic tomatoes *(Lycopersicon esculentum)* ripened on and off vine. J Food Sci. April 2000; 65(3):545-548.

Barretto SA, Cyrillo DC: Analysis of household expenditures with food in the city of S. Paulo in the 1990s. Rev Saude Publica. February 2001; 35(1):52-59. [Article in Portuguese.]

Casey PH, Szeto K, Lensing S, Bogle M, Weber J: Children in food-insufficient, low-income families: prevalence, health, and nutrition status. Arch Pediatr Adolesc Med. April 2001; 155(4):508-514.

Chakravarty I, Ghosh K: Micronutrient malnutrition—present status and future remedies. J Indian Med Assoc. September 2000; 98(9):539-542.

Combs GF Jr: Food system-based approaches to improving micronutrient nutrition: the case for selenium. Biofactors. 2000; 12(1-4):39-43.

Dixon LB, Winkleby MA, Radimer KL: Dietary intakes and serum nutrients differ between adults from food-insufficient and food-sufficient families: Third National Health and Nutrition Examination Survey, 1988-1994. J Nutr. April 2001; 131(4):1232-1246.

Dreeben O: Health status of African Americans. J Health Soc Policy. 2001; 14(1):1-17.

Efroymson D, Ahmed S, Townsend J, Alam SM, Dey AR, Saha R, Dhar B, Sujon AI, Ahmed KU, Rahman O: Hungry for tobacco: an analysis of the economic impact of tobacco consumption on the poor in Bangladesh. Tob Control. September 2001; 10(3):212-217.

Gilbert C, Foster A: Childhood blindness in the context of VISION 2020—the right to sight. Bull World Health Organ. 2001; 79(3):227-232.

Guyer B, Freedman MA, Strobino DM, Sondik EJ: Annual summary of vital statistics: trends in the health of Americans during the twentieth century. Pediatrics. December 2000; 106(6):1307-1317.

Harris SS, Soteriades E, Dawson-Hughes B: Framingham Heart Study, Boston Low-Income Elderly Osteoporosis Study: Secondary hyperparathyroidism and bone turnover in elderly blacks and whites. J Clin Endocrinol Metab. August 2001; 86(8):3801-3804.

Hogan C, Lunney J, Gabel J, Lynn J: Medicare beneficiaries' costs of care in the last year of life. Health Aff (Millwood). July-August 2001; 20(4):188-195.

Jacobs Starkey L, Kuhnlein HV: Montreal food bank users' intakes compared with recommendations of Canada's Food Guide to Healthy Eating. Can J Diet Pract Res. 2000; 61(2):73-75.

Johnson FC, Hotchkiss DR, Mock NB, McCandless P, Karolak M: The impact of the AFDC and Food Stamp programs on child nutrition: empirical evidence from New Orleans. J Health Care Poor Underserved. August 1999; 10(3):298-312.

Kwok T, Woo J, Kwan M: Does low-lactose milk powder improve the nutritional intake and nutritional status of frail older Chinese people living in nursing homes? J Nutr Health Aging. 2001; 5(1):17-21.

Maeda T, Taguchi H, Minami H, Sato K, Shiga T, Kosaka H, Yoshikawa K: Vitamin B_6 phototoxicity induced by UVA radiation. Arch Dermatol Res. November 2000; 292(11):562-567.

Perez-Escamilla R, Ferris AM, Drake L, Haldeman L, Peranick J, Campbell M, Peng YK, Burke G, Bernstein B: Food stamps are associated with food security and dietary intake of inner-city preschoolers from Hartford, Connecticut. J Nutr. November 2000; 130(11):2711-2717.

Schlech WF III: Foodborne listeriosis. Clin Infect Dis. September 2000; 31(3):770-775.

Thompson D, Brown JB, Nichols GA, Elmer PJ, Oster G: Body mass index and future healthcare costs: a retrospective cohort study. Obes Res. March 2001; 9(3):210-218.

Toshima Y, Ojima M, Yamada H, Mori H, Tonomura M, Hioki Y, Koya E: Observation of everyday hand-washing behavior of Japanese, and effects of antibacterial soap. Int J Food Microbiol. August 15, 2001; 68(1-2):83-91.

Townsend MS, Peerson J, Love B, Achterberg C, Murphy SP: Food insecurity is positively related to overweight in women. J Nutr. June 2001; 131(6):1738-1745.

Visscher TL, Seidell JC: The public health impact of obesity. Annu Rev Public Health. 2001; 22:355-75.

APPENDIXES

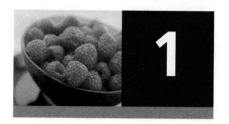

1 Sources of Nutrition Information

American Association of Family and Consumer Services
1555 King Street
Alexandria, VA 22314
Tel.: 703-706-4600
Fax.: 703-706-4663
Internet: www.aafcs.org

American Dental Association
211 East Chicago Avenue
Chicago, IL 60611
Tel.: 800-621-8099
Internet: www.ada.org

American Diabetes Association
1660 Duke Street
Alexandria, VA 22314
Tel.: 800-342-2383
Diabetes Forecast (bimonthly)
Internet: www.diabetes.org

American Dietetic Association (ADA)
216 West Jackson Boulevard, Suite 800
Chicago, IL 60606-6995
Tel.: 800-877-1600
Journal of the American Dietetic Association (monthly)
Internet: www.eatright.org

American Heart Association (AHA)
7272 Greenville Avenue
Dallas, TX 75231-4596
Tel.: 800-242-8721
Internet: www.americanheart.org

American Institute of Nutrition (AIN)
9650 Rockville Pike
Bethesda, MD 20014
Tel.: 301-530-7050
Journal of Nutrition (monthly)
Internet: www.faseb.org/asns

American Medical Association (AMA)
515 North State Street
Chicago, IL 60610
Tel.: 312-464-4543
Journal of the American Medical Association (weekly)
Internet: www.amafoundation.org

American Society of Clinical Nutrition, Inc. (ASCN)
9650 Rockville Pike
Bethesda, MD 20814-3998
Tel.: 301-530-7110
The American Journal of Clinical Nutrition (monthly)

American Society for Parenteral and Enteral Nutrition (ASPEN)
8630 Fenton Street, Suite 412
Silver Spring, MD 20910-3805
Tel.: 301-587-6315
Fax.: 301-587-2365
Journal of Parenteral and Enteral Nutrition (bimonthly)
ASPEN Update (monthly newspaper)
Internet: www.nutritioncare.org

Cancer Information Service
Office of Cancer Communications
National Cancer Institute
Building 31, Room 10A16
9000 Rockville Pike
Bethesda, MD 20892
Internet: www.cis.nci.nih.gov

Center for Nutrition Policy and Promotion, USDA
1120 Twentieth Street, NW, Suite 200, North Lobby
Washington, DC 20036
Internet: www.usda.gov/cnpp

Centers for Disease Control and Prevention
1600 Clifton Road
Atlanta, GA 30333
Internet: www.cdc.gov

Food and Drug Administration (FDA)
Regulatory Affairs
5600 Fishers Lane, No. 1490
Rockville, MD 20857
Tel.: 301-827-3101
Internet: www.fda.com

Food and Nutrition Information Center
National Agricultural Library, USDA
10301 Baltimore Boulevard, Room 304
Beltsville, MD 20705-2351
Internet: www.nal.usda.gov/fnic

Food Safety and Inspection Service, USDA
Food Safety Education Staff
1400 Independence Avenue, SW
Room 2942S
Washington, DC 20250
Internet: www.fsis.usda.gov

Gateway to Government Food Safety Information
Internet: www.foodsafety.gov

healthfinder®—Gateway to Reliable Consumer Health Information
National Health Information Center
U.S. Department of Health and Human Services
P.O. Box 1133
Washington, DC 20013-1133
Internet: www.healthfinder.gov

National Aging Information Center
Administration on Aging
330 Independence Avenue, SW
Room 4656
Washington, DC 20201
Internet: www.aoa.gov/elderpage.html

National Dairy Council
10255 West Itiggins Road, Suite 900
Rosemont, IL 60018-5616
Tel.: 847-803-2000
Dairy Council Digest (bimonthly newsletter)

National Heart, Lung, and Blood Institute Information Center
P.O. Box 30105
Bethesda, MD 20824-0105
Internet: www.nhlbi.nih.gov

National Institute of Diabetes and Digestive and Kidney Diseases
Office of Communications and Public Liaison
31 Center Drive, MSC 2560
Bethesda, MD 20892-2560
Internet: www.niddk.nih.gov

National Institute on Alcohol Abuse and Alcoholism
600 Executive Boulevard, Suite 409
Bethesda, MD 20892-7003
Internet: www.niaaa.nih.gov

Contact your county extension home economist (cooperative extension system) or a nutrition professional in your local public health department, hospital, American Red Cross, dietetic association, diabetes association, heart association, or cancer society.

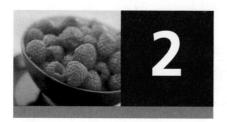

2 Nutrition Materials

Del Monte
Consumer Affairs Dept.
P.O. Box 193
San Francisco, CA 94119-3575
Tel.: 800-543-3090
Fax.: 415-242-3080

General Foods Consumer Center
250 North Street
White Plains, NY 10625
Tel.: 914-335-2500
Internet: www.kraftfoods.com

General Mills, Inc.
1 General Mills Boulevard
Minneapolis, MN 55426
Tel.: 612-540-2311
(Maxwell Division: 914-335-2500)

Kellogg Company
1 Kellogg Square
Battle Creek, MI 49016-3599
Tel.: 616-961-2000 or 800-961-1413
Fax.: 616-961-2871
Internet: www.kellogg.com

Kraft Foods, Inc.
1 Kraft Court
Glenview, IL 60025
Tel.: 800-323-0768
Internet: www.kraftfoods.com

McDonald's Corporation
2111 McDonald's Drive
Oakbrook, IL 60523
Internet: www.mcdonalds.com

Mead Johnson Nutritional Division
2400 West Lloyd Expressway
Evansville, IN 47721
Tel.: 800-457-3550

National Cattleman's Beef Association
Nutrition Research Department
444 North Michigan Avenue
Chicago, IL 60611
Tel.: 800-368-3138
Internet: www.beef.org

National Peanut Council (NPC)
1500 King Street, Suite 301
Alexandria, VA 22314
Tel.: 703-838-9500
Fax.: 703-838-9089
Internet: www.peanutsusa.com

Nestlé Food Company (Carnation)
800 North Brand Boulevard
Glendale, CA 91203
Tel.: 800-242-5200 or 818-549-6000
Internet: www.verybestbaby.com

Nestlé Food Company (Evaporated Milk Association)
800 North Brand Boulevard
Glendale, CA 91203
Tel.: 800-854-8935
Internet: www.verybestbaking.com

Novartis (previously Sandoz Nutrition Corps.)
5100 Gamble Drive
Saint Louis Park
Minneapolis, MN 55416
Tel.: 800-333-3785
Internet: www.novartisnutrition.com

The Quaker Oats Company
321 North Clark Street
Quaker Tower
Chicago, IL 60610
Tel.: 312-222-7111
Internet: www.quakeroats.com

Ralston Purina Company
Checkerboard Square
P.O. Box 618
St. Louis, MO 63188-0618
Tel.: 800-725-7866
Fax.: 314-877-7022
Internet: www.ralcorpholding.com

Ross Laboratories
625 Cleveland Avenue
Columbus, OH 43215
Tel.: 800-624-7677 or 800-727-5767

Sunkist Growers
P.O. Box 7888
Van Nuys, CA 91409
Tel.: 818-986-4800
Internet: www.sunkist.com

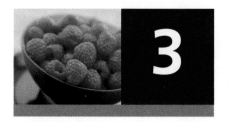

3 Metric Conversions and Equivalents

■ EQUIVALENTS

1 oz = 30 g (approximate)	1 c = 16 tbsp = 240 mL
1 lb = 454 g	1 L = 1000 mL
1 g = 1 mL	1 mg = 1000 μg

■ METRIC MEASUREMENT CONVERSIONS

SYMBOL	WHEN YOU KNOW	MULTIPLY BY	TO FIND	SYMBOL
LENGTH				
in	inches	2.54	centimeters	cm
ft	feet	30	centimeters	cm
yd	yards	0.9	meters	m
mi	miles	1.6	kilometers	km
mm	millimeters	0.04	inches	in
cm	centimeters	0.4	inches	in
m	meters	3.3	feet	ft
m	meters	1.1	yards	yd
km	kilometers	0.6	miles	mi
MASS (WEIGHT)				
oz	ounces	28	grams	g
lb	pounds	0.45	kilograms	kg
g	grams	0.035	ounces	oz
kg	kilograms	2.2	pounds	lb
	stones (British)	14	pounds	lb
VOLUME				
tsp	teaspoons	5	milliliters	mL
tbsp	tablespoons	15	milliliters	mL
fl oz	fluid ounces	30	milliliters	mL
c	cups	0.24	liters	L
pt	pints	0.47	liters	L
qt	quarts	0.95	liters	L
gal (U.S.)	gallons (U.S.)	3.8	liters	L
gal (Imp)	gallons (Imperial)	4.5	liters	L

Continued

■ METRIC MEASUREMENT CONVERSIONS—cont'd

SYMBOL	WHEN YOU KNOW	MULTIPLY BY	TO FIND	SYMBOL
VOLUME—cont'd				
ft³	cubic feet	0.028	cubic meters	m³
yd³	cubic yards	0.76	cubic meters	m³
mL	milliliters	0.03	fluid ounces	fl oz
L	liters	2.1	pints	pt
L	liters	1.06	quarts	qt
L	liters	0.26	gallons (U.S.)	gal (U.S.)
L	liters	0.22	gallons (Imperial)	gal (Imp)

TEMPERATURE

$°C = (°F − 32) × 0.555$

$°F = (°C × 1.8) + 32$

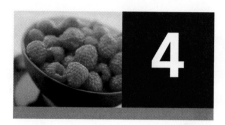

4 Nutritive Values for Selected Fast Foods

■ ARBY'S®

	SERVING OUNCES	SERVING GRAMS (g)	CALORIES	% CALORIES FROM FAT	TOTAL FAT (g)	SATURATED FAT (g)
ROAST BEEF SANDWICHES						
Arby's Melt w/Cheddar	5.2	150	340	41%	15	5
Arby-Q®	6.4	186	360	36%	14	4
Beef 'N Cheddar	6.9	198	480	46%	24	8
Big Montana®	11	313	630	46%	32	15
Giant Roast Beef	7.9	228	480	43%	23	10
Junior Roast Beef	4.4	129	310	39%	13	4.5
Regular Roast Beef	5.4	157	350	43%	16	6
Super Roast Beef	8.5	245	470	44%	23	7
OTHER SANDWICHES						
Chicken Bacon 'N Swiss	7.4	213	610	48%	33	8
Chicken Breast Fillet	7.2	208	540	49%	30	5
Chicken Cordon Bleu	8.4	242	620	49%	35	8
Grilled Chicken Deluxe	8.7	252	440	44%	22	4
Roast Chicken Club	8.4	278	520	50%	28	7
Hot Ham 'N Swiss	5.9	170	340	35%	13	4.5
SUB SANDWICHES						
French Dip	10	285	440	36%	18	8
Hot Ham 'N Swiss	9.7	278	530	45%	27	8
Italian	11	312	780	60%	53	15
Philly Beef 'N Swiss	10.8	311	700	54%	42	15
Roast Beef	11.6	334	760	56%	48	16
Turkey	10.6	306	630	52%	37	9
MARKET FRESH™ SANDWICHES						
Roast Beef & Swiss	12.5	360	810	47%	42	13
Roast Ham & Swiss	12.5	360	730	42%	34	8
Roast Chicken Caesar	12.7	363	820	41%	38	9
Roast Turkey & Swiss	12.5	360	760	39%	33	6
MARKET FRESH™ SALADS						
Turkey Club Salad (dressing not included)	12	325	350	54%	21	10
Caesar Salad (dressing not included)	8	223	90	38%	4	2.5
Grilled Chicken Caesar (dressing not included)	12	338	230	30%	8	3.5
Chicken Finger Salad (dressing not included)	13	367	570	54%	34	9
Caesar Side Salad	5	137	45	44%	2	1
LIGHT MENU						
Light Grilled Chicken	7.5	174	280	17%	5	1.5
Light Roast Chicken Deluxe	7.2	194	260	17%	5	1
Light Roast Turkey Deluxe	7.2	194	260	17%	5	0.5

CHOLESTEROL (mg)	PROTEIN (g)	CARBOHYDRATE (g)	DIETARY FIBER (g)	SODIUM (mg)	VITAMIN C % RDI	CALCIUM % RDI	IRON % RDI
70	16	36	2	890	0%	8%	15%
70	16	40	2	1530	8%	8%	20%
90	23	43	2	1240	2%	10%	20%
155	47	41	3	2080	0%	8%	40%
110	32	41	3	1440	0%	6%	30%
70	16	34	2	740	0%	6%	15%
85	21	34	2	950	0%	6%	20%
85	22	47	3	1130	2%	8%	20%
110	31	49	2	1550	4%	15%	15%
90	24	47	2	1160	6%	8%	15%
120	34	47	2	1820	6%	15%	15%
110	29	37	2	1050	2%	8%	15%
115	29	38	2	1440	4%	15%	15%
90	23	35	1	1450	2%	15%	15%
100	28	42	2	1680	2%	8%	25%
110	29	45	3	1860	6%	30%	20%
120	29	49	3	2450	4%	30%	15%
130	36	46	4	1940	15%	30%	25%
130	35	47	3	2230	6%	30%	25%
100	26	51	2	2170	4%	20%	2%
130	37	73	5	1780	4%	20%	15%
125	36	74	5	2180	6%	20%	8%
140	43	75	5	2160	15%	4%	8%
130	43	75	5	1920	4%	20%	0%
90	33	9	3	920	70%	35%	10%
10	7	8	3	170	70%	20%	10%
80	33	8	3	920	70%	20%	10%
65	30	39	3	1300	70%	6%	10%
5	4	4	2	95	45%	4%	6%
55	29	30	3	1170	0%	8%	10%
40	23	33	3	1010	4%	10%	15%
40	23	33	3	980	2%	8%	10%

Continued

■ ARBY'S®—cont'd

	SERVING OUNCES	SERVING GRAMS (g)	CALORIES	% CALORIES FROM FAT	TOTAL FAT (g)	SATURATED FAT (g)
SALADS						
Roast Chicken Salad	14.8	420	160	13%	2.5	0
Grilled Chicken Salad	16.3	464	210	19%	4.5	1.5
Garden Salad	12.3	349	70	7%	1	0
Side Salad	5.7	161	25	0%	0	0
SIDE ITEMS						
Cheddar Curly Fries	6	170	460	48%	24	6
Curly Fries—Small	3.8	99	310	45%	15	3.5
Curly Fries—Medium	4.5	128	400	45%	20	5
Curly Fries—Large	7	198	620	44%	30	7
Homestyle Fries—Child-size	3	85	220	39%	10	2.5
Homestyle Fries—Small	4	113	300	40%	13	3.5
Homestyle Fries—Medium	5	142	370	38%	16	4
Homestyle Fries—Large	7.5	213	560	39%	24	6
Potato Cakes (2)	3.5	100	250	56%	16	4
Jalapeno Bites™	4	111	330	57%	21	9
Mozzarella Sticks	4.8	137	470	55%	29	14
Onion Petals	4	113	410	54%	24	3.5
Chicken Finger Snack	6.4	181	580	50%	32	7
Chicken Finger—4-Pack	6.77	192	640	55%	38	8
Baked Potato with Butter and Sour Cream	11.2	320	500	42%	24	15
Broccoli 'N Cheddar Baked Potato	14	384	540	39%	24	12
Deluxe Baked Potato	13	361	650	48%	34	20
DESSERTS						
Apple Turnover (Iced)	4.5	128	420	33%	16	4.5
Cherry Turnover (Iced)	4.5	128	410	34%	16	4.5
BREAKFAST ITEMS						
Biscuit with Butter	2.9	82	280	54%	17	4
Biscuit with Ham	4.3	125	330	55%	20	5
Biscuit with Sausage	4.2	122	460	65%	33	9
Biscuit with Bacon	3.4	96	360	61%	24	7
Croissant with Ham	3.7	105	310	55%	19	11
Croissant with Sausage	3.6	102	440	66%	32	15
Croissant with Bacon	2.7	76	340	62%	23	13
Sourdough with Ham	6.1	173	390	12%	6	1
Sourdough with Sausage	5.9	170	520	33%	19	5
Sourdough with Bacon	5.1	144	420	21%	10	2.5
Add Egg	2	57	110	72%	9	2
Add Slice Swiss Cheese	0.5	14	45	68%	3	2
French Toastix (no syrup)	4.4	124	370	41%	17	4
CONDIMENTS						
Arby's Sauce® Packet	0.5	14	15	0%	0	0
BBQ Dipping Sauce	1	28	40	0%	0	0

CHOLESTEROL (mg)	PROTEIN (g)	CARBOHYDRATE (g)	DIETARY FIBER (g)	SODIUM (mg)	VITAMIN C % RDI	CALCIUM % RDI	IRON % RDI
40	20	15	6	700	70%	8%	10%
65	30	14	6	800	70%	8%	10%
0	4	14	6	45	70%	8%	8%
0	2	5	2	20	15%	2%	4%
5	6	54	4	1290	25%	6%	10%
0	4	39	3	770	20%	0%	8%
0	5	50	4	990	25%	0%	10%
0	8	78	7	1540	35%	0%	15%
0	3	32	3	430	20%	0%	4%
0	3	42	3	570	25%	0%	4%
0	4	53	4	710	35%	0%	6%
0	6	79	6	1070	50%	0%	10%
0	2	26	3	490	10%	0%	4%
40	7	30	2	670	2%	4%	4%
60	18	34	2	1330	2%	40%	4%
0	4	43	2	300	0%	4%	4%
35	19	55	3	1450	15%	0%	15%
70	31	42	0	1590	0%	2%	15%
55	8	65	6	170	50%	10%	20%
50	12	71	7	680	120%	25%	20%
90	20	67	6	750	60%	10%	20%
0	4	65	2	230	5%	1%	10%
0	4	63	1	250	11%	1%	9%
0	5	27	0.5	780	0%	4%	0%
30	12	28	1	830	0%	4%	4%
25	12	28	1	300	0%	0%	4%
10	9	27	1	220	0%	4%	2%
50	13	29	0	1130	N/A	N/A	19%
45	13	29	0	600	0%	0%	4%
30	10	28	1	520	0%	0%	21%
30	19	67	2	1570	0%	8%	10%
25	19	67	2	1040	0%	8%	14%
10	16	66	3	960	0%	8%	12%
175	5	2	0	170	0%	2%	4%
10	3	0	0	220	0%	10%	0%
0	7	48	4	440	0%	7%	10%
0	0	4	0	180	2%	0%	0%
0	0	10	0	350	4%	0%	2%

Continued

■ ARBY'S®—cont'd

	SERVING OUNCES	SERVING GRAMS (g)	CALORIES	% CALORIES FROM FAT	TOTAL FAT (g)	SATURATED FAT (g)
CONDIMENTS—cont'd						
Au Jus Sauce	3	85	5	0%	0.05	.02
BBQ Vinaigrette Dressing	2	57	140	71%	11	1.5
Bleu Cheese Dressing	2	57	300	93%	31	6
Bronco Berry Sauce™	1.5	43	90	0%	0	0
Buttermilk Ranch Dressing	2	57	360	97%	39	6
Buttermilk Ranch Dressing Reduced Calorie	2	57	60	0%	0	0
Caesar Dressing	2	57	310	100%	34	5
Croutons, Cheese and Garlic	0.63	17.7	100	53%	6.25	N/A
Croutons, Seasoned	0.25	7	30	33%	1	0
German Mustard Packet	0.25	5	5	0%	0	0
Honey French Dressing	2	57	290	72%	24	4
Honey Mustard Sauce	1	28	130	85%	12	1.5
Horsey Sauce® Packet	0.5	14	60	75%	5	0.5
Italian Dressing, Reduced Calorie	2	57	25	40%	1	1
Italian Parmesan Dressing	2	57	240	92%	24	4
Ketchup Packet	0.32	9	10	0%	0	0
French Toast Syrup	0.5	43	130	0%	0	0
Mayonnaise Packet	0.44	12	90	100%	10	1.5
Mayonnaise Packet Light, Cholesterol-Free	0.44	12	20	75%	1.5	0
Marinara Sauce	1.5	43	35	33%	1	0
Tangy Southwest Sauce™	1.5	43	250	96%	26	4.5
Thousand Island Dressing	2	57	290	86%	28	4.5
BEVERAGES						
Milk	8	227	120	36%	5	3
Hot Chocolate	8.6	244	110	10%	1	0.5
Orange Juice	10	283	140	0%	0	0
Vanilla Shake	14	397	470	30%	15	7
Chocolate Shake	14	397	480	31%	16	8
Strawberry Shake	14	397	500	24%	13	8
Jamocha Shake	14	397	470	30%	15	7

CALORIE AND SODIUM RANGES FOR POPULAR SOFT DRINKS AND BEVERAGES

BEVERAGE	CALORIE RANGE (KCAL)	SODIUM RANGE
Cola Beverages	185-215	45-65
Non-Cola Carbonated Beverages	185-225	55-95
Diet Sodas	0	55-90
Orange Sodas	260-280	75-80
Black Coffee (8 oz)	0	0
Iced Tea (16 oz)	0	0

Information is based on 20-oz drink with ice (~16 oz actual drink). Additional nutrients are not reported because of insignificant levels.

CHOLESTEROL (mg)	PROTEIN (g)	CARBOHYDRATE (g)	DIETARY FIBER (g)	SODIUM (mg)	VITAMIN C % RDI	CALCIUM % RDI	IRON % RDI
0	0.30	0.89	0.02	386	0%	0%	0%
0	0	9	0	660	0%	0%	2%
45	2	3	0	580	0%	2%	0%
0	0	23	0	35	4%	0%	0%
5	1	2	0	490	0%	2%	0%
0	1	13	1	750	0%	0%	0%
60	1	1	0	470	2%	0%	0%
N/A	2.5	10	0	138	N/A	N/A	N/A
0	1	5	1	70	0%	0%	2%
0	0	0	0	60	0%	0%	0%
0	0	18	<1	410	0%	0%	0%
10	0	5	0	160	0%	0%	0%
5	0	3	0	150	0%	0%	2%
0	0	3	<1	1030	0%	0%	0%
0	1	4	0	950	2%	2%	0%
0	0	2	0	100	0%	0%	0%
0	0	32	0	45	0%	0%	0%
10	0	0	0	65	0%	0%	0%
0	0	1	0	110	0%	0%	0%
0	1	4	0	260	10%	0%	4%
30	0	3	0	290	0%	0%	0%
35	1	9	0	480	0%	0%	0%
20	8	12	0	120	4%	30%	2%
0	2	23	0	120	0%	5%	0%
0	1	34	0	0	130%	0%	0%
45	10	83	0	360	4%	50%	6%
45	10	84	0	370	4%	50%	4%
15	11	87	0	340	2%	35%	2%
45	10	82	0	390	4%	50%	4%

Nutritional information contained in this Arby's, Inc. brochure was obtained from independent laboratory analysis; Genesis Nutrition and Diet Software; supplier information; and the USDA Handbook #8. Information on Arby's products contained herein is based on laboratory and calculated analysis of Arby's ingredients as of July 25, 2001. Actual nutritional information may differ, based on regional variability in product availability and in individual unit compliance with Arby's Standard Operating Procedures. Information is not to be used by individuals with special dietary needs in lieu of professional medical advice.

■ BURGER KING®

	SERVING SIZE (g)	CALORIES	CALORIES FROM FAT	TOTAL FAT (g)	SATURATED FAT	TOTAL TRANS. FAT (g)
BURGERS						
Whopper® Sandwich	304	760	410	46	14	1.2
without Mayo	283	600	250	28	12	1.1
Whopper® with Cheese Sandwich	329	850	480	53	20	1.5
without Mayo	308	690	320	36	17	1.4
Double Whopper® Sandwich	401	1060	620	69	25	2.2
without Mayo	380	900	460	51	22	2.1
Double Whopper® with Cheese Sandwich	426	1150	690	76	30	2.5
without Mayo	405	990	530	59	28	2.4
Whopper Jr.® Sandwich	158	390	200	22	7	0.5
without Mayo	147	310	120	13	5	0.5
Whopper Jr.® with Cheese Sandwich	160	440	230	26	9	0.7
without Mayo	149	360	150	17	8	0.6
BK Homestyle™ Griller	242	480	240	27	11	0
BK Smokehouse Cheddar™ Griller	241	720	440	48	19	0
King Supreme™ Sandwich	196	550	310	34	14	1.2
BK ¼ lb. Burger™	210	490	190	21	8	0.7
Hamburger	121	310	120	13	5	0.5
Cheeseburger	133	360	160	17	8	0.7
Double Hamburger	164	450	210	24	10	0.9
Double Cheeseburger	189	540	280	31	15	1.3
Bacon Double Cheeseburger	193	580	310	34	17	1.3
SANDWICHES						
BK Big Fish® Sandwich	262	710	350	39	15	2.1
Chicken Whopper®	272	580	240	26	5	0.5
without Mayo	251	420	80	9	2.5	0.4
Chicken Whopper Jr.®	165	350	130	14	2.5	0.3
without Mayo	155	270	50	6	1.5	0.2
Specialty Chicken Sandwich	204	560	260	28	6	2.2
without Mayo	190	460	150	17	4.5	2.2
Chicken Tenders®—4 pieces	62	170	90	9	2.5	2
Chicken Tenders®—5 pieces	77	210	110	12	3.5	2.3
Chicken Tenders®—6 pieces	92	250	130	14	4	2.7
Chicken Tenders®—8 pieces	123	340	170	19	5	3.6
BK Veggie™ Burger	173	330	90	10	1.5	0.1
with Reduced Fat Mayo	162	290	60	7	1	0.1
French Fries—Small (salted)	74	230	100	11	3	3
French Fries—Small (no salt)	74	230	100	11	3	3
French Fries—Medium (salted)	117	360	160	18	5	4.7

BURGER KING® trade marks, trade name, and Nutritional Guide are reproduced with permission from Burger King Brands, Inc.

CHOLESTEROL (mg)	SODIUM (mg)	CARBOHYDRATE (g)	DIETARY FIBER (g)	TOTAL SUGARS (g)	PROTEIN (g)	VITAMIN A % DV	VITAMIN C % DV	CALCIUM % DV	IRON % DV
100	1000	52	4	11	35	20	15	15	40
85	870	52	4	11	34	10	15	15	40
120	1430	53	4	11	39	25	15	25	40
110	1310	53	4	11	39	15	15	25	40
185	1100	52	4	11	59	20	15	20	50
175	980	52	4	11	59	10	15	20	50
210	1530	53	4	11	64	25	15	30	50
195	1410	53	4	11	64	15	15	30	50
45	570	32	2	6	17	10	6	8	20
40	510	31	2	6	17	4	6	8	20
55	790	32	2	6	19	10	6	15	20
50	730	32	2	6	19	8	6	15	20
75	760	35	2	5	26	10	10	6	25
125	1240	32	2	3	39	6	6	20	25
100	790	32	2	6	30	4	2	15	25
60	950	50	3	10	26	4	4	10	30
40	580	31	2	6	17	2	2	8	20
50	790	31	2	6	19	6	2	15	20
75	620	31	2	6	28	2	2	10	25
100	1050	32	2	6	32	10	2	25	25
110	1240	32	2	6	35	10	2	25	25
50	1160	66	4	7	24	2	0	8	20
75	1370	48	3	7	39	15	10	8	45
60	1250	47	3	7	38	6	10	8	45
45	900	30	2	4	25	6	6	6	30
40	840	30	2	4	25	2	6	6	30
60	1270	52	3	5	25	8	0	6	15
55	1190	52	3	5	25	2	0	6	15
25	420	10	0	0	11	0	0	0	2
30	530	13	<1	0	14	0	0	2	2
35	630	15	<1	0	16	2	0	2	4
50	840	20	<1	0	22	2	0	2	4
0	770	45	4	6	14	8	10	6	35
0	690	44	4	6	14	8	10	6	35
0	410	29	2	0	3	0	8	2	2
0	240	29	2	0	3	0	8	2	2
0	640	46	4	1	4	0	15	2	4

Continued

■ **BURGER KING®—cont'd**

	SERVING SIZE (g)	CALORIES	CALORIES FROM FAT	TOTAL FAT (g)	SATURATED FAT	TOTAL TRANS. FAT (g)
SANDWICHES—cont'd						
French Fries—Medium (no salt)	116	360	160	18	5	4.7
French Fries—Large (salted)	160	500	220	25	7	6.4
French Fries—Large (no salt)	159	500	220	25	7	6.4
French Fries—King Size (salted)	194	600	270	30	8	7.8
French Fries—King Size (no salt)	193	600	270	30	8	7.8
Onion Rings—Small	51	180	80	9	2	2
Onion Rings—Medium	91	320	140	16	4	3.6
Onion Rings—Large	137	480	210	23	6	5.4
Onion Rings—King Size	159	550	240	27	7	6
SALADS						
Chicken Caesar (without dressing and croutons)	257	160	50	6	3	0
Garden Salad (without dressing)	142	25	0	0	0	0
DESSERTS						
Dutch Apple Pie	113	340	130	14	3	3
Hershey®'s Sundae Pie	79	310	160	18	13	2
Hot fudge brownie royale	113	440	170	19	6	2.1
Fresh baked cookies	96	440	190	21	7	N/A
BREAKFAST						
Croissan'wich® with Sausage, Egg & Cheese	157	520	350	39	14	2.5
Croissan'wich® with Sausage & Cheese	107	420	280	31	11	2.4
Croissan'wich® with Egg & Cheese	112	320	170	19	7	2
Egg'wich™ with Canadian Bacon, Egg, & Cheese	155	420	210	23	7	0.6
Egg'wich™ with Canadian Bacon & Egg	142	380	170	19	4	0.4
Egg'wich™ with Egg and Cheese	140	410	210	23	7	0.6
French Toast Sticks—5 Sticks	112	390	180	20	4.5	4.5
Cini-minis—4 rolls (without Vanilla Icing)	108	440	210	23	6	N/A
Hash Brown Rounds—Small	75	230	130	15	4	4.9
Hash Brown Rounds—Large	128	390	230	25	7	8.4
DRINKS						
Vanilla Shake—Small	305	560	290	32	21	1.5
Vanilla Shake—Medium	397	720	370	41	27	2.0
Chocolate Shake—Small (Syrup added)	333	620	290	32	21	1.5
Chocolate Shake—Medium (Syrup added)	425	790	380	42	27	2.0
Strawberry Shake—Small (Syrup added)	333	620	290	32	21	1.5
Strawberry Shake—Medium (Syrup added)	425	780	370	41	27	2.0

CHOLESTEROL (mg)	SODIUM (mg)	CARBOHYDRATE (g)	DIETARY FIBER (g)	TOTAL SUGARS (g)	PROTEIN (g)	VITAMIN A % DV	VITAMIN C % DV	CALCIUM % DV	IRON % DV
0	380	46	4	1	4	0	15	2	4
0	880	63	5	1	6	0	20	2	6
0	510	63	5	1	6	0	20	2	6
0	1070	76	6	1	7	0	20	2	6
0	620	76	6	1	7	0	20	2	6
0	260	22	2	3	2	0	0	6	0
0	460	40	3	5	4	0	0	10	0
0	690	60	5	7	7	0	0	15	0
5	800	70	5	8	8	0	0	20	0
40	730	5	3	3	25	15	10	10	20
0	15	5	2	3	1	50	25	2	4
1	470	52	1	23	2	2	0	0	8
10	135	33	<1	20	3	0	0	4	8
50	250	62	6	46	6	8	0	4	50
15	390	57	2	32	4	8	0	2	10
210	1090	24	1	4	19	10	0	30	25
45	840	23	<1	4	14	4	0	10	20
185	730	24	<1	3	12	8	0	30	20
140	900	36	3	3	18	8	0	25	20
125	680	35	3	3	15	4	0	15	20
130	760	36	3	3	15	8	0	25	20
0	440	46	2	11	6	0	0	6	10
25	710	51	1	20	6	20	2	6	15
0	450	23	2	0	2	0	2	0	2
0	760	38	4	0	3	0	2	2	4
95	220	56	1	46	11	25	0	30	2
125	280	73	1	60	15	30	0	40	2
95	310	72	2	61	12	25	0	35	6
125	380	89	2	75	15	30	0	45	6
95	230	71	1	61	11	25	0	35	2
125	300	88	1	75	15	30	0	45	2

Continued

■ BURGER KING®—cont'd

	SERVING SIZE (g)	CALORIES	CALORIES FROM FAT	TOTAL FAT (g)	SATURATED FAT	TOTAL TRANS FAT (g)
DRINKS—cont'd						
Coca Cola® Classic—Kids	282	120	0	0	0	0
Coca Cola® Classic—Small	376	160	0	0	0	0
Coca Cola® Classic—Medium	518	230	0	0	0	0
Coca Cola® Classic—Large	753	330	0	0	0	0
Coca Cola® Classic—King	988	430	0	0	0	0
Diet Coke®—Kids	282	0	0	0	0	0
Diet Coke®—Small	376	0	0	0	0	0
Diet Coke®—Medium	518	0	0	0	0	0
Diet Coke®—Large	753	0	0	0	0	0
Diet Coke®—King	988	0	0	0	0	0
Sprite®—Kids	282	120	0	0	0	0
Sprite®—Small	376	160	0	0	0	0
Sprite®—Medium	518	220	0	0	0	0
Sprite®—Large	753	320	0	0	0	0
Sprite®—King	988	420	0	0	0	0
Dr. Pepper®—Kids	282	120	0	0	0	0
Dr. Pepper®—Small	376	160	0	0	0	0
Dr. Pepper®—Medium	518	220	0	0	0	0
Dr. Pepper®—Large	753	320	0	0	0	0
Dr. Pepper®—King	988	410	0	0	0	0
Frozen Coca Cola® Classic—Medium	439	370	0	0	0	0
Frozen Coca Cola® Classic—Large	539	460	0	0	0	0
Frozen Minute Maid® Cherry—Medium	439	370	0	0	0	0
Frozen Minute Maid® Cherry—Large	539	460	0	0	0	0
Minute Maid® Pure Orange Juice	284	140	0	0	0	0
Coffee—Small	244	0	0	0	0	0
Coffee—Medium	366	5	0	0	0	0
Coffee—Large	488	10	0	0	0	0
Reduced Fat Milk—1% Milk Fat	244	110	25	2.5	1.5	N/A

CHOLESTEROL (mg)	SODIUM (mg)	CARBOHYDRATE (g)	DIETARY FIBER (g)	TOTAL SUGARS (g)	PROTEIN (g)	VITAMIN A % DV	VITAMIN C % DV	CALCIUM % DV	IRON % DV
0	N/A	31	0	31	0	0	0	0	0
0	N/A	41	0	41	0	0	0	0	0
0	N/A	56	0	56	0	0	0	0	0
0	N/A	82	0	82	0	0	0	0	0
0	N/A	108	0	108	0	0	0	0	0
0	N/A	0	0	0	0	0	0	0	0
0	N/A	0	0	0	0	0	0	0	0
0	N/A	0	0	0	0	0	0	0	0
0	N/A	0	0	0	0	0	0	0	0
0	N/A	30	0	30	0	0	0	0	0
0	N/A	40	0	40	0	0	0	0	0
0	N/A	55	0	55	0	0	0	0	0
0	N/A	80	0	80	0	0	0	0	0
0	N/A	105	0	105	0	0	0	0	0
0	N/A	30	0	30	0	0	0	0	0
0	N/A	39	0	39	0	0	0	0	0
0	N/A	54	0	54	0	0	0	0	0
0	N/A	79	0	79	0	0	0	0	0
0	N/A	104	0	104	0	0	0	0	0
0	N/A	92	0	92	0	0	0	0	0
0	N/A	116	0	116	0	0	0	0	0
0	N/A	92	0	92	0	0	0	0	0
0	N/A	116	0	116	0	0	0	0	0
0	25	33	0	30	0	0	70	2	0
0	0	<1	0	0	0	0	0	0	0
0	5	<1	0	0	0	0	0	0	0
0	10	2	0	0	0	0	0	0	0
10	125	12	0	11	8	10	4	30	0

■ KFC

	SERVING SIZE (g)	SERVING SIZE (oz)	CALORIES	FAT CALORIES	TOTAL FAT (g)	TOTAL FAT % DV	SATU-RATED FAT (g)	SATU-RATED FAT % DV	CHOLES-TEROL (mg)
CHICKEN									
Original Recipe Chicken— Whole Wing	47	1.6	140	90	10	15%	2.5	12%	55
Original Recipe Chicken— Breast	153	5.4	400	220	24	38%	6	31%	135
Original Recipe Chicken— Drumstick	61	2.2	140	80	9	13%	2	10%	75
Original Recipe Chicken— Thigh	91	3.2	250	160	18	28%	4.5	23%	95
Extra Crispy Chicken— Whole Wing	55	1.9	220	140	15	23%	4	16%	55
Extra Crispy Chicken— Breast	168	5.9	470	240	28	42%	8	40%	160
Extra Crispy Chicken— Drumstick	67	2.4	195	110	12	19%	3	14%	77
Extra Crispy Chicken— Thigh	118	4.2	380	250	27	41%	7	35%	118
Hot & Spicy Chicken— Whole Wing	55	1.9	210	130	25	23%	4	18%	55
Hot & Spicy Chicken— Breast	180	6.5	505	270	29	44%	8	42%	162
Hot & Spicy Chicken— Drumstick	64	2.3	175	90	10	17%	3	14%	77
Hot & Spicy Chicken— Thigh	107	3.8	355	225	26	40%	7	33%	126
SANDWICHES									
Original Recipe Sandwich with sauce	200	7.3	450	200	22	34%	5	25%	70
Original Recipe Sandwich without sauce	187	6.6	360	120	13	20%	3.5	18%	60
Triple Crunch Sandwich with sauce	189	6.6	490	260	29	45%	6	30%	70
Triple Crunch Sandwich without sauce	176	6.5	390	140	15	23%	4.5	23%	50
Triple Crunch Zinger Sandwich with sauce	210	7.4	550	290	32	49%	7	35%	85
Triple Crunch Zinger Sandwich without sauce	176	6.2	390	140	15	23%	4.5	23%	50
Tender Roast Sandwich with sauce	211	7.4	350	130	15	23%	3	15%	75
Tender Roast Sandwich without sauce	177	6.2	270	45	5	8%	1.5	8%	65

CHOLES-TEROL % DV	SODIUM (mg)	SODIUM % DV	TOTAL CARBOHY-DRATES (g)	TOTAL CARBOHY-DRATES % DV	DIETARY FIBER (g)	DIETARY FIBER % DV	SUGARS (g)	PROTEIN (g)	% DAILY VALUE			
									VITA-MIN A	VITA-MIN C	CALCIUM	IRON
18%	414	17%	5	2%	0	0%	0	9	**	**	**	2%
45%	1116	47%	16	5%	1	4%	0	29	**	**	4%	6%
25%	422	18%	4	1%	0	0%	0	13	**	**	**	4%
32%	747	31%	6	2%	1	0%	0	16	**	**	2%	4%
18%	415	17%	10	3%	<1	0%	0	10	**	**	**	2%
54%	874	37%	17	6%	<1	0%	0	39	**	**	2%	6%
25%	375	15%	7	2%	<1	0%	0	15	**	**	**	4%
39%	625	26%	14	5%	<1	0%	0	21	**	**	2%	6%
17%	350	14%	9	3%	<1	0%	0	10	**	**	2%	4%
53%	1170	48%	23	8%	1	9%	9	38	**	**	6%	6%
26%	360	14%	9	3%	<1	0%	0	13	**	**	**	4%
41%	630	27%	13	4%	1	5%	0	19	**	**	2%	4%
23%	940	39%	33	17%	2	8%	0	29	2%	**	4%	10%
20%	890	37%	21	11%	<1	0%	<1	29	2%	**	4%	10%
23%	710	30%	39	13%	2	8%	0	28	2%	**	4%	10%
17%	650	27%	29	10%	2	8%	0	25	**	**	4%	15%
28%	830	35%	39	13%	2	8%	3	28	6%	**	4%	10%
17%	650	27%	36	12%	2	8%	0	25	**	**	4%	10%
25%	880	37%	26	9%	1	4%	1	32	4%	**	4%	10%
22%	690	29%	23	8%	1	4%	<1	31	**	**	4%	10%

Continued

■ KFC—cont'd

	SERVING SIZE (g)	SERVING SIZE (oz)	CALORIES	FAT CALORIES	TOTAL FAT (g)	TOTAL FAT % DV	SATU- RATED FAT (g)	SATU- RATED FAT % DV	CHOLES- TEROL (mg)
SANDWICHES—cont'd									
Honey BBQ Flavored Sandwich	178	5.3	310	50	6	9%	2	10%	125
Twister	240	8.5	600	300	34	52%	7	35%	50
Crispy Caesar Twister	270	8.5	744	357	41	64%	9	47%	55
Honey BBQ Crunch Melt	231	8.1	556	235	26	40%	5	25%	60
CRISPY STRIPS									
Colonels Crispy Strips (3)	115	4.1	300	125	16	24%	4	21%	56
Spicy Crispy Strips (3)	115	4.1	335	140	15	22%	4	22%	70
Honey BBQ Strips (3)	178	5.3	377	139	15	23%	4	22%	45
POPCORN CHICKEN									
Popcorn Chicken—Small	99	3.5	362	207	23	35%	6	30%	43
Popcorn Chicken—Large	170	6.0	620	356	40	32%	10	50%	73
POT PIE									
Chunky Chicken Pot Pie (after baking)	368	13.0	770	378	42	65%	13	65%	70
WINGS									
Hot Wings Pieces (6)	135	4.8	471	297	33	51%	8	40%	150
Honey BBQ Pieces (6)	189	6.7	607	343	38	59%	10	50%	193
VEGETABLES									
Mashed Potatoes with Gravy	136	4.8	120	50	6	9%	1	5%	<1
Potato Wedges	135	4.8	280	120	13	20%	4	20%	5
Macaroni and Cheese	153	5.4	180	70	8	12%	3	15%	10
Corn on the Cob	162	5.7	150	15	1.5	3%	0	0%	0
BBQ Baked Beans	156	5.5	190	25	3	5%	1	5%	5
Cole Slaw	142	5.0	232	121	13.5	21%	2	11%	8
Potato Salad	160	5.6	230	130	14	22%	2	10%	15
Green Beans	132	4.7	45	15	1.5	2%	0.5	2%	5
Mean Greens	152	5.4	70	30	3	5%	1	5%	10
BREADS									
Biscuit (1)	56	2.0	180	80	10	14%	2.5	12%	0
DESSERTS									
Double Choc. Chip Cake	76	2.7	320	140	16	25%	4	20%	55
Little Bucket Parfait— Fudge Brownie	99	3.5	280	90	10	15%	3.5	18%	145

CHOLES-TEROL % DV	SODIUM (mg)	SODIUM % DV	TOTAL CARBOHY-DRATES (g)	TOTAL CARBOHY-DRATES % DV	DIETARY FIBER (g)	DIETARY FIBER % DV	SUGARS (g)	PROTEIN (g)	% DAILY VALUE			
									VITA-MIN A	VITA-MIN C	CALCIUM	IRON
42%	560	23%	37	12%	2	8%	7	28	6%	**	6%	10%
17%	1430	60%	52	17%	4	16%	4	22	2%	*	10%	10%
19%	1616	69%	66	22%	5	19%	4	27	8%	–	17%	14%
20%	1010	40%	48	16%	2	8%	7	33	**	**	4%	10%
20%	1165	48%	18	6%	1	0%	1	26	2%	**	**	6%
22%	1140	47%	23	8%	<1	0%	<1	25	2%	**	2%	5%
15%	1709	71%	33	11%	4	16%	12	27	2%	**	4%	2%
15%	610	25%	21	7%	0.2	0%	0	17	0%	0%	0%	2%
25%	1046	44%	36	12%	0	0%	0	30	0%	0%	2%	4%
23%	2160	90%	69	23%	5	20%	8	29	80%	2%	10%	10%
50%	1230	51%	18	6%	2	8%	0	27	**	**	4%	8%
63%	1145	47%	33	11%	1	4%	18	33	8%	8%	4%	8%
0%	440	18%	17	6%	2	8%	0	1	**	**	**	2%
2%	750	31%	28	9%	5	20%	1	5	**	2%	2%	10%
3%	860	30%	21	7%	2	8%	2	7	20%	**	15%	**
0%	20	1%	35	12%	2	7%	8	5	2%	6%	**	**
2%	760	32%	33	11%	6	24%	13	6	8%	**	8%	10%
3%	284	12%	26	9%	3	12%	20	2	9%	57%	3%	**
5%	540	22%	23	8%	3	12%	9	4	10%	**	2%	15%
2%	730	30%	7	2%	3	12%	3	1	4%	4%	4%	4%
3%	650	27%	11	4%	5	20%	1	4	60%	10%	20%	10%
0%	560	23%	20	7%	<1	0%	2	4	**	**	2%	6%
18%	230	10%	41	14%	1	4%	28	4	0%	0%	4%	10%
48%	190	8%	44	15%	1	4%	35	3	2%	0%	2%	6%

Continued

■ KFC—cont'd

	SERVING SIZE (g)	SERVING SIZE (oz)	CALORIES	FAT CALORIES	TOTAL FAT (g)	TOTAL FAT % DV	SATU-RATED FAT (g)	SATU-RATED FAT % DV	CHOLES-TEROL (mg)
DESSERTS—cont'd									
Little Bucket Parfait—Lemon Creme	127	4.5	410	130	14	22%	8	40%	20
Little Bucket Parfait—Chocolate Cream	113	4.0	290	130	15	23%	11	55%	15
Little Bucket Parfait—Strawberry Shortcake	99	3.5	200	60	7	11%	6	30%	10
Colonel's Pies—Pecan Pie Slice	113	4.0	490	200	23	35%	5	25%	65
Colonel's Pies—Apple Pie Slice	113	4.0	310	130	14	22%	3	15%	0
Colonel's Pies—Strawberry Creme Pie Slice	78	2.7	280	130	15	23%	8	40%	15

CHOLES-TEROL % DV	SODIUM (mg)	SODIUM % DV	TOTAL CARBOHY-DRATES (g)	TOTAL CARBOHY-DRATES % DV	DIETARY FIBER (g)	DIETARY FIBER % DV	SUGARS (g)	PROTEIN (g)	% DAILY VALUE			
									VITA-MIN A	VITA-MIN C	CALCIUM	IRON
7%	290	12%	62	21%	4	16%	50	7	2%	4%	20%	4%
5%	330	14%	37	12%	2	8%	25	3	**	0%	4%	6%
3%	220	9%	33	11%	1	4%	26	1	**	8%	2%	4%
22%	510	21%	66	22%	2	8%	31	5	4%	0%	2%	8%
0%	280	12%	44	15%	0	0%	23	2	0%	0%	0%	6%
5%	130	5%	32	11%	2	8%	22	4	2%	4%	0%	4%

■ WENDY'S

	SERVING SIZE	WEIGHT (g)	CALORIES	CALORIES FROM FAT	TOTAL FAT (g)	SATURATED (g)
SANDWICHES						
Classic Single® with Everything	1 ea	218	410	170	19	7
Big Bacon Classic®	1 ea	282	580	270	30	12
Jr. Hamburger	1 ea	117	270	80	9	3
Jr. Cheeseburger	1 ea	129	310	110	12	6
Jr. Bacon Cheeseburger	1 ea	165	380	170	19	7
Jr. Cheeseburger Deluxe	1 ea	179	350	140	16	6
Hamburger, Kids' Meal	1 ea	110	270	80	9	3
Cheeseburger, Kids' Meal	1 ea	122	310	110	12	6
Grilled Chicken Sandwich	1 ea	188	300	60	7	1.5
Chicken Breast Fillet Sandwich	1 ea	207	430	150	16	3
Chicken Club Sandwich	1 ea	215	470	180	20	4.5
Spicy Chicken® Sandwich	1 ea	212	410	120	14	2.5
SANDWICH COMPONENTS						
¼ lb Hamburger Patty	¼ lb	74	200	120	14	6
2 oz Hamburger Patty	2 oz	37	100	60	7	3
Grilled Chicken Fillet	1 pc	82	110	30	3.5	1
Breaded Chicken Fillet	1 pc	99	230	100	11	2
Spicy Chicken® Fillet	1 pc	104	210	80	9	1.5
Kaiser Bun	1 ea	71	200	20	2.5	0.5
Sandwich Bun	1 ea	58	160	15	2	0
American Cheese	1 sl	18	70	50	6	3.5
American Cheese Jr.	1 sl	12	45	35	3.5	2.5
Bacon	1 pc	4	20	15	1.5	0.5
Honey Mustard Reduced Calorie	1 tsp	7	25	15	1.5	0
Ketchup	1 tsp	7	10	0	0	0
Lettuce	1 lea	15	0	0	0	0
Mayonnaise	1 ½ tsp	9	30	30	3	0
Mustard	½ tsp	5	5	0	0	0
Onion	4 rings	13	5	0	0	0
Pickles	4 sl	11	0	0	0	0
Tomatoes	1 sl	26	5	0	0	0
FRENCH FRIES						
Kids' Meal	3.2 oz	91	270	120	13	2
Medium	5.0 oz	142	420	180	20	3
Biggie®	5.6 oz	159	470	200	23	3.5
Great Biggie®	6.7 oz	190	570	240	27	4

CHOLESTEROL (mg)	SODIUM (mg)	TOTAL CARBO-HYDRATES (g)	DIETARY FIBER (g)	SUGARS (g)	PROTEIN (g)	% RECOMMENDED DAILY INTAKE			
						VITAMIN A	VITAMIN C	CALCIUM	IRON
70	920	37	2	8	25	6	15	10	25
100	1460	46	3	10	34	15	25	25	30
30	620	34	2	6	14	2	6	10	20
45	800	34	2	6	17	4	6	15	20
55	870	34	2	5	20	8	15	15	20
50	860	36	2	7	18	10	15	15	20
30	620	33	1	6	14	2	6	10	20
45	800	33	2	6	17	4	6	15	20
55	740	36	2	8	24	4	15	8	15
55	750	46	2	6	27	4	20	10	15
65	940	47	2	6	30	4	20	10	15
65	1280	43	2	5	28	4	15	10	15
65	290	0	0	0	19	0	0	2	13
30	150	0	0	0	9	0	0	1	7
55	400	1	0	0	19	0	2	0	4
50	390	13	0	0	22	0	8	0	2
60	920	10	0	0	22	0	2	1	3
0	340	38	1	6	6	0	4	8	10
0	300	31	1	4	5	0	4	8	10
15	260	0	0	0	4	4	0	10	0
10	170	0	0	0	3	4	0	8	0
5	90	0	0	0	1	0	0	0	0
0	40	2	0	2	0	0	0	0	0
0	80	2	0	1	0	2	0	0	0
0	0	0	0	0	0	0	0	0	0
5	60	1	0	0	0	0	0	0	0
0	50	0	0	0	0	0	0	0	0
0	0	1	0	1	0	0	2	0	0
0	140	0	0	0	0	0	0	0	0
0	0	1	0	1	0	4	8	0	0
0	85	35	3	0	4	0	8	1	4
0	130	55	5	0	6	0	10	2	6
0	150	61	6	0	7	0	15	3	7
0	180	73	7	1	8	0	15	3	8

Continued

■ WENDY'S—cont'd

	SERVING SIZE	WEIGHT (g)	CALORIES	CALORIES FROM FAT	TOTAL FAT (g)	SATURATED (g)
HOT STUFFED BAKED POTATOES™						
Plain	10 oz	284	310	0	0	0
Bacon & Cheese	1 ea	380	530	160	17	4
Broccoli and Cheese	1 ea	411	470	130	14	3
Sour Cream & Chive	1 ea	312	370	50	5	4
Whipped Margarine	1 pkt	14	70	60	7	1.5
CHILI						
Small	8 oz	227	210	60	7	2.5
Large	12 oz	340	310	90	10	3.5
Cheddar Cheese, shredded	2 tbsp	17	70	50	6	3.5
Saltine Crackers	2 ea	6	25	5	0.5	0
CRISPY CHICKEN NUGGETS™						
5 Piece	5	75	230	140	16	3
4 Piece Kids' Meal	4	60	190	120	13	2.5
Barbecue Sauce	1 pkt	28	45	0	0	0
Honey Mustard Sauce	1 pkt	28	130	100	12	2
Sweet and Sour Sauce	1 pkt	28	50	0	0	0

						NUTRITION FACTS
	SERVING SIZE	WEIGHT (g)	CALORIES	CALORIES FROM FAT	TOTAL FAT (g)	SATURATED (g)	CHOLESTEROL (mg)
SALADS							
Caesar Side Salad (Romaine, Parmesan Cheese, Bacon Pieces)	1 ea	99	70	40	4	2	15
Homestyle Garlic Croutons	1 pkt	14	70	25	2.5	0	0
Caesar Dressing	1 pkt	28	150	150	16	2.5	20
Side Salad (Iceberg, Romaine, Cucumbers, Grape Tomatoes, Red Onions, Carrots)	1 ea	167	35	0	0	0	0
Chicken BLT Salad (Iceberg, Romaine, Spring Salad Mix, Cucumbers, Grape Tomatoes, Cheddar Cheese, Bacon Pieces, Diced Chicken)	1 ea	376	310	150	16	8	60
Homestyle Garlic Croutons	1 pkt	14	70	25	2.5	0	0
Honey Mustard Dressing	1 pkt	71	310	260	29	4.5	25

CHOLESTEROL (mg)	SODIUM (mg)	TOTAL CARBO-HYDRATES (g)	DIETARY FIBER (g)	SUGARS (g)	PROTEIN (g)	% RECOMMENDED DAILY INTAKE			
						VITAMIN A	VITAMIN C	CALCIUM	IRON
0	25	72	6	5	7	0	60	2	20
25	820	78	7	5	16	10	60	10	25
5	470	80	9	6	9	35	120	15	25
15	75	72	7	5	7	4	60	6	20
0	115	0	0	0	0	10	0	0	0
30	800	21	5	5	15	8	6	8	16
45	1190	32	7	8	23	10	10	12	24
15	110	1	0	0	4	4	0	10	0
0	80	4	0	0	1	0	0	0	2
30	470	11	0	0	11	0	2	2	2
25	380	9	0	0	9	0	2	2	2
0	160	10	0	7	1	0	0	0	4
10	220	6	0	5	0	0	0	0	0
0	120	12	0	10	0	0	2	0	0

SODIUM (mg)	POTASSIUM (mg)	TOTAL CARBO-HYDRATES (g)	DIETARY FIBER (g)	SUGARS (g)	PROTEIN (g)	% DAILY VALUE			
						VITAMIN A	VITAMIN C	CALCIUM	IRON
250	280	2	1	1	7	45	35	15	6
120	15	9	0	0	1	0	0	0	2
240	5	1	0	0	1	0	0	0	0
20	350	7	3	4	2	140	30	4	4
1100	610	10	4	4	33	50	50	30	10
120	15	9	0	0	1	0	0	0	2
410	10	12	0	11	1	0	0	0	0

Continued

■ WENDY'S—cont'd

	SERVING SIZE	WEIGHT (g)	CALORIES	CALORIES FROM FAT	TOTAL FAT (g)	SATURATED (g)	CHOLESTEROL (mg)
							NUTRITION FACTS
SALADS—cont'd							
Mandarin Chicken™ Salad (Iceberg, Romaine, Spring Salad Mix, Mandarin Oranges, Diced Chicken)	1 ea	348	150	15	1.5	0	10
Roasted Almonds	1 pkt	21	130	110	12	1	0
Crispy Rice Noodles	1 pkt	14	60	20	2	0.5	0
Oriental Sesame Dressing	1 pkt	71	280	190	21	3	0
Spring Mix Salad (Iceberg, Romaine, Spring Salad Mix, Cucumbers, Grape Tomatoes, Red Onions, Carrots, Cheddar Cheese)	1 ea	315	180	100	11	6	30
Honey Roasted Pecans	1 pkt	20	130	110	13	1	0
House Vinaigrette Dressing	1 pkt	71	220	180	20	3	0
Taco Supremo Salad (Iceberg, Romaine, Tomatoes, Red Onions, Cheddar Cheese, Wendy's Chili)	1 ea	495	360	150	17	9	65
Taco Chips	1 pkt	43	220	100	11	2	0
Sour Cream	1 pkt	28	60	50	6	3.5	15
Salsa	1 ea	85	30	0	0	0	0
ADDITIONAL SALAD DRESSINGS							
Blue Cheese	1 pkt	71	290	270	30	6	45
Creamy Ranch	1 pkt	71	250	230	25	4.5	15
Fat Free French Style	1 pkt	71	90	0	0	0	0
Low Fat Honey Mustard	1 pkt	71	120	30	3.5	0	0
Reduced Fat Creamy Ranch	1 pkt	71	110	80	9	1.5	15

	SERVING SIZE	WEIGHT (g)	CALORIES	CALORIES FROM FAT	TOTAL FAT (g)	SATURATED (g)
FROSTY™						
Junior, 6 oz cup	1 ea	113	170	40	4	2.5
Small, 12 oz cup	1 ea	227	330	80	8	5
Medium, 16 oz cup	1 ea	298	440	100	11	7

Soft drink serving size reflects the amount of liquid in a medium (20 oz) beverage cup. To determine nutritional information for a Kids' size (12 oz) soft drink, multiply by 0.6; Small (16 oz) soft drink, multiply by 0.8; Biggie® (32 oz) soft drink, multiply by 1.6.

SODIUM (mg)	POTASSIUM (mg)	TOTAL CARBO-HYDRATES (g)	DIETARY FIBER (g)	SUGARS (g)	PROTEIN (g)	% DAILY VALUE			
						VITAMIN A	VITAMIN C	CALCIUM	IRON
650	420	17	3	11	20	35	50	6	10
70	150	4	2	1	4	0	0	6	4
180	15	10	0	1	1	0	0	0	2
620	40	21	0	19	2	0	2	2	4
230	620	12	5	5	11	170	50	30	10
65	65	5	2	3	2	0	0	2	2
830	5	9	0	8	0	0	2	0	0
1090	950	29	8	8	27	50	45	35	20
150	95	25	2	0	3	0	0	6	4
15	40	1	0	0	1	4	0	4	0
440	15	6	0	4	1	8	10	6	2
870	25	3	0	1	2	2	0	6	6
640	70	5	0	3	1	0	0	6	0
240	10	21	1	18	0	0	0	0	4
370	15	23	0	18	0	0	0	0	0
610	80	7	1	3	1	0	0	6	0

CHOLESTEROL (mg)	SODIUM (mg)	TOTAL CARBO-HYDRATES (g)	DIETARY FIBER (g)	SUGARS (g)	PROTEIN (g)	% RECOMMENDED DAILY INTAKE			
						VITAMIN A	VITAMIN C	CALCIUM	IRON
20	100	26	0	21	4	8	0	16	3
35	200	56	0	43	8	15	0	31	6
50	260	73	0	56	11	20	0	41	8

Continued

■ WENDY'S—cont'd

	SERVING SIZE	WEIGHT (g)	CALORIES	CALORIES FROM FAT	TOTAL FAT (g)	SATURATED (g)
BEVERAGES						
Cola Soft Drink	11 oz	312	130	0	0	0
Diet Cola Soft Drink	11 oz	312	0	0	0	0
Lemon-Lime Soft Drink	11 oz	312	130	0	0	0

Soft drink serving size reflects the amount of liquid in a medium (20 oz) beverage cup. To determine nutritional information for a Kids' size (12 oz) soft drink, multiply by 0.6; Small (16 oz) soft drink, multiply by 0.8; Biggie (32 oz) soft drink, multiply by 1.6.

CHOLESTEROL (mg)	SODIUM (mg)	TOTAL CARBO-HYDRATES (g)	DIETARY FIBER (g)	SUGARS (g)	PROTEIN (g)	% RECOMMENDED DAILY INTAKE			
						VITAMIN A	VITAMIN C	CALCIUM	IRON
0	10	36	0	36	0	0	0	0	0
0	15	0	0	0	0	0	0	0	0
0	30	34	0	34	0	0	0	0	0

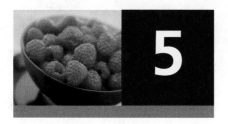

5 Nutritive Values of Various Foods

FOODS, APPROXIMATE MEASURES, UNITS, AND WEIGHT (WEIGHT OF EDIBLE PORTION ONLY)		GRAMS	WATER (g)	FOOD ENERGY (CALORIES)	PROTEIN (g)	FAT (g)	FATTY ACIDS	
							SATURATED (g)	MONO- UNSATURATED (g)

BEVERAGES

Alcoholic

  Beer

Regular	12 fl oz	360	92	150	1	0	0.0	0.0
Light	12 fl oz	355	95	95	1	0	0.0	0.0
Gin, rum, vodka, whiskey 80-proof	1½ fl oz	42	67	95	0	0	0.0	0.0
Table wine								
Red	3½ fl oz	102	88	75	tr	0	0.0	0.0
White	3½ fl oz	102	87	80	tr	0	0.0	0.0
Carbonated[2]								
Club soda	12 fl oz	355	100	0	0	0	0.0	0.0
Cola type								
Regular	12 fl oz	369	89	160	0	0	0.0	0.0
Diet, artificially sweetened	12 fl oz	355	100	tr	0	0	0.0	0.0
Ginger ale	12 fl oz	366	91	125	0	0	0.0	0.0
Coffee								
Brewed	6 fl oz	180	100	tr	tr	tr	tr	tr
Instant, prepared (2 tsp powder plus 6 fl oz water)	6 fl oz	182	99	tr	tr	tr	tr	tr
Fruit drinks, noncarbonated								
Canned								
Fruit punch drink	6 fl oz	190	88	85	tr	0	0.0	0.0
Tea								
Brewed	8 fl oz	240	100	tr	tr	tr	tr	tr
Instant, powder, prepared:								
Unsweetened (1 tsp powder plus 8 fl oz water)	8 fl oz	241	100	tr	tr	tr	tr	tr
Sweetened (3 tsp powder plus 8 fl oz water)	8 fl oz	262	91	85	tr	tr	tr	tr

DAIRY PRODUCTS

Butter. See Fats and Oils

Cheese

  Natural

Blue	1 oz	28	42	100	6	8	5.3	2.2
Camembert (3 wedges per 4-oz container)	1 wedge	38	52	115	8	9	5.8	2.7
Cheddar								
Cut pieces	1 oz	28	37	115	7	9	6.0	2.7
	1 cu in	17	37	70	4	6	3.6	1.6
Shredded	1 c	113	37	455	28	37	23.8	10.6

From Nutritive Value of Foods, U.S. Department of Agriculture, Home and Garden Bulletin No. 72.
tr = nutrient present in trace amounts.
[1]Value not determined.
[2]Mineral content varies depending on water source.
[3]Blend of aspartame and saccharin; if only sodium saccharin is used, sodium is 75 mg; if only aspartame is used, sodium is 23 mg.
[4]With added ascorbic acid.

POLY-UNSATURATED (g)	CHOLES-TEROL (mg)	CARBO-HYDRATE (g)	CALCIUM (mg)	PHOS-PHORUS (mg)	IRON (mg)	POTASSIUM (mg)	SODIUM (mg)	VITAMIN A VALUES		THIAMIN (mg)	RIBO-FLAVIN (mg)	NIACIN (mg)	ASCORBIC ACID (mg)
								IU	RE				
0.0	0	13	14	50	0.1	115	18	0	0	0.02	0.09	1.8	0
0.0	0	5	14	43	0.1	64	11	0	0	0.03	0.11	1.4	0
0.0	0	tr	tr	tr	tr	1	tr	0	0	tr	tr	tr	0
0.0	0	3	8	18	0.4	113	5	(1)	(1)	0.00	0.03	0.1	0
0.0	0	3	9	14	0.3	83	5	(1)	(1)	0.00	0.01	0.1	0
0.0	0	0	18	0	tr	0	78	0	0	0.00	0.00	0.0	0
0.0	0	41	11	52	0.2	7	18	0	0	0.00	0.00	0.0	0
0.0	0	tr	14	39	0.2	7	32[3]	0	0	0.00	0.00	0.0	0
0.0	0	32	11	0	0.1	4	29	0	0	0.00	0.00	0.0	0
tr	0	tr	4	2	tr	124	2	0	0	0.00	0.02	0.4	0
tr	0	1	2	6	0.1	71	tr	0	0	0.00	0.03	0.6	0
0.0	0	22	15	2	0.4	48	15	20	2	0.03	0.04	tr	61[4]
tr	0	tr	0	2	tr	36	1	0	0	0.00	0.03	tr	0
tr	0	1	1	4	tr	61	1	0	0	0.00	0.02	0.1	0
tr	0	22	1	3	tr	49	tr	0	0	0.00	0.04	0.1	0
0.2	21	1	150	110	0.1	73	396	200	65	0.01	0.11	0.3	0
0.3	27	tr	147	132	0.1	71	320	350	96	0.01	0.19	0.2	0
0.3	30	tr	204	145	0.2	28	176	300	86	0.01	0.11	tr	0
0.2	18	tr	123	87	0.1	17	105	180	52	tr	0.06	tr	0
1.1	119	1	815	579	0.8	111	701	1200	342	0.03	0.42	0.1	0

Continued

FOODS, APPROXIMATE MEASURES, UNITS, AND WEIGHT (WEIGHT OF EDIBLE PORTION ONLY)		GRAMS	WATER (g)	FOOD ENERGY (CALORIES)	PROTEIN (g)	FAT (g)	FATTY ACIDS	
							SATURATED (g)	MONO-UNSATURATED (g)
DAIRY PRODUCTS—cont'd								
Cottage (curd not pressed down)								
Creamed (cottage cheese, 4% fat)								
Large curd	1 c	225	79	235	28	10	6.4	2.9
Small curd	1 c	210	79	215	26	9	6.0	2.7
With fruit	1 c	226	72	280	22	8	4.9	2.2
Lowfat (2%)	1 c	226	79	205	31	4	2.8	1.2
Uncreamed (cottage cheese dry curd, less than ½% fat)	1 c	145	80	125	25	1	0.4	0.2
Cream	1 oz	28	54	100	2	10	6.2	2.8
Feta	1 oz	28	55	75	4	6	4.2	1.3
Mozzarella, made with								
Whole milk	1 oz	28	54	80	6	6	3.7	1.9
Part skim milk (low moisture)	1 oz	28	49	80	8	5	3.1	1.4
Muenster	1 oz	28	42	105	7	9	5.4	2.5
Parmesan, grated								
Cup, not pressed down	1 c	100	18	455	42	30	19.1	8.7
Tablespoon	1 tbsp	5	18	25	2	2	1.0	0.4
Ounce	1 oz	28	18	130	12	9	5.4	2.5
Provolone	1 oz	28	41	100	7	8	4.8	2.1
Ricotta, made with								
Whole milk	1 c	246	72	430	28	32	20.4	8.9
Part skim milk	1 c	246	74	340	28	19	12.1	5.7
Swiss	1 oz	28	37	105	8	8	5.0	2.1
Pasteurized process cheese								
American	1 oz	28	39	105	6	9	5.6	2.5
Swiss	1 oz	28	42	95	7	7	4.5	2.0
Pasteurized process cheese food, American	1 oz	28	43	95	6	7	4.4	2.0
Pasteurized process cheese spread, American	1 oz	28	48	80	5	6	3.8	1.8
Cream, sweet								
Half-and-half (cream and milk)	1 c	242	81	315	7	28	17.3	8.0
	1 tbsp	15	81	20	tr	2	1.1	0.5
Light, coffee, or table	1 c	240	74	470	6	46	28.8	13.4
	1 tbsp	15	74	30	tr	3	1.8	0.8
Whipping, unwhipped (volume about double when whipped)								
Light	1 c	239	64	700	5	74	46.2	21.7
	1 tbsp	15	64	45	tr	5	2.9	1.4
Heavy	1 c	238	58	820	5	88	54.8	25.4
	1 tbsp	15	58	50	tr	6	3.5	1.6
Whipped topping, (pressurized)	1 c	60	61	155	2	13	8.3	3.9
	1 tbsp	3	61	10	tr	1	0.4	0.2

tr = nutrient present in trace amounts.

NUTRIENTS IN INDICATED QUANTITY													
POLY-UNSATURATED (g)	CHOLES-TEROL (mg)	CARBO-HYDRATE (g)	CALCIUM (mg)	PHOS-PHORUS (mg)	IRON (mg)	POTASSIUM (mg)	SODIUM (mg)	VITAMIN A VALUES IU	RE	THIAMIN (mg)	RIBO-FLAVIN (mg)	NIACIN (mg)	ASCORBIC ACID (mg)
0.3	34	6	135	297	0.3	190	911	370	108	0.05	0.37	0.3	tr
0.3	31	6	126	277	0.3	177	850	340	101	0.04	0.34	0.3	tr
0.2	25	30	108	236	0.2	151	915	280	81	0.04	0.29	0.2	tr
0.1	19	8	155	340	0.4	217	918	160	45	0.05	0.42	0.3	tr
tr	10	3	46	151	0.3	47	19	40	12	0.04	0.21	0.2	0
0.4	31	1	23	30	0.3	34	84	400	124	tr	0.06	tr	0
0.2	25	1	140	96	0.2	18	316	130	36	0.04	0.24	0.3	0
0.2	22	1	147	105	0.1	19	106	220	68	tr	0.07	tr	0
0.1	15	1	207	149	0.1	27	150	180	54	0.01	0.10	tr	0
0.2	27	tr	203	133	0.1	38	178	320	90	tr	0.09	tr	0
0.7	79	4	1376	807	1.0	107	1861	700	173	0.05	0.39	0.3	0
tr	4	tr	69	40	tr	5	93	40	9	tr	0.02	tr	0
0.2	22	1	390	229	0.3	30	528	200	49	0.01	0.11	0.1	0
0.2	20	1	214	141	0.1	39	248	230	75	0.01	0.09	tr	0
0.9	124	7	509	389	0.9	257	207	1210	330	0.03	0.48	0.3	0
0.6	76	13	669	449	1.1	307	307	1060	278	0.05	0.46	0.2	0
0.3	26	1	272	171	tr	31	74	240	72	0.01	0.10	tr	0
0.3	27	tr	174	211	0.1	46	406	340	82	0.01	0.10	tr	0
0.2	24	1	219	216	0.2	61	338	230	65	tr	0.08	tr	0
0.2	18	2	163	130	0.2	79	337	260	62	0.01	0.13	tr	0
0.2	16	2	159	202	0.1	69	381	220	54	0.01	0.12	tr	0
1.0	89	10	254	230	0.2	314	98	1050	259	0.08	0.36	0.2	2
0.1	6	1	16	14	tr	19	6	70	16	0.01	0.02	tr	tr
1.7	159	9	231	192	0.1	292	95	1730	437	0.08	0.36	0.1	2
0.1	10	1	14	12	tr	18	6	110	27	tr	0.02	tr	tr
2.1	265	7	166	146	0.1	231	82	2690	705	0.06	0.30	0.1	1
0.1	17	tr	10	9	tr	15	5	170	44	tr	0.02	tr	tr
3.3	326	7	154	149	0.1	179	89	3500	1002	0.05	0.26	0.1	1
0.2	21	tr	10	9	tr	11	6	220	63	tr	0.02	tr	tr
0.5	46	7	61	54	tr	88	78	550	124	0.02	0.04	tr	0
tr	2	tr	3	3	tr	4	4	30	6	tr	tr	tr	0

Continued

FOODS, APPROXIMATE MEASURES, UNITS, AND WEIGHT (WEIGHT OF EDIBLE PORTION ONLY)		GRAMS	WATER (g)	FOOD ENERGY (CALORIES)	PROTEIN (g)	FAT (g)	FATTY ACIDS	
							SATURATED (g)	MONO-UNSATURATED (g)
DAIRY PRODUCTS—cont'd								
Cream, sour	1 c	230	71	495	7	48	30.0	13.9
	1 tbsp	12	71	25	tr	3	1.6	0.7
Milk								
Fluid								
Whole (3.3% fat)	1 c	244	88	150	8	8	5.1	2.4
Lowfat (2%)								
No milk solids added	1 c	244	89	120	8	5	2.9	1.4
Milk solids added, label claim less than 10 g of protein per cup	1 c	245	89	125	9	5	2.9	1.4
Lowfat (1%)								
No milk solids added	1 c	244	90	100	8	3	1.6	0.7
Milk solids added, label claim less than 10 g of protein per cup	1 c	245	90	105	9	2	1.5	0.7
Nonfat (skim)								
No milk solids added	1 c	245	91	85	8	tr	0.3	0.1
Milk solids added, label claim less than 10 g of protein per cup	1 c	245	90	90	9	1	0.4	0.2
Buttermilk	1 c	245	90	100	8	2	1.3	0.6
Milk desserts, frozen								
Ice cream, vanilla								
Regular (about 11% fat)								
Hardened	½ gal	1064	61	2155	38	115	71.3	33.1
	1 c	133	61	270	5	14	8.9	4.1
	3 fl oz	50	61	100	2	5	3.4	1.6
Soft serve (frozen custard)	1 c	173	60	375	7	23	13.5	6.7
Rich (about 16% fat), hardened	½ gal	1188	59	2805	33	190	118.3	54.9
	1 c	148	59	350	4	24	14.7	6.8
Ice milk, vanilla								
Hardened (about 4% fat)	½ gal	1048	69	1470	41	45	28.1	13.0
	1 c	131	69	185	5	6	3.5	1.6
Soft serve (about 3% fat)	1 c	175	70	225	8	5	2.9	1.3
Sherbet (about 2% fat)	½ gal	1542	66	2160	17	31	19.0	8.8
	1 c	193	66	270	2	4	2.4	1.1
EGGS								
Eggs, large (24 oz per dozen)								
Raw								
Whole, without shell	1 egg	50	75	80	6	6	1.7	2.2
White	1 white	33	88	15	3	tr	0.0	0.0
Yolk	1 yolk	17	49	65	3	6	1.7	2.2

tr = nutrient present in trace amounts.

NUTRIENTS IN INDICATED QUANTITY

POLY-UNSATURATED (g)	CHOLES-TEROL (mg)	CARBO-HYDRATE (g)	CALCIUM (mg)	PHOS-PHORUS (mg)	IRON (mg)	POTASSIUM (mg)	SODIUM (mg)	VITAMIN A VALUES		THIAMIN (mg)	RIBO-FLAVIN (mg)	NIACIN (mg)	ASCORBIC ACID (mg)
								IU	RE				
1.8	102	10	268	195	0.1	331	123	1820	448	0.08	0.34	0.2	2
0.1	5	1	14	10	tr	17	6	90	23	tr	0.02	tr	tr
0.3	33	11	291	228	0.1	370	120	310	76	0.09	0.40	0.2	2
0.2	18	12	297	232	0.1	377	122	500	139	0.10	0.40	0.2	2
0.2	18	12	313	245	0.1	397	128	500	140	0.10	0.42	0.2	2
0.1	10	12	300	235	0.1	381	123	500	144	0.10	0.41	0.2	2
0.1	10	12	313	245	0.1	397	128	500	145	0.10	0.42	0.2	2
tr	4	12	302	247	0.1	406	126	500	149	0.09	0.34	0.2	2
tr	5	12	316	255	0.1	418	130	500	149	0.10	0.43	0.2	2
0.1	9	12	285	219	0.1	371	257	80	20	0.08	0.38	0.1	2
4.3	476	254	1406	1075	1.0	2052	929	4340	1064	0.42	2.63	1.1	6
0.5	59	32	176	134	0.1	257	116	540	133	0.05	0.33	0.1	1
0.2	22	12	66	51	tr	96	44	200	50	0.02	0.12	0.1	tr
1.0	153	38	236	199	0.4	338	153	790	199	0.8	0.45	0.2	1
7.1	703	256	1213	927	0.8	1771	868	7200	1758	0.36	2.27	0.9	5
0.9	88	32	151	115	0.1	221	108	900	219	0.04	0.28	0.1	1
1.7	146	232	1409	1035	1.5	2117	836	1710	419	0.61	2.78	0.9	6
0.2	18	29	176	129	0.2	265	105	210	52	0.08	0.35	0.1	1
0.2	13	38	274	202	0.3	412	163	175	44	0.12	0.54	0.2	1
1.1	113	469	827	594	2.5	1585	706	1480	308	0.26	0.71	1.0	31
0.1	14	59	103	74	0.3	198	88	190	39	0.03	0.09	0.1	4
0.7	274	1	28	90	1.0	65	69	260	78	0.04	0.15	tr	0
0.0	0	tr	4	4	tr	45	50	0	0	tr	0.09	tr	0
0.7	272	tr	26	86	0.9	15	8	310	94	0.04	0.07	tr	0

Continued

FOODS, APPROXIMATE MEASURES, UNITS, AND WEIGHT (WEIGHT OF EDIBLE PORTION ONLY)		GRAMS	WATER (g)	FOOD ENERGY (CALORIES)	PROTEIN (g)	FAT (g)	FATTY ACIDS	
							SATURATED (g)	MONO-UNSATURATED (g)
FATS AND OILS								
Butter (4 sticks per lb)								
Stick	½ c	113	16	810	1	92	57.1	26.4
Tablespoon (⅛ stick)	1 tbsp	14	16	100	tr	11	7.1	3.3
Pat (1 in square, ⅓ in high; 90 per lb)	1 pat	5	16	35	tr	4	2.5	1.2
Fats, cooking (vegetable shortenings)	1 c	205	0	1810	0	205	51.3	91.2
	1 tbsp	13	0	115	0	13	3.3	5.8
Lard	1 c	205	0	1850	0	205	80.4	92.5
	1 tbsp	13	0	115	0	13	5.1	5.9
Oils, salad or cooking								
Corn	1 c	218	0	1925	0	218	27.7	52.8
	1 tbsp	14	0	125	0	14	1.8	3.4
Olive	1 c	216	0	1910	0	216	29.2	159.2
	1 tbsp	14	0	125	0	14	1.9	10.3
Peanut	1 c	216	0	1910	0	216	36.5	99.8
	1 tbsp	14	0	125	0	14	2.4	6.5
Safflower	1 c	218	0	1925	0	218	19.8	26.4
	1 tbsp	14	0	125	0	14	1.3	1.7
Soybean oil, hydrogenated	1 c	218	0	1925	0	218	32.5	93.7
(partially hardened)	1 tbsp	14	0	125	0	14	2.1	6.0
Soybean-cottonseed oil blend,	1 c	218	0	1925	0	218	39.2	64.3
hydrogenated	1 tbsp	14	0	125	0	14	2.5	4.1
Sunflower	1 c	218	0	1925	0	218	22.5	42.5
	1 tbsp	14	0	125	0	14	1.4	2.7
Salad dressings								
Commercial								
Blue cheese	1 tbsp	15	32	75	1	8	1.5	1.8
French								
Regular	1 tbsp	16	35	85	tr	9	1.4	4.0
Low calorie	1 tbsp	16	75	25	tr	2	0.2	0.3
Italian								
Regular	1 tbsp	15	34	80	tr	9	1.3	3.7
Low calorie	1 tbsp	15	86	5	tr	tr	tr	tr
Mayonnaise								
Regular	1 tbsp	14	15	100	tr	11	1.7	3.2
Imitation	1 tbsp	15	63	35	tr	3	0.5	0.7
Prepared from home recipe								
Cooked type[7]	1 tbsp	16	69	25	1	2	0.5	0.6
Vinegar and oil	1 tbsp	16	47	70	0	8	1.5	2.4

tr = nutrient present in trace amounts.
[5]For salted butter; unsalted butter contains 12 mg sodium per stick, 2 mg per tbsp, or 1 mg per pat.
[6]Values for vitamin A are year-round average.
[7]Fatty acid values apply to product made with regular margarine.

NUTRIENTS IN INDICATED QUANTITY

POLY-UNSATURATED (g)	CHOLES-TEROL (mg)	CARBO-HYDRATE (g)	CALCIUM (mg)	PHOS-PHORUS (mg)	IRON (mg)	POTASSIUM (mg)	SODIUM (mg)	VITAMIN A VALUES		THIAMIN (mg)	RIBO-FLAVIN (mg)	NIACIN (mg)	ASCORBIC ACID (mg)
								IU	RE				
3.4	247	tr	27	26	0.2	29	933[5]	13,460[6]	852[6]	0.01	0.04	tr	0
0.4	31	tr	3	3	tr	4	116[5]	430[6]	106[6]	tr	tr	tr	0
0.2	11	tr	1	1	tr	1	41[5]	150[6]	38[6]	tr	tr	tr	0
53.5	0	0	0	0	0.0	0	0	0	0	0.00	0.00	0.0	0
3.4	0	0	0	0	0.0	0	0	0	0	0.00	0.00	0.0	0
23.0	195	0	0	0	0.0	0	0	0	0	0.00	0.00	0.0	0
1.5	12	0	0	0	0.0	0	0	0	0	0.00	0.00	0.0	0
128.0	0	0	0	0	0.0	0	0	0	0	0.00	0.00	0.0	0
8.2	0	0	0	0	0.0	0	0	0	0	0.00	0.00	0.0	0
18.1	0	0	0	0	0.0	0	0	0	0	0.00	0.00	0.0	0
1.2	0	0	0	0	0.0	0	0	0	0	0.00	0.00	0.0	0
69.1	0	0	0	0	0.0	0	0	0	0	0.00	0.00	0.0	0
4.5	0	0	0	0	0.0	0	0	0	0	0.00	0.00	0.0	0
162.4	0	0	0	0	0.0	0	0	0	0	0.00	0.00	0.0	0
10.4	0	0	0	0	0.0	0	0	0	0	0.00	0.00	0.0	0
82.0	0	0	0	0	0.0	0	0	0	0	0.00	0.00	0.0	0
5.3	0	0	0	0	0.0	0	0	0	0	0.00	0.00	0.0	0
104.9	0	0	0	0	0.0	0	0	0	0	0.00	0.00	0.0	0
6.7	0	0	0	0	0.0	0	0	0	0	0.00	0.00	0.0	0
143.2	0	0	0	0	0.0	0	0	0	0	0.00	0.00	0.0	0
9.2	0	0	0	0	0.0	0	0	0	0	0.00	0.00	0.0	0
4.2	3	1	12	11	tr	6	164	30	10	tr	0.02	tr	tr
3.5	0	1	2	1	tr	2	188	tr	tr	tr	tr	tr	tr
1.0	0	2	6	5	tr	3	306	tr	tr	tr	tr	tr	tr
3.2	0	1	1	1	tr	5	162	30	3	tr	tr	tr	tr
tr	0	2	1	1	tr	4	136	tr	tr	tr	tr	tr	tr
5.8	8	tr	3	4	0.1	5	80	40	12	0.00	0.00	tr	0
1.6	4	2	tr	tr	0.0	2	75	0	0	0.00	0.00	0.0	0
0.3	9	2	13	14	0.1	19	117	70	20	0.01	0.02	tr	tr
3.9	0	tr	0	0	0.0	1	tr	0	0	0.00	0.00	0.0	0

Continued

FOODS, APPROXIMATE MEASURES, UNITS, AND WEIGHT (WEIGHT OF EDIBLE PORTION ONLY)		GRAMS	WATER (g)	FOOD ENERGY (CALORIES)	PROTEIN (g)	FAT (g)	FATTY ACIDS	
							SATURATED (g)	MONO-UNSATURATED (g)
FISH AND SHELLFISH								
Clams								
Raw, meat only	3 oz	85	82	65	11	1	0.3	0.3
Canned, drained solids	3 oz	85	77	85	13	2	0.5	0.5
Crabmeat, canned	1 c	135	77	135	23	3	0.5	0.8
Fish sticks, frozen, reheated, (stick, 4 by 1 by ½ in)	1 stick	28	52	70	6	3	0.8	1.4
Flounder or Sole, baked, with lemon juice								
With butter	3 oz	85	73	120	16	6	3.2	1.5
With margarine	3 oz	85	73	120	16	6	1.2	2.3
Without added fat	3 oz	85	78	80	17	1	0.3	0.2
Haddock, breaded, fried[8]	3 oz	85	61	175	17	9	2.4	3.9
Halibut, broiled, with butter and lemon juice	3 oz	85	67	140	20	6	3.3	1.6
Herring, pickled	3 oz	85	59	190	17	13	4.3	4.6
Ocean perch, breaded, fried[8]	1 fillet	85	59	185	16	11	2.6	4.6
Oysters								
Raw, meat only (13-19 medium Selects)	1 c	240	85	160	20	4	1.4	0.5
Breaded, fried[8]	1 oyster	45	65	90	5	5	1.4	2.1
Salmon								
Canned (pink), solids and liquid	3 oz	85	71	120	17	5	0.9	1.5
Baked (red)	3 oz	85	67	140	21	5	1.2	2.4
Smoked	3 oz	85	59	150	18	8	2.6	3.9
Sardines, Atlantic, canned in oil, drained solids	3 oz	85	62	175	20	9	2.1	3.7
Scallops, breaded, frozen, reheated	6 scallops	90	59	195	15	10	2.5	4.1
Shrimp								
Canned, drained solids	3 oz	85	70	100	21	1	0.2	0.2
French fried (7 medium)[10]	3 oz	85	55	200	16	10	2.5	4.1
Trout, broiled, with butter and lemon juice	3 oz	85	63	175	21	9	4.1	2.9
Tuna, canned, drained solids								
Oil pack, chunk light	3 oz	85	61	165	24	7	1.4	1.9
Water pack, solid white	3 oz	85	63	135	30	1	0.3	0.2
Tuna salad[11]	1 c	205	63	375	33	19	3.3	4.9

tr = nutrient present in trace amounts.
[8]Dipped in egg, milk, and breadcrumbs; fried in vegetable shortening.
[9]If bones are discarded, value for calcium will be greatly reduced.
[10]Dipped in egg, breadcrumbs, and flour; fried in vegetable shortening.
[11]Made with drained chunk light tuna, celery, onion, pickle relish, and mayonnaise-type salad dressing.

NUTRIENTS IN INDICATED QUANTITY

POLY-UNSATURATED (g)	CHOLES-TEROL (mg)	CARBO-HYDRATE (g)	CALCIUM (mg)	PHOS-PHORUS (mg)	IRON (mg)	POTASSIUM (mg)	SODIUM (mg)	VITAMIN A VALUES		THIAMIN (mg)	RIBO-FLAVIN (mg)	NIACIN (mg)	ASCORBIC ACID (mg)
								IU	RE				
0.3	43	2	59	138	2.6	154	102	90	26	0.09	0.15	1.1	9
0.4	54	2	47	116	3.5	119	102	90	26	0.01	0.09	0.9	3
1.4	135	1	61	246	1.1	149	1350	50	14	0.11	0.11	2.6	0
0.8	26	4	11	58	0.3	94	53	20	5	0.03	0.05	0.6	0
0.5	68	tr	13	187	0.3	272	145	210	54	0.05	0.08	1.6	1
1.9	55	tr	14	187	0.3	273	151	230	69	0.05	0.08	1.6	1
0.4	59	tr	13	197	0.3	286	101	30	10	0.05	0.08	1.7	1
2.4	75	7	34	183	1.0	270	123	70	20	0.06	0.10	2.9	0
0.7	62	tr	14	206	0.7	441	103	610	174	0.06	0.07	7.7	1
3.1	85	0	29	128	0.9	85	850	110	33	0.04	0.18	2.8	0
2.8	66	7	31	191	1.2	241	138	70	20	0.10	0.11	2.0	0
1.4	120	8	226	343	15.6	290	175	740	223	0.34	0.43	6.0	24
1.4	35	5	49	73	3.0	64	70	150	44	0.07	0.10	1.3	4
2.1	34	0	167[9]	243	0.7	307	443	60	18	0.03	0.15	6.8	0
1.4	60	0	26	269	0.5	305	55	290	87	0.18	0.14	5.5	0
0.7	51	0	12	208	0.8	327	1700	260	77	0.17	0.17	6.8	0
2.9	85	0	371[9]	424	2.6	349	425	190	56	0.03	0.17	4.6	0
2.5	70	10	39	203	2.0	369	298	70	21	0.11	0.11	1.6	0
0.4	128	1	98	224	1.4	104	1955	50	15	0.01	0.03	1.5	0
2.6	168	11	61	154	2.0	189	384	90	26	0.06	0.09	2.8	0
1.6	71	tr	26	259	1.0	297	122	230	60	0.07	0.07	2.3	1
3.1	55	0	7	199	1.6	298	303	70	20	0.04	0.09	10.1	0
0.3	48	0	17	202	0.6	255	468	110	32	0.03	0.10	13.4	0
9.2	80	19	31	281	2.5	531	877	230	53	0.06	0.14	13.3	6

Continued

FOODS, APPROXIMATE MEASURES, UNITS, AND WEIGHT (WEIGHT OF EDIBLE PORTION ONLY)		GRAMS	WATER (g)	FOOD ENERGY (CALORIES)	PROTEIN (g)	FAT (g)	FATTY ACIDS	
							SATURATED (g)	MONO-UNSATURATED (g)
FRUITS AND FRUIT JUICES								
Apples								
Raw								
Unpeeled, without cores								
2¾-in diam. (about 3 per lb with cores)	1 apple	138	84	80	tr	tr	0.1	tr
3¼-in diam. (about 2 per lb with cores)	1 apple	212	84	125	tr	1	0.1	tr
Peeled, sliced	1 c	110	84	65	tr	tr	0.1	tr
Dried, sulfured	10 rings	64	32	155	1	tr	tr	tr
Apple juice, bottled or canned[13]	1 c	248	88	115	tr	tr	tr	tr
Applesauce, canned								
Sweetened	1 c	255	80	195	tr	tr	0.1	tr
Unsweetened	1 c	244	88	105	tr	tr	tr	tr
Apricots								
Raw, without pits (about 12 per lb with pits	3 apricots	106	86	50	1	tr	tr	0.2
Canned (fruit and liquid)								
Heavy syrup pack	1 c	258	78	215	1	tr	tr	0.1
	3 halves	85	78	70	tr	tr	tr	tr
Juice pack	1 c	248	87	120	2	tr	tr	tr
	3 halves	84	87	40	1	tr	tr	tr
Dried								
Uncooked (28 large or 37 medium halves per cup)	1 c	130	31	310	5	1	tr	0.3
Cooked, unsweetened, fruit and liquid	1 c	250	76	210	3	tr	tr	0.2
Apricot nectar, canned	1 c	251	85	140	1	tr	tr	0.1
Avocados, raw, whole, without skin and seed								
California (about 2 per lb with skin and seed)	1 avocado	173	73	305	4	30	4.5	19.4
Florida (about 1 per lb with skin and seed)	1 avocado	304	80	340	5	27	5.3	14.8
Bananas, raw, without peel								
Whole (about 2½ per lb with peel)	1 banana	114	74	105	1	1	0.2	tr
Sliced	1 c	150	74	140	2	1	0.3	0.1
Blackberries, raw	1 c	144	86	75	1	1	0.2	0.1
Blueberries								
Raw	1 c	145	85	80	1	1	tr	0.1
Frozen, sweetened	10 oz	284	77	230	1	tr	tr	0.1
	1 c	230	77	185	1	tr	tr	tr

tr = nutrient present in trace amounts.
[12]Sodium bisulfite used to preserve color; unsulfited product would contain less sodium.

| NUTRIENTS IN INDICATED QUANTITY | | | | | | | | | | | | | |

POLY-UNSATURATED (g)	CHOLES-TEROL (mg)	CARBO-HYDRATE (g)	CALCIUM (mg)	PHOS-PHORUS (mg)	IRON (mg)	POTASSIUM (mg)	SODIUM (mg)	VITAMIN A VALUES		THIAMIN (mg)	RIBO-FLAVIN (mg)	NIACIN (mg)	ASCORBIC ACID (mg)
								IU	RE				
0.1	0	21	10	10	0.2	159	tr	70	7	0.02	0.02	0.1	8
0.2	0	32	15	15	0.4	244	tr	110	11	0.04	0.03	0.2	12
0.1	0	16	4	8	0.1	124	tr	50	5	0.02	0.01	0.1	4
0.1	0	42	9	24	0.9	288	56[12]	0	0	0.00	0.10	0.6	2
0.1	0	29	17	17	0.9	295	7	tr	tr	0.05	0.04	0.2	2[14]
0.1	0	51	10	18	0.9	156	8	30	3	0.03	0.07	0.5	4[14]
tr	0	28	7	17	0.3	183	5	70	7	0.03	0.06	0.5	3[14]
0.1	0	12	15	20	0.6	314	1	2770	277	0.03	0.04	0.6	11
tr	0	55	23	31	0.8	361	10	3170	317	0.05	0.06	1.0	8
tr	0	18	8	10	0.3	119	3	1050	105	0.02	0.02	0.3	3
tr	0	31	30	50	0.7	409	10	4190	419	0.04	0.05	0.9	12
tr	0	10	10	17	0.3	139	3	1420	142	0.02	0.02	0.3	4
0.1	0	80	59	152	6.1	1791	13	9410	941	0.01	0.20	3.9	3
0.1	0	55	40	103	4.2	1222	8	5910	591	0.02	0.08	2.4	4
tr	0	36	18	23	1.0	286	8	3300	330	0.02	0.04	0.7	2[14]
3.5	0	12	19	73	2.0	1097	21	1060	106	0.19	0.21	3.3	14
4.5	0	27	33	119	1.6	1484	15	1860	186	0.33	0.37	5.8	24
0.1	0	27	7	23	0.4	451	1	90	9	0.05	0.11	0.6	10
0.1	0	35	9	30	0.5	594	2	120	12	0.07	0.15	0.8	14
0.1	0	18	46	30	0.8	282	tr	240	24	0.04	0.06	0.6	30
0.3	0	20	9	15	0.2	129	9	150	15	0.07	0.07	0.5	19
0.2	0	62	17	20	1.1	170	3	120	12	0.06	0.15	0.7	3
0.1	0	50	14	16	0.9	138	2	100	10	0.05	0.12	0.6	2

[13]Also applies to pasteurized apple cider.
[14]Without added ascorbic acid; for value with added ascorbic acid, refer to label.

Continued

FOODS, APPROXIMATE MEASURES, UNITS, AND WEIGHT (WEIGHT OF EDIBLE PORTION ONLY)		GRAMS	WATER (g)	FOOD ENERGY (CALORIES)	PROTEIN (g)	FAT (g)	FATTY ACIDS	
							SATURATED (g)	MONO-UNSATURATED (g)
FRUITS AND FRUIT JUICES—cont'd								
Cantaloupe. See Melons								
Cherries								
Sour, red, pitted, canned, water pack	1 c	244	90	90	2	tr	0.1	0.1
Sweet, raw, without pits and stems	10 cherries	68	81	50	1	1	0.1	0.2
Cranberry juice cocktail, bottled, sweetened	1 c	253	85	145	tr	tr	tr	tr
Cranberry sauce, sweetened, canned, strained	1 c	277	61	420	1	tr	tr	0.1
Dates								
Whole, without pits	10 dates	83	23	230	2	tr	0.1	0.1
Chopped	1 c	178	23	490	4	1	0.3	0.2
Figs, dried	10 figs	187	28	475	6	2	0.4	0.5
Fruit cocktail, canned, fruit and liquid								
Heavy syrup pack	1 c	255	80	185	1	tr	tr	tr
Juice pack	1 c	248	87	115	1	tr	tr	tr
Grapefruit								
Raw, without peel, membrane and seeds (3¾-in diam., 1 lb 1 oz, whole, with refuse)	½ grapefruit	120	91	40	1	tr	tr	tr
Canned, sections with syrup	1 c	254	84	150	1	tr	tr	tr
Grapefruit juice								
Raw	1 c	247	90	95	1	tr	tr	tr
Canned								
Unsweetened	1 c	247	90	95	1	tr	tr	tr
Sweetened	1 c	250	87	115	1	tr	tr	tr
Frozen concentrate, unsweetened								
Undiluted	6 fl oz	207	62	300	4	1	0.1	0.1
Diluted with 3 parts water by volume	1 c	247	89	100	1	tr	tr	tr
Grapes, European type (adherent skin), raw								
Thompson Seedless	10 grapes	50	81	35	tr	tr	0.1	tr
Tokay and Emperor, seeded types	10 grapes	57	81	40	tr	tr	0.1	tr
Grape juice								
Canned or bottled	1 c	253	84	155	1	tr	0.1	tr
Frozen concentrate, sweetened								
Undiluted	6 fl oz	216	54	385	1	1	0.2	tr
Diluted with 3 parts water by volume	1 c	250	87	125	tr	tr	0.1	tr

tr = nutrient present in trace amounts.
[14]Without added ascorbic acid; for value with added ascorbic acid, refer to label.

NUTRIENTS IN INDICATED QUANTITY

POLY-UNSATURATED (g)	CHOLES-TEROL (mg)	CARBO-HYDRATE (g)	CALCIUM (mg)	PHOS-PHORUS (mg)	IRON (mg)	POTASSIUM (mg)	SODIUM (mg)	VITAMIN A VALUES IU	VITAMIN A VALUES RE	THIAMIN (mg)	RIBO-FLAVIN (mg)	NIACIN (mg)	ASCORBIC ACID (mg)
0.1	0	22	27	24	3.3	239	17	1840	184	0.04	0.10	0.4	5
0.2	0	11	10	13	0.3	152	tr	150	15	0.03	0.04	0.3	5
0.1	0	38	8	3	0.4	61	10	10	1	0.01	0.04	0.1	108[15]
0.2	0	108	11	17	0.6	72	80	60	6	0.04	0.06	0.3	6
tr	0	61	27	33	1.0	541	2	40	4	0.07	0.08	1.8	0
tr	0	131	57	71	2.0	1161	5	90	9	0.16	0.18	3.9	0
1.0	0	122	269	127	4.2	1331	21	250	25	0.13	0.16	1.3	1
0.1	0	48	15	28	0.7	224	15	520	52	0.05	0.05	1.0	5
tr	0	29	20	35	0.5	236	10	760	76	0.03	0.04	1.0	7
tr	0	10	14	10	0.1	167	tr	10[16]	1[16]	0.04	0.02	0.3	41
0.1	0	39	36	25	1.0	328	5	tr	tr	0.10	0.05	0.6	54
0.1	0	23	22	37	0.5	400	2	20	2	0.10	0.05	0.5	94
0.1	0	22	17	27	0.5	378	2	20	2	0.10	0.05	0.6	72
0.1	0	28	20	28	0.9	405	5	20	2	0.10	0.06	0.8	67
0.2	0	72	56	101	1.0	1002	6	60	6	0.30	0.16	1.6	248
0.1	0	24	20	35	0.3	336	2	20	2	0.10	0.05	0.5	83
0.1	0	9	6	7	0.1	93	1	40	4	0.05	0.03	0.2	5
0.1	0	10	6	7	0.1	105	1	40	4	0.05	0.03	0.2	6
0.1	0	38	23	28	0.6	334	8	20	2	0.07	0.09	0.7	tr[14]
0.2	0	96	28	32	0.8	160	15	60	6	0.11	0.20	0.9	179[15]
0.1	0	32	10	10	0.3	53	5	20	2	0.04	0.07	0.3	60[15]

[15]With added ascorbic acid.
[16]For white grapefruit; pink grapefruit have about 310 IU or 31 RE.

Continued

FOODS, APPROXIMATE MEASURES, UNITS, AND WEIGHT (WEIGHT OF EDIBLE PORTION ONLY)		GRAMS	WATER (g)	FOOD ENERGY (CALORIES)	PROTEIN (g)	FAT (g)	FATTY ACIDS	
							SATURATED (g)	MONO-UNSATURATED (g)
FRUITS AND FRUIT JUICES—cont'd								
Kiwifruit, raw, without skin (about 5 per lb with skin)	1 kiwifruit	76	83	45	1	tr	tr	0.1
Lemons, raw, without peel and seeds (about 4 per lb with peel and seeds)	1 lemon	58	89	15	1	tr	tr	tr
Lemon juice								
Raw	1 c	244	91	60	1	tr	tr	tr
Canned or bottled, unsweetened	1 c	244	92	50	1	1	0.1	tr
	1 tbsp	15	92	5	tr	tr	tr	tr
Frozen, single-strength, unsweetened	6 fl oz	244	92	55	1	1	0.1	tr
Lime juice								
Raw	1 c	246	90	65	1	tr	tr	tr
Canned, unsweetened	1 c	246	93	50	1	1	0.1	0.1
Mangos, raw, without skin and seed (about 1½ per lb with skin and seed)	1 mango	207	82	135	1	1	0.1	0.2
Melons, raw, without rind and cavity contents								
Cantaloupe, orange-fleshed (5-in diam., 2⅓ lb, whole, with rind and cavity contents)	½ melon	267	90	95	2	1	0.1	0.1
Honeydew (6½-in diam., 5¼ lb, whole, with rind and cavity contents)	¹⁄₁₀ melon	129	90	45	1	tr	tr	tr
Nectarines, raw, without pits (about 3 per lb with pits)	1 nectarine	136	86	65	1	1	0.1	0.2
Oranges, raw								
Whole, without peel and seeds (2⅝-in diam., about 2½ per lb, with peel and seeds)	1 orange	131	87	60	1	tr	tr	tr
Sections without membranes	1 c	180	87	85	2	tr	tr	tr
Orange juice								
Raw, all varieties	1 c	248	88	110	2	tr	0.1	0.1
Canned, unsweetened	1 c	249	89	105	1	tr	tr	0.1
Chilled	1 c	249	88	110	2	1	0.1	0.1
Frozen concentrate								
Undiluted	6 fl oz	213	58	340	5	tr	0.1	0.1
Diluted with 3 parts water by volume	1 c	249	88	110	2	tr	tr	tr
Orange and grapefruit juice, canned	1 c	247	89	105	1	tr	tr	tr

tr = nutrient present in trace amounts.
[17]Sodium benzoate and sodium bisulfite added as preservatives.

NUTRIENTS IN INDICATED QUANTITY													
POLY-UNSATURATED (g)	CHOLES-TEROL (mg)	CARBO-HYDRATE (g)	CALCIUM (mg)	PHOS-PHORUS (mg)	IRON (mg)	POTASSIUM (mg)	SODIUM (mg)	VITAMIN A VALUES IU	VITAMIN A VALUES RE	THIAMIN (mg)	RIBO-FLAVIN (mg)	NIACIN (mg)	ASCORBIC ACID (mg)
0.1	0	11	20	30	0.3	252	4	130	13	0.02	0.04	0.4	74
0.1	0	5	15	9	0.3	80	1	20	2	0.02	0.01	0.1	31
tr	0	21	17	15	0.1	303	2	50	5	0.07	0.02	0.2	112
0.2	0	16	27	22	0.3	249	51[17]	40	4	0.10	0.02	0.5	61
tr	0	1	2	1	tr	15	3[17]	tr	tr	0.01	tr	tr	4
0.2	0	16	20	20	0.3	217	2	30	3	0.14	0.03	0.3	77
0.1	0	22	22	17	0.1	268	2	20	2	0.05	0.02	0.2	72
0.2	0	16	30	25	0.6	185	39[17]	40	4	0.08	0.01	0.4	16
0.1	0	35	21	23	0.3	323	4	8060	806	0.12	0.12	1.2	57
0.3	0	22	29	45	0.6	825	24	8610	861	0.10	0.06	1.5	113
0.1	0	12	8	13	0.1	350	13	50	5	0.10	0.02	0.8	32
0.3	0	16	7	22	0.2	288	tr	1000	100	0.02	0.06	1.3	7
tr	0	15	52	18	0.1	237	tr	270	27	0.11	0.05	0.4	70
tr	0	21	72	25	0.2	326	tr	370	37	0.16	0.07	0.5	96
0.1	0	26	27	42	0.5	496	2	500	50	0.22	0.07	1.0	124
0.1	0	25	20	35	1.1	436	5	440	44	0.15	0.07	0.8	86
0.2	0	25	25	27	0.4	473	2	190	19	0.28	0.05	0.7	82
0.1	0	81	68	121	0.7	1436	6	590	59	0.60	0.14	1.5	294
tr	0	27	22	40	0.2	473	2	190	19	0.20	0.04	0.5	97
tr	0	25	20	35	1.1	390	7	290	29	0.14	0.07	0.8	72

Continued

FOODS, APPROXIMATE MEASURES, UNITS, AND WEIGHT (WEIGHT OF EDIBLE PORTION ONLY)		GRAMS	WATER (g)	FOOD ENERGY (CALORIES)	PROTEIN (g)	FAT (g)	FATTY ACIDS	
							SATURATED (g)	MONO- UNSATURATED (g)
FRUITS AND FRUIT JUICES—cont'd								
Papayas, raw, ½-in cubes	1 c	140	86	65	1	tr	0.1	0.1
Peaches								
Raw								
Whole, 2½-in diam., peeled, pitted (about 4 per lb with peels and pits)	1 peach	87	88	35	1	tr	tr	tr
Sliced	1 c	170	88	75	1	tr	tr	0.1
Canned, fruit and liquid								
Heavy syrup pack	1 c	256	79	190	1	tr	tr	0.1
	1 half	81	79	60	tr	tr	tr	tr
Juice pack	1 c	248	87	110	2	tr	tr	tr
	1 half	77	87	35	tr	tr	tr	tr
Dried								
Uncooked	1 c	160	32	380	6	1	0.1	0.4
Cooked, unsweetened, fruit and liquid	1 c	258	78	200	3	1	0.1	0.2
Frozen, sliced, sweetened	10 oz	284	75	265	2	tr	tr	0.1
	1 c	250	75	235	2	tr	tr	0.1
Pears								
Raw, with skin, cored								
Bartlett, 2½-in diam. (about 2½ per lb with cores and stems)	1 pear	166	84	100	1	1	tr	0.1
Bosc, 2½-in diam. (about 3 per lb with cores and stems)	1 pear	141	84	85	1	1	tr	0.1
D'Anjou, 3-in diam. (about 2 per lb with cores and stems)	1 pear	200	84	120	1	1	tr	0.2
Canned, fruit and liquid								
Heavy syrup pack	1 c	255	80	190	1	tr	tr	0.1
	1 half	79	80	60	tr	tr	tr	tr
Juice pack	1 c	248	86	125	1	tr	tr	tr
	1 half	77	86	40	tr	tr	tr	tr
Pineapple								
Raw, diced	1 c	155	87	75	1	1	tr	0.1
Canned, fruit and liquid								
Heavy syrup pack								
Crushed, chunks, tidbits	1 c	255	79	200	1	tr	tr	tr
Slices	1 slice	58	79	45	tr	tr	tr	tr
Juice pack								
Chunks or tidbits	1 c	250	84	150	1	tr	tr	tr
Slices	1 slice	58	84	35	tr	tr	tr	tr

tr = nutrient present in trace amounts.
[18]With added ascorbic acid.

NUTRIENTS IN INDICATED QUANTITY

POLY-UNSATURATED (g)	CHOLES-TEROL (mg)	CARBO-HYDRATE (g)	CALCIUM (mg)	PHOS-PHORUS (mg)	IRON (mg)	POTASSIUM (mg)	SODIUM (mg)	VITAMIN A VALUES		THIAMIN (mg)	RIBO-FLAVIN (mg)	NIACIN (mg)	ASCORBIC ACID (mg)
								IU	RE				
tr	0	17	35	12	0.3	247	9	400	40	0.04	0.04	0.5	92
tr	0	10	4	10	0.1	171	tr	470	47	0.01	0.04	0.9	6
0.1	0	19	9	20	0.2	335	tr	910	91	0.03	0.07	1.7	11
0.1	0	51	8	28	0.7	236	15	850	85	0.03	0.06	1.6	7
tr	0	16	2	9	0.2	75	5	270	27	0.01	0.02	0.5	2
tr	0	29	15	42	0.7	317	10	940	94	0.02	0.04	1.4	9
tr	0	9	5	13	0.2	99	3	290	29	0.01	0.01	0.4	3
0.6	0	98	45	190	6.5	1594	11	3460	346	tr	0.34	7.0	8
0.3	0	51	23	98	3.4	826	5	510	51	0.01	0.05	3.9	10
0.2	0	68	9	31	1.1	369	17	810	81	0.04	0.10	1.9	268[18]
0.2	0	60	8	28	0.9	325	15	710	71	0.03	0.09	1.6	236[18]
0.2	0	25	18	18	0.4	208	tr	30	3	0.03	0.07	0.2	7
0.1	0	21	16	16	0.4	176	tr	30	3	0.03	0.06	0.1	6
0.2	0	30	22	22	0.5	250	tr	40	4	0.04	0.08	0.2	8
0.1	0	49	13	18	0.6	166	13	10	1	0.03	0.06	0.6	3
tr	0	15	4	6	0.2	51	4	tr	tr	0.01	0.02	0.2	1
tr	0	32	22	30	0.7	238	10	10	1	0.03	0.03	0.5	4
tr	0	10	7	9	0.2	74	3	tr	tr	0.01	0.01	0.2	1
0.2	0	19	11	11	0.6	175	2	40	4	0.14	0.06	0.7	24
0.1	0	52	36	18	1.0	265	3	40	4	0.23	0.06	0.7	19
tr	0	12	8	4	0.2	60	1	10	1	0.05	0.01	0.2	4
0.1	0	39	35	15	0.7	305	3	100	10	0.24	0.05	0.7	24
tr	0	9	8	3	0.2	71	1	20	2	0.06	0.01	0.2	6

Continued

FOODS, APPROXIMATE MEASURES, UNITS, AND WEIGHT (WEIGHT OF EDIBLE PORTION ONLY)		GRAMS	WATER (g)	FOOD ENERGY (CALORIES)	PROTEIN (g)	FAT (g)	FATTY ACIDS	
							SATURATED (g)	MONO-UNSATURATED (g)
FRUITS AND FRUIT JUICES—cont'd								
Pineapple juice, unsweetened, canned	1 c	250	86	140	1	tr	tr	tr
Plantains, without peel								
Raw	1 plantain	179	65	220	2	1	0.3	0.1
Cooked, boiled, sliced	1 c	154	67	180	1	tr	0.1	tr
Plums, without pits								
Raw								
2⅛-in diam. (about 6½ per lb with pits)	1 plum	66	85	35	1	tr	tr	0.3
1½-in diam. (about 15 per lb with pits)	1 plum	28	85	15	tr	tr	tr	0.1
Canned, purple, fruit and liquid								
Heavy syrup pack	1 c	258	76	230	1	tr	tr	0.2
	3 plums	133	76	120	tr	tr	tr	0.1
Juice pack	1 c	252	84	145	1	tr	tr	tr
	3 plums	95	84	55	tr	tr	tr	tr
Prunes, dried								
Uncooked	4 extra large or 5 large prunes	49	32	115	1	tr	tr	0.2
Cooked, unsweetened, fruit and liquid	1 c	212	70	225	2	tr	tr	0.3
Prune juice, canned or bottled	1 c	256	81	180	2	tr	tr	0.1
Raisins, seedless								
Cup, not pressed down	1 c	145	15	435	5	1	0.2	tr
Packet, ½ oz (1½ tbsp)	1 packet	14	15	40	tr	tr	tr	tr
Raspberries								
Raw	1 c	123	87	60	1	1	tr	0.1
Frozen, sweetened	10 oz	284	73	295	2	tr	tr	tr
	1 c	250	73	255	2	tr	tr	tr
Rhubarb, cooked, added sugar	1 c	240	68	280	1	tr	tr	tr
Strawberries								
Raw, capped, whole	1 c	149	92	45	1	1	tr	0.1
Frozen, sweetened, sliced	10 oz	284	73	275	2	tr	tr	0.1
	1 c	255	73	245	1	tr	tr	tr
Tangerines								
Raw, without peel and seeds (2⅜-in diam., about 4 per lb, with peel and seeds)	1 tangerine	84	88	35	1	tr	tr	tr
Canned, light syrup, fruit and liquid	1 c	252	83	155	1	tr	tr	tr
Tangerine juice, canned, sweetened	1 c	249	87	125	1	tr	tr	tr

tr = nutrient present in trace amounts.

NUTRIENTS IN INDICATED QUANTITY

POLY-UNSATURATED (g)	CHOLES-TEROL (mg)	CARBO-HYDRATE (g)	CALCIUM (mg)	PHOS-PHORUS (mg)	IRON (mg)	POTASSIUM (mg)	SODIUM (mg)	VITAMIN A VALUES IU	RE	THIAMIN (mg)	RIBO-FLAVIN (mg)	NIACIN (mg)	ASCORBIC ACID (mg)
0.1	0	34	43	20	0.7	335	3	10	1	0.14	0.06	0.6	27
0.1	0	57	5	61	1.1	893	7	2020	202	0.09	0.10	1.2	33
0.1	0	48	3	43	0.9	716	8	1400	140	0.07	0.08	1.2	17
0.1	0	9	3	7	0.1	114	tr	210	21	0.03	0.06	0.3	6
tr	0	4	1	3	tr	48	tr	90	9	0.01	0.03	0.1	3
0.1	0	60	23	34	2.2	235	49	670	67	0.04	0.10	0.8	1
tr	0	31	12	17	1.1	121	25	340	34	0.02	0.05	0.4	1
tr	0	38	25	38	0.9	388	3	2540	254	0.06	0.15	1.2	7
tr	0	14	10	14	0.3	146	1	960	96	0.02	0.06	0.4	3
0.1	0	31	25	39	1.2	365	2	970	97	0.04	0.08	1.0	2
0.1	0	60	49	74	2.4	708	4	650	65	0.05	0.21	1.5	6
tr	0	45	31	64	3.0	707	10	10	1	0.04	0.18	2.0	10
0.2	0	115	71	141	3.0	1089	17	10	1	0.23	0.13	1.2	5
tr	0	11	7	14	0.3	105	2	tr	tr	0.02	0.01	0.1	tr
0.4	0	14	27	15	0.7	187	tr	160	16	0.04	0.11	1.1	31
0.3	0	74	43	48	1.8	324	3	170	17	0.05	0.13	0.7	47
0.2	0	65	38	43	1.6	285	3	150	15	0.05	0.11	0.6	41
0.1	0	75	348	19	0.5	230	2	170	17	0.04	0.06	0.5	8
0.3	0	10	21	28	0.6	247	1	40	4	0.03	0.10	0.3	84
0.2	0	74	31	37	1.7	278	9	70	7	0.05	0.14	1.1	118
0.2	0	66	28	33	1.5	250	8	60	6	0.04	0.13	1.0	106
tr	0	9	12	8	0.1	132	1	770	77	0.09	0.02	0.1	26
0.1	0	41	18	25	0.9	197	15	2120	212	0.13	0.11	1.1	50
0.1	0	30	45	35	0.5	443	2	1050	105	0.15	0.05	0.2	55

Continued

FOODS, APPROXIMATE MEASURES, UNITS, AND WEIGHT (WEIGHT OF EDIBLE PORTION ONLY)		GRAMS	WATER (g)	FOOD ENERGY (CALORIES)	PROTEIN (g)	FAT (g)	FATTY ACIDS	
							SATURATED (g)	MONO-UNSATURATED (g)
FRUITS AND FRUIT JUICES—cont'd								
Watermelon, raw, without rind and seeds								
Piece (4 by 8 in wedge with rind and seeds; 1/16 of 32 2/3-lb melon, 10 by 16 in)	1 piece	482	92	155	3	2	0.3	0.2
Diced	1 c	160	92	50	1	1	0.1	0.1
GRAIN PRODUCTS								
Bagels, plain or water, enriched, 3 1/2-in diam.[19]	1 bagel	68	29	200	7	2	0.3	0.5
Barley, pearled, light, uncooked	1 c	200	11	700	16	2	0.3	0.2
Biscuits, baking powder, 2-in diam. (enriched flour, vegetable shortening)								
From home recipe	1 biscuit	28	28	100	2	5	1.2	2.0
From mix	1 biscuit	28	29	95	2	3	0.8	1.4
From refrigerated dough	1 biscuit	20	30	65	1	2	0.6	0.9
Breadcrumbs, enriched								
Dry, grated	1 c	100	7	390	13	5	1.5	1.6
Soft. See White bread								
Breads								
Boston brown bread, canned, slice, 3 1/4 in by 1/2 in[20]	1 slice	45	45	95	2	1	0.3	0.1
Cracked-wheat bread (3/4 enriched wheat flour, 1/4 cracked wheat flour)[20]								
Loaf, 1 lb	1 loaf	454	35	1190	42	16	3.1	4.3
Slice (18 per loaf)	1 slice	25	35	65	2	1	0.2	0.2
Toasted	1 slice	21	26	65	2	1	0.2	0.2
French or Vienna bread, enriched[20]								
Loaf, 1 lb	1 loaf	454	34	1270	43	18	3.8	5.7
Slice								
French, 5 by 2 1/2 by 1 in	1 slice	35	34	100	3	1	0.3	0.4
Vienna, 4 3/4 by 4 by 1/2 in	1 slice	25	34	70	2	1	0.2	0.3
Italian bread, enriched								
Loaf, 1 lb	1 loaf	454	32	1255	41	4	0.6	0.3
Slice, 4 1/2 by 3 1/4 by 3/4 in	1 slice	30	32	85	3	tr	tr	tr
Mixed grain bread, enriched[20]								
Loaf, 1 lb	1 loaf	454	37	1165	45	17	3.2	4.1
Slice (18 per loaf)	1 slice	25	37	65	2	1	0.2	0.2
Toasted	1 slice	23	27	65	2	1	0.2	0.2

tr = nutrient present in trace amounts.
[19]Egg bagels have 44 mg cholesterol and 22 IU or 7 RE vitamin A per bagel.

NUTRIENTS IN INDICATED QUANTITY

POLY-UNSATURATED (g)	CHOLES-TEROL (mg)	CARBO-HYDRATE (g)	CALCIUM (mg)	PHOS-PHORUS (mg)	IRON (mg)	POTASSIUM (mg)	SODIUM (mg)	VITAMIN A VALUES		THIAMIN (mg)	RIBO-FLAVIN (mg)	NIACIN (mg)	ASCORBIC ACID (mg)
								IU	RE				
1.0	0	35	39	43	0.8	559	10	1760	176	0.39	0.10	1.0	46
0.3	0	11	13	14	0.3	186	3	590	59	0.13	0.03	0.3	15
0.7	0	38	29	46	1.8	50	245	0	0	0.26	0.20	2.4	0
0.9	0	158	32	378	4.2	320	6	0	0	0.24	0.10	6.2	0
1.3	tr	13	47	36	0.7	32	195	10	3	0.08	0.08	0.8	tr
0.9	tr	14	58	128	0.7	56	262	20	4	0.12	0.11	0.8	tr
0.6	1	10	4	79	0.5	18	249	0	0	0.08	0.05	0.7	0
1.0	5	73	122	141	4.1	152	736	0	0	0.35	0.35	4.8	0
0.1	3	21	41	72	0.9	131	113	0[21]	0[21]	0.06	0.04	0.7	0
5.7	0	227	295	581	12.1	608	1966	tr	tr	1.73	1.73	15.3	tr
0.3	0	12	16	32	0.7	34	106	tr	tr	0.10	0.09	0.8	tr
0.3	0	12	16	32	0.7	34	106	tr	tr	0.07	0.09	0.8	tr
5.9	0	230	499	386	14.0	409	2633	tr	tr	2.09	1.59	18.2	tr
0.5	0	18	39	30	1.1	32	203	tr	tr	0.16	0.12	1.4	tr
0.3	0	13	28	21	0.8	23	145	tr	tr	0.12	0.09	1.0	tr
1.6	0	256	77	350	12.7	336	2656	0	0	1.80	1.10	15.0	0
0.1	0	17	5	23	0.8	22	176	0	0	0.12	0.07	1.0	0
6.5	0	212	472	962	14.8	990	1870	tr	tr	1.77	1.73	18.9	tr
0.4	0	12	27	55	0.8	56	106	tr	tr	0.10	0.10	1.1	tr
0.4	0	12	27	55	0.8	56	106	tr	tr	0.08	0.10	1.1	tr

[20]Made with vegetable shortening.

[21]Made with white cornmeal. If made with yellow cornmeal, value is 32 IU or 3 RE.

Continued

FOODS, APPROXIMATE MEASURES, UNITS, AND WEIGHT (WEIGHT OF EDIBLE PORTION ONLY)		GRAMS	WATER (g)	FOOD ENERGY (CALORIES)	PROTEIN (g)	FAT (g)	FATTY ACIDS	
							SATURATED (g)	MONO- UNSATURATED (g)
GRAIN PRODUCTS—cont'd								
Breads—cont'd								
Oatmeal bread, enriched[22]								
Loaf, 1 lb	1 loaf	454	37	1145	38	20	3.7	7.1
Slice (18 per loaf)	1 slice	25	37	65	2	1	0.2	0.4
Toasted	1 slice	23	30	65	2	1	0.2	0.4
Pita bread, enriched, white, 6½-in diam.	1 pita	60	31	165	6	1	0.1	0.1
Pumpernickel (⅔ rye flour, ⅓ enriched wheat flour)[22]								
Loaf, 1 lb	1 loaf	454	37	1160	42	16	2.6	3.6
Slice, 5 by 4 by ⅜ in	1 slice	32	37	80	3	1	0.2	0.3
Toasted	1 slice	29	28	80	3	1	0.2	0.3
Raisin bread, enriched[22]								
Loaf, 1 lb	1 loaf	454	33	1260	37	18	4.1	6.5
Slice (18 per loaf)	1 slice	25	33	65	2	1	0.2	0.3
Toasted	1 slice	21	24	65	2	1	0.2	0.3
Rye bread, light (⅔ enriched wheat flour, ⅓ rye flour)[22]								
Loaf, 1lb	1 loaf	454	37	1190	38	17	3.3	5.2
Slice, 4¾ by 3¾ by ⁷⁄₁₆ in	1 slice	25	37	65	2	1	0.2	0.3
Toasted	1 slice	22	28	65	2	1	0.2	0.3
Wheat bread, enriched[22]								
Loaf, 1 lb	1 loaf	454	37	1160	43	19	3.9	7.3
Slice (18 per loaf)	1 slice	25	37	65	2	1	0.2	0.4
Toasted	1 slice	23	28	65	3	1	0.2	0.4
White bread, enriched[22]								
Loaf, 1 lb	1 loaf	454	37	1210	38	18	5.6	6.5
Slice (18 per loaf)	1 slice	25	37	65	2	1	0.3	0.4
Toasted	1 slice	22	28	65	2	1	0.3	0.4
Slice (22 per loaf)	1 slice	20	37	55	2	1	0.2	0.3
Toasted	1 slice	17	28	55	2	1	0.2	0.3
Cubes	1 c	30	37	80	2	1	0.4	0.4
Crumbs, soft	1 c	45	37	120	4	2	0.6	0.6
Whole-wheat bread[22]								
Loaf, 1 lb	1 loaf	454	38	1110	44	20	5.8	6.8
Slice (16 per loaf)	1 slice	28	38	70	3	1	0.4	0.4
Toasted	1 slice	25	29	70	3	1	0.4	0.4
Bread stuffing (from enriched bread), prepared from mix								
Dry type	1 c	140	33	500	9	31	6.1	13.3
Moist type	1 c	203	61	420	9	26	5.3	11.3
Buckwheat flour, light, sifted	1 c	98	12	340	6	1	0.2	0.4

tr = nutrient present in trace amounts.
[22]Made with vegetable shortening.

NUTRIENTS IN INDICATED QUANTITY													
POLY-UNSATURATED (g)	CHOLES-TEROL (mg)	CARBO-HYDRATE (g)	CALCIUM (mg)	PHOS-PHORUS (mg)	IRON (mg)	POTASSIUM (mg)	SODIUM (mg)	VITAMIN A VALUES IU	VITAMIN A VALUES RE	THIAMIN (mg)	RIBO-FLAVIN (mg)	NIACIN (mg)	ASCORBIC ACID (mg)
8.2	0	212	267	563	12.0	707	2231	0	0	2.09	1.20	15.4	0
0.5	0	12	15	31	0.7	39	124	0	0	0.12	0.07	0.9	0
0.5	0	12	15	31	0.7	39	124	0	0	0.09	0.07	0.9	0
0.4	0	33	49	60	1.4	71	339	0	0	0.27	0.12	2.2	0
6.4	0	218	322	990	12.4	1966	2461	0	0	1.54	2.36	15.0	0
0.5	0	16	23	71	0.9	141	177	0	0	0.11	0.17	1.1	0
0.5	0	16	23	71	0.9	141	177	0	0	0.09	0.17	1.1	0
6.7	0	239	463	395	14.1	1058	1657	tr	tr	1.50	2.81	18.6	tr
0.4	0	13	25	22	0.8	59	92	tr	tr	0.08	0.15	1.0	tr
0.4	0	13	25	22	0.8	59	92	tr	tr	0.06	0.15	1.0	tr
5.5	0	218	363	658	12.3	926	3164	0	0	1.86	1.45	15.0	0
0.3	0	12	20	36	0.7	51	175	0	0	0.10	0.08	0.8	0
0.3	0	12	20	36	0.7	51	175	0	0	0.08	0.08	0.8	0
4.5	0	213	572	835	15.8	627	2447	tr	tr	2.09	1.45	20.5	tr
0.3	0	12	32	47	0.9	35	138	tr	tr	0.12	0.08	1.2	tr
0.3	0	12	32	47	0.9	35	138	tr	tr	0.10	0.08	1.2	tr
4.2	0	222	572	490	12.9	508	2334	tr	tr	2.13	1.41	17.0	tr
0.2	0	12	32	27	0.7	28	129	tr	tr	0.12	0.08	0.9	tr
0.2	0	12	32	27	0.7	28	129	tr	tr	0.09	0.08	0.9	tr
0.2	0	10	25	21	0.6	22	101	tr	tr	0.09	0.06	0.7	tr
0.2	0	10	25	21	0.6	22	101	tr	tr	0.07	0.06	0.7	tr
0.3	0	15	38	32	0.9	34	154	tr	tr	0.14	0.09	1.1	tr
0.4	0	22	57	49	1.3	50	231	tr	tr	0.21	0.14	1.7	tr
5.2	0	206	327	1180	15.5	799	2887	tr	tr	1.59	0.95	17.4	tr
0.3	0	13	20	74	1.0	50	180	tr	tr	0.10	0.06	1.1	tr
0.3	0	13	20	74	1.0	50	180	tr	tr	0.08	0.06	1.1	tr
9.6	0	50	92	136	2.2	126	1254	910	273	0.17	0.20	2.5	0
8.0	67	40	81	134	2.0	118	1023	850	256	0.10	0.18	1.6	0
0.4	0	78	11	86	1.0	314	2	0	0	0.08	0.04	0.4	0

Continued

FOODS, APPROXIMATE MEASURES, UNITS, AND WEIGHT (WEIGHT OF EDIBLE PORTION ONLY)		GRAMS	WATER (g)	FOOD ENERGY (CALORIES)	PROTEIN (g)	FAT (g)	FATTY ACIDS	
							SATURATED (g)	MONO-UNSATURATED (g)
GRAIN PRODUCTS—cont'd								
Bulgur, uncooked	1 c	170	10	600	19	3	1.2	0.3
Cakes prepared from cake mixes with enriched flour[23]								
Angel food								
Whole cake, 9¾-in diam. tube cake	1 cake	635	38	1510	38	2	0.4	0.2
Piece, 1/12 of cake	1 piece	53	38	125	3	tr	tr	tr
Coffee cake, crumb								
Whole cake, 7¾ by 5⅝ by 1¼ in	1 cake	430	30	1385	27	41	11.8	16.7
Piece, 1/6 of cake	1 piece	72	30	230	5	7	2.0	2.8
Devil's food with chocolate frosting								
Whole, 2-layer cake, 8- or 9-in diam.	1 cake	1107	24	3755	49	136	55.6	51.4
Piece, 1/16 of cake	1 piece	69	24	235	3	8	3.5	3.2
Cupcake, 2½-in diam.	1 cupcake	35	24	120	2	4	1.8	1.6
Gingerbread								
Whole cake, 8 in square	1 cake	570	37	1575	18	39	9.6	16.4
Piece, 1/9 of cake	1 piece	63	37	175	2	4	1.1	1.8
Cheesecake								
Whole cake, 9-in diam.	1 cake	1110	46	3350	60	213	119.9	65.5
Piece, 1/12 of cake	1 piece	92	46	280	5	18	9.9	5.4
Cookies made with enriched flour								
Brownies with nuts								
Commercial, with frosting, 1½ by 1¾ by ⅞ in	1 brownie	25	13	100	1	4	1.6	2.0
From home recipe, 1¾ by 1¾ by ⅞ in[24]	1 brownie	20	10	95	1	6	1.4	2.8
Chocolate chip								
Commercial, 2¼-in diam., ⅜ in thick	4 cookies	42	4	180	2	9	2.9	3.1
Cornmeal								
Whole-ground, unbolted, dry form	1 c	122	12	435	11	5	0.5	1.1
Bolted (nearly whole-grain), dry form	1 c	122	12	440	11	4	0.5	0.9
Degermed, enriched								
Dry form	1 c	138	12	500	11	2	0.2	0.4
Cooked	1 c	240	88	120	3	tr	tr	0.1

tr = nutrient present in trace amounts.
[23]Excepting angel food cake, cakes made from mixes containing vegetable shortening and frostings made with margarine.
[24]Made with vegetable oil.

NUTRIENTS IN INDICATED QUANTITY

POLY-UNSATURATED (g)	CHOLES-TEROL (mg)	CARBO-HYDRATE (g)	CALCIUM (mg)	PHOS-PHORUS (mg)	IRON (mg)	POTASSIUM (mg)	SODIUM (mg)	VITAMIN A VALUES IU	VITAMIN A VALUES RE	THIAMIN (mg)	RIBO-FLAVIN (mg)	NIACIN (mg)	ASCORBIC ACID (mg)
1.2	0	129	49	575	9.5	389	7	0	0	0.48	0.24	7.7	0
1.0	0	342	527	1086	2.7	845	3226	0	0	0.32	1.27	1.6	0
0.1	0	29	44	91	0.2	71	269	0	0	0.03	0.11	0.1	0
9.6	279	225	262	748	7.3	469	1853	690	194	0.82	0.90	7.7	1
1.6	47	38	44	125	1.2	78	310	120	32	0.14	0.15	1.3	tr
19.7	598	645	653	1162	22.1	1439	2900	1660	498	1.11	1.66	10.0	1
1.2	37	40	41	72	1.4	90	181	100	31	0.07	0.10	0.6	tr
0.6	19	20	21	37	0.7	46	92	50	16	0.04	0.05	0.3	tr
10.5	6	291	513	570	10.8	1562	1733	0	0	0.86	1.03	7.4	1
1.2	1	32	57	63	1.2	173	192	0	0	0.09	0.11	0.8	tr
14.4	2053	317	622	977	5.3	1088	2464	2820	833	0.33	1.44	5.1	56
1.2	170	26	52	81	0.4	90	204	230	69	0.03	0.12	0.4	5
0.6	14	16	13	26	0.6	50	59	70	18	0.08	0.07	0.3	tr
1.2	18	11	9	26	0.4	35	51	20	6	0.05	0.05	0.3	tr
2.6	5	28	13	41	0.8	68	140	50	15	0.10	0.23	1.0	tr
2.5	0	90	24	312	2.2	346	1	620	62	0.46	0.13	2.4	0
2.2	0	91	21	272	2.2	303	1	590	59	0.37	0.10	2.3	0
0.9	0	108	8	137	5.9	166	1	610	61	0.61	0.36	4.8	0
0.2	0	26	2	34	1.4	38	0	140	14	0.14	0.10	1.2	0

Continued

FOODS, APPROXIMATE MEASURES, UNITS, AND WEIGHT (WEIGHT OF EDIBLE PORTION ONLY)		GRAMS	WATER (g)	FOOD ENERGY (CALORIES)	PROTEIN (g)	FAT (g)	FATTY ACIDS	
							SATURATED (g)	MONO-UNSATURATED (g)
GRAIN PRODUCTS—cont'd								
Crackers[25]								
Cheese								
Plain, 1 in square	10 crackers	10	4	50	1	3	0.9	1.2
Sandwich type (peanut butter)	1 sandwich	8	3	40	1	2	0.4	0.8
Graham, plain, 2½ in square	2 crackers	14	5	60	1	1	0.4	0.6
Melba toast, plain	1 piece	5	4	20	1	tr	0.1	0.1
Rye wafers, whole-grain, 1⅞ by 3½ in	2 wafers	14	5	55	1	1	0.3	0.4
Saltines[26]	4 crackers	12	4	50	1	1	0.5	0.4
Snack-type, standard	1 round cracker	3	3	15	tr	1	0.2	0.4
Wheat, thin	4 crackers	8	3	35	1	1	0.5	0.5
Whole-wheat wafers	2 crackers	8	4	35	1	2	0.5	0.6
Croissants, made with enriched flour, 4½ by 4 by 1¾ in	1 croissant	57	22	235	5	12	3.5	6.7
Danish pastry, made with enriched flour								
Plain without fruit or nuts								
Packaged ring, 12 oz	1 ring	340	27	1305	21	71	21.8	28.6
Round piece, about 4¼-in diam., 1 in high	1 pastry	57	27	220	4	12	3.6	4.8
Ounce	1 oz	28	27	110	2	6	1.8	2.4
Fruit, round piece	1 pastry	65	30	235	4	13	3.9	5.2
Doughnuts, made with enriched flour								
Cake type, plain, 3¼-in diam., 1 in high	1 doughnut	50	21	210	3	12	2.8	5.0
Yeast-leavened, glazed, 3¾-in diam., 1¼ in high	1 doughnut	60	27	235	4	13	5.2	5.5
English muffins, plain, enriched	1 muffin	57	42	140	5	1	0.3	0.2
Toasted	1 muffin	50	29	140	5	1	0.3	0.2
Pies, piecrust made with enriched flour, vegetable shortening, 9-in diam.								
Apple								
Whole	1 pie	945	48	2420	21	105	27.4	44.4
Piece, ⅙ of pie	1 piece	158	48	405	3	18	4.6	7.4
Blueberry								
Whole	1 pie	945	51	2285	23	102	25.5	44.4
Piece, ⅙ of pie	1 piece	158	51	380	4	17	4.3	7.4

tr = nutrient present in trace amounts.
[25]Crackers made with enriched flour except for rye wafers and whole wheat wafers.
[26]Made with lard.

NUTRIENTS IN INDICATED QUANTITY

POLY-UNSATURATED (g)	CHOLES-TEROL (mg)	CARBO-HYDRATE (g)	CALCIUM (mg)	PHOS-PHORUS (mg)	IRON (mg)	POTASSIUM (mg)	SODIUM (mg)	VITAMIN A VALUES IU	VITAMIN A VALUES RE	THIAMIN (mg)	RIBO-FLAVIN (mg)	NIACIN (mg)	ASCORBIC ACID (mg)
0.3	6	6	11	17	0.3	17	112	20	5	0.05	0.04	0.4	0
0.3	1	5	7	25	0.3	17	90	tr	tr	0.04	0.03	0.6	0
0.4	0	11	6	20	0.4	36	86	0	0	0.02	0.03	0.6	0
0.1	0	4	6	10	0.1	11	44	0	0	0.01	0.01	0.1	0
0.3	0	10	7	44	0.5	65	115	0	0	0.06	0.03	0.5	0
0.2	4	9	3	12	0.5	17	165	0	0	0.06	0.05	0.6	0
0.1	0	2	3	6	0.1	4	30	tr	tr	0.01	0.01	0.1	0
0.4	0	5	3	15	0.3	17	69	tr	tr	0.04	0.03	0.4	0
0.4	0	5	3	22	0.2	31	59	0	0	0.02	0.03	0.4	0
1.4	13	27	20	64	2.1	68	452	50	13	0.17	0.13	1.3	0
15.6	292	152	360	347	6.5	316	1302	360	99	0.95	1.02	8.5	tr
2.6	49	26	60	58	1.1	53	218	60	17	0.16	0.17	1.4	tr
1.3	24	13	30	29	0.5	26	109	30	8	0.08	0.09	0.7	tr
2.9	56	28	17	80	1.3	57	233	40	11	0.16	0.14	1.4	tr
3.0	20	24	22	111	1.0	58	192	20	5	0.12	0.12	1.1	tr
0.9	21	26	17	55	1.4	64	222	tr	tr	0.28	0.12	1.8	0
0.3	0	27	96	67	1.7	331	378	0	0	0.26	0.19	2.2	0
0.3	0	27	96	67	1.7	331	378	0	0	0.23	0.19	2.2	0
26.5	0	360	76	208	9.5	756	2844	280	28	1.04	0.76	9.5	9
4.4	0	60	13	35	1.6	126	476	50	5	0.17	0.13	1.6	2
27.4	0	330	104	217	12.3	945	2533	850	85	1.04	0.85	10.4	38
4.6	0	55	17	36	2.1	158	423	140	14	0.17	0.14	1.7	6

Continued

FOODS, APPROXIMATE MEASURES, UNITS, AND WEIGHT (WEIGHT OF EDIBLE PORTION ONLY)		GRAMS	WATER (g)	FOOD ENERGY (CALORIES)	PROTEIN (g)	FAT (g)	FATTY ACIDS	
							SATURATED (g)	MONO-UNSATURATED (g)
GRAIN PRODUCTS—cont'd								
Pies—cont'd								
Cherry								
Whole	1 pie	945	47	2465	25	107	28.4	46.3
Piece, ⅙ of pie	1 piece	158	47	410	4	18	4.7	7.7
Creme								
Whole	1 pie	910	43	2710	20	139	90.1	23.7
Piece, ⅙ of pie	1 piece	152	43	455	3	23	15.0	4.0
Custard								
Whole	1 pie	910	58	1985	56	101	33.7	40.0
Piece, ⅙ of pie	1 piece	152	58	330	9	17	5.6	6.7
Lemon meringue								
Whole	1 pie	840	47	2140	31	86	26.0	34.4
Piece, ⅙ of pie	1 piece	140	47	355	5	14	4.3	5.7
Peach								
Whole	1 pie	945	48	2410	24	101	24.6	43.5
Piece, ⅙ of pie	1 piece	158	48	405	4	17	4.1	7.3
Pecan								
Whole	1 pie	825	20	3450	42	189	28.1	101.5
Piece, ⅙ of pie	1 piece	138	20	575	7	32	4.7	17.0
Pumpkin								
Whole	1 pie	910	59	1920	36	102	38.2	40.0
Piece, ⅙ of pie	1 piece	152	59	320	6	17	6.4	6.7
Pies, fried								
Apple	1 pie	85	43	255	2	14	5.8	6.6
Cherry	1 pie	85	42	250	2	14	5.8	6.7
Popcorn, popped								
Air-popped, unsalted	1 c	8	4	30	1	tr	tr	0.1
Popped in vegetable oil, salted	1 c	11	3	55	1	3	0.5	1.4
Sugar syrup coated	1 c	35	4	135	2	1	0.1	0.3
Pretzels, made with enriched flour								
Stick, 2¼ in long	10 pretzels	3	3	10	tr	tr	tr	tr
Twisted, dutch, 2¾ by 2⅝ in	1 pretzel	16	3	65	2	1	0.1	0.2
Twisted, thin, 3¼ by 2¼ by ¼ in	10 pretzels	60	3	240	6	2	0.4	0.8
Rice								
Brown, cooked, served hot	1 c	195	70	230	5	1	0.3	0.3
White, enriched								
Commercial varieties, all types								
Raw	1 c	185	12	670	12	1	0.2	0.2
Cooked, served hot	1 c	205	73	225	4	tr	0.1	0.1
Wheat flours								
All-purpose or family flour, enriched								
Sifted, spooned	1 c	115	12	420	12	1	0.2	0.1
Unsifted, spooned	1 c	125	12	455	13	1	0.2	0.1

tr = nutrient present in trace amounts.

NUTRIENTS IN INDICATED QUANTITY

POLY-UNSATURATED (g)	CHOLES-TEROL (mg)	CARBO-HYDRATE (g)	CALCIUM (mg)	PHOS-PHORUS (mg)	IRON (mg)	POTASSIUM (mg)	SODIUM (mg)	VITAMIN A VALUES IU	RE	THIAMIN (mg)	RIBO-FLAVIN (mg)	NIACIN (mg)	ASCORBIC ACID (mg)
27.4	0	363	132	236	9.5	992	2873	4160	416	1.13	0.85	9.5	0
4.6	0	61	22	40	1.6	166	480	700	70	0.19	0.14	1.6	0
6.4	46	351	273	919	6.8	796	2207	1250	391	0.36	0.89	6.4	0
1.1	8	59	46	154	1.1	133	369	210	65	0.06	0.15	1.1	0
19.1	1010	213	874	1028	9.1	1247	2612	2090	573	0.82	1.91	5.5	0
3.2	169	36	146	172	1.5	208	436	350	96	0.14	0.32	0.9	0
17.6	857	317	118	412	8.4	420	2369	1430	395	0.59	0.84	5.0	25
2.9	143	53	20	69	1.4	70	395	240	66	0.10	0.14	0.8	4
26.5	0	361	95	274	11.3	1408	2533	6900	690	1.04	0.95	14.2	28
4.4	0	60	16	46	1.9	235	423	1150	115	0.17	0.16	2.4	5
47.0	569	423	388	850	27.2	1015	1823	1320	322	1.82	0.99	6.6	0
7.9	95	71	65	142	4.6	170	305	220	54	0.30	0.17	1.1	0
18.2	655	223	464	628	8.2	1456	1947	22,480	2493	0.82	1.27	7.3	0
3.0	109	37	78	105	1.4	243	325	3750	416	0.14	0.21	1.2	0
0.6	14	31	12	34	0.9	42	326	30	3	0.09	0.06	1.0	1
0.6	13	32	11	41	0.7	61	371	190	19	0.06	0.06	0.6	1
0.2	0	6	1	22	0.2	20	tr	10	1	0.03	0.01	0.2	0
1.2	0	6	3	31	0.3	19	86	20	2	0.01	0.02	0.1	0
0.6	0	30	2	47	0.5	90	tr	30	3	0.13	0.02	0.4	0
tr	0	2	1	3	0.1	3	48	0	0	0.01	0.01	0.1	0
0.2	0	13	4	15	0.3	16	258	0	0	0.05	0.04	0.7	0
0.6	0	48	16	55	1.2	61	966	0	0	0.19	0.15	2.6	0
0.4	0	50	23	142	1.0	137	0	0	0	0.18	0.04	2.7	0
0.3	0	149	44	174	5.4	170	9	0	0	0.81	0.06	6.5	0
0.1	0	50	21	57	1.8	57	0	0	0	0.23	0.02	2.1	0
0.5	0	88	18	100	5.1	109	2	0	0	0.73	0.46	6.1	0
0.5	0	95	20	109	5.5	119	3	0	0	0.80	0.50	6.6	0

Continued

FOODS, APPROXIMATE MEASURES, UNITS, AND WEIGHT (WEIGHT OF EDIBLE PORTION ONLY)		GRAMS	WATER (g)	FOOD ENERGY (CALORIES)	PROTEIN (g)	FAT (g)	FATTY ACIDS	
							SATURATED (g)	MONO-UNSATURATED (g)
GRAIN PRODUCTS—cont'd								
Wheat flours—cont'd								
Cake or pastry flour, enriched, sifted, spooned	1 c	96	12	350	7	1	0.1	0.1
Self-rising, enriched, unsifted, spooned	1 c	125	12	440	12	1	0.2	0.1
Whole wheat, from hard wheats, stirred	1 c	120	12	400	16	2	0.3	0.3
LEGUMES, NUTS, AND SEEDS								
Almonds, shelled								
Slivered, packed	1 c	135	4	795	27	70	6.7	45.8
Whole	1 oz	28	4	165	6	15	1.4	9.6
Beans, dry								
Cooked, drained								
Black	1 c	171	66	225	15	1	0.1	0.1
Great Northern	1 c	180	69	210	14	1	0.1	0.1
Lima	1 c	190	64	260	16	1	0.2	0.1
Pea (navy)	1 c	190	69	225	15	1	0.1	0.1
Pinto	1 c	180	65	265	15	1	0.1	0.1
Canned, solids and liquid								
White with								
Frankfurters (sliced)	1 c	255	71	365	19	18	7.4	8.8
Pork and tomato sauce	1 c	255	71	310	16	7	2.4	2.7
Pork and sweet sauce	1 c	255	66	385	16	12	4.3	4.9
Red kidney	1 c	255	76	230	15	1	0.1	0.1
Black-eyed peas, dry, cooked (with residual cooking liquid)	1 c	250	80	190	13	1	0.2	tr
Brazil nuts, shelled	1 oz	28	3	185	4	19	4.6	6.5
Carob flour	1 c	140	3	255	6	tr	tr	0.1
Cashew nuts, salted								
Dry roasted	1 c	137	2	785	21	63	12.5	37.4
	1 oz	28	2	165	4	13	2.6	7.7
Roasted in oil	1 c	130	4	750	21	63	12.4	36.9
	1 oz	28	4	165	5	14	2.7	8.1
Chestnuts, European (Italian), roasted, shelled	1 c	143	40	350	5	3	0.6	1.1
Chickpeas, cooked, drained	1 c	163	60	270	15	4	0.4	0.9
Coconut								
Raw								
Piece, about 2 by 2 by ½ in	1 piece	45	47	160	1	15	13.4	0.6
Shredded or grated	1 c	80	47	285	3	27	23.8	1.1
Dried, sweetened, shredded	1 c	93	13	470	3	33	29.3	1.4

tr = nutrient present in trace amounts.
[27]Cashews without salt contain 21 mg sodium per cup or 4 mg per oz.

NUTRIENTS IN INDICATED QUANTITY

POLY-UNSATURATED (g)	CHOLES-TEROL (mg)	CARBO-HYDRATE (g)	CALCIUM (mg)	PHOS-PHORUS (mg)	IRON (mg)	POTASSIUM (mg)	SODIUM (mg)	VITAMIN A VALUES IU	RE	THIAMIN (mg)	RIBO-FLAVIN (mg)	NIACIN (mg)	ASCORBIC ACID (mg)
0.3	0	76	16	70	4.2	91	2	0	0	0.58	0.38	5.1	0
0.5	0	93	331	583	5.5	113	1349	0	0	0.80	0.50	6.6	0
1.1	0	85	49	446	5.2	444	4	0	0	0.66	0.14	5.2	0
14.8	0	28	359	702	4.9	988	15	0	0	0.28	1.05	4.5	1
3.1	0	6	75	147	1.0	208	3	0	0	0.06	0.22	1.0	tr
0.5	0	41	47	239	2.9	608	1	tr	tr	0.43	0.05	0.9	0
0.6	0	38	90	266	4.9	749	13	0	0	0.25	0.13	1.3	0
0.5	0	49	55	293	5.9	1163	4	0	0	0.25	0.11	1.3	0
0.7	0	40	95	281	5.1	790	13	0	0	0.27	0.13	1.3	0
0.5	0	49	86	296	5.4	882	3	tr	tr	0.33	0.16	0.7	0
0.7	30	32	94	303	4.8	668	1374	330	33	0.18	0.15	3.3	tr
0.7	10	48	138	235	4.6	536	1181	330	33	0.20	0.08	1.5	5
1.2	10	54	161	291	5.9	536	969	330	33	0.15	0.10	1.3	5
0.6	0	42	74	278	4.6	673	968	10	1	0.13	0.10	1.5	0
0.3	0	35	43	238	3.3	573	20	30	3	0.40	0.10	1.0	0
6.8	0	4	50	170	1.0	170	1	tr	tr	0.28	0.03	0.5	tr
0.1	0	126	390	102	5.7	1275	24	tr	tr	0.07	0.07	2.2	tr
10.7	0	45	62	671	8.2	774	877[27]	0	0	0.27	0.27	1.9	0
2.2	0	9	13	139	1.7	160	181[27]	0	0	0.06	0.06	0.4	0
10.6	0	37	53	554	5.3	689	814[28]	0	0	0.55	0.23	2.3	0
2.3	0	8	12	121	1.2	150	177[28]	0	0	0.12	0.05	0.5	0
1.2	0	76	41	153	1.3	847	3	30	3	0.35	0.25	1.9	37
1.9	0	45	80	273	4.9	475	11	tr	tr	0.18	0.09	0.9	0
0.2	0	7	6	51	1.1	160	9	0	0	0.03	0.01	0.2	1
0.3	0	12	11	90	1.9	285	16	0	0	0.05	0.02	0.4	3
0.4	0	44	14	99	1.8	313	244	0	0	0.03	0.02	0.4	1

[28]Cashews without salt contain 22 mg sodium per cup or 5 mg per oz.

Continued

FOODS, APPROXIMATE MEASURES, UNITS, AND WEIGHT (WEIGHT OF EDIBLE PORTION ONLY)		GRAMS	WATER (g)	FOOD ENERGY (CALORIES)	PROTEIN (g)	FAT (g)	FATTY ACIDS	
							SATURATED (g)	MONO-UNSATURATED (g)
LEGUMES, NUTS, AND SEEDS—cont'd								
Filberts (hazelnuts), chopped	1 c	115	5	725	15	72	5.3	56.5
	1 oz	28	5	180	4	18	1.3	13.9
Lentils, dry, cooked	1 c	200	72	215	16	1	0.1	0.2
Macadamia nuts, roasted in oil, salted	1 c	134	2	960	10	103	15.4	80.9
	1 oz	28	2	205	2	22	3.2	17.1
Mixed nuts, with peanuts, salted								
Dry roasted	1 oz	28	2	170	5	15	2.0	8.9
Roasted in oil	1 oz	28	2	175	5	16	2.5	9.0
Peanuts, roasted in oil, salted	1 c	145	2	840	39	71	9.9	35.5
	1 oz	28	2	165	8	14	1.9	6.9
Peanut butter	1 tbsp	16	1	95	5	8	1.4	4.0
Peas, split, dry, cooked	1 c	200	70	230	16	1	0.1	0.1
Pecans, halves	1 c	108	5	720	8	73	5.9	45.5
	1 oz	28	5	190	2	19	1.5	12.0
Pine nuts (pinyons), shelled	1 oz	28	6	160	3	17	2.7	6.5
Pistachio nuts, dried, shelled	1 oz	28	4	165	6	14	1.7	9.3
Pumpkin and squash kernels, dry, hulled	1 oz	28	7	155	7	13	2.5	4.0
Refried beans, canned	1 c	290	72	295	18	3	0.4	0.6
Sesame seeds, dry, hulled	1 tbsp	8	5	45	2	4	0.6	1.7
Soybeans, dry, cooked, drained	1 c	180	71	235	20	10	1.3	1.9
Soy products								
Miso	1 c	276	53	470	29	13	1.8	2.6
Tofu, piece 2½ by 2¾ by 1 in	1 piece	120	85	85	9	5	0.7	1.0
Sunflower seeds, dry, hulled	1 oz	28	5	160	6	14	1.5	2.7
Tahini	1 tbsp	15	3	90	3	8	1.1	3.0
Walnuts								
Black, chopped	1 c	125	4	760	30	71	4.5	15.9
	1 oz	28	4	170	7	16	1.0	3.6
English or Persian, pieces or chips	1 c	120	4	770	17	74	6.7	17.0
	1 oz	28	4	180	4	18	1.6	4.0
MEAT AND MEAT PRODUCTS								
Beef, cooked[32]								
Cuts braised, simmered, or pot roasted								
Relatively fat such as chuck blade								
Lean and fat, piece, 2½ by 2½ by ¾ in	3 oz	85	43	325	22	26	10.8	11.7
Lean only	2.2 oz	62	53	170	19	9	3.9	4.2

tr = nutrient present in trace amounts.
[29]Macadamia nuts without salt contain 9 mg sodium per cup or 2 mg per oz.
[30]Mixed nuts without salt contain 3 mg sodium per oz.

NUTRIENTS IN INDICATED QUANTITY

POLY-UNSATURATED (g)	CHOLES-TEROL (mg)	CARBO-HYDRATE (g)	CALCIUM (mg)	PHOS-PHORUS (mg)	IRON (mg)	POTASSIUM (mg)	SODIUM (mg)	VITAMIN A VALUES		THIAMIN (mg)	RIBO-FLAVIN (mg)	NIACIN (mg)	ASCORBIC ACID (mg)
								IU	RE				
6.9	0	18	216	359	3.8	512	3	80	8	0.58	0.13	1.3	1
1.7	0	4	53	88	0.9	126	1	20	2	0.14	0.03	0.3	tr
0.5	0	38	50	238	4.2	498	26	40	4	0.14	0.12	1.2	0
1.8	0	17	60	268	2.4	441	348[29]	10	1	0.29	0.15	2.7	0
0.4	0	4	13	57	0.5	93	74[29]	tr	tr	0.06	0.03	0.6	0
3.1	0	7	20	123	1.0	169	190[30]	tr	tr	0.06	0.06	1.3	0
3.8	0	6	31	131	0.9	165	185[30]	10	1	0.14	0.06	1.4	tr
22.6	0	27	125	734	2.8	1019	626[31]	0	0	0.42	0.15	21.5	0
4.4	0	5	24	143	0.5	199	122[31]	0	0	0.08	0.03	4.2	0
2.5	0	3	5	60	0.3	110	75	0	0	0.02	0.02	2.2	0
0.3	0	42	22	178	3.4	592	26	80	8	0.30	0.18	1.8	0
18.1	0	20	39	314	2.3	423	1	140	14	0.92	0.14	1.0	2
4.7	0	5	10	83	0.6	111	tr	40	4	0.24	0.04	0.3	1
7.3	0	5	2	10	0.9	178	20	10	1	0.35	0.06	1.2	1
2.1	0	7	38	143	1.9	310	2	70	7	0.23	0.05	0.3	tr
5.9	0	5	12	333	4.2	229	5	110	11	0.06	0.09	0.5	tr
1.4	0	51	141	245	5.1	1141	1228	0	0	0.14	0.16	1.4	17
1.9	0	1	11	62	0.6	33	3	10	1	0.06	0.01	0.4	0
5.3	0	19	131	322	4.9	972	4	50	5	0.38	0.16	1.1	0
7.3	0	65	188	853	4.7	922	8142	110	11	0.17	0.28	0.8	0
2.9	0	3	108	151	2.3	50	8	0	0	0.07	0.04	0.1	0
9.3	0	5	33	200	1.9	195	1	10	1	0.65	0.07	1.3	tr
3.5	0	3	21	119	0.7	69	5	10	1	0.24	0.02	0.8	1
46.9	0	15	73	580	3.8	655	1	370	37	0.27	0.14	0.9	tr
10.6	0	3	16	132	0.9	149	tr	80	8	0.06	0.03	0.2	tr
47.0	0	22	113	380	2.9	602	12	150	15	0.46	0.18	1.3	4
11.1	0	5	27	90	0.7	142	3	40	4	0.11	0.04	0.3	1
0.9	87	0	11	163	2.5	163	53	tr	tr	0.06	0.19	2.0	0
0.3	66	0	8	146	2.3	163	44	tr	tr	0.05	0.17	1.7	0

[31]Peanuts without salt contain 22 mg sodium per cup or 4 mg per oz.
[32]Outer layer of fat was removed to within approximately ½ in of the lean. Deposits of fat within the cut were not removed.

Continued

FOODS, APPROXIMATE MEASURES, UNITS, AND WEIGHT (WEIGHT OF EDIBLE PORTION ONLY)	GRAMS	WATER (g)	FOOD ENERGY (CALORIES)	PROTEIN (g)	FAT (g)	FATTY ACIDS SATURATED (g)	FATTY ACIDS MONO-UNSATURATED (g)
MEAT AND MEAT PRODUCTS—cont'd							
Beef, cooked[32]—cont'd							
Relatively lean, such as bottom round							
Lean and fat, piece, 4⅛ by 2¼ by ½ in	3 oz	85	54	220	25	13	4.8	5.7
Lean only	2.8 oz	78	57	175	25	8	2.7	3.4
Ground beef, broiled, patty, 3 by ⅝ in							
Lean	3 oz	85	56	230	21	16	6.2	6.9
Regular	3 oz	85	54	245	20	18	6.9	7.7
Heart, lean, braised	3 oz	85	65	150	24	5	1.2	0.8
Liver, fried, slice, 6½ by 2⅜ by ⅜ in[33]	3 oz	85	56	185	23	7	2.5	3.6
Roast, oven cooked, no liquid added							
Relatively fat, such as rib							
Lean and fat, 2 pieces, 4⅛ by 2¼ by ¼ in	3 oz	85	46	315	19	26	10.8	11.4
Lean only	2.2 oz	61	57	150	17	9	3.6	3.7
Relatively lean, such as eye of round							
Lean and fat, 2 pieces, 2½ by 2½ by ⅜ in	3 oz	85	57	205	23	12	4.9	5.4
Lean only	2.6 oz	75	63	135	22	5	1.9	2.1
Steak							
Sirloin, broiled							
Lean and fat, piece, 2½ by 2½ by ¾ in	3 oz	85	53	240	23	15	6.4	6.9
Lean only from item 587	2.5 oz	72	59	150	22	6	2.6	2.8
Beef, canned, corned	3 oz	85	59	185	22	10	4.2	4.9
Beef, dried, chipped	2.5 oz	72	48	145	24	4	1.8	2.0
Lamb, cooked							
Chops, (3 per lb with bone)							
Arm, braised							
Lean and fat	2.2 oz	63	44	220	20	15	6.9	6.0
Lean only	1.7 oz	48	49	135	17	7	2.9	2.6
Loin, broiled							
Lean and fat	2.8 oz	80	54	235	22	16	7.3	6.4
Lean only	2.3 oz	64	61	140	19	6	2.6	2.4
Leg, roasted							
Lean and fat, 2 pieces, 4⅛ by 2¼ by ¼ in	3 oz	85	59	205	22	13	5.6	4.9
Lean only	2.6 oz	73	64	140	20	6	2.4	2.2

tr = nutrient present in trace amounts.

[32]Outer layer of fat was removed to within approximately ½ in of the lean. Deposits of fat within the cut were not removed.

[33]Fried in vegetable shortening.

[34]Value varies widely.

POLY-UNSATURATED (g)	CHOLES-TEROL (mg)	CARBO-HYDRATE (g)	CALCIUM (mg)	PHOS-PHORUS (mg)	IRON (mg)	POTASSIUM (mg)	SODIUM (mg)	VITAMIN A VALUES		THIAMIN (mg)	RIBO-FLAVIN (mg)	NIACIN (mg)	ASCORBIC ACID (mg)
								IU	RE				
0.5	81	0	5	217	2.8	248	43	tr	tr	0.06	0.21	3.3	0
0.3	75	0	4	212	2.7	240	40	tr	tr	0.06	0.20	3.3	0
0.6	74	0	9	134	1.8	256	65	tr	tr	0.04	0.18	4.4	0
0.7	76	0	9	144	2.1	248	70	tr	tr	0.03	0.16	4.9	0
1.6	164	0	5	213	6.4	198	54	tr	tr	0.12	1.31	3.4	5
1.3	410	7	9	392	5.3	309	90	30,690[34]	9120[34]	0.18	3.52	12.3	23
0.9	72	0	8	145	2.0	246	54	tr	tr	0.06	0.16	3.1	0
0.3	49	0	5	127	1.7	218	45	tr	tr	0.05	0.13	2.7	0
0.5	62	0	5	177	1.6	308	50	tr	tr	0.07	0.14	3.0	0
0.2	52	0	3	170	1.5	297	46	tr	tr	0.07	0.13	2.8	0
0.6	77	0	9	186	2.6	306	53	tr	tr	0.10	0.23	3.3	0
0.3	64	0	8	176	2.4	290	48	tr	tr	0.09	0.22	3.1	0
0.4	80	0	17	90	3.7	51	802	tr	tr	0.02	0.20	2.9	0
0.2	46	0	14	287	2.3	142	3053	tr	tr	0.05	0.23	2.7	0
0.9	77	0	16	132	1.5	195	46	tr	tr	0.04	0.16	4.4	0
0.4	59	0	12	111	1.3	162	36	tr	tr	0.03	0.13	3.0	0
1.0	78	0	16	162	1.4	272	62	tr	tr	0.09	0.21	5.5	0
0.4	60	0	12	145	1.3	241	54	tr	tr	0.08	0.18	4.4	0
0.8	78	0	8	162	1.7	273	57	tr	tr	0.09	0.24	5.5	0
0.4	65	0	6	150	1.5	247	50	tr	tr	0.08	0.20	4.6	0

Continued

FOODS, APPROXIMATE MEASURES, UNITS, AND WEIGHT (WEIGHT OF EDIBLE PORTION ONLY)		GRAMS	WATER (g)	FOOD ENERGY (CALORIES)	PROTEIN (g)	FAT (g)	FATTY ACIDS	
							SATURATED (g)	MONO-UNSATURATED (g)
MEAT AND MEAT PRODUCTS—cont'd								
Lamb, cooked—cont'd								
Rib, roasted								
Lean and fat, 3 pieces, 2½ by 2½ by ¼ in	3 oz	85	47	315	18	26	12.1	10.6
Lean only	2 oz	57	60	130	15	7	3.2	3.0
Pork, cured, cooked								
Bacon								
Regular	3 medium slices	19	13	110	6	9	3.3	4.5
Canadian-style	2 slices	46	62	85	11	4	1.3	1.9
Ham, light cure, roasted								
Lean and fat, 2 pieces, 4⅛ by 2¼ by ¼ in	3 oz	85	58	205	18	14	5.1	6.7
Lean only	2.4 oz	68	66	105	17	4	1.3	1.7
Ham, canned, roasted, 2 pieces, 4⅛ by 2¼ by ¼ in	3 oz	85	67	140	18	7	2.4	3.5
Luncheon meat								
Canned, spiced or unspiced, slice, 3 by 2 by ½ in	2 slices	42	52	140	5	13	4.5	6.0
Chopped ham (8 slices per 6-oz pkg)	2 slices	42	64	95	7	7	2.4	3.4
Cooked ham (8 slices per 8-oz pkg)								
Regular	2 slices	57	65	105	10	6	1.9	2.8
Extra lean	2 slices	57	71	75	11	3	0.9	1.3
Pork, fresh, cooked								
Chop, loin (cut 3 per lb with bone)								
Broiled								
Lean and fat	3.1 oz	87	50	275	24	19	7.0	8.8
Lean only	2.5 oz	72	57	165	23	8	2.6	3.4
Pan fried								
Lean and fat	3.1 oz	89	45	335	21	27	9.8	12.5
Lean only	2.4 oz	67	54	180	19	11	3.7	4.8
Ham (leg), roasted								
Lean and fat, piece, 2½ by 2½ by ¾ in	3 oz	85	53	250	21	18	6.4	8.1
Lean only	2.5 oz	72	60	160	20	8	2.7	3.6
Rib, roasted								
Lean and fat, piece, 2½ by ¾ in	3 oz	85	51	270	21	20	7.2	9.2
Lean only	2.5 oz	71	57	175	20	10	3.4	4.4
Shoulder cut, braised								
Lean and fat, 3 pieces, 2½ by 2½ by ¼ in	3 oz	85	47	295	23	22	7.9	10.0
Lean only	2.4 oz	67	54	165	22	8	2.8	3.7

tr = nutrient present in trace amounts.
[35]Contains added sodium ascorbate. If sodium ascorbate is not added, ascorbic acid content is negligible.

NUTRIENTS IN INDICATED QUANTITY

POLY-UNSATURATED (g)	CHOLES-TEROL (mg)	CARBO-HYDRATE (g)	CALCIUM (mg)	PHOS-PHORUS (mg)	IRON (mg)	POTASSIUM (mg)	SODIUM (mg)	VITAMIN A VALUES IU	RE	THIAMIN (mg)	RIBO-FLAVIN (mg)	NIACIN (mg)	ASCORBIC ACID (mg)
1.5	77	0	19	139	1.4	224	60	tr	tr	0.08	0.18	5.5	0
0.5	50	0	12	111	1.0	179	46	tr	tr	0.05	0.13	3.5	0
1.1	16	tr	2	64	0.3	92	303	0	0	0.13	0.05	1.4	6
0.4	27	1	5	136	0.4	179	711	0	0	0.38	0.09	3.2	10
1.5	53	0	6	182	0.7	243	1009	0	0	0.51	0.19	3.8	0
0.4	37	0	5	154	0.6	215	902	0	0	0.46	0.17	3.4	0
0.8	35	tr	6	188	0.9	298	908	0	0	0.82	0.21	4.3	19[35]
1.5	26	1	3	34	0.3	90	541	0	0	0.15	0.08	1.3	tr
0.9	21	0	3	65	0.3	134	576	0	0	0.27	0.09	1.6	8[35]
0.7	32	2	4	141	0.6	189	751	0	0	0.49	0.14	3.0	16[35]
0.3	27	1	4	124	0.4	200	815	0	0	0.53	0.13	2.8	15[35]
2.2	84	0	3	184	0.7	312	61	10	3	0.87	0.24	4.3	tr
0.9	71	0	4	176	0.7	302	56	10	1	0.83	0.22	4.0	tr
3.1	92	0	4	190	0.7	323	64	10	3	0.91	0.24	4.6	tr
1.3	72	0	3	178	0.7	305	57	10	1	0.84	0.22	4.0	tr
2.0	79	0	5	210	0.9	280	50	10	2	0.54	0.27	3.9	tr
1.0	68	0	5	202	0.8	269	46	10	1	0.50	0.25	3.6	tr
2.3	69	0	9	190	0.8	313	37	10	3	0.50	0.24	4.2	tr
1.2	56	0	8	182	0.7	300	33	10	2	0.45	0.22	3.8	tr
2.4	93	0	6	162	1.4	286	75	10	3	0.46	0.26	4.4	tr
1.0	76	0	5	151	1.3	271	68	10	1	0.40	0.24	4.0	tr

FOODS, APPROXIMATE MEASURES, UNITS, AND WEIGHT (WEIGHT OF EDIBLE PORTION ONLY)		GRAMS	WATER (g)	FOOD ENERGY (CALORIES)	PROTEIN (g)	FAT (g)	FATTY ACIDS	
							SATURATED (g)	MONO-UNSATURATED (g)
MEAT AND MEAT PRODUCTS—cont'd								
Sausages (See also Luncheon meats)								
Bologna, slice (8 per 8-oz pkg)	2 slices	57	54	180	7	16	6.1	7.6
Braunschweiger, slice (6 per 6-oz pkg)	2 slices	57	48	205	8	18	6.2	8.5
Brown and serve (10–11 per 8-oz pkg), browned	1 link	13	45	50	2	5	1.7	2.2
Frankfurter (10 per 1-lb pkg), cooked (reheated)	1 frankfurter	45	54	145	5	13	4.8	6.2
Pork link (16 per 1-lb pkg), cooked[36]	1 link	13	45	50	3	4	1.4	1.8
Salami								
Cooked type, slice (8 per 8-oz pkg)	2 slices	57	60	145	8	11	4.6	5.2
Dry type, slice (12 per 4-oz pkg)	2 slices	20	35	85	5	7	2.4	3.4
Sandwich spread (pork, beef)	1 tbsp	15	60	35	1	3	0.9	1.1
Vienna sausage (7 per 4-oz can)	1 sausage	16	60	45	2	4	1.5	2.0
Veal, medium fat, cooked, bone removed								
Cutlet, 4⅛ by 2¼ by ½ in, braised or broiled	3 oz	85	60	185	23	9	4.1	4.1
Rib, 2 pieces, 4⅛ by 2¼ by ¼ in, roasted	3 oz	85	55	230	23	14	6.0	6.0
POULTRY AND POULTRY PRODUCTS								
Chicken								
Fried, flesh, with skin[37]								
Batter dipped								
Breast, ½ breast (5.6 oz with bones)	4.9 oz	140	52	365	35	18	4.9	7.6
Drumstick (3.4 oz with bones)	2.5 oz	72	53	195	16	11	3.0	4.6
Flour coated								
Breast, ½ breast (4.2 oz with bones)	3.5 oz	98	57	220	31	9	2.4	3.4
Drumstick (2.6 oz with bones)	1.7 oz	49	57	120	13	7	1.8	2.7
Roasted, flesh only								
Breast, ½ breast (4.2 oz with bones and skin)	3.0 oz	86	65	140	27	3	0.9	1.1
Drumstick, (2.9 oz with bones and skin)	1.6 oz	44	67	75	12	2	0.7	0.8
Stewed, flesh only, light and dark meat, chopped or diced	1 c	140	67	250	38	9	2.6	3.3

tr = nutrient present in trace amounts.
[35]Contains added sodium ascorbate. If sodium ascorbate is not added, ascorbic acid content is negligible.

POLY-UNSATURATED (g)	CHOLES-TEROL (mg)	CARBO-HYDRATE (g)	CALCIUM (mg)	PHOS-PHORUS (mg)	IRON (mg)	POTASSIUM (mg)	SODIUM (mg)	VITAMIN A VALUES		THIAMIN (mg)	RIBO-FLAVIN (mg)	NIACIN (mg)	ASCORBIC ACID (mg)
								IU	RE				
1.4	31	2	7	52	0.9	103	581	0	0	0.10	0.08	1.5	12[35]
2.1	89	2	5	96	5.3	113	652	8010	2405	0.14	0.87	4.8	6[35]
0.5	9	tr	1	14	0.1	25	105	0	0	0.05	0.02	0.4	0
1.2	23	1	5	39	0.5	75	504	0	0	0.09	0.05	1.2	12[35]
0.5	11	tr	4	24	0.2	47	168	0	0	0.10	0.03	0.6	tr
1.2	37	1	7	66	1.5	113	607	0	0	0.14	0.21	2.0	7[35]
0.6	16	1	2	28	0.3	76	372	0	0	0.12	0.06	1.0	5[35]
0.4	6	2	2	9	0.1	17	152	10	1	0.03	0.02	0.3	0
0.3	8	tr	2	8	0.1	16	152	0	0	0.01	0.02	0.3	0
0.6	109	0	9	196	0.8	258	56	tr	tr	0.06	0.21	4.6	0
1.0	109	0	10	211	0.7	259	57	tr	tr	0.11	0.26	6.6	0
4.3	119	13	28	259	1.8	281	385	90	28	0.16	0.20	14.7	0
2.7	62	6	12	106	1.0	134	194	60	19	0.08	0.15	3.7	0
1.9	87	2	16	228	1.2	254	74	50	15	0.08	0.13	13.5	0
1.6	44	1	6	86	0.7	112	44	40	12	0.04	0.11	3.0	0
0.7	73	0	13	196	0.9	220	64	20	5	0.06	0.10	11.8	0
0.6	41	0	5	81	0.6	108	42	30	8	0.03	0.10	2.7	0
2.2	116	0	20	210	1.6	252	98	70	21	0.07	0.23	8.6	0

[36]One patty (8 per pound) of bulk sausage is equivalent to 2 links.
[37]Fried in vegetable shortening.

Continued

FOODS, APPROXIMATE MEASURES, UNITS, AND WEIGHT (WEIGHT OF EDIBLE PORTION ONLY)		GRAMS	WATER (g)	FOOD ENERGY (CALORIES)	PROTEIN (g)	FAT (g)	FATTY ACIDS	
							SATURATED (g)	MONO-UNSATURATED (g)
POULTRY AND POULTRY PRODUCTS—cont'd								
Chicken liver, cooked	1 liver	20	68	30	5	1	0.4	0.3
Duck, roasted, flesh only	½ duck	221	46	445	52	25	9.2	8.2
Turkey, roasted, flesh only								
Dark meat, piece, 2½ by 1⅝ by ¼ in	4 pieces	85	63	160	24	6	2.1	1.4
Light meat, piece, 4 by 2 by ¼ in	2 pieces	85	66	135	25	3	0.9	0.5
Light and dark meat								
Chopped or diced	1 c	140	65	240	41	7	2.3	1.4
Pieces (1 slice white meat, 4 by 2 by ¼ in and 2 slices dark meat, 2½ by 1⅝ by ¼ in)	3 pieces	85	65	145	25	4	1.4	0.9
Poultry food products								
Chicken								
Canned, boneless	5 oz	142	69	235	31	11	3.1	4.5
Frankfurter (10 per 1-lb pkg)	1 frankfurter	45	58	115	6	9	2.5	3.8
Roll, light (6 slices per 6 oz pkg)	2 slices	57	69	90	11	4	1.1	1.7
Turkey								
Gravy and turkey, frozen	5 oz	142	85	95	8	4	1.2	1.4
Ham, cured turkey thigh meat (8 slices per 8-oz pkg)	2 slices	57	71	75	11	3	1.0	0.7
Loaf, breast meat (8 slices per 6-oz pkg)	2 slices	42	72	45	10	1	0.2	0.2
Patties, breaded, battered, fried (2.25 oz)	1 patty	64	50	180	9	12	3.0	4.8
Roast, boneless, frozen, seasoned, light and dark meat, cooked	3 oz	85	68	130	18	5	1.6	1.0
SUGARS AND SWEETS								
Sugars								
Brown, pressed down	1 c	220	2	820	0	0	0.0	0.0
White								
Granulated	1 c	200	1	770	0	0	0.0	0.0
	1 tbsp	12	1	45	0	0	0.0	0.0
	1 packet	6	1	25	0	0	0.0	0.0
Powdered, sifted, spooned into cup	1 c	100	1	385	0	0	0.0	0.0
Syrups								
Chocolate-flavored syrup or topping								
Thin type	2 tbsp	38	37	85	1	tr	0.2	0.1
Fudge type	2 tbsp	38	25	125	2	5	3.1	1.7

tr = nutrient present in trace amounts.
[38]If sodium ascorbate is used, product contains 11 mg ascorbic acid.

NUTRIENTS IN INDICATED QUANTITY

POLY-UNSATURATED (g)	CHOLES-TEROL (mg)	CARBO-HYDRATE (g)	CALCIUM (mg)	PHOS-PHORUS (mg)	IRON (mg)	POTASSIUM (mg)	SODIUM (mg)	VITAMIN A VALUES		THIAMIN (mg)	RIBO-FLAVIN (mg)	NIACIN (mg)	ASCORBIC ACID (mg)
								IU	RE				
0.2	126	tr	3	62	1.7	28	10	3270	983	0.03	0.35	0.9	3
3.2	197	0	27	449	6.0	557	144	170	51	0.57	1.04	11.3	0
1.8	72	0	27	173	2.0	246	67	0	0	0.05	0.21	3.1	0
0.7	59	0	16	186	1.1	259	54	0	0	0.05	0.11	5.8	0
2.0	106	0	35	298	2.5	417	98	0	0	0.09	0.25	7.6	0
1.2	65	0	21	181	1.5	253	60	0	0	0.05	0.15	4.6	0
2.5	88	0	20	158	2.2	196	714	170	48	0.02	0.18	9.0	3
1.8	45	3	43	48	0.9	38	616	60	17	0.03	0.05	1.4	0
0.9	28	1	24	89	0.6	129	331	50	14	0.04	0.07	3.0	0
0.7	26	7	20	115	1.3	87	787	60	18	0.03	0.18	2.6	0
0.9	32	tr	6	108	1.6	184	565	0	0	0.03	0.14	2.0	0
0.1	17	0	3	97	0.2	118	608	0	0	0.02	0.05	3.5	0[38]
3.0	40	10	9	173	1.4	176	512	20	7	0.06	0.12	1.5	0
1.4	45	3	4	207	1.4	253	578	0	0	0.04	0.14	5.3	0
0.0	0	212	187	56	4.8	757	97	0	0	0.02	0.07	0.2	0
0.0	0	199	3	tr	0.1	7	5	0	0	0.00	0.00	0.0	0
0.0	0	12	tr	tr	tr	tr	tr	0	0	0.00	0.00	0.0	0
0.0	0	6	tr	tr	tr	tr	tr	0	0	0.00	0.00	0.0	0
0.0	0	100	1	tr	tr	4	2	0	0	0.00	0.00	0.0	0
0.1	0	22	6	49	0.8	85	36	tr	tr	tr	0.02	0.1	0
0.2	0	21	38	60	0.5	82	42	40	13	0.02	0.08	0.1	0

Continued

FOODS, APPROXIMATE MEASURES, UNITS, AND WEIGHT (WEIGHT OF EDIBLE PORTION ONLY)		GRAMS	WATER (g)	FOOD ENERGY (CALORIES)	PROTEIN (g)	FAT (g)	FATTY ACIDS	
							SATURATED (g)	MONO-UNSATURATED (g)
SUGARS AND SWEETS—cont'd								
Molasses, cane, blackstrap	2 tbsp	40	24	85	0	0	0.0	0.0
Table syrup (corn and maple)	2 tbsp	42	25	122	0	0	0.0	0.0
VEGETABLES AND VEGETABLE PRODUCTS								
Alfalfa seeds, sprouted, raw	1 c	33	91	10	1	tr	tr	tr
Artichokes, globe or French, cooked, drained	1 artichoke	120	87	55	3	tr	tr	tr
Asparagus, green								
Cooked, drained								
From raw								
Cuts and tips	1 c	180	92	45	5	1	0.1	tr
Spears, ½-in diam. at base	4 spears	60	92	15	2	tr	tr	tr
From frozen								
Cuts and tips	1 c	180	91	50	5	1	0.2	tr
Spears, ½-in diam. at base	4 spears	60	91	15	2	tr	0.1	tr
Canned, spears, ½-in diam. at base	4 spears	80	95	10	1	tr	tr	tr
Bamboo shoots, canned, drained	1 c	131	94	25	2	1	0.1	tr
Beans								
Lima, immature seeds, frozen, cooked, drained								
Thick-seeded types (Ford-hooks)	1 c	170	74	170	10	1	0.1	tr
Thin-seeded types (baby limas)	1 c	180	72	190	12	1	0.1	tr
Snap								
Cooked, drained								
From raw (cut and French style)	1 c	125	89	45	2	tr	0.1	tr
From frozen (cut)	1 c	135	92	35	2	tr	tr	tr
Canned, drained solids (cut)	1 c	135	93	25	2	tr	tr	tr
Beans, mature. See Beans, dry and Black-eyed peas, dry.								
Bean sprouts (mung)								
Raw	1 c	104	90	30	3	tr	tr	tr
Cooked, drained	1 c	124	93	25	3	tr	tr	tr
Beets								
Cooked, drained								
Diced or sliced	1 c	170	91	55	2	tr	tr	tr
Whole beets, 2-in diam.	2 beets	100	91	30	1	tr	tr	tr
Canned, drained solids, diced or sliced	1 c	170	91	55	2	tr	tr	tr
Beet greens, leaves and stems, cooked, drained	1 c	144	89	40	4	tr	tr	0.1

tr = nutrient present in trace amounts.
[39]For regular pack; special dietary pack contains 3 mg sodium.
[40]For green varieties; yellow varieties contain 101 IU or 10 RE.
[41]For green varieties; yellow varieties contain 151 IU or 15 RE

| NUTRIENTS IN INDICATED QUANTITY | | | | | | | | | | | | | |

POLY-UNSATURATED (g)	CHOLES-TEROL (mg)	CARBO-HYDRATE (g)	CALCIUM (mg)	PHOS-PHORUS (mg)	IRON (mg)	POTASSIUM (mg)	SODIUM (mg)	VITAMIN A VALUES IU	RE	THIAMIN (mg)	RIBO-FLAVIN (mg)	NIACIN (mg)	ASCORBIC ACID (mg)
0.0	0	22	274	34	10.1	1171	38	0	0	0.04	0.08	0.8	0
0.0	0	32	1	4	tr	7	19	0	0	0.00	0.00	0.0	0
0.1	0	1	11	23	0.3	26	2	50	5	0.03	0.04	0.2	3
0.1	0	12	47	72	1.6	316	79	170	17	0.07	0.06	0.7	9
0.2	0	8	43	110	1.2	558	7	1490	149	0.18	0.22	1.9	49
0.1	0	3	14	37	0.4	186	2	500	50	0.06	0.07	0.6	16
0.3	0	9	41	99	1.2	392	7	1470	147	0.12	0.19	1.9	44
0.1	0	3	14	33	0.4	131	2	490	49	0.04	0.06	0.6	15
0.1	0	2	11	30	0.5	122	278[39]	380	38	0.04	0.07	0.7	13
0.2	0	4	10	33	0.4	105	9	10	1	0.03	0.03	0.2	1
0.3	0	32	37	107	2.3	694	90	320	32	0.13	0.10	1.8	22
0.3	0	35	50	202	3.5	740	52	300	30	0.13	0.10	1.4	10
0.2	0	10	58	49	1.6	374	4	830[40]	83[40]	0.09	0.12	0.8	12
0.1	0	8	61	32	1.1	151	18	710[41]	71[41]	0.06	0.10	0.6	11
0.1	0	6	35	26	1.2	147	339[42]	470[43]	47[43]	0.02	0.08	0.3	6
0.1	0	6	14	56	0.9	155	6	20	2	0.09	0.13	0.8	14
tr	0	5	15	35	0.8	125	12	20	2	0.06	0.13	1.0	14
tr	0	11	19	53	1.1	530	83	20	2	0.05	0.02	0.5	9
tr	0	7	11	31	0.6	312	49	10	1	0.03	0.01	0.3	6
0.1	0	12	26	29	3.1	252	466[44]	20	2	0.02	0.07	0.3	7
0.1	0	8	164	59	2.7	1309	347	7340	734	0.17	0.42	0.7	36

[42]For regular pack; special dietary pack contains 3 mg sodium.
[43]For green varieties; yellow varieties contain 142 IU or 14 RE.
[44]For regular pack; special dietary pack contains 78 mg sodium.

Continued

FOODS, APPROXIMATE MEASURES, UNITS, AND WEIGHT (WEIGHT OF EDIBLE PORTION ONLY)		GRAMS	WATER (g)	FOOD ENERGY (CALORIES)	PROTEIN (g)	FAT (g)	FATTY ACIDS	
							SATURATED (g)	MONO-UNSATURATED (g)
VEGETABLES AND VEGETABLE PRODUCTS—cont'd								
Black-eyed peas, immature seeds, cooked and drained								
From raw	1 c	165	72	180	13	1	0.3	0.1
From frozen	1 c	170	66	225	14	1	0.3	0.1
Broccoli								
Raw	1 spear	151	91	40	4	1	0.1	tr
Cooked, drained								
From raw								
Spear, medium	1 spear	180	90	50	5	1	0.1	tr
Spears, cut into ½-in pieces	1 c	155	90	45	5	tr	0.1	tr
From frozen								
Piece, 4½ to 5 in long	1 piece	30	91	10	1	tr	tr	tr
Chopped	1 c	185	91	50	6	tr	tr	tr
Brussels sprouts, cooked, drained								
From raw, 7-8 sprouts, 1¼- to 1½-in diam.	1 c	155	87	60	4	1	0.2	0.1
From frozen	1 c	155	87	65	6	1	0.1	tr
Cabbage, common varieties								
Raw, coarsely shredded or sliced	1 c	70	93	15	1	tr	tr	tr
Cooked, drained	1 c	150	94	30	1	tr	tr	tr
Cabbage, Chinese								
Pak-choi, cooked, drained	1 c	170	96	20	3	tr	tr	tr
Pe-tsai, raw, 1-in pieces	1 c	76	94	10	1	tr	tr	tr
Cabbage, red, raw, coarsely shredded or sliced	1 c	70	92	20	1	tr	tr	tr
Cabbage, savoy, raw, coarsely shredded or sliced	1 c	70	91	20	1	tr	tr	tr
Carrots								
Raw, without crowns and tips, scraped								
Whole, 7½ by 1⅛ in, or strips, 2½ to 3 in long	1 carrot or 18 strips	72	88	30	1	tr	tr	tr
Grated	1 c	110	88	45	1	tr	tr	tr
Cooked, sliced, drained								
From raw	1 c	156	87	70	2	tr	0.1	tr
From frozen	1 c	146	90	55	2	tr	tr	tr
Canned, sliced, drained solids	1 c	146	93	35	1	tr	0.1	tr
Cauliflower								
Raw (flowerets)	1 c	100	92	25	2	tr	tr	tr
Cooked, drained								
From raw (flowerets)	1 c	125	93	30	2	tr	tr	tr
From frozen (flowerets)	1 c	180	94	35	3	tr	0.1	tr

tr = nutrient present in trace amounts.
[45]For regular pack; special dietary pack contains 61 mg sodium.

NUTRIENTS IN INDICATED QUANTITY

POLY-UNSATURATED (g)	CHOLES-TEROL (mg)	CARBO-HYDRATE (g)	CALCIUM (mg)	PHOS-PHORUS (mg)	IRON (mg)	POTASSIUM (mg)	SODIUM (mg)	VITAMIN A VALUES IU	RE	THIAMIN (mg)	RIBO-FLAVIN (mg)	NIACIN (mg)	ASCORBIC ACID (mg)
0.6	0	30	46	196	2.4	693	7	1050	105	0.11	0.18	1.8	3
0.5	0	40	39	207	3.6	638	9	130	13	0.44	0.11	1.2	4
0.3	0	8	72	100	1.3	491	41	2330	233	0.10	0.18	1.0	141
0.2	0	10	205	86	2.1	293	20	2540	254	0.15	0.37	1.4	113
0.2	0	9	177	74	1.8	253	17	2180	218	0.13	0.32	1.2	97
tr	0	2	15	17	0.2	54	7	570	57	0.02	0.02	0.1	12
0.1	0	10	94	102	1.1	333	44	3500	350	0.10	0.15	0.8	74
0.4	0	13	56	87	1.9	491	33	1110	111	0.17	0.12	0.9	96
0.3	0	13	37	84	1.1	504	36	910	91	0.16	0.18	0.8	71
0.1	0	4	33	16	0.4	172	13	90	9	0.04	0.02	0.2	33
0.2	0	7	50	38	0.6	308	29	130	13	0.09	0.08	0.3	36
0.1	0	3	158	49	1.8	631	58	4370	437	0.05	0.11	0.7	44
0.1	0	2	59	22	0.2	181	7	910	91	0.03	0.04	0.3	21
0.1	0	4	36	29	0.3	144	8	30	3	0.04	0.02	0.2	40
tr	0	4	25	29	0.3	161	20	700	70	0.05	0.02	0.2	22
0.1	0	7	19	32	0.4	233	25	20,250	2025	0.07	0.04	0.7	7
0.1	0	11	30	48	0.6	355	39	30,940	3094	0.11	0.06	1.0	10
0.1	0	16	48	47	1.0	354	103	38,300	3830	0.05	0.09	0.8	4
0.1	0	12	41	38	0.7	231	86	25,850	2585	0.04	0.05	0.6	4
0.1	0	8	37	35	0.9	261	352[45]	20,110	2011	0.03	0.04	0.8	4
0.1	0	5	29	46	0.6	355	15	20	2	0.08	0.06	0.6	72
0.1	0	6	34	44	0.5	404	8	20	2	0.08	0.07	0.7	69
0.2	0	7	31	43	0.7	250	32	40	4	0.07	0.10	0.6	56

Continued

FOODS, APPROXIMATE MEASURES, UNITS, AND WEIGHT (WEIGHT OF EDIBLE PORTION ONLY)		GRAMS	WATER (g)	FOOD ENERGY (CALORIES)	PROTEIN (g)	FAT (g)	FATTY ACIDS	
							SATURATED (g)	MONO-UNSATURATED (g)
VEGETABLES AND VEGETABLE PRODUCTS—cont'd								
Celery, pascal type, raw								
Stalk, large outer, 8 by 1½ in (at root end)	1 stalk	40	95	5	tr	tr	tr	tr
Pieces, diced	1 c	120	95	20	1	tr	tr	tr
Collards, cooked, drained								
From raw (leaves without stems)	1 c	190	96	25	2	tr	0.1	tr
From frozen (chopped)	1 c	170	88	60	5	1	0.1	0.1
Corn, sweet								
Cooked, drained								
From raw, ear 5 by 1¾ in	1 ear	77	70	85	3	1	0.2	0.3
From frozen								
Ear, trimmed to about 3½ in long	1 ear	63	73	60	2	tr	0.1	0.1
Kernels	1 c	165	76	135	5	tr	tr	tr
Canned								
Cream style	1 c	256	79	185	4	1	0.2	0.3
Whole kernel, vacuum pack	1 c	210	77	165	5	1	0.2	0.3
Cowpeas. See Black-eyed peas, immature, mature								
Cucumber, with peel, slices, ⅛ in thick (large, 2⅛-in diam.; small, 1¾-in diam.)	6 large or 8 small slices	28	96	5	tr	tr	tr	tr
Dandelion greens, cooked, drained	1 c	105	90	35	2	1	0.1	tr
Eggplant, cooked, steamed	1 c	96	92	25	1	tr	tr	tr
Endive, curly (including escarole), raw, small pieces	1 c	50	94	10	1	tr	tr	tr
Jerusalem-artichoke, raw, sliced	1 c	150	78	115	3	tr	0.0	tr
Kale, cooked, drained								
From raw, chopped	1 c	130	91	40	2	1	0.1	tr
From frozen, chopped	1 c	130	91	40	4	1	0.1	tr
Kohlrabi, thickened bulb-like stems, cooked, drained, diced	1 c	165	90	50	3	tr	tr	tr
Lettuce, raw								
Butterhead, as Boston types								
Head, 5-in diam	1 head	163	96	20	2	tr	tr	tr
Leaves	1 outer or 2 inner leaves	15	96	tr	tr	tr	tr	tr
Crisphead, as iceberg								
Head, 6-in diam	1 head	539	96	70	5	1	0.1	tr
Wedge, ¼ of head	1 wedge	135	96	20	1	tr	tr	tr
Pieces, chopped or shredded	1 c	55	96	5	1	tr	tr	tr

tr = nutrient present in trace amounts.
[46]For yellow varieties; white varieties contain only a trace of vitamin A.

NUTRIENTS IN INDICATED QUANTITY

POLY-UNSATURATED (g)	CHOLES-TEROL (mg)	CARBO-HYDRATE (g)	CALCIUM (mg)	PHOS-PHORUS (mg)	IRON (mg)	POTASSIUM (mg)	SODIUM (mg)	VITAMIN A VALUES IU	RE	THIAMIN (mg)	RIBO-FLAVIN (mg)	NIACIN (mg)	ASCORBIC ACID (mg)
tr	0	1	14	10	0.2	144	35	50	5	0.01	0.01	0.1	3
0.1	0	4	43	31	0.6	341	106	150	15	0.04	0.04	0.4	8
0.2	0	5	148	19	0.8	177	36	4220	422	0.03	0.08	0.4	19
0.4	0	12	357	46	1.9	427	85	10,170	1017	0.08	0.20	1.1	45
0.5	0	19	2	79	0.5	192	13	170[46]	17[46]	0.17	0.06	1.2	5
0.2	0	14	2	47	0.4	158	3	130[48]	13[48]	0.11	0.04	1.0	3
0.1	0	34	3	78	0.5	229	8	410[48]	41[48]	0.11	0.12	2.1	4
0.5	0	46	8	131	1.0	343	730[47]	250[48]	25[48]	0.06	0.14	2.5	12
0.5	0	41	11	134	0.9	391	571[48]	510[48]	51[48]	0.09	0.15	2.5	17
tr	0	1	4	5	0.1	42	1	10	1	0.01	0.01	0.1	1
0.3	0	7	147	44	1.9	244	46	12,290	1229	0.14	0.18	0.5	19
0.1	0	6	6	21	0.3	238	3	60	6	0.07	0.02	0.6	1
tr	0	2	26	14	0.4	157	11	1030	103	0.04	0.04	0.2	3
tr	0	26	21	117	5.1	644	6	30	3	0.30	0.09	2.0	6
0.3	0	7	94	36	1.2	296	30	9620	962	0.07	0.09	0.7	53
0.3	0	7	179	36	1.2	417	20	8260	826	0.06	0.15	0.9	33
0.1	0	11	41	74	0.7	561	35	60	6	0.07	0.03	0.6	89
0.2	0	4	52	38	0.5	419	8	1580	158	0.10	0.10	0.5	13
tr	0	tr	5	3	tr	39	1	150	15	0.01	0.01	tr	1
0.5	0	11	102	108	2.7	852	49	1780	178	0.25	0.16	1.0	21
0.1	0	3	26	27	0.7	213	12	450	45	0.06	0.04	0.3	5
0.1	0	1	10	11	0.3	87	5	180	18	0.03	0.02	0.1	2

[47]For regular pack; special dietary pack contains 8 mg sodium.
[48]For regular pack; special dietary pack contains 6 mg sodium.

Continued

FOODS, APPROXIMATE MEASURES, UNITS, AND WEIGHT (WEIGHT OF EDIBLE PORTION ONLY)		GRAMS	WATER (g)	FOOD ENERGY (CALORIES)	PROTEIN (g)	FAT (g)	FATTY ACIDS	
							SATURATED (g)	MONO-UNSATURATED (g)
VEGETABLES AND VEGETABLE PRODUCTS—cont'd								
Lettuce, raw—cont'd								
Looseleaf (bunching varieties including romaine or cos), chopped or shredded pieces	1 c	56	94	10	1	tr	tr	tr
Mushrooms								
Raw, sliced or chopped	1 c	70	92	20	1	tr	tr	tr
Cooked, drained	1 c	156	91	40	3	1	0.1	tr
Canned, drained solids	1 c	156	91	35	3	tr	0.1	tr
Mustard greens, without stems and midribs, cooked, drained	1 c	140	94	20	3	tr	tr	0.2
Okra pods, 3 by 5/8 in, cooked	8 pods	85	90	25	2	tr	tr	tr
Onions								
Raw								
Chopped	1 c	160	91	55	2	tr	0.1	0.1
Sliced	1 c	115	91	40	1	tr	0.1	tr
Cooked (whole or sliced), drained	1 c	210	92	60	2	tr	0.1	tr
Onions, spring, raw, bulb (3/8-in diam.) and white portion of top	6 onions	30	92	10	1	tr	tr	tr
Onion rings, breaded, pan-fried, frozen, prepared	2 rings	20	29	80	1	5	1.7	2.2
Parsley								
Raw	10 sprigs	10	88	5	tr	tr	tr	tr
Freeze-dried	1 tbsp	0.4	2	tr	tr	tr	tr	tr
Parsnips, cooked (diced or 2-in lengths), drained	1 c	156	78	125	2	tr	0.1	0.2
Peas, edible pod, cooked, drained	1 c	160	89	65	5	tr	0.1	tr
Peas, green								
Canned, drained solids	1 c	170	82	115	8	1	0.1	0.1
Frozen, cooked, drained	1 c	160	80	125	8	tr	0.1	tr
Peppers								
Hot chili, raw	1 pepper	45	88	20	1	tr	tr	tr
Sweet (about 5 per lb, whole), stem and seeds removed								
Raw	1 pepper	74	93	20	1	tr	tr	tr
Cooked, drained	1 pepper	73	95	15	tr	tr	tr	tr
Potatoes, cooked								
Baked (about 2 per lb, raw)								
With skin	1 potato	202	71	220	5	tr	0.1	tr
Flesh only	1 potato	156	75	145	3	tr	tr	tr

tr = nutrient present in trace amounts.
[49]For regular pack; special dietary pack contains 3 mg sodium.
[50]For red peppers; green peppers contain 350 IU or 35 RE.
[51]For green peppers; red peppers contain 4220 IU or 422 RE.

NUTRIENTS IN INDICATED QUANTITY

POLY-UNSATURATED (g)	CHOLES-TEROL (mg)	CARBO-HYDRATE (g)	CALCIUM (mg)	PHOS-PHORUS (mg)	IRON (mg)	POTASSIUM (mg)	SODIUM (mg)	VITAMIN A VALUES IU	RE	THIAMIN (mg)	RIBO-FLAVIN (mg)	NIACIN (mg)	ASCORBIC ACID (mg)
0.1	0	2	38	14	0.8	148	5	1060	106	0.03	0.04	0.2	10
0.1	0	3	4	73	0.9	259	3	0	0	0.07	0.31	2.9	2
0.3	0	8	9	136	2.7	555	3	0	0	0.11	0.47	7.0	6
0.2	0	8	17	103	1.2	201	663	0	0	0.13	0.03	2.5	0
0.1	0	3	104	57	1.0	283	22	4240	424	0.06	0.09	0.6	35
tr	0	6	54	48	0.4	274	4	490	49	0.11	0.05	0.7	14
0.2	0	12	40	46	0.6	248	3	0	0	0.10	0.02	0.2	13
0.1	0	8	29	33	0.4	178	2	0	0	0.07	0.01	0.1	10
0.1	0	13	57	48	0.4	319	17	0	0	0.09	0.02	0.2	12
tr	0	2	18	10	0.6	77	1	1500	150	0.02	0.04	0.1	14
1.0	0	8	6	16	0.3	26	75	50	5	0.06	0.03	0.7	tr
tr	0	1	13	4	0.6	54	4	520	52	0.01	0.01	0.1	9
tr	0	tr	1	2	0.2	25	2	250	25	tr	0.01	tr	1
0.1	0	30	58	108	0.9	573	16	0	0	0.13	0.08	1.1	20
0.2	0	11	67	88	3.2	384	6	210	21	0.20	0.12	0.9	77
0.3	0	21	34	114	1.6	294	372[49]	1310	131	0.21	0.13	1.2	16
0.2	0	23	38	144	2.5	269	139	1070	107	0.45	0.16	2.4	16
tr	0	4	8	21	0.5	153	3	4840[50]	484[50]	0.04	0.04	0.4	109
0.2	0	4	4	16	0.9	144	2	390[51]	39[51]	0.06	0.04	0.4	95[52]
0.1	0	3	3	11	0.6	94	1	280[53]	28[53]	0.04	0.03	0.3	81[54]
0.1	0	51	20	115	2.7	844	16	0	0	0.22	0.07	3.3	26
0.1	0	34	8	78	0.5	610	8	0	0	0.16	0.03	2.2	20

[52]For green peppers; red peppers contain 141 mg ascorbic acid.
[53]For green peppers; red peppers contain 2740 IU or 274 RE.
[54]For green peppers; red peppers contain 121 mg ascorbic acid.

Continued

FOODS, APPROXIMATE MEASURES, UNITS, AND WEIGHT (WEIGHT OF EDIBLE PORTION ONLY)		GRAMS	WATER (g)	FOOD ENERGY (CALORIES)	PROTEIN (g)	FAT (g)	FATTY ACIDS	
							SATURATED (g)	MONO-UNSATURATED (g)
VEGETABLES AND VEGETABLE PRODUCTS—cont'd								
Potatoes, cooked—cont'd								
Boiled (about 3 per lb, raw)								
Peeled after boiling	1 potato	136	77	120	3	tr	tr	tr
Peeled before boiling	1 potato	135	77	115	2	tr	tr	tr
French fried, strip, 2 to 3½ in long, frozen								
Oven heated	10 strips	50	53	110	2	4	2.1	1.8
Fried in vegetable oil	10 strips	50	38	160	2	8	2.5	1.6
Potato products, prepared								
Au gratin								
From dry mix	1 c	245	79	230	6	10	6.3	2.9
From home recipe	1 c	245	74	325	12	19	11.6	5.3
Hashed brown, from frozen	1 c	156	56	340	5	18	7.0	8.0
Mashed								
From home recipe								
Milk added	1 c	210	78	160	4	1	0.7	0.3
Milk and margarine added	1 c	210	76	225	4	9	2.2	3.7
From dehydrated flakes (without milk), water, milk, butter, and salt added	1 c	210	76	235	4	12	7.2	3.3
Potato salad, made with mayonnaise	1 c	250	76	360	7	21	3.6	6.2
Scalloped								
From dry mix	1 c	245	79	230	5	11	6.5	3.0
From home recipe	1 c	245	81	210	7	9	5.5	2.5
Potato chips	10 chips	20	3	105	1	7	1.8	1.2
Pumpkin								
Cooked from raw, mashed	1 c	245	94	50	2	tr	0.1	tr
Canned	1 c	245	90	85	3	1	0.4	0.1
Radishes, raw, stem ends, rootlets cut off	4 radishes	18	95	5	tr	tr	tr	tr
Sauerkraut, canned, solids and liquid	1 c	236	93	45	2	tr	0.1	tr
Seaweed								
Kelp, raw	1 oz	28	82	10	tr	tr	0.1	tr
Spirulina, dried	1 oz	28	5	80	16	2	0.8	0.2
Southern peas. See Black-eyed peas, immature, mature								
Spinach								
Raw, chopped	1 c	55	92	10	2	tr	tr	tr
Cooked, drained								
From raw	1 c	180	91	40	5	tr	0.1	tr
From frozen (leaf)	1 c	190	90	55	6	tr	0.1	tr
Canned, drained solids	1 c	214	92	50	6	1	0.2	tr

tr = nutrient present in trace amounts.
[55]Value not determined.
[56]With added salt; if none is added, sodium content is 58 mg.

POLY-UNSATURATED (g)	CHOLES-TEROL (mg)	CARBO-HYDRATE (g)	CALCIUM (mg)	PHOS-PHORUS (mg)	IRON (mg)	POTASSIUM (mg)	SODIUM (mg)	VITAMIN A VALUES		THIAMIN (mg)	RIBO-FLAVIN (mg)	NIACIN (mg)	ASCORBIC ACID (mg)
								IU	RE				
0.1	0	27	7	60	0.4	515	5	0	0	0.14	0.03	2.0	18
0.1	0	27	11	54	0.4	443	7	0	0	0.13	0.03	1.8	10
0.3	0	17	5	43	0.7	229	16	0	0	0.06	0.02	1.2	5
3.8	0	20	10	47	0.4	366	108	0	0	0.09	0.01	1.6	5
0.3	12	31	203	233	0.8	537	1076	520	76	0.05	0.20	2.3	8
0.7	56	28	292	277	1.6	970	1061	650	93	0.16	0.28	2.4	24
2.1	0	44	23	112	2.4	680	53	0	0	0.17	0.03	3.8	10
0.1	4	37	55	101	0.6	628	636	40	12	0.18	0.08	2.3	14
2.5	4	35	55	97	0.5	607	620	360	42	0.18	0.08	2.3	13
0.5	29	32	103	118	0.5	489	697	380	44	0.23	0.11	1.4	20
9.3	170	28	48	130	1.6	635	1323	520	83	0.19	0.15	2.2	25
0.5	27	31	88	137	0.9	497	835	360	51	0.05	0.14	2.5	8
0.4	29	26	140	154	1.4	926	821	330	47	0.17	0.23	2.6	26
3.6	0	10	5	31	0.2	260	94	0	0	0.03	tr	0.8	8
tr	0	12	37	74	1.4	564	2	2650	265	0.08	0.19	1.0	12
tr	0	20	64	86	3.4	505	12	54,040	5404	0.06	0.13	0.9	10
tr	0	1	4	3	0.1	42	4	tr	tr	tr	0.01	0.1	4
0.1	0	10	71	47	3.5	401	1560	40	4	0.05	0.05	0.3	35
tr	0	3	48	12	0.8	25	66	30	3	0.01	0.04	0.1	(55)
0.6	0	7	34	33	8.1	386	297	160	16	0.67	1.04	3.6	3
0.1	0	2	54	27	1.5	307	43	3690	369	0.04	0.10	0.4	15
0.2	0	7	245	101	6.4	839	126	14,740	1474	0.17	0.42	0.9	18
0.2	0	10	277	91	2.9	566	163	14,790	1479	0.11	0.32	0.8	23
0.4	0	7	272	94	4.9	740	683[56]	18,780	1878	0.03	0.30	0.8	31

Continued

FOODS, APPROXIMATE MEASURES, UNITS, AND WEIGHT (WEIGHT OF EDIBLE PORTION ONLY)		GRAMS	WATER (g)	FOOD ENERGY (CALORIES)	PROTEIN (g)	FAT (g)	FATTY ACIDS	
							SATURATED (g)	MONO-UNSATURATED (g)
VEGETABLES AND VEGETABLE PRODUCTS—cont'd								
Spinach souffle	1 c	136	74	220	11	18	7.1	6.8
Squash, cooked								
Summer (all varieties), sliced, drained	1 c	180	94	35	2	1	0.1	tr
Winter (all varieties), baked, cubes	1 c	205	89	80	2	1	0.3	0.1
Sunchoke. See Jerusalem-artichoke								
Sweet potatoes								
Cooked (raw, 5 by 2 in; about 2½ per lb)								
Baked in skin, peeled	1 potato	114	73	115	2	tr	tr	tr
Boiled, without skin	1 potato	151	73	160	2	tr	0.1	tr
Candied, 2½ by 2-in piece	1 piece	105	67	145	1	3	1.4	0.7
Canned								
Solid pack (mashed)	1 c	255	74	260	5	1	0.1	tr
Vacuum pack, piece 2¾ by 1 in	1 piece	40	76	35	1	tr	tr	tr
Tomatoes								
Raw, 2⅗-in diam. (3 per 12 oz pkg.)	1 tomato	123	94	25	1	tr	tr	tr
Canned, solids and liquid	1 c	240	94	50	2	1	0.1	0.1
Tomato juice, canned	1 c	244	94	40	2	tr	tr	tr
Tomato products, canned								
Paste	1 c	262	74	220	10	2	0.3	0.4
Puree	1 c	250	87	105	4	tr	tr	tr
Sauce	1 c	245	89	75	3	tr	0.1	0.1
Turnips, cooked, diced	1 c	156	94	30	1	tr	tr	tr
Turnip greens, cooked, drained								
From raw (leaves and stems)	1 c	144	93	30	2	tr	0.1	tr
From frozen (chopped)	1 c	164	90	50	5	1	0.2	tr
Vegetable juice cocktail, canned	1 c	242	94	45	2	tr	tr	tr
Vegetables, mixed								
Canned, drained solids	1 c	163	87	75	4	tr	0.1	tr
Frozen, cooked, drained	1 c	182	83	105	5	tr	0.1	tr
Waterchestnuts, canned	1 c	140	86	70	1	tr	tr	tr

tr = nutrient present in trace amounts.
[57]For regular pack; special dietary pack contains 31 mg sodium.
[58]With added salt; if none is added, sodium content is 24 mg.
[59]With no added salt; if salt is added, sodium content is 2070 mg.
[60]With no added salt; if salt is added, sodium content is 998 mg.
[61]With salt added.

NUTRIENTS IN INDICATED QUANTITY

POLY-UNSATURATED (g)	CHOLES-TEROL (mg)	CARBO-HYDRATE (g)	CALCIUM (mg)	PHOS-PHORUS (mg)	IRON (mg)	POTASSIUM (mg)	SODIUM (mg)	VITAMIN A VALUES		THIAMIN (mg)	RIBO-FLAVIN (mg)	NIACIN (mg)	ASCORBIC ACID (mg)
								IU	RE				
3.1	184	3	230	231	1.3	201	763	3460	675	0.09	0.30	0.5	3
0.2	0	8	49	70	0.6	346	2	520	52	0.08	0.07	0.9	10
0.5	0	18	29	41	0.7	896	2	7290	729	0.17	0.05	1.4	20
0.1	0	28	32	63	0.5	397	11	24,880	2488	0.08	0.14	0.7	28
0.2	0	37	32	41	0.8	278	20	25,750	2575	0.08	0.21	1.0	26
0.2	8	29	27	27	1.2	198	74	4400	440	0.02	0.04	0.4	7
0.2	0	59	77	133	3.4	536	191	38,570	3857	0.07	0.23	2.4	13
tr	0	8	9	20	0.4	125	21	3190	319	0.01	0.02	0.3	11
0.1	0	5	9	28	0.6	255	10	1390	139	0.07	0.06	0.7	22
0.2	0	10	62	46	1.5	530	391[57]	1450	145	0.11	0.07	1.8	36
0.1	0	10	22	46	1.4	537	881[58]	1360	136	0.11	0.08	1.6	45
0.9	0	49	92	207	7.8	2442	170[59]	6470	647	0.41	0.50	8.4	111
0.1	0	25	38	100	2.3	1050	50[60]	3400	340	0.18	0.14	4.3	88
0.2	0	18	34	78	1.9	909	1482[61]	2400	240	0.16	0.14	2.8	32
0.1	0	8	34	30	0.3	211	78	0	0	0.04	0.04	0.5	18
0.1	0	6	197	42	1.2	292	42	7920	792	0.06	0.10	0.6	39
0.3	0	8	249	56	3.2	367	25	13,080	1308	0.09	0.12	0.8	36
0.1	0	11	27	41	1.0	467	883	2830	283	0.10	0.07	1.8	67
0.2	0	15	44	68	1.7	474	243	18,990	1899	0.08	0.08	0.9	8
0.1	0	24	46	93	1.5	308	64	7780	778	0.13	0.22	1.5	6
tr	0	17	6	27	1.2	165	11	10	1	0.02	0.03	0.5	2

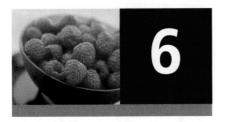

6 Dietary Fiber Content and Composition of Typical Servings of U.S. Foods

FOOD	SERVING SIZE HOUSEHOLD	WT	SOLUBLE HC	P	TOTAL	INSOLUBLE C	HC	P	KL	TOTAL	TOTAL
FRUITS											
Category 1											
Apple pie filling, canned	⅛ of 9-in pie	71	0.1	0.1	0.2	0.2	0.1	0.1	tr	0.5	0.7
Cantaloupe, fresh	½ c cubed	80	tr	0.1	0.1	0.3	0.1	0.1	tr	0.5	0.6
Cherries, tart, canned	½ c	89	0.1	0.1	0.2	0.1	0.1	0.2	0.2	0.6	0.8
Cherry pie filling, canned	⅛ of 9-in pie	106	0.5	tr	0.5	0.1	0.1	0.1	0.1	0.4	0.9
Cranberry sauce, canned	¼ c	69	tr	0.1	0.2	0.2	0.1	tr	0.2	0.5	0.7
Fruit cocktail, canned	½ c	84	0.1	0.1	0.2	0.2	0.2	0.1	0.2	0.7	0.9
Grapes, fresh, black, red, Thompson (3)	10	50	tr	tr	tr	0.1	0.1	0.1	0.2	0.5	0.5
Honeydew melon, fresh	½ c cubed	85	tr	0.1	0.1	0.2	0.1	0.1	tr	0.4	0.5
Lemon, fresh, peeled	1 wedge (¼ fruit)	15	tr	tr	tr	0.1	tr	0.1	tr	0.2	0.2
Lemonade, with pulp	1 c	244	0.0	0.0	0.0	0.0	0.0	0.0	0.0	0.0	0.0
Orange, mandarin, canned	½ c	107	tr	tr	tr	tr	0.1	0.1	tr	0.2	0.3
Pineapple, canned or fresh (2)	2 slices (3-in diameter, ⁵⁄₁₆ in thick) or ½ c diced	78	tr	tr	0.1	0.3	0.3	tr	tr	0.6	0.7
Plum, Friar, fresh, unpeeled	1 (2⅛-in diameter)	66	0.1	0.2	0.3	0.2	0.1	0.1	0.1	0.5	0.8
Plum, prune, fresh, unpeeled	1 (1½-in diameter)	28	tr	0.1	0.1	0.1	0.1	0.1	0.1	0.4	0.5
Plum, canned	*3*	*65*	*0.1*	*0.3*	*0.4*	*0.3*	*0.3*	*0.1*	*0.1*	*0.8*	*1.2*
Watermelon, fresh	½ c cubed	80	tr	tr	tr	0.1	0.1	0.1	tr	0.3	0.3
Category 2											
Applesauce, canned	½ c	122	0.1	0.2	0.3	0.5	0.4	0.2	0.1	1.2	1.5
Apricot, canned or fresh, unpeeled (2)	4 halves canned or 2 fresh	75	0.1	0.3	0.4	0.4	0.3	0.1	0.1	0.9	1.3
Apricot, dried	*4 halves*	*14*	*0.1*	*0.2*	*0.3*	*0.3*	*0.2*	*0.1*	*0.1*	*0.7*	*1.0*
Banana	1 (8¾ in long)	114	0.2	0.3	0.5	0.3	0.2	0.2	0.6	1.3	1.8
Grapefruit, fresh, with membrane (4)	½ (3⁹⁄₁₆-in diameter)	100	0.1	0.2	0.3	0.3	0.3	0.5	tr	1.1	1.4

From Marlette JA, Cheung T: Database and quick methods of assessing typical dietary fiber intakes using data for 228 commonly consumed foods. JADA, October 1997; 97(10):1142–1147.
tr = nutrient present in trace amounts.

Continued

FOOD	SERVING SIZE		DIETARY FIBER COMPONENTS (G/SERVING FRESH WT)									
			SOLUBLE			INSOLUBLE						
	HOUSEHOLD	WT	HC	P	TOTAL	C	HC	P	KL	TOTAL	TOTAL
FRUITS—cont'd												
Category 2—cont'd												
Grapefruit, fresh, without membrane (3)	*½ (3⁹⁄₁₆-in diameter)*	*100*	*0.1*	*0.1*	*0.1*	*0.1*	*0.1*	*0.1*	*tr*	*0.3*	*0.4*
Kiwi fruit	1 medium	76	0.1	0.2	0.3	0.3	0.2	0.1	0.6	1.2	1.5
Nectarine, fresh, unpeeled	1 (2½-in diameter)	136	0.2	0.3	0.6	0.4	0.3	0.2	0.1	1.0	1.6
Papaya, fresh	½ c cubed	70	tr	tr	0.1	0.6	0.3	0.5	tr	1.4	1.5
Peach, canned or fresh, peeled (2)	2 halves canned or 1 fresh (2½-in diameter)	100	0.2	0.3	0.5	0.3	0.2	0.1	0.1	0.8	1.3
Peach, fresh, unpeeled	1	100	0.2	0.4	0.6	0.5	0.4	0.1	0.1	1.1	1.7
Raisins, seedless	¼ c	37	0.1	0.1	0.2	0.3	0.2	0.2	0.7	1.4	1.6
Rhubarb, fresh, cooked with sugar	½ c	135	tr	0.2	0.2	0.5	0.2	0.1	0.1	0.9	1.1
Strawberries, fresh or frozen (2)	½ c	75	0.1	0.2	0.3	0.3	0.2	0.1	0.4	1.0	1.3
Tangerine, fresh	1 medium (2⅜-in diameter)	84	0.1	0.2	0.3	0.4	0.3	0.4	0.1	1.2	1.5
Category 3												
Apple, unpeeled, Granny Smith, McIntosh, Red Delicious (3)	1 (2¾-in diameter)	138	0.1	0.3	0.4	1.0	0.8	0.5	0.3	2.6	3.0
Apple, fresh, peeled	*1 (2¾-in diameter)*	*128*	*tr*	*0.2*	*0.2*	*0.7*	*0.5*	*0.4*	*0.1*	*1.7*	*1.9*
Blueberries, fresh or frozen (2)	½ c	73	0.1	0.1	0.2	0.4	0.5	0.3	0.7	1.9	2.1
Orange, fresh, Florida, navel, Temple, Valencia (4)	1 (2⅝-in diameter)	131	0.2	0.3	0.5	0.5	0.5	0.6	0.1	1.7	2.2
Raspberries, red, fresh	½ c	62	0.1	0.2	0.3	0.4	0.4	0.1	1.4	2.3	2.6
Category 4												
Avocado (2)	½	95	0.4	0.8	1.2	1.3	0.9	0.3	0.1	2.6	3.8
Blackberries, frozen	½ c	76	0.1	0.3	0.4	0.9	0.9	0.4	2.3	4.5	4.9
Dates, dried	3	25	0.0	0.1	0.1	0.9	0.9	0.4	2.0	4.2	4.3
Figs, dried	3	62	0.2	0.3	0.5	1.0	0.8	1.1	1.5	4.4	4.9
Pear, Bartlett, fresh, unpeeled	1 (2½-in diameter, 3½ in long)	166	0.3	0.4	0.7	1.2	1.4	0.7	0.6	3.9	4.6
Pear, canned	*2 halves*	*102*	*0.1*	*0.2*	*0.3*	*0.6*	*0.6*	*0.1*	*0.2*	*1.5*	*1.8*
Prunes, dried	5	42	0.4	0.7	1.1	0.5	0.7	0.3	0.5	2.0	3.1

tr = nutrient present in trace amounts.

FOOD	SERVING SIZE HOUSEHOLD	WT	SOLUBLE HC	P	TOTAL	INSOLUBLE C	HC	P	KL	TOTAL	TOTAL
VEGETABLES											
Category 1											
Bamboo shoots, canned	½ c sliced	66	0.1	tr	0.1	0.5	0.3	tr	0.1	0.9	1.0
Bean sprouts, mung, raw, canned or cooked (3)	½ c	60	tr	tr	tr	0.3	0.3	0.1	0.1	0.8	0.8
Cabbage, Chinese, fresh	½ c shredded	38	tr	tr	tr	0.2	0.1	0.1	tr	0.4	0.4
Cabbage, green or red, raw (2)	½ c shredded	35	tr	tr	tr	0.3	0.2	0.2	tr	0.7	0.7
Cabbage, green, cooked	*½ c shredded*	*73*	*tr*	*0.1*	*0.1*	*0.6*	*0.5*	*0.4*	*0.1*	*1.6*	*1.7*
Cucumber, unpeeled	½ c	52	tr	tr	tr	0.2	0.1	0.1	0.1	0.5	0.5
Cucumber, peeled	½ c	70	tr	tr	tr	0.2	0.1	0.1	tr	0.4	0.4
Endive, fresh	½ c chopped	25	tr	tr	tr	0.2	0.1	0.3	0.1	0.7	0.7
Escarole, fresh	½ c pieces	25	tr	tr	tr	0.1	0.1	0.1	0.1	0.4	0.4
Ketchup	2½-oz packets or 2 tbsp	14	tr	tr	0.1	0.1	tr	tr	tr	0.1	0.2
Lettuce, fresh, leaf, romaine or iceberg (4)	1 c shredded or 4 to 6 leaves	56	tr	tr	tr	0.3	0.1	0.2	0.1	0.7	0.7
Mushrooms, fresh	½ c pieces or 2	35	0.1	tr	0.1	0.1	tr	tr	0.1	0.2	0.3
Mushrooms, canned	¼ c	39	0.1	tr	0.1	0.7	0.1	0.1	tr	0.9	1.0
Olives, green with pimento, or black (2)	5 large	20	tr	tr	tr	0.1	0.1	0.1	0.1	0.4	0.4
Onion, green, raw	1 stalk (10½ in long) or 2 tbsp chopped	13	tr	tr	tr	0.1	0.1	0.1	tr	0.3	0.3
Pickle, dill or bread and butter chips (2)	2 slices (1½-in diameter, ¼ in thick)	13	tr	tr	tr	0.1	tr	tr	tr	0.1	0.1
Pickle relish	1 tbsp	15	tr	tr	tr	0.1	tr	tr	tr	0.2	0.2
Radish, red or white, fresh (2)	10 (¾- to 1-in diameter) or ½ c sliced	50	tr	tr	tr	0.3	0.1	0.2	tr	0.6	0.6
Soup, cream of mushroom, canned	1 c prepared	244	0.1	tr	0.2	0.2	0.1	tr	0.0	0.3	0.5
Soup, cream of tomato, canned	1 c prepared	244	0.1	0.1	0.2	0.4	0.2	tr	0.1	0.7	0.9
Squash, yellow zucchini, cooked or raw (2)	½ c sliced	80	tr	tr	0.1	0.2	0.2	0.2	tr	0.6	0.7
Tomato, canned or fresh (3)	½ c or 1 whole (2⅗-in diameter)	100	tr	0.1	0.2	0.3	0.1	0.1	0.1	0.6	0.8
Water chestnuts, canned	½ c sliced	70	tr	tr	tr	0.5	0.3	tr	tr	0.8	0.8
Category 2											
Asparagus, canned or fresh, cooked (2)	½ c or 6 spears (6½ in long, ½-in diameter)	100	0.2	0.1	0.3	0.5	0.5	0.2	0.2	1.4	1.7

Continued

FOOD	SERVING SIZE HOUSEHOLD	WT	SOLUBLE HC	SOLUBLE P	SOLUBLE TOTAL	INSOLUBLE C	INSOLUBLE HC	INSOLUBLE P	INSOLUBLE KL	INSOLUBLE TOTAL	TOTAL
VEGETABLES—cont'd											
Category 2—cont'd											
Beans, green, or yellow wax, canned, cooked, or raw (5)	½ c	65	0.1	0.1	0.3	0.5	0.4	0.3	0.1	1.2	1.5
Beets, canned or fresh, cooked (2)	½ c sliced	85	0.2	0.3	0.5	0.6	0.4	0.2	tr	1.2	1.6
Beet greens, fresh, cooked	½ c (1-in pieces)	72	0.1	0.2	0.3	0.6	0.4	0.2	0.1	1.3	1.6
Bok choy, fresh, cooked	½ c shredded	85	tr	tr	0.1	0.4	0.2	0.4	0.1	1.1	1.2
Broccoli, cooked or raw or frozen (3)	2 stalks (4½ to 5 in long)	60	0.1	0.1	0.2	0.6	0.5	0.4	0.1	1.7	1.8
Carrot, canned, cooked, or raw (3)	1 (1⅛-in diameter, 7½-in long) or ½ c sliced	70	0.2	0.2	0.4	0.6	0.4	0.4	0.1	1.5	1.9
Cauliflower, cooked or raw (2)	½ c (1-in pieces)	55	0.1	0.1	0.2	0.4	0.4	0.2	tr	1.0	1.2
Celery, cooked or raw (2)	½ c diced or 3 stalks (5 in long, ¾-in diameter)	62	tr	tr	0.1	0.5	0.2	0.3	tr	1.0	1.1
Corn, creamed, canned	½ c	128	0.4	tr	0.4	0.4	0.6	tr	0.2	1.2	1.6
Corn, whole kernel, canned or frozen (2)	½ c	82	0.1	tr	0.1	0.5	0.7	0.2	0.1	1.5	1.6
Corn, cooked on cob	*1 ear (3½-in diameter)*	*77*	*tr*	*tr*	*0.1*	*0.3*	*0.5*	*0.1*	*tr*	*0.9*	*1.0*
Eggplant, fresh, cooked	½ c cubed	48	0.1	0.2	0.2	0.4	0.3	0.1	0.1	0.9	1.2
Kohlrabi, fresh, cooked	½ c sliced	82	0.1	0.1	0.2	0.6	0.4	0.3	tr	1.4	1.6
Onion rings, frozen, cooked	7 rings	70	0.2	0.2	0.4	0.7	0.4	0.1	0.1	1.3	1.7
Onion, red, white, or yellow, raw or cooked (4)	½ c chopped	80	tr	0.1	0.1	0.4	0.4	0.3	tr	1.1	1.2
Pea pods, fresh, cooked	½ c	80	0.1	0.2	0.2	0.8	0.4	0.4	0.1	1.6	1.8
Pepper, green or chili, canned or raw (2)	1 green or 2 canned chilis or ½ c chopped	62	tr	0.1	0.1	0.3	0.2	0.1	0.1	0.8	0.9
Potato chips	*1 bag*	*28*	*0.1*	*0.1*	*0.2*	*0.3*	*0.4*	*0.1*	*0.0*	*0.8*	*0.9*
Potato, french fries	10 strips	50	0.1	0.1	0.2	0.5	0.3	0.1	tr	0.9	1.1
Potato, red, peeled, boiled	1 (2½-in diameter)	135	0.2	0.2	0.4	0.4	0.3	0.1	tr	0.8	1.2
Potato, red, unpeeled, boiled	*1 (2½-in diameter)*	*150*	*0.3*	*0.3*	*0.6*	*0.8*	*0.6*	*0.2*	*0.2*	*1.8*	*2.4*
Potato, white, peeled, boiled, or baked without skin (6)	*1 (2½-in diameter)*	*135*	*0.2*	*0.2*	*0.4*	*0.8*	*0.6*	*0.3*	*tr*	*1.7*	*2.1*

tr = nutrient present in trace amounts.

			DIETARY FIBER COMPONENTS (G/SERVING FRESH WT)									
	SERVING SIZE		SOLUBLE			INSOLUBLE						
FOOD	HOUSEHOLD	WT	HC	P	TOTAL	C	HC	P	KL	TOTAL	TOTAL
VEGETABLES—cont'd											
Category 2—cont'd											
Potato, white, unpeeled, baked	*1 (2½-in diameter)*	*170*	*0.6*	*0.4*	*1.0*	*1.7*	*0.8*	*0.2*	*0.5*	*3.1*	*4.1*
Potato hash, with corned beef, canned	1 c	225	0.5	0.2	0.7	0.9	0.2	0.1	0.1	1.3	2.0
Potato salad, American, peeled	½ c	125	0.2	0.2	0.4	0.6	0.3	0.1	tr	1.1	1.5
Potato, scalloped, frozen, cooked	½ c	*122*	*0.1*	*0.1*	*0.2*	*0.4*	*0.2*	*0.1*	*tr*	*0.7*	*0.9*
Rutabaga, fresh, cooked	½ c cubed	85	0.1	0.2	0.3	0.6	0.4	0.5	0.1	1.6	1.9
Sauerkraut, canned	½ c	73	0.1	0.1	0.2	0.7	0.4	0.5	tr	1.7	1.9
Soup, vegetable and beef, canned	1 c prepared	251	0.3	0.1	0.4	0.7	0.2	0.1	0.2	1.1	1.6
Squash, acorn or butternut, cooked (2)	½ c cubed	102	0.1	0.3	0.3	0.9	0.3	0.3	tr	1.6	1.9
Sweet potato, canned or baked, peeled (2)	½ c or 1 whole (5 in long, 2-in diameter)	106	0.2	0.3	0.5	0.8	0.4	0.2	0.1	1.4	1.9
Category 3											
Collard, frozen, cooked	½ c chopped	85	0.1	0.1	0.2	1.0	0.7	0.8	0.2	2.7	2.9
Kale, fresh, cooked	½ c	65	0.1	0.2	0.3	0.7	0.7	0.7	0.2	2.2	2.5
Mustard greens, frozen, cooked	½ c chopped	75	tr	0.2	0.2	0.8	0.5	0.6	0.1	2.0	2.2
Okra, frozen, cooked	½ c sliced	92	0.3	0.3	0.6	0.4	0.3	0.2	0.6	1.5	2.1
Parsnip, fresh, cooked	½ c sliced	78	0.2	0.4	0.6	0.9	0.9	0.5	0.1	2.4	3.0
Soup, vegetarian vegetable, canned	1 c prepared	241	0.3	0.2	0.6	0.9	0.4	0.1	0.1	1.6	2.1
Spaghetti sauce, meatless	½ c	125	0.1	0.4	0.6	0.9	0.4	0.3	0.8	2.4	3.0
Spinach, canned, cooked or raw (3)	½ c canned or cooked, or 2 c raw	100	0.1	0.2	0.3	0.8	0.5	0.3	0.3	2.0	2.3
Swiss chard, fresh, cooked	½ c chopped	88	0.1	0.2	0.3	0.7	0.5	0.3	0.2	1.8	2.1
Turnip greens, frozen	½ c chopped	82	tr	0.1	0.1	0.7	0.5	0.6	0.1	1.9	2.1
Category 4											
Artichoke, fresh, cooked	1 medium	120	3.0	0.5	3.5	1.2	1.0	0.7	0.1	2.9	6.4
Brussels sprouts, frozen, cooked	½ c	78	0.1	0.3	0.4	1.0	1.2	0.6	0.1	2.8	3.2
Pumpkin, canned	½ c	122	0.2	0.5	0.6	1.8	0.4	0.5	0.2	2.9	3.5
GRAIN PRODUCTS											
Category 1											
Biscuit, baking powder (2)	1 (2-in diameter, 1¼ in high)	28	0.1	tr	0.1	0.1	0.2	tr	tr	0.4	0.5

Continued

FOOD	SERVING SIZE HOUSEHOLD	WT	DIETARY FIBER COMPONENTS (G/SERVING FRESH WT) SOLUBLE HC	P	TOTAL	INSOLUBLE C	HC	P	KL	TOTAL	TOTAL
GRAIN PRODUCTS—cont'd											
Category 1—cont'd											
Bread, French	2 small slices (2½ in wide, 2 in high, ½ in thick)	30	0.2	tr	0.2	0.3	0.2	tr	tr	0.6	0.8
Bread, raisin without icing	1 slice	25	0.1	tr	0.2	0.1	0.1	tr	0.2	0.5	0.7
Bread, white or Italian (4)	1 slice	25	0.2	tr	0.2	0.2	0.2	tr	0.2	0.6	0.8
Bread, rye	1 slice	25	0.2	tr	0.2	0.1	0.3	tr	0.1	0.5	0.7
Brownie, plain	1 (1¾-in square)	20	0.1	tr	0.1	tr	0.1	tr	0.2	0.3	0.4
Brownie, with nuts	1 (1¾-in square)	20	0.1	tr	0.1	0.1	0.1	tr	0.3	0.5	0.6
Bun, hamburger	1	40	0.3	tr	0.3	0.3	0.3	tr	0.1	0.7	1.0
Cake, pound or sponge (3)	¹⁄₁₅ of 1-lb loaf	30	0.1	tr	0.1	0.1	0.1	tr	0.1	0.2	0.4
Cake, gingerbread	1 piece (2¾-in square)	63	0.2	tr	0.2	0.2	0.3	tr	0.2	0.6	0.9
Cake, coffee (2)	⅛ of 8-in round cake	58	0.2	tr	0.2	0.1	0.3	tr	0.1	0.5	0.8
Cake, white or yellow (4)	3-in square sheet cake or ¹⁄₁₂ of 9-in 2-layer cake	80	0.3	tr	0.3	0.2	0.2	tr	0.1	0.5	0.8
Cake, coconut, frozen	¹⁄₁₀ of 6-in square, 3-layer cake	48	0.1	tr	0.1	tr	0.3	tr	tr	0.3	0.4
Cake, Twinkies	1 piece	42	0.1	tr	0.1	0.1	0.1	tr	tr	0.2	0.3
Cereal, Corn Chex	1 c	28	tr	tr	tr	0.3	0.1	tr	0.4	0.8	0.8
Cereal, Total, cornflakes	1 c	28	tr	0.0	tr	0.3	0.1	tr	0.5	0.8	0.9
Cereal, Golden Grahams	1 c	28	0.1	tr	0.1	0.3	0.3	tr	0.1	0.7	0.8
Cereal, puffed rice	1 c	14	tr	0.0	tr	tr	tr	tr	0.1	0.1	0.2
Cereal, puffed wheat	1 c	14	0.3	tr	0.3	0.2	0.3	tr	0.1	0.6	0.9
Cereal, Rice Krispies	1 c	28	0.1	tr	0.1	0.1	0.1	tr	0.2	0.4	0.5
Cereal, Special K	1 c	28	tr	tr	0.1	0.2	0.2	tr	0.2	0.7	0.7
Cereal, Smacks	¾ c	28	0.2	tr	0.2	0.2	0.2	tr	tr	0.5	0.7
Cereal, sugar-frosted cornflakes	¾ c	28	tr	tr	tr	0.3	0.1	tr	0.1	0.5	0.5
Cookies, gingersnap	4	28	0.2	tr	0.2	0.1	0.2	0.0	0.1	0.4	0.5
Cookies, oatmeal (2)	1 large	28	0.1	tr	0.3	0.1	0.2	tr	0.2	0.6	0.9
Cookies, oatmeal and raisin (2)	2	24	0.1	tr	0.3	0.1	0.2	tr	0.2	0.6	1.0
Cookies, peanut	1 large	26	0.1	tr	0.1	0.2	0.3	0.1	tr	0.5	0.6
Cookies, plain sugar	1	20	0.1	0.0	0.1	tr	0.1	tr	tr	0.1	0.2
Cookies, macaroon	2	30	0.1	tr	0.1	0.1	0.3	tr	tr	0.3	0.5
Cookies, shortbread (2)	4	30	0.2	tr	0.2	0.1	0.2	tr	0.0	0.3	0.4
Cookies, sugar wafer, cream filled	8	28	0.1	tr	0.1	0.1	0.1	tr	tr	0.2	0.3
Crackers, cheese, snack	13 small	14	0.1	tr	0.1	0.1	0.1	tr	tr	0.2	0.3
Crackers, graham	2 pieces (2½-in square)	14	0.1	tr	0.1	0.1	0.1	tr	0.1	0.3	0.4

tr = nutrient present in trace amounts.

| | SERVING SIZE | | DIETARY FIBER COMPONENTS (G/SERVING FRESH WT) | | | | | | | | |
| | | | SOLUBLE | | | INSOLUBLE | | | | | |
FOOD	HOUSEHOLD	WT	HC	P	TOTAL	C	HC	P	KL	TOTAL	TOTAL
GRAIN PRODUCTS—cont'd											
Category 1—cont'd											
Crackers, peanut butter and cheese squares	2 sandwiches	14	0.1	tr	0.1	0.2	0.2	tr	0.1	0.4	0.5
Crackers, Ritz	4 crackers	14	0.1	0.0	0.1	tr	0.1	0.0	tr	0.2	0.3
Crackers, saltine	4	11	0.1	tr	0.1	0.1	0.1	tr	0.1	0.2	0.3
Crackers, Waverly	4	14	0.1	tr	0.1	0.1	0.1	tr	tr	0.2	0.3
Croutons, seasoned	¼ c	8	0.1	0.0	0.1	0.1	0.1	0.0	tr	0.1	0.2
Doughnut, jelly	1	65	0.3	tr	0.3	0.1	0.2	tr	0.1	0.4	0.7
Doughnut, plain (2)	1	25	0.1	tr	0.1	0.1	0.1	tr	tr	0.2	0.3
Flour, white, wheat, all purpose	1 tbsp	8	0.1	tr	0.1	tr	0.1	0.0	tr	0.2	0.2
Hominy, white, cooked	½ c	80	tr	tr	tr	0.4	0.1	tr	tr	0.5	0.5
Ice cream cone, Comet cup	1	5	tr	0.0	tr	tr	0.1	0.0	tr	0.1	0.1
Muffin, blueberry (2)	1 small	40	0.2	tr	0.2	0.2	0.2	tr	0.3	0.6	0.8
Muffin, plain (2)	1 small	40	0.2	tr	0.2	0.1	0.2	tr	0.1	0.4	0.6
Pancake	2 (4-in diameter)	54	0.2	tr	0.2	0.3	0.3	tr	0.1	0.7	0.8
Pancake, buckwheat	*2 (4-in diameter)*	*54*	*0.3*	*tr*	*0.3*	*0.8*	*0.7*	*tr*	*0.9*	*2.3*	*2.6*
Piecrust (3)	⅛ of 9-in pie	23	0.1	tr	0.1	0.1	0.2	tr	0.1	0.4	0.5
Rice, medium grain, regular, cooked	½ c	102	tr	tr	tr	0.1	0.1	tr	0.1	0.3	0.4
Roll, dinner (3)	1 small	28	0.3	tr	0.3	0.2	0.2	tr	0.1	0.5	0.8
Roll, hard	1 small	25	0.2	0.0	0.2	0.1	0.2	tr	0.3	0.6	0.8
Taco shell	1	11	tr	tr	tr	0.3	0.3	tr	0.1	0.7	0.7
Tortilla, flour	1	30	0.1	0.0	0.1	0.1	0.1	0.0	0.1	0.3	0.4
Waffle (3)	1 (4½-in square)	50	0.2	tr	0.2	0.1	0.2	tr	0.2	0.5	0.7
Category 2											
Cake, devil's food	3-in square sheet cake or ¹⁄₁₂ of 9-in 2-layer cake	81	0.2	0.1	0.2	0.3	0.2	0.1	0.8	1.3	1.6
Cereal, Product 19	¾ c	28	0.1	tr	0.1	0.5	0.4	0.1	0.4	1.4	1.5
Cereal, Cream of Wheat, quick, cooked	¾ c	179	0.3	tr	0.3	0.5	0.4	tr	0.2	1.1	1.4
Cereal, cornflakes	1 c	28	0.1	tr	0.1	0.6	0.3	tr	0.2	1.1	1.2
Cereal, Grapenuts	¼ c	28	0.4	tr	0.4	0.4	0.9	tr	0.2	1.6	2.0
Cereal, granola	¼ c	28	0.2	tr	0.5	0.3	0.9	0.1	0.1	1.4	1.9
Cookies, date (2)	2	30	0.1	p	0.1	0.2	0.2	0.1	0.5	1.0	1.1
Cookies, fig	2	30	0.2	0.2	0.4	0.2	0.2	0.3	0.3	1.0	1.4
Crackers, Triscuits	3	14	0.1	tr	0.1	0.4	0.7	tr	0.1	1.2	1.3
Cream puff, fresh, without filling	1	50	0.2	tr	0.2	0.3	0.4	0.0	0.3	1.0	1.2
Doughnut, glazed	1	64	0.3	tr	0.3	0.2	0.3	tr	0.3	0.8	1.1

Continued

FOOD	SERVING SIZE HOUSEHOLD	WT	SOLUBLE HC	P	TOTAL	INSOLUBLE C	HC	P	KL	TOTAL	DIETARY FIBER COMPONENTS (G/SERVING FRESH WT) TOTAL
GRAIN PRODUCTS—cont'd											
Category 2—cont'd											
Éclair, frozen	1	100	0.7	tr	0.7	0.2	0.2	tr	0.5	1.0	1.7
Hush puppies, fresh	3	45	0.2	tr	0.2	0.3	0.5	0.1	0.2	1.1	1.3
Muffin, English	1	57	0.3	tr	0.3	0.5	0.5	tr	0.4	1.3	1.7
Noodles, chow mein	1 c	45	0.4	tr	0.4	0.4	0.6	tr	tr	1.1	1.5
Pasta, macaroni, spaghetti, shells, egg noodles, or vermicelli (8)	1 c	130	0.4	tr	0.4	0.5	0.7	tr	0.3	1.6	2.0
Pie, apple	⅛ of 9-in pie	118	0.5	0.1	0.5	0.3	0.4	0.1	0.1	0.9	1.5
Pie, cherry	⅛ of 9-in pie	118	0.6	tr	0.6	0.2	0.2	0.1	0.1	0.6	1.2
Pie, pecan	⅛ of 9-in pie	103	0.2	tr	0.3	0.2	0.4	0.1	0.2	0.9	1.2
Pie, rhubarb	⅛ of 9-in pie	118	0.3	0.2	0.6	0.6	0.4	0.1	0.1	1.1	1.7
Pie, strawberry	⅛ of 9-in pie	93	0.4	0.1	0.5	0.2	0.2	tr	0.2	0.6	1.1
Roll, submarine	½ of 11½-in roll	68	0.5	tr	0.5	0.3	0.5	tr	0.6	1.4	1.9
Roll, sweetened, cinnamon (2)	1	56	0.3	tr	0.3	0.3	0.3	tr	0.2	0.8	1.1
Roll, sweetened, with raisins	1	53	0.3	tr	0.3	0.2	0.3	tr	0.3	0.8	1.1
Roll, sweetened, with nuts (2)	1	73	0.4	tr	0.4	0.4	0.4	0.1	0.2	1.0	1.4
Stuffing, cornbread	½ c	90	0.2	tr	0.2	0.5	0.2	0.1	0.1	0.9	1.1
Category 3											
Bread, whole wheat	1 slice	28	0.3	tr	0.3	0.6	1.2	tr	0.4	2.2	2.5
Cereal, Frosted Mini Wheats	4 biscuits	31	0.2	0.0	0.2	0.8	1.2	0.1	0.3	2.3	2.5
Cereal, Grape Nut Flakes	⅛ c	28	0.4	tr	0.4	0.6	1.0	tr	0.2	1.9	2.3
Cereal, Life	⅔ c	28	0.2	tr	0.7	0.2	0.6	tr	0.5	1.4	2.2
Cereal, oatmeal, cooked	¾ c	175	0.2	tr	1.2	0.2	0.5	tr	0.6	1.5	2.7
Cereal, shredded wheat	1 large	24	0.2	tr	0.3	0.8	1.4	tr	0.2	2.4	2.7
Cereal, Wheat Chex	⅔ c	28	0.5	tr	0.5	0.9	1.2	0.1	0.1	2.3	2.8
Cornbread	1 piece (2½-in square)	78	0.2	tr	0.2	1.0	0.8	tr	0.3	2.1	2.3
Muffin, wheat bran, home prepared	1 small	40	0.3	tr	0.3	0.6	1.1	tr	0.3	2.0	2.3
Muffin, wheat bran commercial	1 small	40	0.2	tr	0.2	0.5	0.8	tr	0.2	1.5	1.8
Category 4											
Cereal, 40% bran flakes	¾ c	28	0.5	tr	0.6	1.3	3.0	0.1	0.4	4.9	5.5
Cereal, All Bran	⅓ c	28	0.7	tr	0.7	2.0	4.4	0.2	0.8	7.4	8.1
Cereal, oat bran, uncooked	⅓ c	31	0.5	tr	2.0	0.3	1.1	0.1	1.1	3.3	5.3
Cereal, Wheaties	1 c	28	0.5	tr	0.5	0.8	1.4	0.1	0.4	2.7	3.2
Lasagna, with meat sauce, frozen	½ of package	298	0.4	0.3	0.7	1.4	0.9	0.3	0.8	3.4	4.1
Wheat germ	¼ c	28	0.3	tr	0.3	1.0	2.1	0.2	0.3	3.6	3.9

tr = nutrient present in trace amounts.

FOOD	SERVING SIZE			DIETARY FIBER COMPONENTS (G/SERVING FRESH WT)								
				SOLUBLE			INSOLUBLE					
	HOUSEHOLD	WT		HC	P	TOTAL	C	HC	P	KL	TOTAL	TOTAL
LEGUMES												
Category 1												
Beans, black, dry, cooked	½ c	86		0.1	tr	0.1	1.2	0.9	0.2	0.4	2.7	2.8
Lentils, dry, cooked	½ c	99		0.1	tr	0.1	1.5	0.9	0.2	0.2	2.8	2.9
Peas, black-eyed, dry, cooked	½ c	82		0.1	0.1	0.2	1.4	0.6	0.3	0.3	2.6	2.8
Peas, crowder, canned	½ c	86		0.3	0.1	0.4	0.9	0.5	0.2	0.3	1.9	2.3
Peas, green, canned, or frozen (3)	½ c	85		0.1	0.1	0.3	1.9	0.5	0.3	0.1	2.8	3.0
Peas, prepared pea soup	1 c	244		0.7	0.1	0.8	1.2	0.4	0.2	0.4	2.2	3.0
Category 2												
Baked beans, canned with pork	½ c	126		1.3	0.4	1.7	2.0	1.1	0.4	0.3	3.8	5.5
Beans, great northern, dry, cooked	½ c	88		0.2	0.1	0.3	5.1	2.0	0.6	0.1	7.9	8.2
Beans, lima, canned or dry, cooked (3)	½ c	87		0.3	0.1	0.5	1.5	1.1	0.2	0.1	2.9	3.4
Beans, kidney, canned	½ c	88		0.8	0.2	1.0	1.9	1.0	0.3	0.3	3.5	4.5
Beans, navy, dry, canned	½ c	91		0.2	0.1	0.2	1.2	1.2	0.3	0.1	2.9	3.1
Peas, pigeon, canned	½ c	77		0.1	0.1	0.2	1.9	0.6	0.2	0.8	3.5	3.7
NUTS AND SEEDS												
Category 1												
Coconut, shredded, sweetened	2 tbsp	9		tr	tr	tr	0.1	0.5	tr	0.0	0.6	0.6
Popcorn, white or yellow, popped (2)	1 c	6		tr	tr	tr	0.2	0.4	tr	0.1	0.8	0.8
Pumpkin seeds	1 tbsp	5		tr	tr	tr	0.2	0.1	tr	0.4	0.7	0.8
Category 2												
Cashews, roasted	18 medium	28		tr	tr	0.1	0.4	0.3	0.2	0.3	1.2	1.3
Peanut butter, chunky	2 tbsp	32		tr	tr	0.1	0.5	0.6	0.3	0.1	1.5	1.6
Peanuts, Spanish or Virginia (2)	30 to 40 whole	28		tr	tr	0.1	0.6	0.8	0.4	0.1	1.9	1.9
Pecans	15 halves	28		0.1	tr	0.1	0.4	0.5	0.3	0.4	1.6	1.7
Walnuts, English	14 halves	28		tr	tr	tr	0.3	0.2	0.2	0.2	1.0	1.1
Category 3												
Almonds, roasted, with skin	22 whole	28		tr	tr	0.1	0.5	0.9	0.5	0.5	2.4	2.5

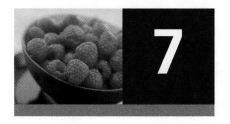

7 Nutritive Value of Selected Ethnic Foods

FOOD	QUANTITY	GRAMS PER SERVING	KCAL	PRO (g)	FAT (g)	CHO (g)	NA (mg)	K (mg)	CHOL (mg)	SAT FATTY ACIDS (g)	MONO FATTY ACIDS (g)	POLY FATTY ACIDS (g)	TOTAL DIETARY FIBER (g)
NAVAJO													
Starch/bread													
Blue corn mush with ash*	¾ c	180	94	2.5	0.5	21.2	32	288	0	—	—	—	—
Flour tortilla, 8-in diameter†‡	¼	34	87	2.5	0.2	19.3	211	29	0	—	—	—	—
Steamed corn hominy, ck†	½ c	115	70	1.8	1.0	13.3	18	108	0	—	—	—	—
Lean meat													
Mutton, flesh, lean only, ck without added fat§	1 oz	28	58	7.9	2.7¶	0	21	96	26	1.0	1.2	0.2	0
High-fat meat													
Mutton, flesh, lean and fat, ck without added fat§	1 oz	28	82	6.7	5.9¶	0	20	87	27	2.5	2.5	0.4	0
Fat													
Piñon nuts in shell	1 tbsp (25 nuts)	9	60	1.3	5.8	0.7	7	67	0	0.8	2.1	2.3	0.4
ALASKAN NATIVE													
Starch/bread													
Pilot bread, 4-in diameter	1	25	104	2.1	2.0	18.2	142	57	—	—	—	—	—
Lean meats													
Caribou, ck	1 oz	28	47	8.3	1.2	0	17	87	31	0.5	0.4	0.2	—
Gumboots (leathery chiton)	2 oz	56	46	9.6	0.9	0	—	—	—	—	—	—	—
Halibut, ck	1 oz	28	39	7.5	0.8	0	20	164	12	0.1	0.3	0.3	—
Herring eggs, plain	0.5 c	85	48	8.2	0.8	3.7	52	—	—	—	—	—	—
Moose, ck	1 oz	28	38	8.2	0.3	0	19	94	22	0.1	0.1	0.1	—
Pike, ck	1 oz	28	33	6.9	0.2	0	13	93	14	0.04	0.1	0.1	—
Seal meat, raw	1 oz	28	41	8.9	0.6	0	—	—	—	0.1	0.1	0.1	—
Venison, ck	1 oz	28	44	8.5	0.9	0	15	94	31	0.4	0.3	0.2	—
Walrus, raw	1 oz	28	56	5.4	3.9	0	—	—	22	0.7	2.4	0.7	—
Whale, bowhead, raw	1 oz	28	37	7.3	0.7	0	17	—	—	0.2	0.4	0.1	—
Medium-fat meats													
Dried fish (king salmon)	0.5 oz	14	60	7.1	5.3	0	—	—	—	—	—	—	—
Muskrat, ck	1 oz	28	67	8.5	3.3	0	27	91	—	—	—	—	—
Salmon, sockeye, ck	1 oz	28	60	7.6	3.1	0	18	105	24	0.5	1.5	0.7	—
High-fat meat													
Hooligan (eulachon), smoked	1 oz	28	86	5.7	6.9	0	—	—	—	—	—	—	—
High-fat meat + 1 fat													
Muktuk, skin and fat	1 × 1 × 2 in	38	138	8	12	0	—	—	—	—	—	—	—

Vegetables													
Fiddlehead fern, raw	1 c	180	34	3.2	0.2	5.0	84	—	—	—	—	—	—
Seaweed, dried black	1 c	13	39	3.7	0.3	5.3	40	—	—	—	—	—	—
Willow greens, ck	0.5 c	28	28	1.7	0.4	5.8	—	—	—	—	—	—	—
Sour dock, ck	0.5 c	55	19	1.3	0.4	3.6	—	—	—	—	—	—	—
Fruits													
Highbush cranberries	1.25 c	119	58	0.5	0.2	15	1	8	0	—	—	—	—
Huckleberries	1 c	150	56	0.6	0.2	13	15	—	—	—	—	—	—
Salmonberries	1.25 c	181	55	1.3	0.1	13	52	—	—	—	—	—	—
Fat													
Seal oil	1 tsp	5	45	0	5	0	—	8	0	0.6	3.0	1.4	—
Free													
Beach asparagus	1 c	55	15	1	0.2	2.4	23	—	—	—	—	—	—
MEXICAN AMERICAN													
Starch/bread													
Bolillo, large, 4.5–5-in long	¼	30	87	2.8	0.9	16.6	174	27	0	0	—	—	0.8
Frijoles cocidos	⅓ c	56	77	4.6	0.3	14.4	1	262	0	0.1	0.1	0.1	3.5
Frijoles refritos, cn	⅓ c	83	89	5.2	0.9	15.9	365	338	0	0.4	0.4	0.1	3.5
Tortilla, corn, 7.5 in across, ready to bake/fry	1	30	69	1.7	0.8	12.8	7	46	0	0.1	0.2	0.5	0.9
Tortilla, flour, 7 in across, ready to bake/fry (Starch/bread 1½)	1	40	118	3.5	2.7	22	164	52	0	0.8	1.3	0.8	0.9
Tortilla, flour, 9 in across, ready to bake/fry	⅓	22	65	1.9	1.5	12	90	28.7	0	0.4	0.7	0.4	0.5

From Ethnic and Regional Food Practices, A Series. Navajo (1998), Alaskan Native (1998), Mexican American (1998), Chinese American (1998), and Hmong American (1999), Jewish (1998), and Soul (1995) Food Practices, Customs, and Holidays. Used with permission from the American Dietetic Association.
*The addition of ash significantly increases the potassium content.
†Although data for flour tortillas and hominy are available from USDA sources, they reflect preparation techniques from other parts of the country. This database contains information from a Navajo-specific study.
‡The 8-inch diameter of the tortilla was chosen to represent the size that is commonly eaten.
§Because of the lack of published data on mutton, the National Live Stock and Meat Board and the New Mexico Cooperative Extension Service recommend substituting lamb nutrient values for mutton, as has been done in this database. However, everyday observation on the Navajo reservation suggests that the untrimmed mutton eaten by many clients is considerably higher in fat than the published data for lean and fat lamb. Thus, trimming mutton might reduce fat and kilocalories beyond the estimates given here.
¶Total fat value includes fatty acids and glycerol.
KEY: CHO = carbohydrate; CHOL = cholesterol; cn = canned; ck = cooked; K = potassium; MONO = monounsaturated; NA = sodium; POLY = polyunsaturated; PRO = protein; SAT = saturated; s + l = small and large.

Continued

FOOD	QUANTITY	GRAMS PER SERVING	KCAL	PRO (g)	FAT (g)	CHO (g)	NA (mg)	K (mg)	CHOL (mg)	SAT FATTY ACIDS (g)	MONO FATTY ACIDS (g)	POLY FATTY ACIDS (g)	TOTAL DIETARY FIBER (g)
MEXICAN AMERICAN—cont'd													
Starch/bread prepared with fat													
Taco shell, 5 in across (corn tortilla, ready to use)	2	24	109	2.0	4.7	15.8	42	58	0	0.7	2.6	1.0	1.2
Lean meat													
Menudo	½ c	—	55	8	1.5	1.8	431	24.5	25	—	—	—	—
Medium-fat meat													
Queso fresco	2 oz or ¼ c	57	80	6.4	4.6	3.0	72	72	18	2.8	1.3	0.1	0
High-fat meat													
Chorizo (High-fat meat 1 + Fat 1)	1 oz	28.5	132	7.2	11.5	—	(367)	(58)	(30)	4.3	5.7	1.0	0
Vegetable													
Chayote, boiled, drained	½ c	80	19	0.5	0.4	4.1	1	138	0	(0)	(0)	(0.2)	(0.6)
Jicama, ck	½ c	(50)	23	0.6	0	5.2	3	90	0	0	0	0	—
Jicama, raw	½ c	60	23	0.8	0.1	5.2	4	105	0	0	0	0	0.4
Nopales, raw	½ c	59	24	0.4	0.3	5.6	3	130	0	0.1	0.1	0.1	2.1
Fruit													
Mango, raw	½ small	104	68	0.5	0.3	17.6	2	161	0	0	0	0	1.5
Papaya, raw	1 c	140	54	0.9	0.2	13.7	4	359	0	0	0	0	1.7
Fat													
Avocado	⅛ medium	25	40	0.5	3.8	1.9	3	150	0	0.6	2.4	0.5	0.5
Free													
Cilantro	¼ c	4	1	0	0	0	1	22	0	0	0	0	—
Jalapeño chili, cn, s + l, chopped	½ c	68	17	0.5	0.4	3.3	995	92	0	(0)	(0)	(0.2)	(1.2)
Salsa de chile	2 tbsp	34	13	0.3	0	3.1	167	46	0	0	0	0	0.7
Verdolagas, ck	½ c	58	10	0.9	0.1	2.1	26	283	0	0	0	0	(1.2)
Occasional													
Pan dulce, 4.5 in across (no frosting or fruit) (Starch/bread 4 + Fat 1)	1	100	384	9.1	11.6	60.8	389	124	?	?	?	?	?
CHINESE AMERICAN													
Starch/bread													
Cellophane or mung bean noodles, ck	¾ c	93	73	—	—	18	—	—	—	—	—	—	—

Food	Amount												
Ginkgo seeds, cn	1/2 c	76	86	1.8	1.2	17.1	238	139	—	0.24	0.46	0.46	—
Lotus root, 1/4-in thick, 2½-in diameter, raw	10 slices	81	45	2.1	0.1	14	33	450	—	—	—	0.08	—
Mung beans or green gram beans, ck	1/3 c	67	71	4.7	0.3	12.7	1	177	—	0.08	0.36	0.08	—
Red beans, ck	1/3 c	58	61	4.1	0.3	11.0	0.9	153	0	0.08	0.36	0.08	—
Rice congee or soup	3/4 c	180	69	1.5	—	15	—	20	—	—	—	—	—
Rice noodles, fresh	1/2 c	49	99	1.3	0.1	23	—	—	—	—	—	—	—
Rice vermicelli, ck	1/2 c	64	56	1	0	13	—	—	—	—	—	—	—
Taro, ck	1/3 c	44	62	0.2	0.1	15	7	210	—	—	—	—	—
Lean meat or substitute													
Beef jerky, 3½-in × 1-in piece	1/2 oz	14	44	6.98	1.3	0.7	(610)	—	—	—	—	—	—
Dried scallop, large	1	13	44	8.6	0.3	1.1	—	205	—	—	—	—	—
Dried shrimp, medium	1 tbsp or 10 shrimp	11	40	6.9	0.4	1.7	0	166	—	—	—	—	—
Soybeans, ck	3 tbsp	32	56	5.4	3	3.2	0	—	0	0.42	0.64	1.62	—
Squid, raw	2 oz	57	52	8.8	0.8	1.8	26	140	132	0.20	0.06	0.24	—
Tripe, beef, raw	2 oz	57	56	8.2	2.2	0	26	154	54	1.16	0.74	0.04	—
Medium-fat meat or substitute													
Beef tongue	1 oz	28	81	6.3	5.9	0.1	17	51	30	2.54	2.70	0.22	—
Tofu or soybean curd, 2½ × 2¾ × 1 in	4 oz or 1/2 c	124	94	10	5.9	2.3	9	150	0	0.86	1.31	3.35	1.5
High-fat meat or substitute													
Salted duck egg	1 whole	68	137	9.8	10.3	0.5	—	171	—	—	—	—	—
Thousand-year-old or preserved limed duck egg	1 whole	63	114	8.8	7.3	2.6	—	323	—	—	—	—	—
High-fat meat + 1 fat													
Chinese sausage (pork and spices)	1 (2 oz)	56	199	11.9	16.4	3.7	493	—	—	6.1	7.5	1.8	—
Chinese sausage (pork, liver, and spices)	1 (2 oz)	56	205	14.9	15.7	—	560	—	—	5.8	7.2	1.7	—
Vegetable													
Amaranth or Chinese spinach, ck	1/2 c	61	14	1.4	0.1	2.7	14	423	—	—	—	—	—
Arrowheads, or fresh corms, large, 3½-in diameter, raw	1	25	25	1.2	0.2	5.0	6	470	—	—	—	—	—
Baby corn, cn	1/2 c	64	13	1.9	0.3	1.9	730	117	—	—	—	—	—
Bamboo shoots, cn	1/2 c	66	25	2.3	0.5	4.2	9	104	—	—	—	—	—
Bitter melon or bitter gourd, raw	1 c	146	28	1.2	0.2	6.6	6	394	—	—	—	—	—

Continued

CHINESE AMERICAN—cont'd

FOOD	QUANTITY	GRAMS PER SERVING	KCAL	PRO (g)	FAT (g)	CHO (g)	NA (mg)	K (mg)	CHOL (mg)	SAT FATTY ACIDS (g)	MONO FATTY ACIDS (g)	POLY FATTY ACIDS (g)	TOTAL DIETARY FIBER (g)
Vegetable—cont'd													
Chayote, raw	1 c	124	32	1.2	0.4	7.2	4	198	—	—	—	—	—
Chinese celery, raw	1 c	120	26	1.6	0.4	5.0	116	392	—	—	—	—	—
Chinese eggplant, white, ck	½ c	87	20	0.9	0.1	4.9	—	—	—	—	—	—	—
Chinese eggplant, purple, ck	½ c	72	17	0.7	0.1	4.0	—	—	—	—	—	—	—
Chinese or black mushrooms, medium, dried	2	8	22	0.7	0.1	5.6	1	115	—	—	—	—	—
Hairy melon or hairy cucumber, raw	1 c	156	22	1.0	—	5.4	—	—	—	—	—	—	—
Leeks, ck	½ c	52	16	0.4	0.1	4.0	6	46	—	—	—	—	—
Luffa, angled, raw	1 c	178	30	1.2	0.2	7.2	2	252	—	—	—	—	—
Luffa, smooth or sponge, raw	1 c	178	34	2.0	0.4	8.0	6	274	—	—	—	—	—
Mung bean sprouts, seed attached, raw	1 c	104	32	3.2	0.2	6.2	6	144	—	—	—	—	—
Mung bean sprouts, seed attached, ck	½ c	62	13	1.3	0.1	2.6	6	63	—	—	—	—	—
Mustard greens, ck	½ c	70	11	1.6	0.2	1.5	11	141	—	—	—	—	—
Peapods or sugar peas, ck	½ c	80	34	2.6	0.2	5.6	3	192	—	—	—	—	—
Soybean sprouts, seed attached, raw	½ c	35	45	4.6	2.4	3.9	5	169	—	0.25	0.26	1.30	—
Soybean sprouts, seed attached, ck	½ c	47	38	4.0	2.1	3.1	10	334	—	0.45	0.47	2.32	—
Straw mushrooms, cn	½ c	66	20	1.5	0.1	3.8	172	47	—	—	—	—	—
Turnip, raw	1 c	110	36	1.2	0.2	8.0	88	248	—	—	—	—	—
Water chestnuts, 1¼–2-in diameter, raw	4 whole	36	38	0.5	0	8.6	5	210	—	—	—	—	—
Water chestnuts, cn (s + l)	½ c	70	35	0.6	0.0	8.7	6	82	—	—	—	—	—
Winter melon or waxed gourd, raw	1 c	132	17	0.5	0.3	4.0	8	14.7	—	—	—	—	(1.3)
Yard-long beans, raw	1 c	90	44	2.6	0.4	7.6	4	218	—	—	—	—	—
Yard-long beans, ck	½ c	52	24	1.3	—	4.8	2	151	—	—	—	—	—
Fruit													
Carambola or star fruit, medium, raw	1½	191	63	1.0	0.6	14.8	2.5	230	—	—	—	—	—
Chinese banana, dwarf, raw	1	100	72	1.8	0.2	18.0	18	435	—	—	—	—	—

Food	Amount												
Guava, medium, raw	1½	135	69	1.2	0.9	15.9	3	384	—	—	—	—	—
Kumquat, medium, raw	5	100	60	1.0	—	16.0	5	220	—	—	—	—	—
Litchi or lychee, raw	10	96	60	0.7	0.4	16.0	0	144	—	—	—	—	—
Litchi or lychee, cn	½ c	77	57	0.2	0.3	14.9	27	52	—	—	—	—	—
Longan, raw	30	96	60	1.2	0	14.4	0	27	—	—	—	—	—
Longan, cn	¾ c	100	68	0.4	0.3	17.6	54	41	—	—	—	—	—
Mango, small, raw	½	104	68	0.5	0.3	17.6	2	161	—	—	—	—	—
Papaya, ripe, 3½-in diameter, 5⅛-in high, raw	½	152	59	0.9	0.2	14.9	4	389	—	—	—	—	—
Persimmon, Japanese (soft type), raw	½	84	59	0.5	0.2	15.6	2.0	135	—	—	—	—	—
Pummelo, raw	¾ c	142	58	1.0	0.4	14.2	1	352	—	—	—	—	—
Milk													
Soybean milk, unsweetened	1 c	240	78	6.6	4.6	4.4	30	338	0	0.52	0.78	2.0	—
Fat													
Coconut milk**	1 tbsp	15	35	0.3	3.6	0.8	2	39	0	3.17	0.15	0.04	—
Sesame paste	1½ tsp	8	48	1.4	4.0	2.0	1	46	0	0.57	1.54	1.78	0.8
Sesame seeds, whole, dried	1 tbsp	9	52	1.6	4.5	2.1	1	42	0	0.63	1.69	1.96	—
Free													
Amaranth or Chinese spinach, raw	1 c	28	7	0.7	0.1	1.1	5	171	—	—	—	—	—
Bok choy, raw	1 c	70	10	1.1	0.1	1.5	46	176	—	—	—	—	—
Bok choy, ck	½ c	85	10	1.3	0.1	1.5	29	315	—	—	—	—	—
Chili pepper, raw	1	45	18	0.9	0.1	4.3	3	153	—	—	—	—	—
Chinese or Peking cabbage, raw	1 c	76	12	0.9	0.2	2.5	7	181	—	—	—	—	—
Chinese or Peking cabbage, ck	½ c	60	8	0.9	0.1	1.4	6	134	—	—	—	—	—
Choy sum or Chinese flowering cabbage, raw	1 c	56	9	1.2	—	1.6	—	—	—	—	—	—	—
Coriander, raw	½ c	8	2	—	—	0.2	2	44	—	—	—	—	—
Garland chrysanthemum, raw	1 c	25	4	0.4	0	1.1	13	143	—	—	—	—	—
Gingerroot, raw	¼ c	24	17	0.4	0.2	3.6	3	100	—	—	—	—	—
Mustard greens, salted and soured	2 tbsp	23	14	0.5	0.1	4.0	—	—	—	—	—	—	—
Oriental radish or daikon, raw	1 c	88	16	0.6	0	1.8	9	—	—	—	—	—	—
Watercress, raw	1 c	34	4	0.8	0	0.4	14	112	—	—	—	—	—
Combination													
Mock duck or wheat gluten, cn	½ c	74	88	14	—	10	—	28	—	—	—	—	—

Continued

**Raw liquid expressed from mixture of grated coconut meat and water.

FOOD	QUANTITY	GRAMS PER SERVING	KCAL	PRO (g)	FAT (g)	CHO (g)	NA (mg)	K (mg)	CHOL (mg)	SAT FATTY ACIDS (g)	MONO FATTY ACIDS (g)	POLY FATTY ACIDS (g)	TOTAL DIETARY FIBER (g)
HMONG AMERICAN													
Starch/bread													
Cellophane or mung bean noodles, ck	¾ c	93	73	—	—	18	—	—	—	—	—	—	—
Rice noodles, fresh	½ c	49	99	1.3	0.1	23	—	—	—	—	—	—	—
Rice soup	¾ c	180	69	1.5	—	15	—	20	—	—	—	—	—
Yard-long beans, pod and seeds, ck	½ c	86	102	7.1	0.4	18.1	4	271	0	0.10	0.03	0.17	—
Medium-fat meat or substitute													
Pig's feet	2½ oz (= 2 exchanges)	71	138	13.6	8.8	0	—	—	71	3.04	4.13	0.96	0
Tofu or soybean curd, 2½ × 2¾ × 1 in	4 oz or ½ c	124	94	10	5.9	2.3	9	150	0	0.86	1.31	3.35	1.5
Vegetables													
Bamboo shoots, cn, drained	½ c	66	13	1.1	0.3	2.1	4	52	0	0.06	0.01	0.11	0.43
Bitter melon, raw	1 c	146	28	1.2	0.2	6.6	6	394	—	—	—	—	—
Cucuzzi squash (spaghetti squash), ck	½ c	78	23	0.5	0.2	5.0	14	91	0	0.05	0.02	0.10	1.09
Luffa gourd/squash, angled, raw	1 c	178	30	1.2	0.2	7.2	2	252	—	—	—	—	—
Luffa gourd/smooth or sponge, raw	1 c	178	34	2	0.4	8	6	274	—	—	—	—	—
Mung bean sprouts, seeds attached, ck	½ c	62	13	1.3	0.1	2.6	6	63	—	—	—	—	—
Pumpkin, ck	½ c	122	24	0.9	0.1	6.0	2	281	0	0.04	0.01	0.00	1.01
Fruits													
Apple pear, raw, 2¼-in high, 2½-in diameter	1	122	51	0.6	0.3	13	0	148	0	0	0	0	—
Guava, medium, raw	1½	135	69	1.2	0.8	15.9	3	384	—	—	—	—	—
Jackfruit	½ c	90	85	1	0.3	22	3	273	0	—	—	—	—
Fats													
Beef tallow	1 tsp	4.3	39	0	4.3	0	0	0	5	2.13	1.77	0.17	0
Chicken fat	1 tsp	4.3	38	0	4.3	0	—	—	4	1.27	1.9	0.9	0
Coconut cream	1 tbsp	19	36	0.5	3.4	1.6	10	19	0	2.99	0.14	0.04	—
Coconut milk, raw	1 tbsp	15	35	0.3	3.6	0.8	2	39	0	3.17	0.15	0.04	—

Food	Amount												
Coconut milk, cn	1 tbsp	15	30	0.3	3.2	0.9	2	33	0	2.89	0.14	0.04	—
Pork lard	1 tsp	4.2	39	0	4.3	0	0	0	4	1.67	1.93	0.47	0
Free													
Coriander (Chinese parsley), raw	1 c	16	4	0.3	0.1	0.4	4	88	—	—	—	—	—
Fish sauce	1 tbsp	16	4	0.8	0.1	0	1088	—	0	—	—	—	0
Pumpkin blossom, ck	1 c	134	20	1.5	0.1	4.4	8	142	0	0.05	0.02	0.01	—
Tender vines and leaves of pumpkin, squash, luffa gourd, and pea plant, ck	1 c	70	14	2	0	2	6	306	0	0	0	0	—
Vinespinach, raw	1 c	56	11	1	0.2	1.9	—	—	0	—	—	—	—
Occasional													
Condensed milk, sweetened	1 fl oz	38.2	123	3.0	3.3	20.8	49	142	13	2.10	0.93	0.13	0
JEWISH													
Starch/bread													
Bagel or bialy	½ sm (1 oz)	28.5	82	3.0	0.7	15.4	99	20	0	0.1	0.3	0.3	0.8
Bulgur, ck	½ c	91	76	2.8	0.2	16.9	4	62	0	0.0	0.0	0.1	(0.5)
Bulke	½ med	28.5	76	2.4	0.9	14	142	29	0	0.2	0.3	0.3	0.4
Farfel, dry	½ c	37.5	90	3.4	0.4	(20.5)	1	42	26	0	0.9	0.8	(1.2)
Hallah	1 slice	28.5	85	2.6	1.8	14.0	140	30	0	0.5	0.9	0.3	0.7
Kasha, ck	½ c	99	91	3.3	0.6	19.7	4	88	0	0.1	0.2	0.2	(2.0)
Kasha, raw	2 tbsp	20.5	71	2.4	0.6	15.4	5	66	0	0.1	0.2	0.2	(1.3)
Lentils	⅓ c	66	77	6.0	0.2	13.3	1	244	0	0	0	0.1	2.4
Matzoh	¾ oz	21	86	2.2	1.4	16.5	135 (160)	26	0	—	0	—	(0.8)
Matzoh meal	2½ tbsp	22.5	86	2.2	0.2	18.2	1	25	0	0	0.0	0.2	(0.8)
Potato starch (flour)	2 tbsp	22.5	79	1.8	0.2	18.0	8	357	0	0.0	0.0	0.1	(0.4)
Pumpernickel bread	1 sl, 5 × 4 × ⅜ in	28	69	2.5	0.4	14.9	159	127	0	—	—	—	3.8
Rye bread	1 sl, 4¾ × 3¾ × 7/16 in	28	68	2.6	0.3	14.6	156	40	0	—	—	—	1.0
Split peas, ck	⅓ c	65	77	5.4	0.2	13.7	1	237	0	0.0	0.1	0.1	3.4
Starch/bread prepared with fat													
Matzoh ball (Starch/bread 1 + Fat 1)	3 balls (1½ oz)	42	134	6	4.6	17	469	62	165	1.3	1.8	0.9	0.7
Potato pancake (Starch/bread 1 + Fat 1)	½ pancake	38	119	2.3	6.3	13.2	194	269	47	1.7	2.7	1.3	(0.4)
Lean meat													
Flanken	1 oz	28.5	57	9.6	1.8	0	18	127	22	0.6	0.8	0.1	0

Continued

FOOD	QUANTITY	GRAMS PER SERVING	KCAL	PRO (g)	FAT (g)	CHO (g)	NA (mg)	K (mg)	CHOL (mg)	SAT FATTY ACIDS (g)	MONO FATTY ACIDS (g)	POLY FATTY ACIDS (g)	TOTAL DIETARY FIBER (g)
JEWISH—cont'd													
Lean meat—cont'd													
Gefilte fish (in broth)	2 oz	57	48	5.2	1	4	299	52	17	0.2	0.5	0.2	0
Herring, smoked	1 oz	28.5	61	7	3.5	0	260	127	23	0.8	1.5	0.8	0
Lox (smoked salmon)	1 oz	28.5	33	5.2	1.2	0	397	50	7	0.3	0.6	0.3	0
Sardines, cn, drained	2 med, 3 × 1 × ½ in	24	50	6	2.8	0	121	95	34	0.4	0.9	1.2	0
Smelts	1 oz	28.5	35	6.4	0.9	0	22	106	26	0.2	0.2	0.3	0
Medium-fat meat													
Beef tongue	1 oz	28.5	81	6.3	5.9	0.1	17	51	30	2.5	2.7	0.2	0
Brisket, beef	1 oz	28.5	69	8.4	3.7	0	21	82	27	1.3	1.6	0.1	0
Chopped liver	¼ c	57	75	7	4.2	3	33	100	195	1.3	1.5	0.7	0.8
Corned beef	1 oz	28.5	72	5.2	5.4	0.1	323	41	28	1.8	2.6	0.2	0
Sablefish, smoked	1 oz	28.5	73	5.0	5.7	0	210	134	18	1.2	3.0	0.8	0
Salmon, cn	¼ c	57	79	11.3	3.4	0	43 (316)	186	(20)	0.9	1.0	1.2	0
High-fat meat													
Pastrami	1 oz	28.5	99	4.9	8.3	0.9	350	65	26	3.0	4.1	0.3	0
Vegetable													
Borscht, beet (no sugar or sour cream)	½ c	—	38	2.0	1.5	4.5	200	173	0	0.3	0.7	0.4	1.4
Sorrel, ck	½ c	72	14	1.3	0.5	2.1	2	231	0	—	—	—	2.4
Cream cheese	1 tbsp	14	49	1.1	4.9	0.4	41	17	15	3.1	1.4	0.2	0
Nondairy liquid creamer	2 tbsp	30	40	0.3	3.0	3.4	24	58	0	variable	variable	variable	0
Nondairy powdered creamer	4 tsp	8	44	0.4	2.8	4.4	16	64	0	variable	variable	variable	0
Schmaltz	1 tsp	5	31	0.2	3.4	0	2	3	3	1.0	1.5	0.7	0
Sour cream	2 tbsp	24	52	0.8	5.0	1.0	12	34	10	3.1	1.5	0.2	0
Free													
Horseradish	1 tbsp	15	6	0.2	0	4.4	14	44	0	0	0	0	1.6
Pickle, dill	1 med	65	7	0.5	0.1	1.4	928	130	0	0.1	0	0.1	0.9
Occasional													
Sweet wine (fat 2)	½ c	118	83	0.2	0	1.7	76	140	0	0	0	0	0
SOUL													
Starch/breads													
Hominy	¾ c	120	86	1.8	1.1	17.1	252	11	0	0.2	0.3	0.5	3.0
Succotash	½ c	85	79	3.7	0.8	17.0	38	225	0	0.1	0.2	0.4	4.6

Food	Portion	Weight (g)	Energy (kcal)	Protein (g)	Fat (g)	Carbohydrate (g)	Sodium (mg)	Potassium (mg)	Cholesterol (mg)	Saturated fat (g)	Monounsaturated fat (g)	Polyunsaturated fat (g)	Fiber (g)
Lean meat													
Hog maw	1 oz	28	45	4.7	2.7	0	15	57	55	—	—	—	0
Pork brains	1 oz	28	39	3.5	2.7	0	26	56	727	0.6	0.5	0.4	0
Pig ear	1 oz (¼ ear)	28	47	4.5	3.1	0	48	11	26	—	—	—	0
Tripe	2 oz	57	56	8.3	2.2	0	26	154	54	1.2	0.7	0.0	0
Opossum	1 oz	28	63	8.6	2.9	0	(27)	(91)	(23)	—	—	—	0
Medium-fat meat													
Neck bones, pork	1 oz	28	66	6.9	4.1	0	20	97	24	1.5	1.8	0.4	0
Pig foot	½ foot	35	68	6.7	4.3	0	(58)	(14)	35	1.5	2.0	0.5	0
Sousemeat (headcheese)	1 oz or 1 sl, 4 × 4 × 1/10 in	28	60	4.6	4.5	0.1	357	9	23	1.4	2.3	0.5	0
Tongue, pork	1 oz (⅓ tongue)	28	77	6.9	5.3	0	31	68	42	1.8	2.5	0.6	0
Pork skin (rind) fried (packaged snack pack or vendor purchased)	1 c medium pieces, not crushed	12	68	7.7	4.3	0	231	—	17	1.7	—	—	0
Oxtail	1 oz	28	72	8.9	3.7	0	20	75	30	1.4	1.6	0.1	0
High-fat meats													
Pig tail	1 oz (⅓ tail)	28	113	4.8	10.2	0	(48)	(11)	37	3.6	4.8	1.1	0
Ham hock	1 oz	28	90	5.7	6.7	1.7	383	98	18	2.0	(1.69)	(0.34)	0
Vienna sausage	2 small 2 × 7/8 in diameter	32	90	3.3	8.1	0.7	304	32	16	3.0	4.0	0.5	0
Vegetables													
Kale, ck	½ c	65	21	1.2	0.3	3.7	15	148	0	0.0	0.0	0.1	1.3
Poke salad, ck	½ c	82	16	1.9	0.3	2.5	—	—	0	—	—	—	1.2
Fruits													
Muscadines	17	85	60	0.6	0.5	15.0	2	156	0	0.2	0.0	0.1	0.7
Saturated fats													
Pork cracklings (Hormel)	1 tbsp	8	57	2.3	5.1	0	18	—	9	1.7	(2.3)	(0.6)	0
Fatback, raw	¼ oz	7	58	0.2	6.3	0	1	5	4	2.3	3.0	0.7	0
Hog jowl	1 oz	28	(54)	1.8	4.8	0	(7)	(41)	(9)	1.6	2.4	0.6	0
Lard	1 tsp	4	38	0	4.3	0	0	0	4	1.7	1.9	0.5	0

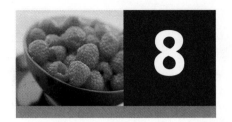

8 Enteral Supplements

PRODUCT	MANUFACTURER	FORM	PROTEIN SOURCE
NUTRITIONAL SUPPLEMENTS, READY TO DRINK			
RESOURCE® Fruit Beverage	Novartis Nutrition	Liquid	Whey protein isolate
RESOURCE® Standard	Novartis Nutrition	Liquid	Sodium and calcium caseinates, soy protein isolate
RESOURCE® Plus	Novartis Nutrition	Liquid	Sodium and calcium caseinates, soy protein isolate
Boost®	Mead Johnson	Liquid	Milk protein concentrate
Boost® High Protein	Mead Johnson	Liquid	Milk protein concentrate, calcium caseinate, sodium caseinate
Boost® Plus	Mead Johnson	Liquid	Milk protein concentrate, calcium and sodium caseinates
Boost® with Fiber	Mead Johnson	Liquid	Milk protein concentrate
Enlive!®	Ross Laboratories	Liquid	Whey protein isolate
Ensure®	Ross Laboratories	Liquid	Calcium caseinate, soy protein isolate, whey protein concentrate
Ensure® Fiber with FOS	Ross Laboratories	Liquid	Sodium and calcium caseinates, soy protein isolate
Ensure® High Protein	Ross Laboratories	Liquid	Calcium and sodium caseinates, soy protein isolate
Ensure Plus®	Ross Laboratories	Liquid	Sodium and calcium caseinates, soy protein isolate
Ensure Plus® HN (Oral Formula)	Ross Laboratories	Liquid	Sodium and calcium caseinates, soy protein isolate
NuBasics®	Nestle Nutrition	Liquid	Calcium caseinate
NuBasics® Juice Drink	Nestle Nutrition	Liquid	Whey protein isolate
NuBasics® Plus	Nestle Nutrition	Liquid	Calcium caseinate
NuBasics® VHP	Nestle Nutrition	Liquid	Calcium-potassium caseinate
NutriFocus™	Ross Laboratories	Liquid	Sodium caseinate, milk protein isolate, soy protein isolate

Reprinted with permission of Novartis Nutrition.

NUTRIENT SOURCE	
FAT SOURCE	**CARBOHYDRATE SOURCE**
N/A	Sugar, corn syrup
High oleic sunflower oil, soybean oil, corn oil	Corn syrup solids, sugar
High oleic sunflower oil, soybean oil, corn oil	Corn syrup solids, sugar
Canola oil, high oleic sunflower oil, corn oil	Corn syrup solids, sugar
Canola oil, high oleic sunflower oil, corn oil	Corn syrup, sugar
Canola oil, high oleic sunflower oil, corn oil	Corn syrup solids, sugar
Vegetable oil (canola, high oleic sunflower, corn oils)	Corn syrup solids, sugar Fiber Source: soy fiber, acacia, cellulose
N/A	Maltodextrin, sugar
High oleic safflower oil, canola oil, corn oil	Sugar, corn syrup, maltodextrin
High oleic safflower oil, canola oil, corn oil	Maltodextrin, sugar Fiber Source: oat fiber, FOS, soy fiber
High oleic safflower oil, soy oil, canola oil	Sugar, maltodextrin
Canola oil, corn oil, high oleic safflower oil	Corn syrup, maltodextrin, sugar
Corn oil	Maltodextrin, sugar
N/A	High fructose corn syrup, maltodextrin, sucrose, apple juice concentrate, strawberry juice concentrate, raspberry juice concentrate
Canola oil, corn oil, soy lecithin	Corn syrup solids, sugar
Canola oil, corn oil, soy lecithin	Corn syrup solids, sugar
Canola oil, high oleic safflower oil, corn oil, lecithin	Corn syrup, sugar Fiber Source: FOS, soy fiber, oat fiber, cellulose
Canola oil, high oleic safflower oil, corn oil, lecithin	Corn syrup, sugar Fiber Source: FOS, soy fiber, oat fiber, cellulose

Continued

				NUTRITIONAL PROFILE			
PRODUCT	CALORIES/ ml	CALORIES (PER SERVING)	PROTEIN (g/SERVING)	CARBO- HYDRATE (g/SERVING)	FAT (g/SERVING)	OSMOLALITY (MOSM/KG WATER)	VOLUME (ml) TO MEET 100% OF THE RDI[1]
NUTRITIONAL SUPPLEMENTS, READY TO DRINK							
RESOURCE® Fruit Beverage	1.0	250	9.0	53.5	0	750	(2)
RESOURCE® Standard	1.06	250	9.0	40	6.0	600	1180
RESOURCE® Plus	1.5	360	13	52	11	870	946
Boost®	1.01	240	10	41	4	610-670	1180
Boost® High Protein	1.01	240	15	33	6	540-605	946
Boost® Plus	1.52	360	14	45	14	720	946
Boost® with Fiber	1.01	240	10	42	4	480	1180
Enlive!®	1.12	300	10	65	0	840	(2)
Ensure®	1.06	250	8.8	40	6.1	590	948
Ensure® Fiber with FOS	1.06	250	8.8	42	6.1	500	948
Ensure® High Protein	0.95	230	12	30.8	6.0	610	948
Ensure Plus®	1.5	355	13	50.1	11.4	680	1185
Ensure Plus® HN (Oral Formula)	1.5	355	14.8	47.3	11.8	650	947
NuBasics®	1.0	250	8.75	33.1	9.2	480-490	2000
NuBasics® Juice Drink	1.0	163	6.5	34	0.1	990	(2)
NuBasics® Plus	1.5	375	13.1	44.1	16.2	620	1333
NuBasics® VHP	1.0	250	15.6	28.2	8.3	480	(2)
NutriFocus™	1.5	355	14.8	50.9	11.7	N/A	(2)

[1]With the exception of chloride.
[2]Not intended as a total feeding.

WATER CONTENT (ml) PER SERVING	NUTRIENT PER SERVING						
	SODIUM mg (mEq)	POTASSIUM mg (mEq)	CHLORIDE mg (mEq)	CALCIUM MG (mEq)	PHOSPHORUS mg (mmol)	MAGNESIUM MG (mEq)	FIBER (g)
196	<80 (<3.5)	<20 (<0.5)	50 (1.4)	10 (0.5)	160 (5.2)	1.0 (<0.1)	—
199	220 (9.6)	350 (9.0)	340 (9.6)	350 (17.5)	250 (8.1)	100 (8.2)	—
181	310 (13.5)	460 (11.8)	340 (9.6)	300 (15)	250 (8.1)	100 (8.2)	—
200	130 (5.7)	400 (10.2)	340 (9.6)	300 (15)	250 (8)	100 (8.2)	—
200	170 (7.4)	380 (9.7)	320 (9)	330 (16)	310 (10)	105 (8.6)	—
185	170 (7.4)	380 (9.7)	320 (9)	330 (16)	310 (10)	105 (8.6)	<1
200	170 (7.4)	380 (9.7)	320 (9)	330 (16)	310 (10)	105 (8.6)	3
191	65 (2.8)	40 (1.0)	340 (9.6)	60 (3.0)	20 (0.6)	8.0 (0.7)	—
200	200 (9)	370 (10)	310 (8.7)	300 (15)	300 (9.7)	100 (8.2)	—
195	200 (9)	370 (10)	320 (9)	350 (18)	300 (9.7)	100 (8.2)	2.8
203	290 (13)	500 (13)	375 (11)	300 (15)	250 (8)	100 (8.2)	—
180	240 (11)	440 (12)	450 (13)	200 (10)	200 (6.5)	100 (8.2)	—
182	280 (12)	430 (11)	410 (11)	250 (13)	250 (8)	100 (8.2)	—
213	219 (10)	312 (8)	300 (8.5)	125 (6.3)	125 (4)	50 (4.1)	—
128	50 (2.2)	50 (1.3)	55 (1.6)	83 (4.2)	166 (5.4)	33.3 (2.7)	—
194	292 (13)	467 (12)	435 (12)	187 (9.4)	187 (6)	75 (6.2)	—
212	219 (9.5)	312 (8.0)	300 (8.5)	145 (7.2)	145 (4.7)	50 (4.1)	—
181	220 (9.5)	400 (10.2)	270 (7.6)	250 (13)	250 (8)	100 (8.2)	5.0

Continued

PRODUCT	MANUFACTURER	FORM	PROTEIN SOURCE
NUTRITIONAL SUPPLEMENTS, POWDER SUPPLEMENTS			
Meritene®	Novartis Nutrition	Powder	Nonfat milk
Boost® High Protein Powder	Mead Johnson	Powder	Nonfat milk
Carnation® Instant Breakfast	Nestle Nutrition	Powder	Nonfat milk
Ensure® Powder	Ross Laboratories	Powder	Sodium and calcium caseinates, soy protein isolate
SCANDISHAKE®	Scandipharm	Powder	Nonfat milk, sodium caseinate

PRODUCT	POWDER MIXED WITH:	SERVING SIZE (ml)	CALORIES/ml	NUTRITIONAL PROFILE CALORIES (PER SERVING)	PROTEIN (g/SERVING)	CARBO-HYDRATE (g/SERVING)
NUTRITIONAL SUPPLEMENTS, POWDER SUPPLEMENTS						
Meritene®	1 c whole milk	260	1.08	280	18	31
Boost® High Protein Powder	1 c skim milk	290	1.09	290	21	48
Carnation® Instant Breakfast	1 c 2% milk	270	0.93	250	12	39
Ensure® Powder	¾ c water	240	1.06	250	9	34
SCANDISHAKE®	1 c soy milk	315	1.65	520	17	56

See Wound-Healing or Immune-Enhancing sections for profile of IMPACT® Recover.

NUTRIENT SOURCE	
FAT SOURCE	**CARBOHYDRATE SOURCE**
Milk fat	Lactose, sugar, corn syrup solids
Butterfat	Lactose, corn syrup solids, sugar
Milk fat	Maltodextrin, sugar, lactose
Corn oil, soy lecithin	Corn syrup, maltodextrin, sugar
Partially hydrogenated vegetable oil	Maltodextrin, sugar, corn syrup solids

			NUTRIENT PER SERVING				
FAT (g/SERVING)	**WATER CONTENT (ml) PER SERVING**	**SODIUM mg (mEq)**	**POTASSIUM mg (mEq)**	**CHLORIDE mg (mEq)**	**CALCIUM mg (mEq)**	**PHOSPHORUS mg (mmol)**	**MAGNESIUM mg (mEq)**
9.0	213	280 (12.2)	730 (18.7)	570 (16.1)	570 (28.5)	500 (16)	100 (8.2)
1	220	320 (13.9)	970 (25)	480 (13.5)	590 (29)	500 (16)	133 (11)
5	217	220 (9.6)	630 (16.2)	—	550 (27.5)	480 (15.5)	110 (9.1)
9	200	200 (8.7)	370 (9.5)	310 (8.7)	125 (6.2)	125 (4)	50 (4.1)
24	224	139 (6)	420 (10.7)	—	70 (3.5)	110 (3.5)	40 (3.3)

Continued

PRODUCT	MANUFACTURER	FORM	PROTEIN SOURCE
STANDARD FORMULAS			
Isosource® Standard	Novartis Nutrition	Liquid	Soy protein isolate
Isosource® HN	Novartis Nutrition	Liquid	Soy protein isolate
Comply®	Mead Johnson	Liquid	Sodium caseinate, calcium caseinate
Ensure Plus HN® (Ross Ready-To-Hang[3])	Ross Laboratories	Liquid	Sodium and calcium caseinates, soy protein isolate
Isocal®	Mead Johnson	Liquid	Calcium caseinate, sodium caseinate, soy protein isolate
Isocal® HN	Mead Johnson	Liquid	Calcium caseinate, sodium caseinate, soy protein isolate
Isocal® HN Plus	Mead Johnson	Liquid	Milk protein concentrate, casein[3]
Nutren® 1.0	Nestle Nutrition	Liquid	Calcium-potassium caseinate
Nutren® 1.5	Nestle Nutrition	Liquid	Calcium-potassium caseinate
Osmolite®	Ross Laboratories	Liquid	Sodium and calcium caseinates, soy protein isolate
Osmolite® HN	Ross Laboratories	Liquid	Sodium and calcium caseinates, soy protein isolate
Osmolite® HN Plus	Ross Laboratories	Liquid	Sodium caseinate, calcium caseinate

PRODUCT	CALORIES/ml	PROTEIN (g/L)	CARBOHY-DRATE (g/L)	FAT (g/L)	OSMOLALITY (mOsm/kg WATER)	NUTRITIONAL PROFILE VOLUME (ml) TO MEET 100% OF THE RDI[5]
STANDARD FORMULAS						
Isosource® Standard	1.2	43	170	39	490	1165
Isosource® HN	1.2	53	160	39	490	1165
Comply®	1.5	60	180	61	460	830
Ensure Plus® HN (Ross Ready-To-Hang)	1.5	62.7	203.6	49.1	525	1000
Isocal®	1.06	34	135	44	270	1890
Isocal® HN	1.06	44	124	45	270	1180
Isocal® HN Plus	1.2	54	156	40	390-400	1000
Nutren® 1.0	1.0	40	127	38	315-370	1500[6]
Nutren® 1.5	1.5	60	169.2	67.6	430-510	1000[6]
Osmolite®	1.06	37.1	151.1	34.7	300	1887
Osmolite® HN	1.06	44.3	143.9	34.7	300	1321
Osmolite® HN Plus	1.2	55.5	157.5	39.3	360	1000

[3]Closed system only.
[4]Flavored product contains sucrose
[5]With the exception of chloride.
[6]With the exception of chloride, chromium, and selenium.

NUTRIENT SOURCE

FAT SOURCE	CARBOHYDRATE SOURCE
Canola oil, MCT oil	Corn syrup, hydrolyzed cornstarch
Canola oil, MCT oil	Corn syrup, hydrolyzed cornstarch
Canola oil, high oleic sunflower oil, MCT oil, corn oil	Maltodextrin
High oleic safflower oil, canola oil, MCT oil, soy lecithin	Maltodextrin
Soy oil, MCT oil, soy lecithin	Maltodextrin
Soy oil, MCT oil	Maltodextrin
Canola oil, MCT oil, high oleic sunflower oil, corn oil	Maltodextrin
Canola oil, MCT oil, corn oil, soy lecithin	Maltodextrin, corn syrup solids[4]
MCT oil, canola oil, corn oil, soy lecithin	Maltodextrin[4]
High oleic safflower oil, canola oil, MCT oil, soy lecithin	Maltodextrin
High oleic safflower oil, canola oil, MCT oil, soy lecithin	Maltodextrin
High oleic safflower oil, canola oil, MCT oil, soy lecithin	Maltodextrin

WATER CONTENT (ml) PER LITER	NUTRIENT PER LITER						
	SODIUM mg (mEq)	POTASSIUM mg (mEq)	CHLORIDE mg (mEq)	CALCIUM mg (mEq)	PHOSPHORUS mg (mmol)	MAGNESIUM mg (mEq)	FIBER (g)
819	1100 (48)	1900 (49)	1100 (31)	1200 (60)	1100 (36)	350 (29)	—
818	1100 (48)	1900 (49)	1100 (31)	1200 (60)	1200 (39)	350 (29)	—
770	1200 (52)	1850 (47)	1700 (48)	1200 (60)	1200 (39)	480 (40)	—
769	1400 (61)	1800 (46)	1700 (48)	1000 (50)	1000 (32)	400 (33)	—
840	530 (23)	1320[3] (34)	1060 (30)	630 (32)	530 (17)	210 (17)	—
850	930 (40)	1610 (41)	1440 (41)	850 (42)	850 (27)	340 (28)	—
810	1350 (59)	1850 (47)	1500 (42)	1000 (50)	1000 (32)	400 (33)	—
852	876 (38)	1248 (32)	1200 (34)	668 (33)	668 (22)	268 (22)	—
775	1168 (51)	1872 (48)	1740 (49)	1000 (50)	1000 (32)	400 (33)	—
841	640 (28)	1020 (26)	850 (24)	535 (26)	535 (17)	215 (17)	—
842	930 (40)	1570 (40)	1440 (41)	760 (38)	760 (25)	305 (25)	—
820	1420 (62)	1940 (50)	1540 (43)	1200 (60)	1200 (39)	400 (33)	—

Continued

PRODUCT	MANUFACTURER	FORM	PROTEIN SOURCE
STANDARD FIBER CONTAINING FORMULAS			
Fibersource Standard™	Novartis Nutrition	Liquid	Soy protein concentrate, soy protein isolate
Fibersource™ HN	Novartis Nutrition	Liquid	Soy protein isolate, soy protein concentrate
Isosource® 1.5 Cal	Novartis Nutrition	Liquid	Sodium and calcium caseinates
Jevity®	Ross Laboratories	Liquid	Sodium and calcium caseinates
Jevity® Plus	Ross Laboratories	Liquid	Sodium and calcium caseinates
Nutren® 1.0 with Fiber	Nestle Nutrition	Liquid	Calcium-potassium caseinate
ProBalance®	Nestle Nutrition	Liquid	Calcium-potassium caseinate
Ultracal®	Mead Johnson	Liquid	Milk protein concentrate, casein
Ultracal® HN Plus	Mead Johnson	Liquid	Milk protein concentrate, casein[9]

PRODUCT	CALORIES/ml	PROTEIN (g/L)	CARBOHY-DRATE (g/L)	FAT (g/L)	NUTRITIONAL PROFILE OSMOLALITY (mOsm/kg WATER)	VOLUME (ml) TO MEET 100% OF THE RDI[10]
STANDARD0 FIBER CONTAINING FORMULAS						
Fibersource™ Standard	1.2	43	170	39	490	1165
Fibersource™ HN	1.2	53	160	39	490	1165
Isosource® 1.5 Ca1[11]	1.5	68	170	65	650	933
Jevity®	1.06	44.3	154.7	34.7	300	1321
Jevity® Plus	1.2	55.5	172.7	39.3	450	1000
Nutren® 1.0 with Fiber	1.0	40	127	38	320-380	1500[12]
ProBalance®	1.2	54	156	40.8	350-450	1000[13]
Ultracal®	1.06	45	142	39	360	1120
Ultracal® HN Plus	1.2	54	156	40	370	1000

[7]Benefiber®, a prebiotic and source of soluble fiber as partially hydrolyzed guar gum.
[8]Flavored product contains sucrose.
[9]Closed system only.
[10]With the exception of chloride.

NUTRIENT SOURCE	
FAT SOURCE	**CARBOHYDRATE SOURCE**
Canola oil, MCT oil	Corn syrup, hydrolyzed cornstarch Fiber Source: Benefiber,®[7] soy fiber
Canola oil, MCT oil	Corn syrup, hydrolyzed cornstarch Fiber Source: Benefiber,®[7] soy fiber
Canola oil, MCT oil, soybean oil	Hydrolyzed cornstarch, sucrose Fiber Source: Benefiber,®[7] soy fiber
High oleic safflower oil, canola oil, MCT oil, soy lecithin	Maltodextrin, corn syrup solids Fiber Source: soy fiber
High oleic safflower oil, canola oil, MCT oil, soy lecithin	Corn syrup, maltodextrin Fiber Source: FOS, oat fiber, soy fiber, gum arabic
Canola oil, MCT oil, corn oil, soy lecithin	Maltodextrin, corn syrup solids[8] Fiber Source: soy polysaccharides
Canola oil, MCT oil, corn oil, soy lecithin	Maltodextrin, corn syrup solids[8] Fiber Source: soy polysaccharides, gum arabic
Canola oil, MCT oil, high oleic sunflower oil, corn oil, soy lecithin	Maltodextrin Fiber Source: cellulose, soy fiber, acacia
Canola oil, MCT oil, high oleic sunflower oil, corn oil, soy lecithin	Maltodextrin Fiber Source: cellulose, soy fiber, acacia

				NUTRIENT PER LITER			
WATER CONTENT (ml) PER LITER	**SODIUM mg (mEq)**	**POTASSIUM mg (mEq)**	**CHLORIDE mg (mEq)**	**CALCIUM mg (mEq)**	**PHOSPHORUS mg (mmol)**	**MAGNESIUM mg (mEq)**	**FIBER (g)**
811	1200 (52)	2000 (51)	900 (25)	1000 (50)	940 (30)	350 (29)	10
814	1200 (52)	2000 (51)	900 (25)	1000 (50)	1000 (32)	350 (29)	10
778	1290 (56)	2250 (58)	1610 (45)	1070 (53)	1070 (35)	430 (35)	8
835	930 (40)	1570 (40)	1310 (37)	910 (45)	760 (25)	305 (25)	14.4
810	1350 (59)	1850 (47)	1500 (42)	1200 (60)	1200 (39)	400 (33)	12
840	876 (38)	1248 (32)	1200 (34)	668 (33)	668 (22)	268 (22)	14
810	764 (33)	1560 (40)	1296 (36.5)	1250 (62)	1000 (32)	400 (33)	10
830	1350 (59)	1850 (47)	1500 (42)	1000 (50)	1000 (32)	400 (33)	14.4
810	1350 (59)	1850 (47)	1500 (42)	1000 (50)	1000 (32)	400 (33)	10

[11]Nutritional profile/nutrient per liter based on product in closed system container.
[13]With the exception of chloride and chromium.
[12]With the exception of chloride, chromium, and selenium.

Continued

PRODUCT	MANUFACTURER	FORM	PROTEIN SOURCE
BLENDERIZED FORMULAS			
COMPLEAT®	Novartis Nutrition	Liquid	Beef, calcium caseinate
COMPLEAT® Pediatric	Novartis Nutrition	Liquid	Beef, sodium and calcium caseinates
Diabetisource®	Novartis Nutrition	Liquid	Beef, calcium caseinate
WOUND-HEALING FORMULAS			
Isosource® VHN	Novartis Nutrition	Liquid	Sodium and calcium caseinates
IMPACT®	Novartis Nutrition	Liquid	Sodium and calcium caseinates, L-arginine
IMPACT® 1.5	Novartis Nutrition	Liquid	Sodium and calcium caseinates, L-arginine
IMPACT® with Fiber	Novartis Nutrition	Liquid	Sodium and calcium caseinates, L-arginine
IMPACT® Glutamine	Novartis Nutrition	Liquid	Wheat protein hydrolysate, sodium caseinate, free amino acids
IMPACT® Recover	Novartis Nutrition	Powder	Whey protein isolate, L-glutamine, L-arginine
Promote®	Ross Laboratories	Liquid	Sodium and calcium caseinates, soy protein isolate
Promote® with Fiber	Ross Laboratories	Liquid	Sodium and calcium caseinates
Protain XL®	Mead Johnson	Liquid	Sodium caseinate, calcium caseinate
Replete®	Nestle Nutrition	Liquid	Calcium-potassium caseinate
Replete® with Fiber	Nestle Nutrition	Liquid	Calcium-potassium caseinate
TraumaCal®	Mead Johnson	Liquid	Calcium caseinate, sodium caseinate

See Wound-Healing section for profile of RESOURCE® Arginaid™ and RESOURCE® Instant Protein Powder.
[14]Benefiber®, a prebiotic and source of soluble fiber as partially hydrolyzed guar gum.

NUTRIENT SOURCE	
FAT SOURCE	**CARBOHYDRATE SOURCE**
Canola oil, beef fat, mono- and diglycerides	Maltodextrin, vegetables, fruits Fiber Source: vegetables, fruits
High oleic sunflower oil, soybean oil, MCT oil, beef fat, mono and diglycerides	Hydrolyzed cornstarch, apple juice, vegetables, fruits Fiber Source: vegetables, fruits
High oleic sunflower oil, canola oil, beef fat	Maltodextrin, fructose, vegetables, fruits Fiber Source: vegetables, fruits
MCT oil, canola oil	Hydrolyzed cornstarch Fiber Source: Benefiber®,[14] soy fiber
Palm kernel oil, sunflower oil, menhaden fish oil	Hydrolyzed cornstarch
MCT oil, palm kernel oil, menhaden fish oil, sunflower oil	Hydrolyzed cornstarch
Palm kernel oil, menhaden fish oil, sunflower oil	Hydrolyzed cornstarch Fiber Source: Benefiber®,[14] soy fiber
Palm kernel oil, menhaden fish oil, sunflower oil	Maltodextrin Fiber Source: Benefiber®,[14] soy fiber
Canola oil, MCT oil	Sugar, hydrolyzed cornstarch Fiber Source: Benefiber®[14]
High oleic safflower oil, canola oil, MCT oil, soy lecithin	Maltodextrin, sugar
High oleic safflower oil, canola oil, MCT oil, soy lecithin	Maltodextrin, sugar Fiber Source: oat fiber, soy fiber
Canola oil, high oleic sunflower oil, MCT oil, corn oil, soy lecithin	Maltodextrin Fiber Source: soy fiber
Canola oil, MCT oil, soy lecithin	Maltodextrin
Canola oil, MCT oil, soy lecithin	Maltodextrin, corn syrup solids Fiber Source: soy polysaccharides
Soybean oil, MCT oil, lecithin	Corn syrup, sugar

Continued

PRODUCT	CALORIES/ml	PROTEIN (g/L)	CARBOHY-DRATE (g/L)	FAT (g/L)	NUTRITIONAL PROFILE OSMOLALITY (mOsm/kg WATER)	VOLUME (mL) TO MEET 100% OF THE RDI[15]
BLENDERIZED FORMULAS—cont'd						
COMPLEAT®	1.07	43	140	37	300	1500
COMPLEAT® Pediatric	1.0	38	130	39	380	Ages 1-10/900[16]
Diabetisource®	1.0	50	90	49	360	1500
WOUND-HEALING FORMULAS—cont'd						
Isosource® VHN[17]	1.0	62	130	29	300	1250
IMPACT®	1.0	56	130	28	375	1500
IMPACT® 1.5	1.5	84	140	69	550	1250
IMPACT® with Fiber	1.0	56	140	28	375	1500
IMPACT® Glutamine	1.3	78	150	43	630	1000
Impact® Recover (per serving)	1.0	17	26	6.6	830-890	1185
Promote®	1.0	62.5	130	26	340	1000
Promote® with Fiber	1.0	62.5	138.3	28.2	380	1000
Protain® XL	1.0	57	145	30	340	1250
Replete®	1.0	62.4	113.2	34	300-350	1000
Replete® with Fiber	1.0	62.4	113.2	34	310-390	1000
TraumaCal®	1.5	82	142	68	560	2000

See Wound-Healing section for profile of RESOURCE® Arginaid™ and RESOURCE® Instant Protein Powder.
[15]With the exception of chloride.
[16]Based on 1989 NRC RDAs.
[17]Nutritional profile/nutrient per liter based on product in closed system container.

WATER CONTENT (ml) PER LITER	NUTRIENT PER LITER						
	SODIUM mg (mEq)	POTASSIUM mg (mEq)	CHLORIDE mg (mEq)	CALCIUM mg (mEq)	PHOSPHORUS mg (mmol)	MAGNESIUM mg (mEq)	FIBER (g)
781	760 (33)	1450 (37)	870 (25)	670 (33)	730 (24)	270 (22)	4.3
844	680 (30)	1500 (38)	720 (20)	1000 (50)	1000 (32)	190 (16)	4.4
849	990 (43)	1600 (41)	1100 (31)	670 (33)	800 (26)	270 (22)	4.3
847	1380 (60)	1800 (46)	1360 (38)	800 (40)	800 (26)	320 (26)	10
853	1100 (48)	1400 (36)	1300 (37)	800 (40)	800 (26)	270 (22)	—
780	1280 (56)	1680 (43)	1600 (45)	960 (48)	960 (31)	320 (26)	—
868	1100 (48)	1400 (36)	1300 (37)	800 (40)	800 (26)	270 (22)	10
807	1200 (52)	1800 (46)	850 (24)	1200 (60)	1200 (39)	400 (33)	10
186	280 (12.2)	350 (9)	330 (9.3)	200 (10)	200 (6.5)	68 (5.5)	3
837	1000 (43)	1980 (51)	1260 (36)	1200 (60)	1200 (39)	400 (33)	—
830	1300 (57)	1980 (51)	1260 (36)	1200 (60)	1200 (39)	400 (33)	14.4
830	920 (40)	1760 (45)	1350 (38)	800 (40)	800 (26)	320 (26)	9.1
845	876 (38)	1500 (38)	1300 (37)	1000 (50)	1000 (32)	400 (33)	—
835	876 (38)	1500 (38)	1300 (37)	1000 (50)	1000 (32)	400 (33)	14
780	1180 (51)	1390 (36)	1610 (45)	750 (38)	750 (24)	200 (16)	—

Continued

PRODUCT	MANUFACTURER	FORM	PROTEIN SOURCE
ELEMENTAL AND SEMI-ELEMENTAL FORMULAS			
IMPACT® Glutamine	Novartis Nutrition	Liquid	Wheat protein hydrolysate, sodium caseinate, free amino acids
Sandosource® Peptide	Novartis Nutrition	Liquid	Casein hydrolysate, free amino acids, sodium caseinate (26% free amino acids, 34% peptide chain length 2-4 amino acids, 40% peptide chain length >4 amino acids)
TOLEREX®	Novartis Nutrition	Powder	Free amino acids (16.8% BCAA, 17.1% glutamine, 8.9% arginine)
VIVONEX® Plus	Novartis Nutrition	Powder	Free amino acids (30% BCAA, 22.2% glutamine, 11.1% arginine)
VIVONEX® RTF	Novartis Nutrition	Liquid	Free amino acids
VIVONEX® T.E.N.	Novartis Nutrition	Powder	Free amino acids (33.2% BCAA, 12.9% glutamine, 7.6% arginine)
AlitraQ®	Ross Laboratories	Powder	Free amino acids, soy hydrolysate, whey protein concentrate, lactalbumin hydrolysate
Criticare® HN	Mead Johnson	Liquid	Casein hydrolysate, free amino acids
Crucial®	Nestle Nutrition	Liquid	Enzymatically hydrolyzed casein, L-arginine
f.a.a.™	Nestle Nutrition	Liquid	Free amino acids
Glutasorb™	Hormel Health Labs	Liquid	Wheat hydrolysate, free amino acids
IntensiCal™	Mead Johnson	Liquid	Casein hydrolysate, L-arginine
Optimental®	Ross Laboratories	Liquid	Soy protein hydrolysate, partially hydrolyzed sodium caseinate, L-arginine
Peptamen®	Nestle Nutrition	Liquid	Enzymatically hydrolyzed whey protein
Peptamen® 1.5	Nestle Nutrition	Liquid	Enzymatically hydrolyzed whey protein
Peptamen® VHP	Nestle Nutrition	Liquid	Enzymatically hydrolyzed whey protein
Perative®	Ross Laboratories	Liquid	Partially hydrolyzed sodium caseinate, lactalbumin hydrolysate, L-arginine
Reabilan®	Nestle Nutrition	Liquid	Enzymatically hydrolyzed casein protein, enzymatically hydrolyzed whey protein
Reabilan® HN	Nestle Nutrition	Liquid	Enzymatically hydrolyzed casein protein, enzymatically hydrolyzed whey protein
Subdue®	Mead Johnson	Liquid	Hydrolyzed whey protein concentrate
Subdue® Plus	Mead Johnson	Liquid	Hydrolyzed whey protein concentrate
Vital® High Nitrogen	Ross Laboratories	Powder	Partially hydrolyzed whey, meat and soy protein, free amino acids

[18]Benefiber, a prebiotic and source of soluble fiber as partially hydrolyzed guar gum.
[19]Flavored product contains sucrose.

NUTRIENT SOURCE

FAT SOURCE	CARBOHYDRATE SOURCE
Palm kernel oil, menhaden fish oil, sunflower oil	Maltodextrin Fiber Source: Benefiber®,[18] soy fiber
MCT oil, soybean oil, hydroxylated lecithin	Hydrolyzed cornstarch
Safflower oil	Maltodextrin, modified cornstarch
Soybean oil	Maltodextrin, modified cornstarch
Soybean oil, MCT oil	Maltodextrin, modified cornstarch
Safflower oil	Maltodextrin, modified cornstarch
MCT oil, safflower oil	Maltodextrin, sugar, fructose
Safflower oil, emulsifiers	Maltodextrin, modified cornstarch
MCT oil, fish oil, soybean oil, soy lecithin	Maltodextrin, cornstarch
Soybean oil, MCT oil, soy lecithin	Maltodextrin, cornstarch
Soybean oil	Maltodextrin, modified starch
MCT oil, canola oil, high oleic sunflower oil, corn oil, menhaden oil	Maltodextrin, modified cornstarch
Structured lipid (sardine oil, MCT oil), canola oil, soy oil	Maltodextrin, sugar
MCT oil, soybean oil, soy lecithin	Maltodextrin, cornstarch
MCT oil, soybean oil, soy lecithin	Maltodextrin, cornstarch
MCT oil, soybean oil, soy lecithin	Maltodextrin, cornstarch
Canola oil, MCT oil, corn oil, soy lecithin	Maltodextrin
MCT oil, soybean oil, canola oil, soy lecithin	Corn syrup solids, cornstarch
MCT oil, soybean oil, canola oil, soy lecithin	Corn syrup solids, cornstarch
MCT oil, canola oil, high oleic sunflower oil, corn oil	Maltodextrin, modified cornstarch[19]
MCT oil, canola oil, high oleic sunflower oil, corn oil	Maltodextrin, modified cornstarch[19]
Safflower oil, MCT oil	Maltodextrin, sugar

Continued

PRODUCT	CALORIES/ml	PROTEIN (g/L)	CARBOHY-DRATE (g/L)	FAT (g/L)	NUTRITIONAL PROFILE OSMOLALITY (mOsm/kg WATER)	VOLUME (ml) TO MEET 100% OF THE RDI[20]
ELEMENTAL AND SEMI-ELEMENTAL FORMULAS—cont'd						
IMPACT® Glutamine	1.3	78	150	43	630	1000
Sandosource® Peptide	1.0	50	160	17	490	1750
TOLEREX®	1.0	21	230	1.5	550	1800
VIVONEX® Plus	1.0	45	190	6.7	650	1800
VIVONEX® RTF	1.0	50	175	12	630	1500
VIVONEX® T.E.N.	1.0	38	210	2.8	630	2000
AlitraQ®	1.0	52.5	165	15.5	575	1500
Criticare® HN	1.06	38	220	5.3	650	1890
Crucial®	1.5	94	135	67.6	490	1000
f.a.a.™	1.0	50	176	11.2	700	1850
Glutasorb™	1.0	52	186	6.7	575	1800
IntensiCal™	1.3	81	150	42	550	1000
Optimental®	1.0	51.3	138.5	28.4	540	1422
Peptamen®	1.0	40	127	39	270	1500[21]
Peptamen® 1.5	1.5	60	191	58.5	450	1000
Peptamen® VHP	1.0	62.5	104.5	39.2	300	1500
Perative®	1.3	66.6	177.2	37.4	385	1155
Reabilan®	1.0	31.5	131.5	40.5	350	2000
Reabilan® HN	1.33	57.9	158	54	490	1500
Subdue®	1.0	50	130	34	330-525	1180
Subdue® Plus	1.5	76	186	51	400	946
Vital® High Nitrogen	1.0	41.7	185	10.8	500	1500

[20]With the exception of chloride.

WATER CONTENT (ml) PER LITER	NUTRIENT PER LITER						
	SODIUM mg (mEq)	POTASSIUM mg (mEq)	CHLORIDE mg (mEq)	CALCIUM mg (mEq)	PHOSPHORUS mg (mmol)	MAGNESIUM mg (mEq)	FIBER (g)
807	1200 (52)	1800 (46)	850 (24)	1200 (60)	1200 (39)	400 (33)	10
840	1200 (52)	1600 (41)	970 (27)	570 (28)	570 (18)	230 (19)	—
864	470 (20)	1170 (30)	950 (27)	560 (28)	560 (18)	220 (18)	—
850	610 (27)	1060 (27)	940 (27)	560 (28)	560 (18)	220 (18)	—
848	670 (29)	800 (20)	800 (23)	670 (33)	670 (22)	270 (22)	—
853	600 (26)	950 (24)	850 (24)	500 (25)	500 (16)	200 (16)	—
846	1000 (43)	1200 (31)	1300 (37)	733 (37)	733 (24)	267 (22)	—
850	630 (27)	1310 (34)	1060 (30)	530 (26)	530 (17)	210 (17)	—
771	1168 (51)	1872 (48)	1740 (49)	1000 (50)	1000 (32)	400 (33)	—
824	560 (24)	1500 (38)	1400 (39)	800 (40)	700 (23)	296 (24)	—
732	600 (26)	1000 (26)	1126 (32)	560 (28)	560 (18)	220 (18)	—
800	1110 (48)	1290 (33)	1470 (41)	1130 (56)	1080 (35)	400 (33)	—
835	1060 (46)	1760 (45)	1340 (38)	1060 (53)	1060 (34)	425 (35)	—
850	560 (24)	1500 (38)	1000 (28)	800 (40)	700 (23)	300 (25)	—
771	1020 (44)	1860 (48)	1740 (49)	1000 (50)	1000 (32)	400 (33)	—
844	560 (24)	1500 (38)	1000 (28)	800 (40)	700 (23)	300 (25)	—
789	1040 (45)	1730 (44)	1650 (47)	870 (43)	870 (28)	350 (29)	—
850	700 (30)	1250 (32)	1880 (52)	500 (25)	500 (16)	250 (21)	—
800	1000 (43)	1662 (43)	2500 (70)	665 (33)	665 (22)	332 (27)	—
840	1100 (48)	1600 (41)	1400 (39)	1100 (55)	1050 (34)	360 (30)	—
760	1180 (51)	2000 (51)	1820 (51)	1390 (69)	1310 (42)	440 (36)	—
867	566 (25)	1400 (36)	1032 (29)	667 (33)	667 (22)	267 (22)	—

[21]With the exception of chloride, chromium, and selenium.

Continued

PRODUCT	MANUFACTURER	FORM	PROTEIN SOURCE
PULMONARY FORMULAS			
Isosource® 1.5 Cal	Novartis Nutrition	Liquid	Sodium and calcium caseinates
Novasource™ Pulmonary	Novartis Nutrition	Liquid	Sodium and calcium caseinates
NutriVent®	Nestle Nutrition	Liquid	Calcium-potassium caseinate
Oxepa®	Ross Laboratories	Liquid	Sodium and calcium caseinates
Pulmocare®	Ross Laboratories	Liquid	Sodium and calcium caseinates
Respalor®	Mead Johnson	Liquid	Calcium caseinate, sodium caseinate
RENAL FORMULAS			
Novasource™ Renal	Novartis Nutrition	Liquid	Sodium and calcium caseinates, L-arginine
Magnacal® Renal	Mead Johnson	Liquid	Calcium caseinate, sodium caseinate
Nepro®	Ross Laboratories	Liquid	Calcium, magnesium and sodium caseinates, milk protein isolate
NutriRenal®	Nestle Nutrition	Liquid	Calcium-potassium caseinate
Renalcal®	Nestle Nutrition	Liquid	Whey protein concentrate, free amino acids
Suplena®	Ross Laboratories	Liquid	Sodium caseinate, calcium caseinate

[22]Benefiber®, a prebiotic and source of soluble fiber as partially hydrolyzed guar gum.
[23]Flavored product contains sucrose.

NUTRIENT SOURCE	
FAT SOURCE	**CARBOHYDRATE SOURCE**
Canola oil, MCT oil, soybean oil	Hydrolyzed cornstarch, sucrose Fiber Source: Benefiber®,[22] soy fiber
Canola oil, MCT oil	Corn syrup, sucrose Fiber Source: Benefiber®,[22] soy fiber
Canola oil, MCT oil, corn oil, soy lecithin	Maltodextrin
Canola oil, MCT oil, sardine oil, borage oil	Sugar, maltodextrin
Canola oil, MCT oil, corn oil, high oleic safflower oil, soy lecithin	Sugar, maltodextrin
Canola oil, MCT oil, high oleic sunflower oil, corn oil, soy lecithin	Maltodextrin[23]
High oleic sunflower oil, corn oil, MCT oil	Corn syrup, fructose
Canola oil, high oleic sunflower oil, MCT oil, corn oil, soy lecithin	Maltodextrin, sugar
High oleic safflower oil, canola oil, soy lecithin	Corn syrup, sucrose
MCT oil, canola oil, corn oil, soy lecithin	Corn syrup solids, maltodextrin, sugar
MCT oil, canola oil, corn oil, soy lecithin	Maltodextrin, modified cornstarch
High oleic safflower oil, soy oil, soy lecithin	Maltodextrin, sugar

Continued

					NUTRITIONAL PROFILE	
PRODUCT	CALORIES/ml	PROTEIN (g/L)	CARBOHY-DRATE (g/L)	FAT (g/L)	OSMOLALITY (mOsm/kg WATER)	VOLUME (ml) TO MEET 100% OF THE RDI
PULMONARY FORMULAS—cont'd						
Isosource® 1.5 Cal[24]	1.5	68	170	65	650	933[25]
Novasource™ Pulmonary[26]	1.5	75	150	68	650	933[25]
NutriVent®	1.5	67.5	100	94	330-450	1000[26]
Oxepa®	1.5	62.5	105.5	93.7	493	947[25]
Pulmocare®	1.5	62.6	105.7	93.3	475	947[25]
Respalor®	1.5	75	146	68	400	1000[25]
RENAL FORMULAS—cont'd						
Novasource™ Renal Brik Pak	2.0	74	200	100	700	1000[27]
Closed System	*2.0*	*74*	*200*	*100*	*960*	*1000[27]*
Magnacal® Renal	2.0	75	200	101	570	1000[27]
Nepro®	2.0	70	222.3	95.6	665	947[27]
NutriRenal®	2.0	70	205	104	650	750[27]
Renalcal®	2.0	34.4	290	82.4	600	1000[27]
Suplena®	2.0	30.0	255.2	95.6	600	947[27]

[24]Nutritional profile/nutrient per liter based on product in closed system containers.
[25]With the exception of chloride.
[26]With the exception of chloride, chromium, and selenium.
[27]With the exception of key vitamins and minerals contraindicated for renal patients.

WATER CONTENT (ml) PER LITER	NUTRIENT PER LITER						
	SODIUM mg (mEq)	POTASSIUM mg (mEq)	CHLORIDE mg (mEq)	CALCIUM mg (mEq)	PHOSPHORUS mg (mmol)	MAGNESIUM mg (mEq)	FIBER (g)
778	1290 (56)	2250 (58)	1610 (45)	1070 (53)	1070 (35)	430 (35)	8
764	1390 (60)	2670 (68)	1500 (42)	1070 (53)	1070 (35)	430 (35)	8
781	1170 (51)	1872 (48)	1740 (49)	1200 (60)	1200 (39)	480 (40)	—
785	1310 (57)	1960 (50)	1690 (48)	1060 (53)	1060 (34)	425 (35)	—
785	1310 (57)	1960 (50)	1690 (48)	1060 (53)	1060 (34)	425 (35)	—
780	1270 (55)	1480 (38)	1690 (48)	1000 (50)	1000 (32)	400 (33)	
709	900 (39)	810 (21)	840 (24)	1300 (65)	650 (21)	200 (17)	—
709	*1600 (70)*	*1100 (28)*	*1000 (28)*	*1300 (65)*	*650 (21)*	*200 (17)*	—
710	800 (35)	1270 (32)	1180 (33)	1010 (50)	800 (26)	200 (17)	—
699	845 (37)	1060 (27)	1010 (28)	1370 (68)	685 (22)	215 (18)	—
704	740 (32)	1256 (32)	1140 (32)	1400 (70)	700 (23)	200 (17)	—
704	—	—	—	—	—	—	—
713	790 (34)	1120 (29)	935 (26)	1430 (71)	730 (24)	215 (18)	—

PRODUCT	MANUFACTURER	FORM	PROTEIN SOURCE
DIABETIC FORMULAS			
Diabetisource®	Novartis Nutrition	Liquid	Beef, calcium caseinate
RESOURCE® Diabetic	Novartis Nutrition	Liquid	Sodium and calcium caseinates, soy protein isolate
Choice DM® Beverage	Mead Johnson	Liquid	Calcium and sodium caseinates, milk protein concentrate
Choice DM® Tube Feeding	Mead Johnson	Liquid	Milk protein concentrate, casein
Glytrol®	Nestle Nutrition	Liquid	Calcium-potassium caseinate
Glucerna®	Ross Laboratories	Liquid	Sodium and calcium caseinates
Glucerna Shake®	Ross Laboratories	Liquid	Sodium and calcium caseinates
IMMUNE-ENHANCING FORMULAS[29]			
IMPACT®	Novartis Nutrition	Liquid	Sodium and calcium caseinates, L-arginine
IMPACT® 1.5	Novartis Nutrition	Liquid	Sodium and calcium caseinates, L-arginine
IMPACT® with Fiber	Novartis Nutrition	Liquid	Sodium and calcium caseinates, L-arginine
IMPACT® Glutamine	Novartis Nutrition	Liquid	Wheat protein hydrolysate, sodium caseinate, free amino acids
IMPACT® Recover	Novartis Nutrition	Powder	Whey protein isolate, L-glutamine, L-arginine
Immun-Aid®	McGaw	Powder	Lactalbumin, L-arginine, L-glutamine, BCAA

[28]Benefiber®, a prebiotic and source of soluble fiber as partially hydrolyzed guar gum.
[29]These formulas have clinical data to support their use as immune-enhancing formulas.

NUTRIENT SOURCE	
FAT SOURCE	**CARBOHYDRATE SOURCE**
High oleic sunflower oil, canola oil, beef fat	Maltodextrin, fructose, vegetables, fruits Fiber Source: vegetables, fruits
High oleic sunflower oil, soybean oil, soy lecithin, monoglycerides	Hydrolyzed cornstarch Fiber Source: Benefiber®,[28] soy fiber
Canola oil, high oleic sunflower oil, corn oil, soy lecithin, mono and diglycerides	Maltodextrin, sugar Fiber Source: soy fiber, acacia, cellulose
Canola oil, high oleic sunflower oil, corn oil, MCT oil, soy lecithin	Maltodextrin Fiber Source: cellulose, soy fiber, acacia
Canola oil, high oleic safflower oil, MCT oil, soy lecithin	Maltodextrin, fructose, modified cornstarch Fiber Source: gum arabic, soy polysaccharides, pectin
High oleic safflower oil, canola oil, soy lecithin	Maltodextrin, fructose Fiber Source: soy fiber
High oleic safflower oil, canola oil, soy lecithin	Maltodextrin, fructose Fiber Source: soy polysaccharide, gum arabic
Palm kernel oil, sunflower oil, menhaden fish oil	Hydrolyzed cornstarch
MCT oil, palm kernel oil, sunflower oil, menhaden fish oil	Hydrolyzed cornstarch
Palm kernel oil, sunflower oil, menhaden fish oil	Hydrolyzed cornstarch Fiber Source: Benefiber®,[28] soy fiber
Palm kernel oil, sunflower oil, menhaden fish oil	Maltodextrin Fiber Source: Benefiber®,[28] soy fiber
Canola oil, MCT oil	Sugar, hydrolyzed cornstarch Fiber Source: Benefiber®[28]
Canola oil, MCT oil	Maltodextrin

					NUTRITIONAL PROFILE[30]	
PRODUCT	CALORIES/ml	PROTEIN (g/L)	CARBOHY-DRATE (g/L)	FAT (g/L)	OSMOLALITY (mOsm/kg WATER)	VOLUME (ml) TO MEET 100% OF THE RDI[31]
DIABETIC FORMULAS—cont'd						
Diabetisource®	1.0	50	90	49	360	1500
RESOURCE® Diabetic	1.06	63	100	47	320	1180
Choice DM® Beverage	0.93	39	101	43	400	1310
Choice DM® Tube Feeding	1.06	45	119	51	300	1120
Glytrol®	1.0	45	100	47.5	380	1400
Glucerna®	1.0	41.8	95.6	54.4	355	1422
Glucerna® Shake	0.93	42.2	92.8	46.4	332	(32)
IMMUNE-ENHANCING FORMULAS[33]—cont'd						
IMPACT®	1.0	56	130	28	375	1500
IMPACT® 1.5	1.5	84	140	69	550	1250
IMPACT® with Fiber	1.0	56	140	28	375	1500
IMPACT® Glutamine	1.3	78	150	43	630	1000
IMPACT® Recover (per serving)	1.0	17	26	6.6	830-890	1185
Immun-Aid®	1.0	80	120	22	460	2000

[30]Nutritional profile/nutrient per liter based on product in closed system containers with the exception of Choice DM® Beverage and Glucerna® Shake.
[31]With the exception of chloride.
[32]Not intended for total feeding.
[33]These formulas have clinical data to support their use as immune-enhancing formulas.

WATER CONTENT (ml) PER LITER	NUTRIENT PER LITER[30]						
	SODIUM mg (mEq)	POTASSIUM mg (mEq)	CHLORIDE mg (mEq)	CALCIUM mg (mEq)	PHOSPHORUS mg (mmol)	MAGNESIUM mg (mEq)	FIBER (g)
849	990 (43)	1600 (41)	1100 (31)	670 (33)	800 (26)	270 (22)	4.3
847	1170 (50)	1780 (46)	930 (26)	1100 (55)	1100 (35)	340 (28)	12.8
850	850 (37)	1820 (47)	1270 (36)	1390 (69)	1310 (42)	440 (36)	11
850	850 (37)	1820 (47)	1270 (36)	1060 (53)	1060 (34)	420 (35)	14.4
847	740 (32)	1400 (36)	1200 (34)	720 (36)	720 (23)	286 (24)	15
853	930 (40)	1570 (40)	1440 (41)	705 (35)	705 (23)	285 (23)	14.1
852	890 (39)	1560 (40)	1400 (42)	1055 (53)	1055 (34)	422 (35)	8.4
853	1100 (48)	1400 (36)	1300 (37)	800 (40)	800 (26)	270 (22)	—
780	1280 (56)	1680 (43)	1600 (45)	960 (48)	960 (31)	320 (26)	—
868	1100 (48)	1400 (36)	1300 (37)	800 (40)	800 (26)	270 (22)	10
807	1200 (52)	1800 (46)	850 (24)	1200 (60)	1200 (39)	400 (33)	10
186	280 (12.2)	350 (9)	330 (9.3)	200 (10)	200 (6.5)	68 (5.6)	3
820	580 (25)	1060 (27)	888 (25)	500 (25)	500 (16)	200 (16)	—

Continued

PRODUCT	MANUFACTURER	FORM	PROTEIN SOURCE
TWO-CALORIE FORMULAS			
Novasource™ 2.0	Novartis Nutrition	Liquid	Calcium and sodium caseinates
RESOURCE® 2.0	Novartis Nutrition	Liquid	Calcium and sodium caseinates
Deliver® 2.0	Mead Johnson	Liquid	Calcium and sodium caseinates
NuBasics® 2.0	Nestle Nutrition	Liquid	Calcium-potassium caseinate
Nutren® 2.0	Nestle Nutrition	Liquid	Calcium-potassium caseinate
TwoCal® HN	Ross Laboratories	Liquid	Calcium and sodium caseinates
PEDIATRIC FORMULAS			
COMPLEAT® Pediatric	Novartis Nutrition	Liquid	Beef, sodium and calcium caseinates
RESOURCE® Just for Kids	Novartis Nutrition	Liquid	Sodium and calcium caseinates, whey protein concentrate
RESOURCE® Just for Kids with Fiber	Novartis Nutrition	Liquid	Sodium and calcium caseinates, whey protein concentrate
VIVONEX® PEDIATRIC	Novartis Nutrition	Powder	Free amino acids (12.9% glutamine, 6.2% arginine, 21.6% BCAA)
EleCare®	Ross Laboratories	Powder	Free amino acids
EnFamil™ Kindercal	Mead Johnson	Liquid	Milk protein concentrate
EnFamil™ Kindercal with Fiber	Mead Johnson	Liquid	Milk protein concentrate
Neocate® One+	SHS North America	Powder	Free amino acids
Nutren Junior®	Nestle Nutrition	Liquid	Milk protein concentrate, whey protein concentrate
Nutren Junior® with Fiber	Nestle Nutrition	Liquid	Milk protein concentrate, whey protein concentrate
PediaSure®	Ross Laboratories	Liquid	Sodium caseinate, whey protein concentrate
PediaSure® with Fiber	Ross Laboratories	Liquid	Sodium caseinate, whey protein concentrate
Peptamen Junior®	Nestle Nutrition	Liquid	Enzymatically hydrolyzed whey protein

[34]Chocolate flavor contains fructose.
[35]Benefiber, a prebiotic and source of soluble fiber as partially hydrolyzed guar gum.
[36]Flavored product contains sucrose.

NUTRIENT SOURCE	
FAT SOURCE	**CARBOHYDRATE SOURCE**
Canola oil, MCT oil, soy lecithin	Corn syrup, sugar, maltodextrin
Canola oil, MCT oil, soy lecithin	Corn syrup, sugar, maltodextrin
Soy oil, MCT oil, soy lecithin	Corn syrup
MCT oil, canola oil, soy lecithin, corn oil	Corn syrup solids, maltodextrin, sugar
MCT oil, canola oil, soy lecithin, corn oil	Corn syrup solids, maltodextrin, sugar
High oleic safflower oil, canola oil, soy lecithin	Corn syrup solids, maltodextrin, sugar
High oleic sunflower oil, soybean oil, MCT oil, beef fat, mono and diglycerides	Hydrolyzed cornstarch, apple juice, vegetables, fruits Fiber Source: vegetables, fruits
High oleic sunflower oil, soybean oil, MCT oil	Hydrolyzed cornstarch, sucrose[34]
High oleic sunflower oil, soybean oil, MCT oil	Hydrolyzed cornstarch, sucrose Fiber Source: Benefiber®,[35] soy fiber
MCT oil, soybean oil	Maltodextrin, modified cornstarch
High oleic safflower oil, MCT oil, soy oil	Corn syrup solids
Canola oil, high oleic sunflower oil, MCT oil, corn oil, soy lecithin	Maltodextrin, sugar
Canola oil, high oleic sunflower oil, MCT oil, corn oil	Maltodextrin, sugar Fiber Source: gum arabic, soy fiber
Fractionated coconut oil, canola oil, safflower oil	Maltodextrin, corn syrup solids, sucrose
Soybean oil, MCT oil, canola oil, soy lecithin	Maltodextrin, sugar
Soybean oil, MCT oil, canola oil, soy lecithin	Maltodextrin, sugar Fiber Source: soy polysaccharides
High oleic safflower oil, soy oil, MCT oil, soy lecithin	Maltodextrin, sugar
High oleic safflower oil, soy oil, MCT oil, soy lecithin	Maltodextrin, sugar Fiber Source: soy fiber
MCT oil, soybean oil, canola oil, soy lecithin	Maltodextrin, cornstarch[36]

					NUTRITIONAL PROFILE	
PRODUCT	CALORIES/ml	PROTEIN (g/L)	CARBOHY-DRATE (g/L)	FAT (g/L)	OSMOLALITY (mOsm/kg WATER)	VOLUME (ml) TO MEET 100% OF THE RDI
TWO-CALORIE FORMULAS—cont'd						
Novasource™ 2.0	2.0	90	220	88	790	948[37]
RESOURCE® 2.0	2.0	90	220	88	790	948[37]
Deliver® 2.0	2.0	75	200	101	640	1000[37]
NuBasics® 2.0	2.0	80	196	106	750	1000[38]
Nutren® 2.0	2.0	80	196	106	745	750[38]
TwoCal® HN	2.0	83.5	219	90.5	730	948[37]
PEDIATRIC FORMULAS—cont'd						
COMPLEAT® Pediatric	1.0	38	130	39	380	Ages 1-10/900[39]
RESOURCE® Just for Kids	1.0	30	110	50	390	Ages 1-10/1000[39]
RESOURCE® Just for Kids with Fiber	1.0	30	110	50	390	Ages 1-10/1000[39]
VIVONEX® Pediatric	0.8	24	130	24	360	Ages 1-6/1000[39] Ages 7-10/1170[39]
EleCare®	1.0	30.1	107	47.6	596	Ages 1-3/1000[39] Ages 4-6/1425[39] Ages 7-10/2025[39]
EnFamil™ Kindercal	1.06	30	135	44	345-520	Ages 7/10/946[39]
EnFamil™ Kindercal with Fiber	1.06	30	139	44	440-520	Ages 7/10/946[39]
Neocate® One⁺	1.0	25	146	35	610	Ages 1-3/1300[39] Ages 4-6/1800[39] Ages 7-10/2000[39]

[37] With the exception of chloride.
[38] With the exception of chloride and chromium.
[39] 1989 National Research Council Recommended Dietary Allowances.

WATER CONTENT (ml) PER LITER	SODIUM mg (mEq)	NUTRIENT PER LITER					
		POTASSIUM mg (mEq)	CHLORIDE mg (mEq)	CALCIUM mg (mEq)	PHOSPHORUS mg (mmol)	MAGNESIUM mg (mEq)	FIBER (g)
700	800 (35)	1520 (39)	1200 (34)	1100 (55)	1100 (36)	420 (35)	—
700	800 (35)	1520 (39)	1200 (34)	1100 (55)	1100 (36)	420 (35)	—
710	800 (35)	1690 (43)	1180 (33)	1010 (50)	1010 (32)	400 (33)	—
700	1300 (57)	1920 (49)	1876 (53)	1340 (67)	1340 (43)	536 (44)	—
700	1300 (57)	1920 (49)	1876 (53)	1340 (67)	1340 (43)	536 (44)	—
701	1460 (63)	2450 (63)	1820 (51)	1055 (53)	1055 (34)	425 (35)	—
844	680 (30)	1500 (38)	720 (20)	1000 (50)	1000 (32)	190 (16)	4.4
853	380 (17)	1300 (33)	850 (24)	1140 (57)	800 (26)	200 (17)	—
853	590 (26)	1140 (29)	510 (14)	1140 (57)	800 (26)	200 (17)	6.0
893	400 (17)	1200 (31)	1000 (28)	970 (48)	800 (26)	200 (17)	—
850	453 (20)	1505 (39)	600 (17)	1084 (54)	811 (26)	84 (7)	—
850	370 (16)	1310 (34)	740 (21)	1010 (50)	850 (27)	210 (17)	—
850	370 (16)	1310 (34)	740 (21)	1010 (50)	850 (27)	210 (17)	6.3
800	200 (9)	930 (24)	350 (10)	620 (31)	620 (20)	90 (7)	—

Continued

					NUTRITIONAL PROFILE	
PRODUCT	CALORIES/ml	PROTEIN (g/L)	CARBOHY-DRATE (g/L)	FAT (g/L)	OSMOLALITY (mOsm/kg WATER)	VOLUME (ml) TO MEET 100% OF THE NRC-RDI[40]
PEDIATRIC FORMULAS—cont'd						
Nutren Junior®	1.0	30	127.5	42	350	1000
Nutren Junior® with Fiber	1.0	30	127.5	42	350	1000
PediaSure®	1.0	30	109.7	49.7	335	Ages 1-6/1000 Ages 7-10/1300
PediaSure® with Fiber	1.0	30	113.5	49.7	345	Ages 1-6/1000 Ages 7-10/1300
Peptamen Junior®	1.0	30	137.6	38.5	260	Ages 7-10/1000

[40]1989 National Research Council Recommended Dietary Allowances.

WATER CONTENT (ml) PER LITER	NUTRIENT PER LITER						
	SODIUM mg (mEq)	POTASSIUM mg (mEq)	CHLORIDE mg (mEq)	CALCIUM mg (mEq)	PHOSPHORUS mg (mmol)	MAGNESIUM mg (mEq)	FIBER (g)
850	460 (20)	1320 (34)	1080 (30)	1000 (50)	800 (26)	200 (17)	—
844	460 (20)	1320 (34)	1080 (30)	1000 (50)	800 (26)	200 (17)	6
844	380 (17)	1310 (34)	1010 (28)	970 (48)	800 (26)	200 (17)	—
844	380 (17)	1310 (34)	1010 (28)	970 (48)	800 (26)	200 (17)	5
850	460 (20)	1320 (34)	1080 (30)	1000 (50)	800 (26)	200 (17)	—

Continued

| PRODUCT | MANU-FACTURER | FORM | NUTRIENT SOURCE | | | CALORIES/ml | CALORIES (PER SERVING) | PROTEIN (g/SERVING) |
			PROTEIN SOURCE	FAT SOURCE	CARBO-HYDRATE SOURCE			
MODULES								
RESOURCE® Arginaid (Serving 1 packet)	Novartis Nutrition	Powder	L-Arginine	—	Citric acid, malic acid	0.15	35	4.5[41]
RESOURCE® Benefiber (Serving 1 packet)	Novartis Nutrition	Powder	—	—	Benefiber®– partially hydrolyzed guar gum	—	16	—
RESOURCE® GlutaSolve (Serving 1 Tbsp.)	Novartis Nutrition	Powder	L-Glutamine	—	Maltodextrin	0.65	90	15[42]
RESOURCE® Instant Protein Powder (Serving 7.0 g)	Novartis Nutrition	Powder	Whey protein isolate	—	—	—	25	6
Hormel™ Instant Soluble Fiber (Serving 8.0 g)	Hormel Health Labs	Powder	—	—	Maltodextrin	—	30	—
HyFiber™ (Serving 1 Tbsp.)	National Nutrition	Powder	—	—	Gum acacia	—	14	—
UniFiber® (Serving 1 Tbsp.)	Niche Pharma-ceuticals	Powder	—	—	Cellulose, corn syrup solids, xanthan gum	—	4	—
Casec® (Serving 1 Tbsp.)	Mead Johnson	Powder	Calcium caseinate	Lecithin	—	—	17	4
Egg/Pro® (Serving 1 Tbsp.)	Nutra/ Balance Products	Powder	Egg albumin	—	—	—	30	6
ProMod® (Serving 6.6 g)	Ross Labo-ratories	Powder	Whey protein concentrate	Lecithin	—	—	28	5
ProPass® (Serving 8.0 g)	AIP	Powder	Whey protein concentrate	Lecithin	—	—	30	6
ProRight® (Serving 8.6 g)	IFP	Powder	Egg albumin	—	—	—	25	6
Restore-X®	Cambridge Nutra-ceuticals	Powder	L-glutamine, N-acetyl-cysteine, L-arginine	—	—	—	75	10[42]

[41]As L-arginine.
[42]As L-glutamine.

NUTRITIONAL PROFILE							NUTRIENT PER SVG		
CARBO-HYDRATE (g/SERVING)	FAT (g/SERVING)	% CAL FROM PROTEIN	% CAL FROM CARBO-HYDRATE	% CAL FROM FAT	OSMOLALITY (mOsm/kg WATER)	WATER CONTENT (ml) PER SERVING	SODIUM mg (mEq)	POTAS-SIUM mg (mEq)	FIBER (g)
4	—	53[41]	47	—	170	237	70 (3.0)	10 (0.3)	—
4	—	—	100	—	—	—	15 (<1)	15 (<1)	3
7	—	68[42]	32	—	—	120	—	—	—
—	—	100	—	—	—	—	35 (1.5)	7 (<1)	—
8	—	—	100	—	—	—	—	—	3
4	—	—	100	—	—	—	15 (<1)	12 (<1)	3
—	—	—	100	—	—	—	—	—	3
—	0.1	>99	—	<1	—	—	4 (<1)	<1 (<1)	—
0.6	—	>90	<10	—	—	—	96 (4.2)	84 (2.2)	—
0.67	0.6	>71	<10	>19	—	—	25 (1.1)	45 (1.2)	—
—	0.5	>80	<20	—	—	—	150 (6.5)	—	—
—	—	100	—	—	—	—	100 (4.3)	90 (2.3)	—
8	—	57[42]	43	—	—	—	—	—	—

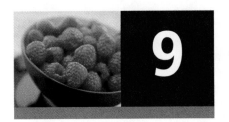

9　The Exchange System

"This material has been modified from Exchange Lists for Meal Planning, which is the basis of a meal planning system designed by a committee of the American Diabetes Association and the American Dietetic Association. While designed primarily for people with diabetes and others who must follow special diets, the Exchange Lists are based on principles of good nutrition that apply to everyone." © 1995 American Diabetes Association, Inc. The American Dietetic Association.

GROUPS/LISTS	CARBOHYDRATE (g)	PROTEIN (g)	FAT (g)	CALORIES
CARBOHYDRATE GROUP				
Starch	15	3	1 or less	80
Fruit	15	—	—	60
Milk				
Skim	12	8	0-3	90
Low-fat	12	8	5	120
Whole	12	8	8	150
Other carbohydrates	15	varies	varies	varies
Vegetables	5	2	—	25
MEAT AND MEAT SUBSTITUTE GROUP				
Very lean	—	7	0-1	35
Lean	—	7	3	55
Medium-fat	—	7	5	75
High-fat	—	7	8	100
FAT GROUP	—	—	5	45

■ STARCH LIST

BREAD

Bagel	½ (1 oz)
Bread, reduced-calorie	2 slices (1½ oz)
Bread, white, whole wheat, pumpernickel, rye	1 slice (1 oz)
Bread sticks, crisp, 4 in long × ½ in	2 (⅔ oz)
English muffin	½
Hot dog or hamburger bun	½ (1 oz)
Pita, 6 in across	½
Roll, plain, small	1 (1 oz)
Raisin bread, unfrosted	1 slice (1 oz)
Tortilla, corn, 6 in across	1
Tortilla, flour, 7-8 in across	1
Waffle, 4½ in square, reduced-fat	1

CEREALS AND GRAINS

Bran cereals	½ c
Bulgur	½ c
Cereals	½ c
Cereals, unsweetened, ready-to-eat	¾ c
Cornmeal (dry)	3 tbsp
Couscous	⅓ c
Flour (dry)	3 tbsp
Granola, low-fat	¼ c
Grape-Nuts	¼ c
Grits	½ c
Kasha	½ c
Millet	¼ c
Muesli	¼ c
Oats	½ c
Pasta	½ c
Puffed cereal	1½ c
Rice milk	½ c
Rice, white or brown	⅓ c
Shredded Wheat	½ c
Sugar-frosted cereal	½ c
Wheat germ	3 tbsp

STARCHY VEGETABLES

Baked beans	⅓ c
Corn	½ c
Corn on cob, medium	1 (5 oz)
Mixed vegetables with corn, peas, or pasta	1 c
Peas, green	½ c

Plantain	½ c
Potato, baked or boiled	1 small (3 oz)
Potato, mashed	½ c
Squash, winter (acorn, butternut)	1 c
Yam, sweet potato, plain	½ c

CRACKERS AND SNACKS

Animal crackers	8
Graham crackers, 2½ in square	3
Matzoh	¾ oz
Melba toast	4 slices
Oyster crackers	24
Popcorn (popped, no fat added or low-fat microwave)	3 c
Pretzels	¾ oz
Rice cakes, 4 in across	2
Saltine-type crackers	6
Snack chips, fat-free (tortilla, potato)	15-20 (¾ oz)
Whole-wheat crackers, no fat added	2-5 (¾ oz)

DRIED BEANS, PEAS, AND LENTILS*

Beans and peas (garbanzo, pinto, kidney, white, split, black-eyed)	½ c
Lima beans	⅔ c
Lentils	½ c
Miso†	3 tbsp

STARCHY FOODS PREPARED WITH FAT‡

Biscuit, 2½ in across	1
Chow mein noodles	½ c
Corn bread, 2 in cube	1 (2 oz)
Crackers, rounded butter type	6
Croutons	1 c
French-fried potatoes	16-25 (3 oz)
Granola	¼ c
Muffin, small	1 (1½ oz)
Pancake, 4 in across	2
Popcorn, microwave	3 c
Sandwich crackers, cheese or peanut butter filling	3
Stuffing, bread (prepared)	⅓ c
Taco shell, 6 in across	2
Waffle, 4½ in square	1
Whole-wheat crackers, fat added	4-6 (1 oz)

*Count as 1 starch exchange, plus 1 very lean meat exchange.
†Contains 400 mg or more of sodium per serving.
‡Count as 1 starch exchange, plus 1 fat exchange.

■ FRUIT LIST

FRUIT			
Apple, unpeeled, small	1 (4 oz)	Papaya	½ fruit (8 oz) or 1 c cubes
Applesauce, unsweetened	½ c	Peach, medium, fresh	1 (6 oz)
Apples, dried	4 rings	Peaches, canned	½ c
Apricots, fresh	4 whole (5½ oz)	Pear, large, fresh	½ (4 oz)
Apricots, dried	8 halves	Pears, canned	½ c
Apricots, canned	½ c	Pineapple, fresh	¾ c
Banana, small	1 (4 oz)	Pineapple, canned	½ c
Blackberries	¾ c	Plums, small	2 (5 oz)
Blueberries	¾ c	Plums, canned	½ c
Cantaloupe, small	⅓ melon (11 oz) or 1 c cubes	Prunes, dried	3
		Raisins	2 tbsp
Cherries, sweet, fresh	12 (3 oz)	Raspberries	1 c
Cherries, sweet, canned	½ c	Strawberries	1¼ c whole berries
Dates	3	Tangerines, small	2 (8 oz)
Figs, fresh	1½ large or 2 medium (3½ oz)	Watermelon	1 slice (13½ oz) or 1¼ c cubes
Figs, dried	1½		
Fruit cocktail	½ c	**FRUIT JUICE**	
Grapefruit, large	½ (11 oz)	Apple juice/cider	½ c
Grapefruit sections, canned	¾ c	Cranberry juice cocktail	⅓ c
		Cranberry juice cocktail, reduced-calorie	1 c
Grapes, small	17 (3 oz)		
Honeydew melon	1 slice (10 oz) or 1 c cubes	Fruit juice blends, 100% juice	⅓ c
Kiwi	1 (3½ oz)	Grape juice	⅓ c
Mandarin oranges, canned	¾ c	Grapefruit juice	½ c
Mango, small	½ fruit (5½ oz) or ½ c	Orange juice	½ c
Nectarine, small	1 (5 oz)	Pineapple juice	½ c
Orange, small	1 (6½ oz)	Prune juice	⅓ c

■ MILK LIST

SKIM AND VERY LOW-FAT MILK*		**LOW-FAT MILK†**	
Skim milk	1 c	2% milk	1 c
½% milk	1 c	Plain low-fat yogurt	¾ c
1% milk	1 c	Sweet acidophilus milk	1 c
Nonfat or low-fat buttermilk	1 c		
Evaporated skim milk	½ c	**WHOLE MILK‡**	
Nonfat dry milk	⅓ c dry	Whole milk	1 c
Plain nonfat yogurt	¾ c	Evaporated whole milk	½ c
Nonfat or low-fat fruit-flavored yogurt sweetened with aspartame or with a nonnutritive sweetener	1 c	Goat's milk	1 c
		Kefir	1 c

*0-3 g of fat per serving.
†5 g of fat per serving.
‡8 g of of fat per serving.

■ OTHER CARBOHYDRATES

FOOD	SERVING SIZE	EXCHANGES PER SERVING
Angel food cake, unfrosted	$\frac{1}{12}$ cake	2 carbohydrates
Brownie, small, unfrosted	2 in square	1 carbohydrate, 1 fat
Cake, unfrosted	2 in square	1 carbohydrate, 1 fat
Cake, frosted	2 in square	2 carbohydrates, 1 fat
Cookie, fat-free	2 small	1 carbohydrate
Cookie or sandwich cookie with creme filling	2 small	1 carbohydrate, 1 fat
Cupcake, frosted	1 small	2 carbohydrates, 1 fat
Cranberry sauce, jellied	$\frac{1}{4}$ c	2 carbohydrates
Doughnut, plain cake	1 medium (1½ oz)	1½ carbohydrates, 2 fats
Doughnut, glazed	3¾ in across (2 oz)	2 carbohydrates, 2 fats
Fruit juice bars, frozen, 100% juice	1 bar (3 oz)	1 carbohydrate
Fruit snacks, chewy (pureed fruit concentrate)	1 roll (¾ oz)	1 carbohydrate
Fruit spreads, 100% fruit	1 tbsp	1 carbohydrate
Gelatin, regular	$\frac{1}{2}$ c	1 carbohydrate
Gingersnaps	3	1 carbohydrate
Granola bar	1 bar	1 carbohydrate, 1 fat
Granola bar, fat-free	1 bar	2 carbohydrates
Hummus	$\frac{1}{3}$ c	1 carbohydrate, 1 fat
Ice cream	$\frac{1}{2}$ c	1 carbohydrate, 2 fats
Ice cream, light	$\frac{1}{2}$ c	1 carbohydrate, 1 fat
Ice cream, fat-free, no sugar added	$\frac{1}{2}$ c	1 carbohydrate
Jam or jelly, regular	1 tbsp	1 carbohydrate
Milk, chocolate, whole	1 c	2 carbohydrates, 1 fat
Pie, fruit, 2 crusts	$\frac{1}{6}$ pie	3 carbohydrates, 2 fats
Pie, pumpkin or custard	$\frac{1}{8}$ pie	1 carbohydrate, 2 fats
Potato chips	12-18 (1 oz)	1 carbohydrate, 2 fats
Pudding, regular (made with low-fat milk)	$\frac{1}{2}$ c	2 carbohydrates
Pudding, sugar-free (made with low-fat milk)	$\frac{1}{2}$ c	1 carbohydrate
Salad dressing, fat-free*	$\frac{1}{4}$ c	1 carbohydrate
Sherbet, sorbet	$\frac{1}{2}$ c	2 carbohydrates
Spaghetti or pasta sauce, canned*	$\frac{1}{2}$ c	1 carbohydrate, 1 fat
Sweet roll or Danish	1 (2½ oz)	2½ carbohydrates, 2 fats
Syrup, light	2 tbsp	1 carbohydrate
Syrup, regular	1 tbsp	1 carbohydrate
Syrup, regular	$\frac{1}{4}$ c	4 carbohydrates
Tortilla chips	6-12 (1 oz)	1 carbohydrate, 2 fats
Yogurt, frozen, low-fat, fat-free	$\frac{1}{3}$ c	1 carbohydrate, 0-1 fat
Yogurt, frozen, fat-free, no sugar added	$\frac{1}{2}$ c	1 carbohydrate
Yogurt, low-fat with fruit	1 c	3 carbohydrates, 0-1 fat
Vanilla wafers	5	1 carbohydrate, 1 fat

*Contains 400 mg or more sodium per exchange.

■ VEGETABLE LIST

Artichoke	Eggplant	Salad greens (endive, escarole,
Artichoke hearts	Green onions or scallions	lettuce, romaine, spinach)
Asparagus	Greens (collard, kale, mustard, turnip)	Sauerkraut*
Beans (green, wax, Italian)	Kohlrabi	Spinach
Bean sprouts	Leeks	Summer squash
Beets	Mixed vegetables (without corn, peas,	Tomato
Broccoli	or pasta)	Tomatoes, canned
Brussels sprouts	Mushrooms	Tomato sauce*
Cabbage	Okra	Tomato/vegetable juice*
Carrots	Onions	Turnips
Cauliflower	Pea pods	Water chestnuts
Celery	Peppers (all varieties)	Watercress
Cucumber	Radishes	Zucchini

*Contains 400 mg or more sodium per exchange.

■ MEAT AND MEAT SUBSTITUTES LIST

VERY LEAN MEAT AND SUBSTITUTES LIST

Poultry	Chicken or turkey (white meat, no skin), Cornish hen (no skin)	1 oz
Fish	Fresh or frozen cod, flounder, haddock, halibut, trout; tuna fresh or canned in water	1 oz
Shellfish	Clams, crab, lobster, scallops, shrimp, imitation shellfish	1 oz
Game	Duck or pheasant (no skin), venison, buffalo, ostrich	1 oz
Cheese	Nonfat or low-fat cottage cheese	¼ c
	Fat-free cheese	1 oz
Other	Processed sandwich meats with 1 g or less fat per ounce, such as deli thin, shaved meats, chipped beef,* turkey ham	1 oz
	Egg whites	2
	Egg substitutes, plain	¼ c
	Hot dogs with 1 g or less fat per ounce*	1 oz
	Kidney (high in cholesterol)	1 oz
	Sausage with 1 g or less fat per ounce	1 oz
	Dried beans, peas, lentils (cooked)†	½ c

LEAN MEAT AND SUBSTITUTES LIST

Beef	USDA Select or Choice grades of lean beef trimmed of fat, such as round, sirloin, and flank steak; tenderloin; roast (rib, chuck, rump); steak (T-bone, porterhouse, cubed), ground round	1 oz
Pork	Lean pork, such as fresh ham; canned, cured, or boiled ham; Canadian bacon*; tenderloin, center loin chop	1 oz
Lamb	Roast, chop, leg	1 oz
Veal	Lean chop, roast	1 oz

*Contains 400 mg or more sodium per exchange.
†Count as one very lean meat and one starch exchange.

Continued

■ MEAT AND MEAT SUBSTITUTES LIST—cont'd

LEAN MEAT AND SUBSTITUTES LIST—cont'd

Poultry	Chicken, turkey (dark meat, no skin), chicken white meat (with skin), domestic duck or goose (well-drained of fat, no skin)	1 oz
Fish	Herring (uncreamed or smoked)	1 oz
	Oysters	6 medium
	Salmon (fresh or canned), catfish	1 oz
	Sardines (canned)	2 medium
	Tuna (canned in oil, drained)	1 oz
Game	Goose (no skin), rabbit	1 oz
Cheese	4.5%-fat cottage cheese	¼ c
	Grated Parmesan	2 tbsp
	Cheeses with 3 g or less fat per ounce	1 oz
Other	Hot dogs with 3 g or less fat per ounce*	1½ oz
	Processed sandwich meat with 3 g or less fat per ounce, such as turkey pastrami or kielbasa	1 oz
	Liver, heart (high in cholesterol)	1 oz

MEDIUM-FAT MEAT AND SUBSTITUTES LIST

Beef	Most beef products fall into this category (ground beef, meatloaf, corned beef, short ribs, Prime grades of meat trimmed of fat, such as prime rib)	1 oz
Pork	Top loin, chop, Boston butt, cutlet	1 oz
Lamb	Rib roast, ground	1 oz
Veal	Cutlet (ground or cubed, unbreaded)	1 oz
Poultry	Chicken dark meat (with skin), ground turkey or ground chicken, fried chicken (with skin)	1 oz
Fish	Any fried fish product	1 oz
Cheese	With 5 g or less fat per ounce	
	Feta	1 oz
	Mozzarella	1 oz
	Ricotta	¼ c (2 oz)
Other	Egg (high in cholesterol, limit to 3 per week)	1
	Sausage with 5 g or less fat per ounce	1 oz
	Soy milk	1 c
	Tempeh	¼ c
	Tofu	4 oz or ½ c

HIGH-FAT MEAT AND SUBSTITUTES LIST

Pork	Spareribs, ground pork, pork sausage	1 oz
Cheese	All regular cheeses, such as American,* cheddar, Monterey Jack, Swiss	1 oz
Other	Processed sandwich meats with 8 g or less fat per ounce, such as bologna, pimento loaf, salami	1 oz
	Sausage, such as bratwurst, Italian, knockwurst, Polish, smoked	1 oz
	Hot dog (turkey or chicken)*	1 (10/lb)
	Bacon	3 slices (20 slices/lb)
	Hot dog (beef, pork, or combination)*‡	1 (10/lb)
	Peanut butter (contains unsaturated fat)‡	2 tbsp

*Contains 400 mg or more sodium per exchange.
†Count as one very lean meat and one starch exchange.
‡Count as one high-fat meat plus one fat exchange.

■ FAT LIST

MONOUNSATURATED FATS LIST

Avocado, medium	$\frac{1}{8}$ (1 oz)
Oil (canola, olive, peanut)	1 tsp
Olives	
Ripe (black)	8 large
Green, stuffed	10 large
Nuts	
Almonds, cashews	6 nuts
Mixed (50% peanuts)	6 nuts
Peanuts	10 nuts
Pecans	4 halves
Peanut butter, smooth or crunchy	2 tsp
Sesame seeds	1 tbsp
Tahini paste	2 tsp

POLYUNSATURATED FATS LIST

Margarine	
Stick, tub, or squeeze	1 tsp
Lower-fat (30% to 50% vegetable oil)	1 tbsp
Mayonnaise	
Regular	1 tsp
Reduced-fat	1 tbsp
Nuts, walnuts, English	4 halves
Oil (corn, safflower, soybean)	1 tsp
Salad dressing	
Regular*	1 tbsp
Reduced-fat	2 tbsp

Miracle Whip Salad Dressing	
Regular	2 tsp
Reduced-fat	1 tbsp
Seeds	
Pumpkin, sunflower	1 tbsp

SATURATED FATS LIST

Bacon, cooked	1 slice (20 slices/lb)
Bacon, grease	1 tsp
Butter	
Stick	1 tsp
Whipped	2 tsp
Reduced-fat	1 tbsp
Chitterlings, boiled	2 tbsp ($\frac{1}{2}$ oz)
Coconut, sweetened, shredded	2 tbsp
Cream, half and half	2 tbsp
Cream cheese	
Regular	1 tbsp ($\frac{1}{2}$ oz)
Reduced-fat	2 tbsp (1 oz)
Fatback or salt pork	
Shortening or lard	1 tsp
Sour cream	
Regular	2 tbsp
Reduced-fat	3 tbsp

*Contains 400 mg or more sodium per exchange.

■ FREE FOODS LIST

FAT-FREE OR REDUCED-FAT FOODS

Cream cheese, fat-free	1 tbsp
Creamers, nondairy, liquid	1 tbsp
Creamers, nondairy, powdered	2 tsp
Mayonnaise, fat-free	1 tbsp
Mayonnaise, reduced-fat	1 tsp
Margarine, fat-free	4 tbsp
Margarine, reduced-fat	1 tsp
Miracle Whip, fat-free	1 tbsp
Miracle Whip, reduced-fat	1 tsp
Nonstick cooking spray	
Salad dressing, fat-free	1 tbsp
Salad dressing, fat-free Italian	2 tbsp
Salsa	¼ c
Sour cream, fat-free, reduced-fat	1 tbsp
Whipped topping, regular or light	2 tbsp

SUGAR-FREE OR LOW-SUGAR FOODS

Candy, hard, sugar-free	1 candy
Gelatin dessert, sugar-free	
Gelatin, unflavored	
Gum, sugar-free	
Jam or jelly, low-sugar or light	2 tsp
Sugar substitutes	
Syrup, sugar-free	2 tbsp

DRINKS

Bouillon, broth, consommé*
Bouillon or broth, low-sodium

Carbonated or mineral water	
Cocoa powder, unsweetened	1 tbsp
Coffee	
Club soda	
Diet soft drinks, sugar-free	
Drink mixes, sugar-free	
Tea	
Tonic water, sugar-free	

CONDIMENTS

Catsup	1 tbsp
Horseradish	
Lemon juice	
Lime juice	
Mustard	
Pickles, dill*	1½ large
Soy sauce, regular or light*	
Taco sauce	1 tbsp
Vinegar	

SEASONINGS

Flavoring extracts
Garlic
Herbs, fresh or dried
Pimento
Spices
Tabasco or hot pepper sauce
Wine, used in cooking
Worcestershire sauce

*Contains 400 mg or more sodium per choice.

■ COMBINATION FOODS LIST

FOOD	SERVING SIZE	EXCHANGES PER SERVING
ENTREES		
Tuna noodle casserole, lasagna, spaghetti with meatballs, chili with beans, macaroni and cheese*	1 c (8 oz)	2 carbohydrates, 2 medium-fat meats
Chow mein (without noodles or rice)	2 c (16 oz)	1 carbohydrate, 2 lean meats
Pizza, cheese, thin crust*	¼ of 10 in (5 oz)	2 carbohydrates, 2 medium-fat meats, 1 fat
Pizza, meat topping, thin crust*	¼ of 10 in (5 oz)	2 carbohydrates, 2 medium-fat meats, 2 fats
Pot pie*	1 (7 oz)	2 carbohydrates, 1 medium-fat meat, 4 fats
FROZEN ENTREES		
Salisbury steak with gravy, mashed potato*	1 (11 oz)	2 carbohydrates, 3 medium-fat meats, 3-4 fats
Turkey with gravy, mashed potato, dressing*	1 (11 oz)	2 carbohydrates, 2 medium-fat meats, 2 fats
Entree with less than 300 calories*	1 (8 oz)	2 carbohydrates, 3 lean meats
SOUPS		
Bean*	1 c	1 carbohydrate, 1 very lean meat
Cream (made with water)*	1 c (8 oz)	1 carbohydrate, 1 fat
Split pea (made with water)*	½ c (4 oz)	1 carbohydrate
Tomato (made with water)*	1 c (8 oz)	1 carbohydrate
Vegetable beef, chicken noodle, or other broth type*	1 c (8 oz)	1 carbohydrate

*Contains 400 mg or more sodium per exchange.

10 Growth Charts for Boys and Girls from Birth to 18 Years of Age

Take all measurements with the child nude or with minimal clothing and without shoes. Measure length with the infant (under 3 years; use "Birth to 36 months" chart) lying on his or her back fully extended. Two people are needed to measure recumbent length properly. Measure stature with the child (at least 2 years of age; use "2 to 18 years" chart) standing. Use a balance beam to measure weight.

Birth to 36 months: Boys
Length-for-age and Weight-for-age percentiles

Name _____

Record # _____

Age (months)

Birth 3 6 9 12 15 18 21 24 27 30 33 36

Length — in / cm

Weight — kg / lb

Percentile curves labeled: 95, 90, 75, 50, 25, 10, 5

Mother's stature	_____		Gestational		
Father's stature	_____		Age: _____ Weeks		Comment

Date	Age	Weight	Length	Head circ.	
	Birth				

Source: Developed by the National Center for Health Statistics in collaboration with
the National Center for Chronic Disease Prevention and Health Promotion (2000).
http://www.cdc.gov/growthcharts
Published May 30, 2000 (modified 4/20/01).

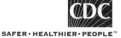

SAFER · HEALTHIER · PEOPLE™

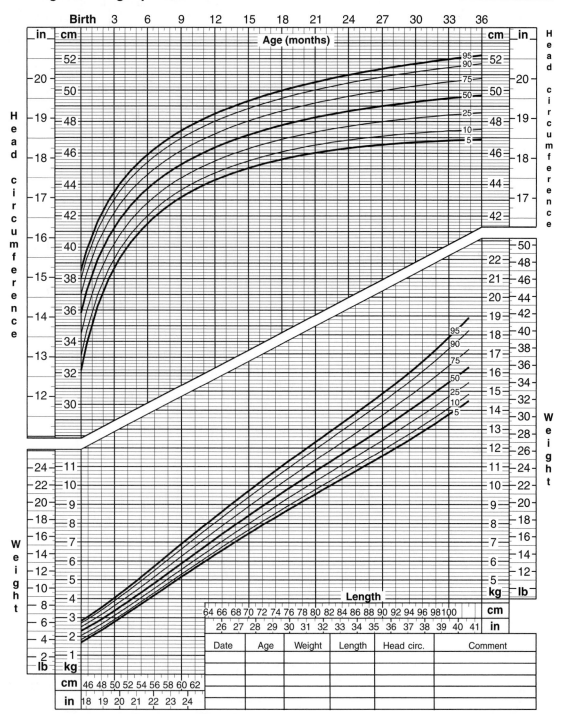

Birth to 36 months: Boys
Head circumference-for-age and
Weight-for-length percentiles

Name _____

Record # _____

Source: Developed by the National Center for Health Statistics in collaboration with
the National Center for Chronic Disease Prevention and Health Promotion (2000).
http://www.cdc.gov/growthcharts
Published May 30, 2000 (modified 4/20/01).

SAFER • HEALTHIER • PEOPLE™

Birth to 36 months: Girls
Length-for-age and Weight-for-age percentiles

Name _____

Record # _____

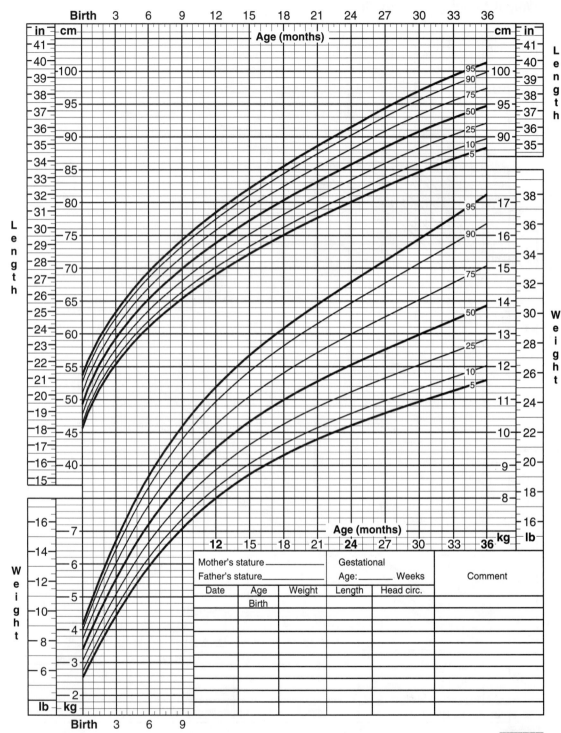

Source: Developed by the National Center for Health Statistics in collaboration with
the National Center for Chronic Disease Prevention and Health Promotion (2000).
http://www.cdc.gov/growthcharts
Published May 30, 2000 (modified 4/20/01).

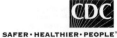

SAFER · HEALTHIER · PEOPLE™

Birth to 36 months: Girls
Head circumference-for-age and
Weight-for-length percentiles

Name _____

Record # _____

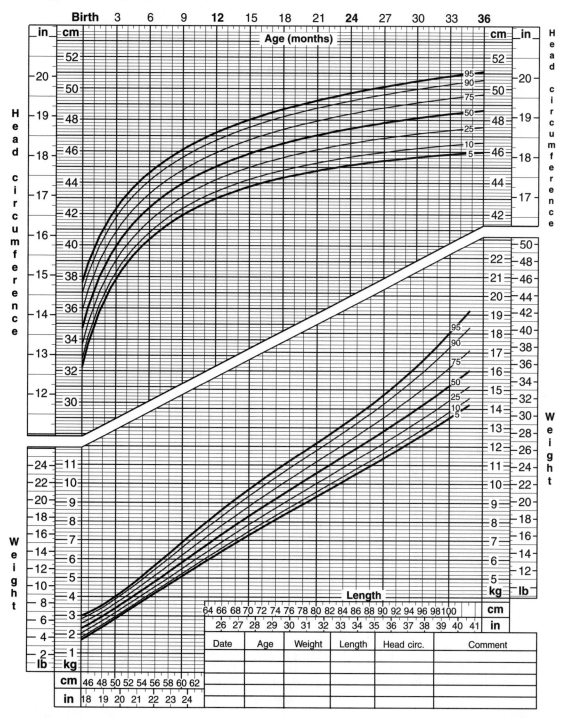

Source: Developed by the National Center for Health Statistics in collaboration with
the National Center for Chronic Disease Prevention and Health Promotion (2000).
http://www.cdc.gov/growthcharts
Published May 30, 2000 (modified 4/20/01).

CDC
SAFER · HEALTHIER · PEOPLE™

CDC Growth Charts: United States

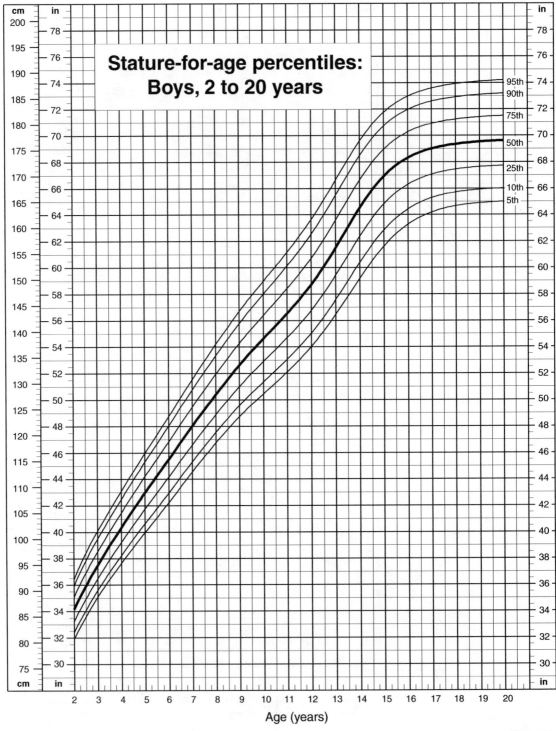

Stature-for-age percentiles:
Boys, 2 to 20 years

Source: Developed by the National Center for Health Statistics in collaboration with
the National Center for Chronic Disease Prevention and Health Promotion (2000).

CDC Growth Charts: United States

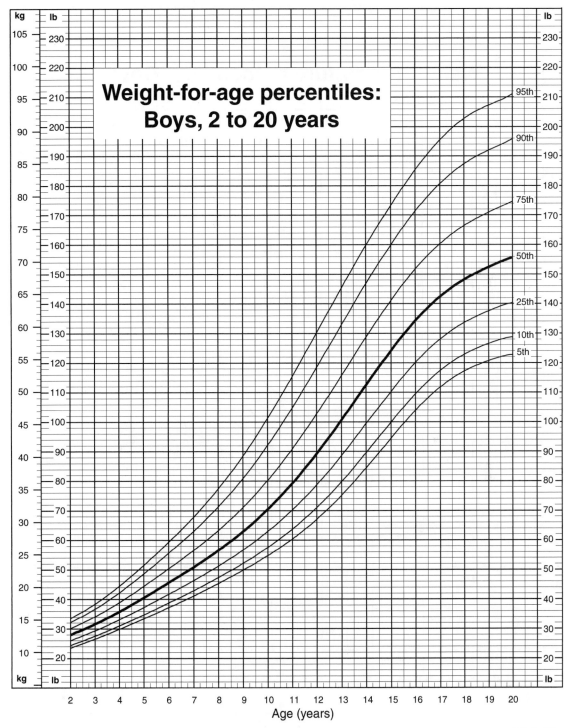

Weight-for-age percentiles: Boys, 2 to 20 years

Age (years)

Source: Developed by the National Center for Health Statistics in collaboration with
the National Center for Chronic Disease Prevention and Health Promotion (2000).

CDC Growth Charts: United States

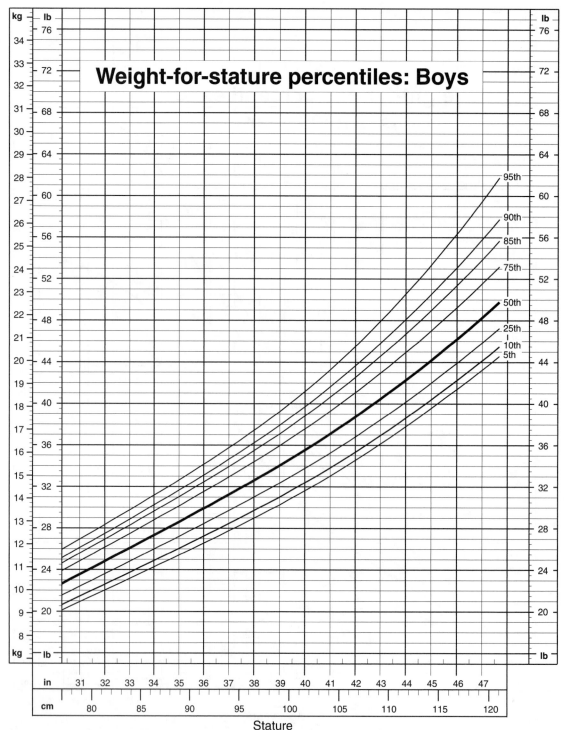

Weight-for-stature percentiles: Boys

Source: Developed by the National Center for Health Statistics in collaboration with
the National Center for Chronic Disease Prevention and Health Promotion (2000).

Revised and corrected November 21, 2000.

CDC Growth Charts: United States

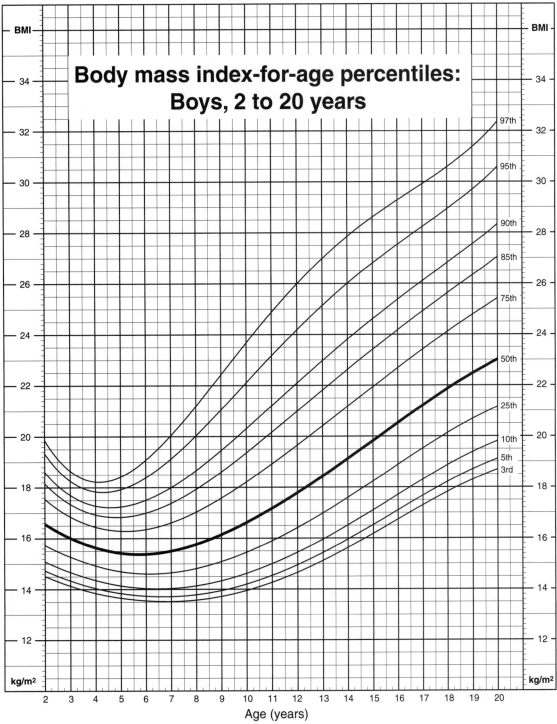

Body mass index-for-age percentiles:
Boys, 2 to 20 years

BMI

97th
95th
90th
85th
75th
50th
25th
10th
5th
3rd

kg/m²

Age (years)

Source: Developed by the National Center for Health Statistics in collaboration with
the National Center for Chronic Disease Prevention and Health Promotion (2000).

CDC
CENTERS FOR DISEASE CONTROL
AND PREVENTION

CDC Growth Charts: United States

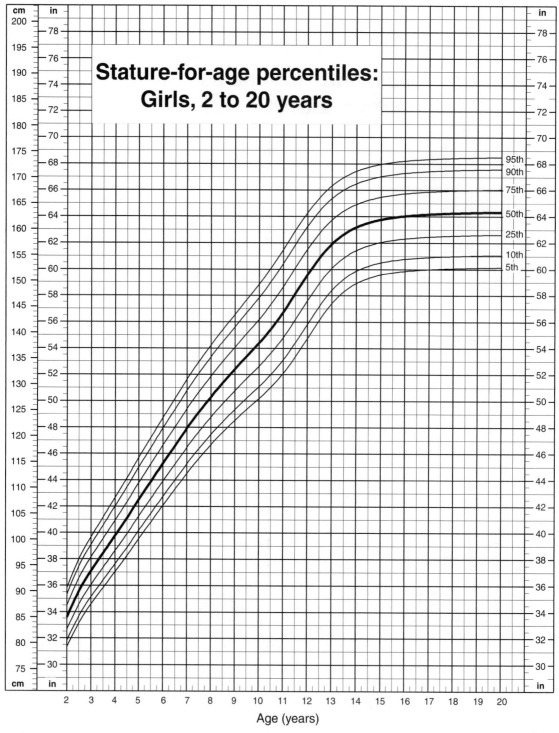

**Stature-for-age percentiles:
Girls, 2 to 20 years**

Age (years)

Source: Developed by the National Center for Health Statistics in collaboration with
the National Center for Chronic Disease Prevention and Health Promotion (2000).

CDC Growth Charts: United States

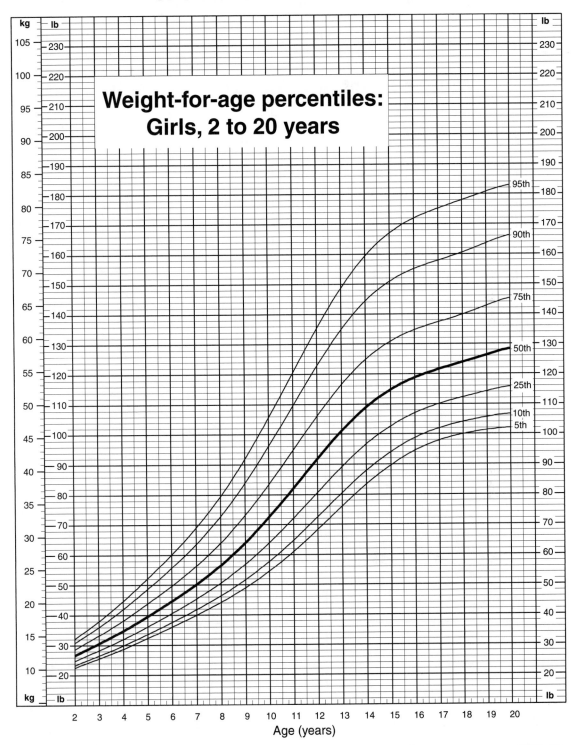

**Weight-for-age percentiles:
Girls, 2 to 20 years**

Age (years)

Source: Developed by the National Center for Health Statistics in collaboration with
the National Center for Chronic Disease Prevention and Health Promotion (2000).

CDC Growth Charts: United States

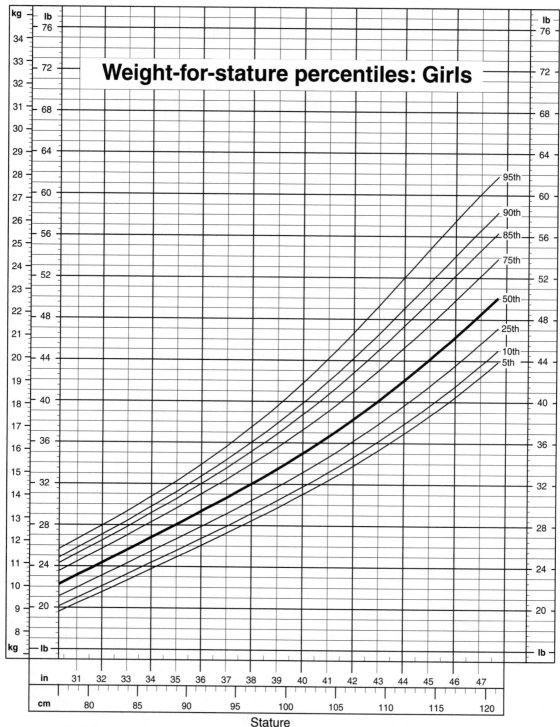

Weight-for-stature percentiles: Girls

Stature

95th
90th
85th
75th
50th
25th
10th
5th

Source: Developed by the National Center for Health Statistics in collaboration with
the National Center for Chronic Disease Prevention and Health Promotion (2000).

Revised and corrected November 21, 2000.

CDC Growth Charts: United States

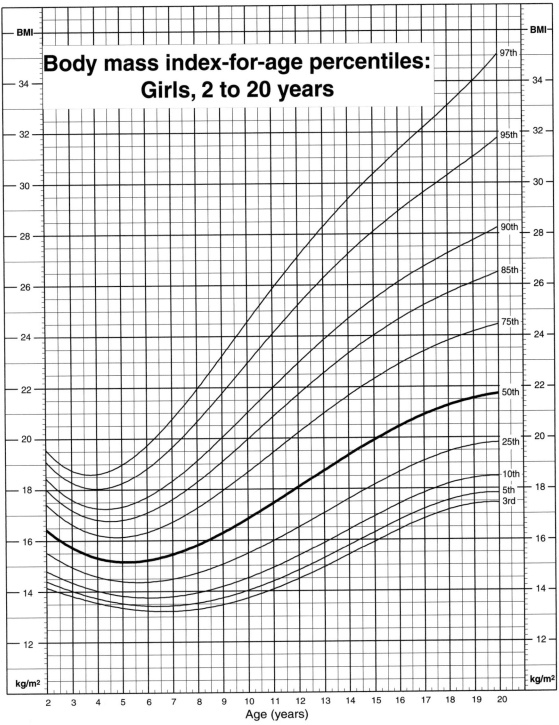

Body mass index-for-age percentiles:
Girls, 2 to 20 years

Source: Developed by the National Center for Health Statistics in collaboration with
the National Center for Chronic Disease Prevention and Health Promotion (2000).

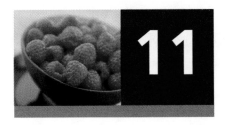

11 Estimating Body Frame Size

1. Frame size may be determined by wrist circumference. Values are affected by variability of soft tissue. Wrist circumference is determined by measuring the smallest part of the wrist distal to the styloid process of the ulna and radius. The "r" value is then determined by this formula:

$$\frac{\text{height in centimeters}}{\text{wrist circumference in centimeters}}$$

Then refer to the following *r* value table to determine frame size:

MEN *r* VALUE	FRAME SIZE	WOMEN *r* VALUE
10.4 or greater	small	11.0 or greater
9.6 to 10.4	medium	10.1 to 11.0
9.6 or less	large	10.1 or less

2. Elbow breadth is measured with the forearm upward at a 90-degree angle. The distance between the outer aspects of the two prominent bones on either side of the elbow is considered to be the elbow breadth. Elbow breadth less than that listed for medium frame indicates a small frame. Elbow breadth greater than that listed for medium frame indicates a large frame.

■ FRAME SIZE FOR WOMEN

HEIGHT IN 1-INCH HEELS	ELBOW BREADTH FOR MEDIUM FRAMES
4'10" to 4'11"	$2\frac{1}{4}$" to $2\frac{1}{2}$"
5'0" to 5'3"	$2\frac{1}{4}$" to $2\frac{1}{2}$"
5'4" to 5'7"	$2\frac{3}{8}$" to $2\frac{5}{8}$"
5'8" to 5'11"	$2\frac{3}{8}$" to $2\frac{5}{8}$"
6'0"	$2\frac{1}{2}$" to $2\frac{3}{4}$"

■ FRAME SIZE FOR MEN

HEIGHT IN 1-IN HEELS	ELBOW BREADTH FOR MEDIUM FRAMES
5'2" to 5'3"	$2\frac{1}{2}$" to $2\frac{7}{8}$"
5'4" to 5'7"	$2\frac{5}{8}$" to $2\frac{7}{8}$"
5'8" to 5'11"	$2\frac{3}{4}$" to 3"
6'0 to 6'3"	$2\frac{3}{4}$" to $3\frac{1}{8}$"
6'4"	$2\frac{7}{8}$" to $3\frac{1}{4}$"

From American Dietetic Association: Manual of clinical dietetics, ed. 6, 2000. Used with permission.

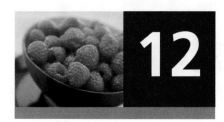

12 Body Mass Index

Measure height to the nearest inch and weight to the nearest pound. Mark them on the body mass index (BMI) nomogram. Then use a straight edge (paper, ruler) to connect the two points and circle the spot where this straight line crosses the center line to obtain the BMI value. *Note:* When computing BMI with the equation weight ÷ height^2, kilograms and meters should be used.

KNOW YOUR BODY MASS INDEX

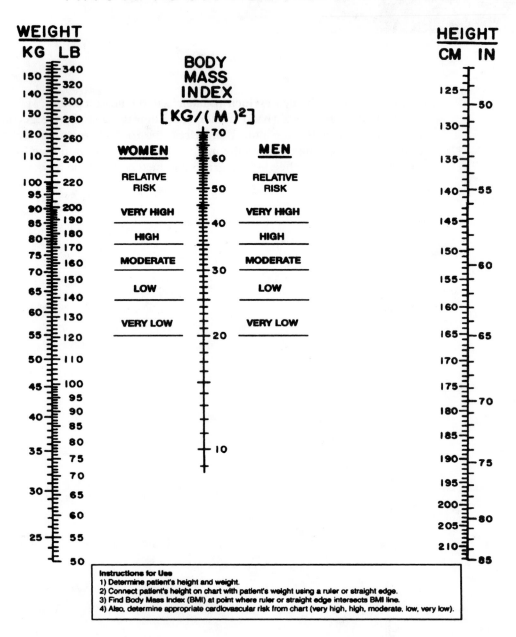

WEIGHT
KG LB

BODY
MASS
INDEX
[KG/(M)²]

HEIGHT
CM IN

WOMEN

RELATIVE RISK

VERY HIGH

HIGH

MODERATE

LOW

VERY LOW

MEN

RELATIVE RISK

VERY HIGH

HIGH

MODERATE

LOW

VERY LOW

Instructions for Use
1) Determine patient's height and weight.
2) Connect patient's height on chart with patient's weight using a ruler or straight edge.
3) Find Body Mass Index (BMI) at point where ruler or straight edge intersects BMI line.
4) Also, determine appropriate cardiovascular risk from chart (very high, high, moderate, low, very low).

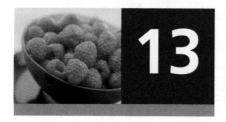

13 Nomogram to Estimate Stature from Knee Height in Persons 60 to 90 Years of Age

An elderly person's stature can be estimated from the following nomogram. To use this nomogram, locate the person's age on the left column and knee height on the middle column, and connect these two points. Mark where the connecting line crosses the stature column for the appropriate sex to find the estimated stature.

A knee-height caliper can be obtained from Ross Laboratory, 1-800-848-2607. In OH, PA, and WV, call 1-800-367-7677 or contact your local Ross representative.

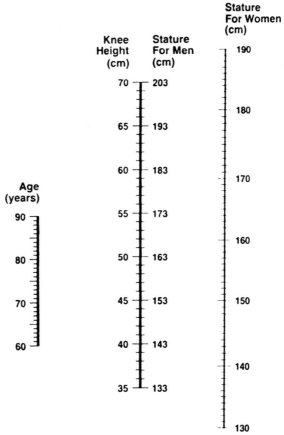

From Consultant Dietitians in Health Care Facilities, A Practice Group of the American Dietetic Association, Pocket Resource for Nutrition Assessment, 1990.

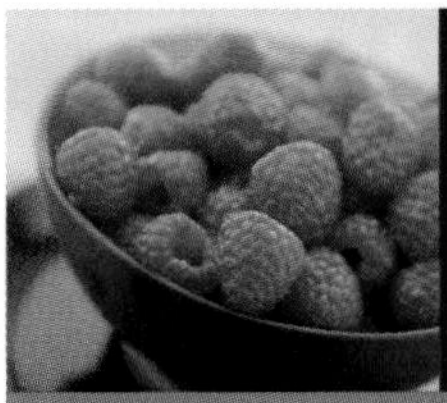

14 Child Care Meal Pattern

BREAKFAST FOR CHILDREN
SELECT ALL THREE COMPONENTS FOR A REIMBURSABLE MEAL

FOOD COMPONENTS	AGES 1-2	AGES 3-5	AGES 6-12*
1 MILK fluid milk	½ c	¾ c	1 c
1 FRUIT/VEGETABLE juice,[†] fruit and/or vegetable	¼ c	½ c	½ c
1 GRAINS/BREAD[‡] bread or	½ slice	½ slice	1 slice
cornbread or biscuit or roll or muffin or	½ serving	½ serving	½ serving
cold dry cereal or	¼ c	⅓ c	¾ c
hot cooked cereal or	¼ c	¼ c	½ c
pasta or noodles or grains	¼ c	¼ c	½ c

*Children age 12 and older may be served larger portions based on their greater food needs. They may not be served less than the minimum quantities listed in this column.
[†]Fruit or vegetable juice must be full strength.
[‡]Breads and grains must be made from whole-grain, enriched meal, or flour. Cereal must be whole-grain, enriched, or fortified.

▎ LUNCH OR SUPPER FOR CHILDREN
▎ SELECT ALL FOUR COMPONENTS FOR A REIMBURSABLE MEAL

FOOD COMPONENTS	AGES 1-2	AGES 3-5	AGES 6-12*
1 MILK			
fluid milk	½ c	¾ c	1 c
2 FRUITS/VEGETABLES			
juice,[†] fruit and/or vegetable	¼ c	½ c	¾ c
1 GRAINS/BREAD[‡]			
bread or	½ slice	½ slice	1 slice
cornbread or biscuit or roll or muffin or	½ serving	½ serving	1 serving
cold dry cereal or	¼ c	⅓ c	¾ c
hot cooked cereal or	¼ c	¼ c	½ c
pasta or noodles or grains	¼ c	¼ c	½ c
1 MEAT/MEAT ALTERNATE			
meat or poultry or fish[§] or	1 oz	1½ oz	2 oz
alternate protein product or	1 oz	1½ oz	2 oz
cheese or	1 oz	1½ oz	2 oz
egg or	½	¾	1
cooked dry beans or peas or	¼ c	⅜ c	½ c
peanut or other nut or seed butters or	2 tbsp	3 tbsp	4 tbsp
nuts and/or seeds[‖] or	½ oz	¾ oz	1 oz
yogurt[¶]	4 oz	6 oz	8 oz

From The Child and Adult Care Food Program (CACFP), USDA, 2001.
*Children age 12 and older may be served larger portions based on their greater food needs. They may not be served less than the minimum quantities listed in this column.
[†]Fruit or vegetable juice must be full strength.
[‡]Breads and grains must be made from whole-grain, enriched meal, or flour. Cereal must be whole-grain, enriched, or fortified.
[§]A serving consists of the edible portion of cooked lean meat or poultry or fish.
[‖]Nuts and seeds may meet only one half of the total meat/meat alternate serving and must be combined with another meat/meat alternate to fulfill the lunch or supper requirement.
[¶]Yogurt may be plain or flavored, unsweetened or sweetened.

Glossary

Absorption The passage of liquids and end products of digestion into the villi of the intestine.

Acanthosis nigricans A skin condition related to obesity and the insulin resistance syndrome that gives the skin a velvety texture and brown color; usually found on the back of the neck or in skinfolds such as the armpits.

Achalasia A condition in which the esophagus and gastrointestinal tract fail to relax, causing a feeling of fullness, vomiting, and possible aspiration of esophageal contents into the respiratory passages.

Acid-base balance A state of equilibrium between acidity and alkalinity of body fluids; problems with acidosis or alkalosis are determined by pH and blood gas analysis.

Acquired immunodeficiency syndrome (AIDS) The condition that develops after exposure to the human immunodeficiency virus (HIV); contracted through exposure to body fluids containing the virus; causes destruction of the immune system.

Active listening A form of communication that uses open-ended questions to help elicit feelings and emotions or more detailed information than can be elicited with yes and no questions.

Activities of daily living (ADL) Activities that the average person performs routinely during a day.

Addison's disease A syndrome related to inadequate hormone secretion of the adrenal glands; may be associated with fluid and electrolyte imbalance and profound hypoglycemia unless treated with steroids.

Adenosine triphosphate (ATP) The form of energy used by the body cells.

Adequate intake (AI) A new term under the umbrella term of Dietary Reference Intake; the level of nutrients presumed to be adequate, but insufficient, research to set an RDA.

Adipose tissue A term for body fat.

Adrenaline A hormone that works to raise blood sugar levels; also causes increased heart rate.

Adult Treatment Panel (ATP III) The Third Report of the Expert Panel on Detection, Evaluation, and Treatment of High Blood Cholesterol in Adults; the panel report sponsored by the National Cholesterol Education Program (NCEP), and the National Heart, Lung, and Blood Institute (NHLBI) of the National Institutes of Health (NIH).

Aerobic exercise Any form of exercise that requires an increased intake of oxygen such as brisk walking or running.

Affective A term that pertains to emotions.

Aging The changes that occur in cellular metabolism related to diminished ability to manufacture new cell growth as related to increasing age.

AIDS enteropathy A condition related to AIDS that causes malabsorption and resultant diarrhea.

AIDS-related complex (ARC) An interim stage between infection with the HIV virus and full-blown AIDS.

Albumin A plasma protein responsible for regulating the osmotic force of blood.

Albuminuria A condition of albumin in the urine.

Alimentary enzymes Enzymes in the digestive tract, such as sucrase, lactase, maltase, lipase, and others.

Alkali A chemical substance with a pH greater than 7.

Allergen A substance that induces hypersensitivity.

Alzheimer's disease An irreversible condition found in aging persons characterized by intellectual decline, changes in personality, and inability to carry out normal daily activities.

Ambulatory care Health care provided generally in the home or outside of an institution such as a hospital.

Amenorrhea The lack of menses.

American Heart Association (AHA) An organization with headquarters in Dallas with 15 affiliate offices in the United States that promotes health initiatives to lower heart disease.

Amino acids The substances that make protein. Essential amino acids must be supplied by the diet; nonessential amino acids can be synthesized by the body.

Amylase An enzyme that hastens the hydrolysis of starch into sugar.

Anabolism The constructive phase of metabolism, resulting in growth and repair; adj. anabolic.

Anaerobic exercise Any exercise that does not increase the intake of oxygen, such as weight lifting.

Anaphylactic shock A condition in which the airways close because of severe inflammation related to an allergic reaction.

Androgens Male hormones such as testosterone.

Anemia A symptom of reduced oxygen delivery to body cells.

Anorexia A condition of loss of appetite.

Anorexia nervosa A serious chronic condition with severe restriction of food intake unrelated to appetite and refusal to accept a normal weight as desirable; often associated with adolescent girls, but also occurs with boys and athletes requiring a low body weight.

Anthropometry The science that deals with body measurements, such as size, weight, and proportion.

Antibodies Substances synthesized in the body that destroy bacteria or antigens.

Antidiuretic hormone A hormone that suppresses the excretion of urine; stored and released by the pituitary gland.

Antigens Substances that react with antibodies or help in the formation of antibodies.

Antioxidants Vitamins and minerals that reduce oxidative injury to body cells; nutrients that decrease the amount of free radicals.

Anuria A condition of lack of urinary excretion.

Arachidonic acid An essential fatty acid which can be produced if there is adequate linoleic acid in the diet.

Arteriosclerosis The hardening and thickening of the walls of the arteries.

Arthralgia A condition of joint pain.

Arthritis A condition related to inflammation of body joints.

Ascites An accumulation of excess fluids in the abdomen.

Aspiration Inhalation of food or liquid into the lungs; can cause pneumonia.

Atherosclerosis A build-up of plaque inside the arteries and blood vessels that leads to heart disease.

Attention deficit hyperactivity disorder (ADHD) The official term of the American Psychiatric Association that relates to a condition generally found in children who have an inability to pay attention and to sustain effort.

Autism A syndrome beginning in infancy characterized by extreme withdrawal from the external environment and an obsessive desire to avoid change; the cause is unknown, and affected children rarely recover.

Autoimmune disease A disease in which the immune system mistakenly attacks healthy tissue.

Autonomic neuropathy Nerve disease of the autonomic or involuntary system, such as the digestive or respiratory system.

Azotemia Abnormally increased levels of nitrogen in the blood.

Baby-bottle tooth decay Also known as nursing-bottle mouth, in which the two upper front teeth are decayed because of frequent exposure to sugars found in milk or other beverages.

Basal metabolism The lowest level of metabolism to support life; does not take into account physical activity.

Beriberi A deficiency disease caused by lack of thiamin.

Beta carotene The precursor to vitamin A which is found in plant products that are deep orange or dark green and leafy. An antioxidant that is believed to lower the risk of cancer and heart disease.

Beta cells The insulin-producing cells in the islets of Langerhans of the pancreas.

Bile A yellow fluid produced by the liver and stored in the gallbladder until needed in the small intestine for digestion of dietary fat.

Biological value of protein Refers to the amount of essential amino acids in relation to the total quantity of protein. Animal protein sources (meat, eggs, milk) have a high biological value of protein.

Biopsychosocial The interplay between forces of biology, psychology, and social factors on one's health and health decisions.

Bipolar disorder Formerly called manic depression, a condition marked by alternating periods of depression and mania (elation and agitation).

Blood urea nitrogen (BUN) The urea nitrogen concentration found in blood; an indicator of renal functioning.

Body Mass Index (BMI) Originally called the Quetelet Index, weight in kilograms divided by the square of the height in meters; felt to give a better indicator for appropriate height and weight measures than Metropolitan Life weight charts.

Bone growth Growth of bones both longitudinally and structurally.

Botulism An often fatal form of food poisoning caused by a poisonous endotoxin.

Bulimarexia A condition vacillating between anorexic and bulimic eating patterns.

Bulimia A condition of overeating with purging or laxative abuse being common.

Cancer A condition of rapid abnormal cell growth leading to tumors and death of healthy cells.

Cancer cachexia A condition of malnutrition associated with cancer.

Capillaries The small blood vessels connecting arteries and veins.

Carbohydrate counting A meal planning strategy used in diabetes management.

Carbohydrate loading A strategy used by athletes to increase the amount of stored glycogen available to the muscles.

Cardiomyopathy A general term referring to heart disease.

Cardiovascular disease Disease of the cardiovascular system.

Cariogenic A substance or factor contributing to dental caries.

Carnitine A substance primarily synthesized in the kidneys with a role in fatty acid oxidation in tissue cells, especially those of cardiac and skeletal muscles.

Carotene Also referred to as beta carotene; the precursor to vitamin A found in dark green leafy and deep orange-colored vegetables and fruits.

Catabolism A destructive process that releases energy; adj. catabolic.

Celiac sprue An inflammatory condition of the villi of the jejunum related to gluten or gliadin found in wheat, American oats, rye, barley, and triticale (a new hybrid grain); found more commonly among persons with British heritage.

Cellulose Structural fiber in fruits, vegetables, and grains.

Central obesity A condition of carrying excess weight in the abdominal area; defined as greater than 35 inches for women or 40 inches for men or a waist-to-hip measure greater than 0.8 for women and 1.0 for men.

Cerebral palsy A motor disorder caused by brain damage beginning in infancy that can involve muscle spasms, uncontrollable movements, or poor balance with a staggering gait.

Cerebrovascular accident (CVA) An embolus or blood clot; often called a "stroke."

Certified diabetes educator (CDE) A health professional who has an advanced degree and 2000 hours of direct patient care related to diabetes and who has passed an exam every five years.

Change agent An individual who facilitates the development of positive health behaviors.

Cheilosis A condition characterized by dry, scaly lips and cracks at the corners of the mouth; seen in riboflavin deficiency.

Chemotherapy A treatment for cancer; the provision of toxic chemicals to the system to destroy cancer cells.

Cholecystikinin A hormone believed to be involved with the recognition of satiety.

Cholecystitis A condition of inflammation of the gallbladder.

Cholelithiasis The presence of gallstones.

Cholesterol A fat-related compound that is produced in the livers of animals; found in animal fats, but does not provide kilocalories.

Chronic disease A disease that can be managed, but cannot be cured.

Chronic renal failure (CRF) A condition of the kidneys in which they have lost most of their function.

Chyme The semiliquid form of digested food that passes from the stomach into the duodenum after undergoing the action of gastric juice.

Cirrhosis A disease of the liver often associated with alcoholism.

Cleft palate A condition in which there is an opening or hole in the roof of the mouth, sometimes extending to the lip, which needs to be surgically repaired.

Clostridium botulinum A form of food poisoning that is usually fatal and that is related to eating canned foods that were inadequately processed to completely destroy the botulism spore.

Clostridium perfringens A type of bacteria that causes food poisoning.

Cognitive Having to do with cognition or ability for the brain to process information.

Colostrum The nutritious substance that precedes breast milk production in the first few days after delivery.

Commodity Supplemental Food Program (CSFP) A government program designed to provide foods to at-risk populations and help farmers.

Communicable disease Any disease that is contagious.

Complete protein Protein containing all of the essential amino acids.

Constipation A condition in which fecal material is too hard to pass easily or in which bowel movements are so infrequent that abdominal discomfort is present.

Continuous ambulatory peritoneal dialysis (CAPD) An alternative form of dialysis used in renal failure to filter toxins from the blood; a dialysis method that a renal patient can do at home in which a dialysate fluid is injected into the abdominal cavity and regularly changed to remove blood toxins

Coronary heart disease (CHD) A term often used interchangeably with cardiovascular disease; relates directly to the heart.

Coronary thrombosis A condition of severe arteriosclerosis that cuts off blood supply to a part or parts of the heart; often fatal.

Cortisol A hormone, produced in the adrenal glands, that works in the opposite manner to insulin to raise blood sugar levels.

Counterregulatory hormones Hormones that work in the opposite manner to insulin; hormones that raise blood sugar levels principally through the release of stored glycogen in the liver or through the inhibition of insulin action.

C-reactive protein (CRP) A protein that can be measured through labs that indicate inflammation.

Creatine A substance naturally found in muscle, and sometimes used by athletes to maintain higher levels of ATP in body cells.

Creatinine A nitrogen compound used in a laboratory test to indicate renal function.

Cretinism A condition of childhood caused by lack of thyroid gland secretion that leads to a dwarf size and is accompanied by mental retardation and sterility if not treated with thyroid extract for life.

Crohn's disease A chronic condition of intermittent inflammation of the terminal portion of the ileum or other portion of the intestinal tract; usually treated with steroids, but attention to good nutrition is important. Also referred to as regional enteritis.

Cystic fibrosis A hereditary disease with dysfunction of the exocrine glands resulting in thick mucus and abnormal secretion of sweat and saliva.

Daily Reference Values (DRV) A system developed for use on food labels to indicate recommended nutrient intakes for 2000 and 2500 kilocalories; also referred to as Daily Values (DV).

DASH diet (Diet Approaches to Stop Hypertension) A recommended diet strategy to prevent and manage hypertension.

Dawn phenomenon Early morning phenomenon involving counterregulatory hormones that results in increased blood glucose levels.

Decalcification The condition in which bone and dental tissue lose calcium.

Decubitus ulcer A bed or pressure sore.

Dementia A state of impaired mental functioning.

Dental caries A term for tooth decay.

Dental enamel The outside hard protective covering of teeth.

Dental erosion The condition of loss of dental enamel.

Dental plaque A calcified coating on teeth that provides a perfect growing medium for bacteria; plaque needs to be removed regularly to prevent dental decay.

Denver Developmental Screening Test A screening test for young children to assess behavioral and cognitive milestones expected based on age.

Deoxyribonucleic acid (DNA) Part of the genetic material of body cells.

Depapillation The smooth appearance of the papilla (elevations on the surface of the tongue containing taste buds) resulting from vitamin B deficiency.

Desirable weight A body mass index (BMI) between 20 and 25; or a realistic weight that allows for good health for an individual.

DETERMINE checklist A tool to identify elderly persons who are at nutritional risk.

Development A term used to describe integration of muscles and body functions.

Developmental disability A condition that is related to impaired development which is present before age 21 years.

Diabetes mellitus Literal meaning, "sweet urine;" a condition related to high blood glucose levels.

Diabetic coma A condition of hyperglycemia with ketonuria; usually found in Type 1 diabetes. Also referred to as diabetic ketoacidosis.

Diabetic retinopathy An eye disease found in persons with long-standing diabetes; prevented through good diabetes management.

Diarrhea Rapid transit of food matter through the gastrointestinal tract; related to watery stools caused by inadequate absorption of water in the large intestine.

Dietary fiber The form of carbohydrate that is virtually indigestible in the human gastrointestinal tract.

Dietary reference intakes (DRIs) An umbrella term that includes a variety of levels of recommended vitamin and mineral intakes for the goal of optimal intake.

Digestion The breakdown of food matter by mechanical and chemical means to allow for absorption of food nutrients.

Diglyceride A form of fat.

Disaccharides The term used to describe double sugars such as sucrose and lactose.

Diuresis The condition of increased excretion of the urine.

Diuretic A substance that promotes urine secretion.

Diverticulitis A condition of inflammation of the diverticula or outpouchings in the intestinal tract.

Diverticulosis A permanent condition of the intestinal tract characterized by small pockets protruding from the intestinal wall; often associated with advancing age.

Down syndrome A congenital condition characterized by physical malformations and some degree of mental retardation; caused by an extra chromosome. Also referred to as trisomy 21 syndrome because of the defect at chromosome 21; formerly referred to as mongolism because persons with this condition have facial characteristics resembling persons of the Mongolian race.

Dumping syndrome A condition characterized by nausea, weakness, sweating, palpitation, fainting, often a warm feeling, and sometimes diarrhea. These symptoms occur after eating in people who have had a partial gastrectomy.

Duodenum The first portion of the small intestine, about 10 in long, connecting the pylorus to the jejunum.

Dysgeusia An impaired sense of taste.

Dyslipidemia A condition of elevated triglycerides with low HDL-cholesterol levels.

Dyspepsia Impaired digestion related to epigastric discomfort after meals.

Dysphagia A condition of difficulty in swallowing.

Edema A condition of excess fluid build-up in the body.

Edentulous Having no teeth.

Electrolyte A mineral that disassociates into ions when fused or in solution so that electricity can be conducted.

Elemental feeding A complete liquid nutrition supplement that does not require digestion.

Elimination diet A diet that restricts foods to a few that are least likely to cause allergic reactions; used as a test for allergens through the addition of foods one at a time to identify tolerance or intolerance.

Embryo The fertilized ovum during the first three months after conception.

Empty kilocalories Foods that provide sugar or fat, but few vitamins, minerals, or protein.

Encopresis Incontinence of fecal material; often caused by a "plug" of solid fecal material that allows liquid fecal material to pass around the solid material.

Endocrine system The glands that secrete hormones directly into the circulation; a major control system of body functioning and metabolism.

Endocrinology The study of hormones.

Endometrial hyperplasia An increase in the thickness of the lining of the uterus.

End stage renal disease (ESRD) A period in which BUN and creatinine levels are very high, with impairment to all body systems. Also known as uremia.

Energy balance The level of energy taken in (kilocalories) that equals that amount of energy expended (basal metabolism plus activity needs).

Enrichment The replacement of nutrients lost in processing.

Enteral nutrition A form of nutrition support usually with liquid nutrition supplements by way of the small intestine.

Enzyme A protein that can hasten or produce a change in a substance.

Epilepsy A group of symptoms related to abnormal electrical activity of the brain resulting in periodic seizure activity.

Epithelial Pertaining to the cellular covering of the internal and external surfaces of the body.

Ergogenic The term used to describe supplements of vitamins, minerals, amino acids, or other substances touted to build muscle or improve athletic performance.

Erythropoietin A hormone produced in the kidneys that stimulates red blood cell production.

Escherichia coli A type of bacteria commonly associated with food poisoning; referred to as *E. coli*.

Esophageal reflux A chronic disease with reflux of the stomach contents; may be associated with hiatal hernia.

Esophageal sphincter The muscular connection between the esophagus and the stomach.

Esophageal varices Enlargement of veins in the esophagus.

Esophagitis Inflammation of the esophagus.

Essential amino acids The substances that are turned into protein that must be supplied in the diet; found in animal protein sources, but can be obtained from plant sources with careful food selection.

Essential fatty acids Forms of fat needed for health that must be supplied by the diet; found in vegetable oils.

Estimated average requirements (EARs) A relatively new term used to describe the average amount of nutrients needed to prevent nutrient deficiency.

Estrogen A female sex hormone produced primarily in ovaries, but also in the adrenal glands and testes of males; allows for implantation of a fertilized egg.

Expanded Food and Nutrition Education Program (EFNEP) A program within Cooperative Extension that assists low-income families in food resource management.

Fad diet A diet that is not meant to be followed long-term, and which is usually imbalanced in nutrient content.

Failure to thrive A medical diagnosis that includes lack of physical growth (below the third percentile for weight and height for age); may be related to maternal deprivation.

Fat-soluble vitamins The vitamins A, D, E, and K; vitamins that require dietary fat for maximum absorption in the small intestines.

Fatty acids An organic compound of carbon, hydrogen, and oxygen that combines with glycerol to form fat.

Female athlete triad A triad of osteoporosis, amenorrhea, and eating disorders that occurs in some female athletes.

Fetal alcohol syndrome A group of symptoms characterized by mental and physical abnormalities of the infant linked to maternal alcohol intake during pregnancy.

Fetus The term used to describe the unborn baby during the second and third trimesters of pregnancy.

Fifteen:fifteen rule (15:15 rule) Treatment and reevaluation of hypoglycemia; treatment with 15 g of carbohydrates for someone who is still conscious, with a recheck of blood sugar levels in 15 minutes (procedure continues if blood sugar remains low).

Fifteen hundred rule (1500 rule) The mathematical formula used to estimate point drop in blood glucose per one unit of regular insulin; the number 1500 divided by the total amount of insulin units regularly injected.

Fluoride A mineral that promotes uptake of calcium by teeth and bones; currently used as a preventive measure against dental caries.

Food additives Additives to food that are used for stabilization or to increase shelf life and safety of food.

Food allergy An abnormal hypersensivity reaction to foods containing protein material called allergens.

Food antigens The protein in various foods that are allergenic.

Food distribution system The system in which food is grown, processed, and delivered to individuals.

Food exchange lists A food guide that groups food based on equivalent amounts of carbohydrates, proteins, and fats.

Food fads Diets or supplements designed to have a "quick-fix" that is not based on scientific theory or appropriate meal planning.

Food insufficiency The term used to describe having inadequate food availability, usually as a result of inadequate purchasing power.

Food intolerance A nonimmune intolerance to certain foods related to poor digestion or other factors.

Food irradiation A process of radiation used to destroy harmful organisms in food to reduce the likelihood of food poisoning.

Food jags A term applied to childhood eating habits in which a few foods are eaten for days or weeks at a time.

Food quack An untrained person who espouses potentially harmful nutritional practices.

Food resource management The management of food choices and preparation to allow maximum nutrient intake for the least amount of food dollars.

Fore milk Breast milk that is released from the front of the breasts; has a lower fat content than hind milk.

Fortification The addition of nutrients to greater than the natural level found in a food; milk and margarine are often fortified.

Free radicals The remnants left after oxygen is used in metabolism, which can cause cellular damage.

GAD antibodies Antibodies associated with the autoimmune destruction of islet cells in the pancreas, which is found with Type 1 diabetes.

Gastritis Inflammation of the stomach.

Gastroparesis A condition in which autonomic neuropathy of the stomach results in partial paralysis such that digestion and the propulsion of food through the digestive tract are impaired.

Gavage feeding A form of feeding by tube.

Generally recognized as safe (GRAS) list The list of substances added to foods such as preservatives and flavoring that are felt to be generally safe.

Genetically modified foods The term used to describe foods that have their genes altered to allow for altered characteristics such as pesticide resistance.

Geriatrics The branch of medicine concerned with the treatment and prevention of diseases affecting elderly individuals.

Gerontology The study of the problems of aging.

Gestational A term that refers to pregnancy.

Gestational diabetes A form of diabetes occurring during pregnancy, usually beginning between the 24th and 28th weeks of gestation.

Gingival The part of the oral lining that covers the tooth bearing border of the jaw; the gums.

Gingivitis An inflammation of the gums.

Gliadin A component of gluten that needs to be avoided in celiac disease.

Glomerular filtration rate (GFR) Amount of glomerular filtrate in milliliters cleared through the kidneys in 1 minute. Rates less than 30 ml/min indicate that kidney disease may be present; lower rates call for aggressive management.

Glucagon A counterregulatory hormone that is given by injection during severe bouts of hypoglycemia in an unconscious diabetic person.

Gluconeogenesis The formation of glucose from protein.

Glucose The term for blood sugar.

Gluten The protein portion of wheat, oats, rye, barley, and triticale (a hybrid grain); complete avoidance is often necessary in the control of celiac disease.

Glycated The process in which glucose attaches to protein throughout body cells.

Glycemia A term for blood glucose level.

Glycemic index A means of rating food based on predictive impact on blood sugar levels; fats have the lowest glycemic index and sugars have the highest.

Glycerol A component of fats.

Glycogen The storage form of carbohydrate found in the liver and muscle tissues; released in the form of sugar as needed for energy or during times of physiological stress.

Glycogen loading A process by which the glycogen stores in the liver are increased beyond normal levels to allow for the demands for endurance in athletic competition.

Glycogenolysis The breakdown of stored carbohydrate in the liver from glycogen to glucose.

Glycosuria Glucose in the urine; an outdated means of diabetes management; sometimes used for a simple means of diabetes screening.

Goiter A swelling of the thyroid gland on the neck caused by iodine deficiency.

Gout A hereditary form of arthritis in which uric acid is built up in the blood and may be deposited in joints and other tissues; usually treated with medication.

GRAS list Generally recognized as safe; standards for acceptable levels of food additives.

Grazing A term applied to a manner of continuous eating throughout the day rather than eating three meals.

Growth Related to the increased size of body components such as organs and bones that occurs with adequate intake of food nutrients and kilocalories.

Growth hormone A substance that stimulates growth; works in the opposite manner to insulin to raise blood sugar levels.

Health A relative state that includes physical, mental, social, and spiritual functioning such that an individual can meet one's full potential.

Health belief model A theory that stresses that an individual's perceived level of health risk and "cost" of behavior change contributes to health decisions.

Heat exhaustion A disorder resulting from excessive loss of body fluids and electrolytes.

Hematocrit The volume percentage of red blood cells in whole blood.

Hematuria The term for blood in the urine.

Heme iron The form of iron found in meat; iron that is readily absorbed.

Hemodialysis A procedure used to remove toxic wastes from the blood of a patient with acute or chronic renal failure.

Hemoglobin The oxygen-carrying pigment of the blood; the principal protein in the red blood cell.

Hemoglobin A_{1c} (HbA_{1c}) A test used to determine long-term diabetes management; indicates an average blood sugar reading over a 3-month time.

Hemorrhage The loss of blood from a ruptured vessel.

Hepatic coma Coma resulting from cerebral damage caused by liver disease.

Hepatitis An inflammatory liver disease that has many forms and causes.

Hiatal hernia Protrusion of part of the stomach through the opening of the esophageal hiatus of the diaphragm.

High-glycemic index A food or meal that raises the blood glucose levels rapidly, primarily being a carbohydrate source.

High-glycemic load Related to glycemic index, but includes total volume of carbohydrate and the rapid rise of glucose.

Hind milk Milk released from the upper part of the breast in response to the hormone oxytocin; very rich in fat.

Hirsutism A condition in which women have male pattern hair growth or loss; commonly found with hyperinsulinemia.

Histidinemia A hereditary metabolic defect marked by excessive histidine in the blood and urine.

Holistic health Having to do with the whole of one's health; considering all factors affecting one's state of health.

Homeostasis The condition in which the body remains at a constant, such as body temperature or blood levels of nutrients and toxins.

Homocysteine A type of protein that is related to cardiovascular risk.

Homocystinuria A lack of enzyme resulting in homocystine in the urine.

Homogenize The process in which fat particles become so finely dispersed that they do not rise in a liquid.

Honeymoon period Usually the first year after diagnosis of insulin-dependent diabetes mellitus; before the complete destruction of the beta cells.

Hormone Chemicals produced by cells of the body to stimulate or retard certain life processes such as growth and reproduction.

Hospices Organizations that support a natural process of death in one's home or in an institutional setting in which death and the grieving process are openly discussed.

Hydrogenated fat A liquid vegetable oil that has the element hydrogen added to make a solid fat.

Hydrolysis The chemical reaction of cellular metabolism involving the addition of water to larger water-based molecules to make them available for cell function.

Hyperalimentation Administration of all nutrients directly into the blood system. Also referred to as total parenteral nutrition (TPN).

Hypercalcemia An excess of calcium in the blood.

Hypercalciuria An excess of calcium in the urine.

Hyperchlorhydria An excess of hydrochloric acid in gastric juice.

Hypercholesterolemia An elevation of cholesterol in the blood.

Hyperemesis A condition of excessive vomiting.

Hyperglycemia An elevation of glucose in the blood; diagnostic of diabetes with two fasting blood sugars over 126 mg/dL.

Hyperglycemic, Hyperosmolar Nonketotic (HHNK) Coma A condition often associated with diabetes in an older person; blood sugars in the 500 mg/dL range or higher, with severe dehydration and confusion evident.

Hyperinsulinemia High levels of insulin in the blood; often associated with obesity and insulin resistance.

Hyperkinesis Abnormally increased motor activity or movement.

Hyperlipidemia An elevation of specific lipoproteins, cholesterol, and triglycerides.

Hyperlipoproteinemia An excess of lipoproteins in the blood.

Hyperosmotic diarrhea A type of diarrhea caused by a high solute load that draws excess water into the intestinal tract.

Hyperparathyroidism Abnormally increased activity of the parathyroid gland.

Hyperphagia An increased hunger.

Hyperplasty A term related to the fat cell theory that describes a situation in which a person has an excess number of fat cells.

Hypertension The term used for high blood pressure.

Hypertriglyceridemia High levels of triglycerides in the blood; often associated with excess alcohol intake or the insulin resistance syndrome.

Hypertrophy A term related to the fat cell theory that describes a situation in which a person has large-sized fat cells.

Hypoalbuminemia Abnormally low levels of albumin in the blood.

Hypochlorhydria A deficiency of hydrochloric acid in gastric juice.

Hypochromic A lack of color in red blood cells as a result of decrease in hemoglobin.

Hypocupremia Low copper levels in the blood.

Hypoglycemia A condition of low blood glucose; defined as blood glucose less than 70 mg/dL.

Hypoglycemic unawareness Low blood sugar without symptoms; generally occurs after years of uncontrolled diabetes.

Hyponatremia Low levels of blood sodium.

Hypoparathyroidism A condition of greatly reduced functioning of the parathyroid glands.

Hypotension The term used for low blood pressure.

Hypothalamus A portion of the thalamus that promotes release or inhibition of pituitary hormones related to the metabolism of carbohydrates, proteins, and fats and to other functions.

IgE antibody The immune factor related to food and other allergies.

Ileum The lower part of the small intestine.

Immunoglobulin A (IgA) Known to have antiviral properties; produced in nonvascular fluids such as saliva and intestinal secretions.

Impaired fasting glucose (IFG) A condition of elevated fasting levels of glucose; defined as fasting glucose greater than 110 mg/dL.

Inborn errors of metabolism Conditions resulting in a lack of a hormone or other metabolic chemical that results in a build-up of toxic by-products in the system; often causes mental retardation unless the diet is altered beginning in infancy.

Incomplete protein Refers to a food that is missing an essential amino acid.

Ingestion The process of eating; taking food into the digestive tract.

Insoluble fiber A form of dietary fiber that does not dissolve in water; referred to as roughage. Whole wheat contains this type of fiber.

Insulin A protein hormone formed in the pancreas and secreted into the blood for the purpose of regulating carbohydrate, lipid, and amino acid metabolism.

Insulin dependent diabetes mellitus (IDDM) A form of diabetes that usually develops in children and young adults; once known as juvenile onset diabetes. Now referred to as Type 1 diabetes (in Arabic numeral rather than Roman numeral form).

Insulin reaction A condition of severe hypoglycemia; usually associated with unconsciousness.

Insulin resistance A condition in which the body cells resist the action of insulin; often found with obesity and with a high saturated fat diet; usually a genetic predisposition exists.

Insulin resistance syndrome A diagnosis is made by correlates, including central obesity, dyslipidemia, hypertension, Type 2 diabetes, gout, and polycystic ovary syndrome.

Insulin shock Excess amounts of injected insulin result in profound hypoglycemia; glucose needed to treat either orally in a conscious state or via a venous route (IV dextrose).

Intermediate care facility (ICF) A group home for persons with developmental disabilities; ICFs were developed in response to the deinstitutionalization of such persons.

International unit (IU) A measure used in describing vitamin content of foods or recommendations of intake.

Intrinsic factor A substance produced in the stomach that helps absorption of vitamin B_{12}.

Iron overload A rare disease of unknown origin characterized by widespread iron deposits in the body; can lead to pancreatic cirrhosis and other problems.

Irritable bowel syndrome (IBS) A noninflammatory condition of the bowel, with altered bowel habits often alternating between diarrhea and constipation and with abdominal pain.

Islets of Langerhans The areas of the pancreas that produce insulin.

"I" versus "You" statements A form of communication in which the speaker uses statements that express personal feelings rather than accusations to another person.

Jaundice A condition related to hyperbilirubinemia, with the deposit of yellow bile pigments causing yellowness of skin.

Jejunostomy A permanent opening performed by surgery between the jejunum and the surface of the abdominal wall.

Jejunum The middle portion of the small intestine connecting the duodenum and the ileum.

Ketoacidosis An accumulation of excess ketones (acid) that changes the pH of the blood; seen in uncontrolled diabetes mellitus.

Ketogenic diet A diet containing large amounts of fat and minimal amounts of protein and carbohydrate; sometimes used in treating certain types of epilepsy in children.

Ketonuria Ketones found in the urine; a test to help with diabetes management during illness, when blood sugar is over 240 mg/dL, or during pregnancy.

Ketosis The accumulation in the blood and tissues of large quantities of ketone bodies as a result of a complete oxidation of fats.

Kilocalorie (kcal) A unit of measure used to describe food energy. One pound of body fat is equivalent to 3500 kcal of food.

Krebs cycle The chemical process found at the cell level that converts food matter into energy.

Kwashiorkor A protein deficiency disease.

Kyphosis Also called hunchback; an abnormal curvature of the spine often related to osteoporosis.

Lactation The breast-feeding period.

Lactobacillus culture A culture containing a beneficial form of bacteria normally found in a healthy intestine; used in making yogurt.

Lactose intolerance The inability to digest the milk sugar lactose because of inadequate amounts of the lactase enzyme; common symptoms are bloating of the abdomen with flatus and diarrhea.

La Leche League An organization usually of women that promotes the art and success of breast-feeding.

Lean tissue A term for muscle tissue.

Learned food aversion An aversion to food that is learned through a negative association such as an illness.

Legumes The fruit or seed of pod-bearing plants such as peas, beans, lentils, and peanuts.

Leptin A hormone believed to help promote satiety, thereby regulating body weight.

Let-down reflex A term used to describe the process whereby the hormone oxytocin allows the hind milk to flow during breast-feeding; characterized by a gentle "pins and needles" sensation.

Linoleic acid The principal essential fatty acid for humans.

Linolenic acid An essential fatty acid.

Lipase An enzyme that hastens the splitting of fats into glycerol and fatty acids.

Lipids A term relating to all forms of fat.

Lipogenesis The formation of adipose tissue or body fat.

Lipogenic Related to substances that induce the promotion of body fat; insulin is a hormone that is lipogenic.

Lipolysis The breakdown of body fat.

Lipoprotein Lipid (fat) attached to protein; lipoproteins are the form of fats found in the blood.

Lipoprotein lipase An enzyme that is needed to break down triglycerides.

Listeria A pathogen that is related to food poisoning.

Macroalbuminuria A condition of large amounts of protein in the urine; associated with chronic renal failure.

Macrobiotic diet A diet progressing in stages and consisting mainly of rice in the last stage. The diet is deficient in many nutrients, including some amino acids.

Macronutrient The energy (kilocalorie) sources in food: carbohydrate, protein, and fat. Alcohol is also an energy source.

Macular degeneration A common cause of old-age blindness in which the macula at the back of the eye degenerates.

Malnutrition A state of inadequate nutrient intake (such as marasmus) or an excess nutrient intake (such as obesity).

Marasmus A condition of protein-calorie malnutrition.

Maturity onset diabetes of youth (MODY) A form of diabetes that resembles Type 2 diabetes.

Meals on Wheels A program of meal delivery to homebound or ill individuals in their homes.

Medical geneology Related to the understanding and recognition of genetically linked health conditions within families.

Medical nutrition therapy A diet modified in nutrients and used as therapy for diabetes, renal and cardiovascular disease, and other diseases and conditions. Previously referred to as diet therapy or therapeutic diet.

Medicare A health program primarily for persons after retirement age.

Medium chain triglycerides (MCT) A type of fat that does not require digestion; often used as a form of enteral nutrition support in conditions of fat malabsorption.

Megadose Large doses; generally ascribed to supplements of vitamins and minerals that are greater than ten times the RDA.

Megaloblastic anemia A form of anemia characterized by megaloblasts in the bone marrow or blood.

Ménière's disease A disorder of the labyrinth of the inner ear that is treated with a low-sodium diet.

Mental retardation An older term used for developmental disability; related to impaired cognition.

Metabolic Having to do with metabolism.

Metabolic obesity A term coined to describe persons who are of normal weight, but who tend to carry excess in the abdominal region.

Metabolic rate The rate at which metabolism occurs; influenced by such factors as exercise and body temperature.

Metabolism The anabolic (constructive) and catabolic (breakdown) processes of the body.

Microalbuminuria Small amount of protein found in the urine; precedes macroalbuminuria.

Micronutrient A substance in food that is needed in small amounts; vitamins and minerals are examples.

Mid-arm circumference A measurement used in anthropometry to help determine body fat percentage.

Milk anemia A form of iron deficiency anemia attributable to an excess intake of milk, which replaces other iron sources such as meat.

Mitochondria The furnaces within body cells where metabolism occurs.

Monoglycerides A form of fat.

Monosaccharides The simplest form of carbohydrate; one unit of sugar molecules; glucose and fructose.

Monounsaturated fats A form of food fat that is referred to as a "good fat"; found in high amounts in olives, olive oil, canola oil, avocados, and most nuts.

Morbidity Sickness rate.

Morbid obesity More than 30% overweight; Body Mass Index greater than 40.

Mortality Death rate.

Myocardial infarction Referred to as MI or heart attack.

Nasogastric A term used in describing the placement of a feeding tube from the nose to the stomach.

Nasojejunal A term used to describe the placement of a feeding tube from the nose to the jejunum.

National Cholesterol Education Program (NCEP) A program that was initiated in 1985 by the National Heart, Lung, and Blood Institute (NHLBI) aimed at reducing illness and death from coronary heart disease through lowering serum cholesterol levels.

Nephron The functional part of the kidney that produces urine; about one million nephrons make up each kidney.

Nephrosis A general term for kidney disease.

Nephrotic syndrome A condition involving edema, proteinuria, hypoalbuminuria, and susceptibility to infections.

Neurologic impairment Impairment related to a low level of consciousness or sensory or motor function.

Neuropathy A condition characterized by functional disturbances and pathologic changes outside the central region of the nervous system.

Neuropeptides Molecules composed of short chains of amino acids.

Nitrogen balance A state in which nitrogen intake through protein ingestion equals the amount being excreted through the kidneys.

Nitrogenous wastes Waste products of the body that contain nitrogen.

Non-insulin–dependent diabetes mellitus (NIDDM) A form of diabetes that is typically found in overweight adults. Insulin injection is sometimes necessary for good blood sugar control, but is not required for survival. Now referred to as Type 2 diabetes (in Arabic numeral rather than Roman numeral form).

Nontropical sprue Another term for celiac disease.

Nonverbal communication Communication done without speech, such as with facial expressions.

Nursing-bottle mouth Another term for baby-bottle tooth decay.

Nursing process A goal-directed series of activities aimed at alleviating or preventing health problems; includes five components: assessment, nursing diagnosis, planning, implementation, and evaluation.

Nutrient A substance found in food that is essential for good health.

Nutrient density The amount of nutrients per kilocalorie; high nutrient density means a large amount of nutrients per serving of food.

Nutrition The sum of the processes by which the body uses food to support health.

Nutritional status The level at which a person meets their nutritional needs without deficiency or excess.

People have good nutritional status when they have met all their nutritional needs.

Nutrition care process Similar to the nursing process excluding the component of diagnosis.

Nutritionist A term that has no legal definition. Registered dietitians are nutritionists in the sense that they are trained in the science of nutrition. Qualified nutritionists include persons with at least a four-year degree in the science of nutrition.

Nutrition Program for the Elderly A federal program designed to provide $\frac{1}{3}$ the RDA of vitamins A and C, calcium, protein, and kilocalories for elderly persons; meals provided in either congregate meal sites such as in churches or other community settings or home-delivered for those in need.

Nutrition Screening Initiative A project of the American Academy of Family Physicians, the American Dietetic Association, and the National Council on the Aging, Inc.; the initiative that developed the nutritional screening tool for older adults called the DETERMINE Checklist.

Nutrition support A term generally ascribed to the provision of enteral and parenteral nutrition; also includes the provision of liquid supplements for weight gain.

Obesity The condition of weighing more than 20% of ideal body weight; a body mass Index greater than 30.

Obstetrician A physician who specializes in the delivery of babies.

Obstipation A condition of intractable constipation.

Older Americans Act Federal legislation that enacted assistance to maintain the health of the elderly population such as the Nutrition Program for the Elderly.

Oliguria A condition of decreased urinary output.

Omega-3 fatty acids The type of fat found in fish oil and some plant products.

Oncology The study of tumors.

Oral glucose tolerance test (OGTT) A test in which a set amount of carbohydrates are consumed in a beverage with hourly monitoring of blood glucose levels up to 3 hours for the diagnosis of diabetes, and occasionally a 6-hour monitoring for the diagnosis of hypoglycemia.

Oral hypoglycemic agents Medication in pill form used to control glucose levels in Type 2 diabetes.

Organic foods Foods that originate from farms certified by the U.S. Department of Agriculture (USDA) that meet guidelines for pesticide use and other chemicals.

Orthostatic hypertension Increased blood pressure that occurs with standing erect.

Osmolality The number of particles dissolved in a solution.

Osteodystrophy A bone disease associated with renal disease, with elevated phosphorus and low or normal calcium levels found in the blood.

Osteomalacia Softening of the bones often associated with vitamin D deficiency; in children the condition is known as rickets.

Osteoporosis A condition characterized by a reduction in the quantity of bone.

Otitis media An ear infection; often a chronic condition in infancy and childhood.

Over-the-counter medications Medications that may be purchased without a prescription.

Overweight An excess of 10% body weight over an ideal weight; body mass index (BMI) greater than 27 is accepted as overweight; some authorities state that overweight is BMI over 24.

Oxidation A chemical process in which oxygen removes electrons from atoms; involved in energy metabolism.

Oxytocin A hormone that causes uterine contraction and promotes the let-down reflex of breast-feeding.

Palliative care Treatment to relieve or lessen pain or other uncomfortable symptoms, but not to effect a cure.

Palmar grasp A hand grasp characterized by use of the palm.

Pancreas A gland behind the stomach that releases insulin, glucagon, and some enzymes of digestion for fats and proteins.

Pancreatitis Inflammation of the pancreas often associated with alcoholism and fat malabsorption.

Paraprofessional "Near" professional; a person who is not a professional, but is trained to do a type of professional work.

Parathyroid glands Small glands situated near the thyroid gland which are the major source of parathyroid hormone that regulate serum calcium levels.

Parenteral nutrition Provision of a liquid nutrition formula directly into the blood system via the subclavian vein or other site.

Parkinson's disease A slowly progressive disease characterized by abnormal involuntary movements and alteration in muscle tone.

Pasteurization The heating of milk or other liquid to a temperature of 60° C (140° F) for 30 minutes,

killing pathogenic bacteria and considerably delaying the development of other bacteria.

Pattern management A term used in diabetes management related to the identification of patterns of hyperglycemia and hypoglycemia.

Peak action A term used to describe the peak action of insulin by injection.

Pediatrician A physician specializing in childhood health and illness.

Pellagra A nutritional deficiency disease caused by long-term lack of niacin, resulting in a number of nervous, digestive, and skin symptoms.

Peptic ulcer A condition of the stomach in which the lining has been eroded.

Periodontal A term to describe the area around or near a tooth.

Periodontal disease Disease of the tissues supporting and surrounding the teeth.

Peripheral Parts of the body away from the interior.

Peripheral nerves Nerves found in the arms, hands, legs, and feet.

Peripheral neuropathy A condition related to damage of peripheral nerves such as in the feet and hands.

Peripheral parenteral nutrition (PPN) Administration of nutrients through peripheral veins.

Peristalsis The worm-like movement by which the digestive tract propels its contents through waves of contraction.

Peritoneal dialysis A form of dialysis in which a dialysis solution is placed directly into the peritoneum surrounding the abdominal cavity and later removed.

Pernicious anemia A form of anemia caused by a lack of the intrinsic factor normally produced by the stomach mucosa, leading to a deficiency in vitamin B_{12}; left untreated can lead to irreversible neurological damage and death.

Phenylketonuria (PKU) A congenital disease resulting from a deficit in the metabolism of the amino acid phenylalanine.

Phospholipids A lipid, or fat, that contains phosphorus; major lipids of cell membranes.

Physiological anemia One form of anemia often found in pregnancy as a result of an increase in plasma volume without an increase in red blood cells.

Phytochemicals A term developed to describe substances in plant-based food that are neither vitamins nor minerals.

Pica An abnormal craving for nonfood substances.

Pincer grasp A hand grasp characterized by use of the thumb and index finger.

Placenta The organ developed prenatally in the uterus that transfers maternal nutrients to the fetus. Also known as afterbirth.

Plant stanols Substances naturally found in plants that resemble cholesterol and compete for absorption in the intestinal tract, thereby lowering serum cholesterol levels.

Podiatrist A physician who specializes in problems of the feet.

Polycystic ovary syndrome (PCOS) A condition that is often found with insulin resistance and hyperinsulinemia; diagnosed based on levels of androgens, hirsutism, menstrual cycle dysfunction, and ovarian cysts.

Polydipsia A condition of excess thirst.

Polyphagia A condition of excess appetite.

Polypharmacy The condition of use of multiple medications.

Polysaccharides The most complex form of carbohydrates; many units of sugar linked together.

Polyunsaturated fatty acids (PUFA) Liquid oils that have less hydrogen than saturated fats.

Polyuria A condition of excessive excretion of urine.

Positive nitrogen balance The condition in which nitrogen intake surpasses nitrogen excretion.

Postpartum blues A period of depression, often brief, related to hormonal changes after pregnancy; often occurs two to three weeks after delivery.

Postpartum psychosis A condition of severe depression following pregnancy in which the woman loses touch with reality.

Postprandial A term that means after meals.

Pouching A term used to describe a person who retains food in the side of his or her mouth; often found in conditions of dementia.

Poverty A financial situation in which the means to meet basic needs such as food and shelter are impaired.

Pradar-Willi syndrome A condition beginning in infancy characterized by hypotonicity and failure to thrive, with hyperphagia beginning in later childhood with a degree of mental retardation; the hyperphagia is often severe enough that food has to be locked away or highly controlled to prevent morbid obesity.

Preconception The time before the conception of pregnancy.

Precursor Something that precedes, such as a substance that is formed into a more active one.

Preeclampsia An older term referring to a condition in late pregnancy related to increased blood pressure, edema, and proteinuria that can lead to eclampsia with convulsions and coma caused by cerebral edema; the current terminology is pregnancy-induced hypertension.

Pregnancy-induced hypertension A condition of pregnancy characterized by elevated blood pressure, proteinuria, and abnormal fluid retention; the cause is unknown, but the condition is associated with poor nutritional status (also known as toxemia).

Premenstrual syndrome (PMS) A condition that occurs after ovulation involving physical and psychological changes that are relieved upon the start of the monthly menstrual cycle.

Prenatal The time preceding birth; also referred to as perinatal.

Preterm milk Breast milk from a mother giving birth to a premature baby.

Products of conception The sources of weight gain in pregnancy, including the weight of the baby, the placenta, increased uterine and breast size, increased blood volume weight, and an expected amount of increased maternal body fat that is equal to a minimum of 15 to 20 lbs.

Prostaglandins A group of chemically related fatty acids that stimulate contraction of the uterus and other smooth muscles and regulate blood pressure, body temperature, platelet aggregation, and inflammation.

Protein-calorie malnutrition Also known as marasmus.

Proteinuria A condition of protein in the urine.

Prothrombin A blood-clotting factor.

Prudent diet A diet that is very low in fat.

P:S ratio The amount of polyunsaturated to saturated fats found in the diet.

Psychomotor Pertaining to physical movements such as with epilepsy.

Public health The field of health sciences concerned with the health of the community as a whole.

Purging A term used in describing bulimic-type actions such as vomiting and laxative abuse.

Purines A compound found in meat and meat extracts; sometimes avoided as a treatment for gout.

Radiation Electromagnetic waves (as in ultraviolet waves, x-rays, gamma rays, and so on).

Radiation therapy The treatment of cancer through the use of radiation to destroy cancer cells.

Radioallergosorbent (RAST) test Used to diagnose food allergies.

Reactive hypoglycemia A form of low blood sugar that may be a precursor to diabetes; characterized by excess, but delayed insulin production in response to simple carbohydrate intake.

Rebound scurvy A type of vitamin C deficiency disease caused by rapid withdrawal from chronic ingestion of megadoses of vitamin C.

Receptor sites The doors or entryways into body cells.

Recommended Dietary Allowances (RDAs) The recommended amount of nutrients to achieve health. The RDAs are felt to easily meet the nutritional needs of 95% of the population.

Refeeding syndrome Also called the nutrition recovery syndrome; occurs when nutritional support is undertaken too aggressively, resulting in decreased serum lab values as the cells increase their intake of minerals such as phosphorus.

Reference dietary intake (RDI) A term developed for use with food labels; average amounts of the updated RDAs.

Renal insufficiency A stage of diminishing renal function when the glomerular filtration rate is reduced to about 30 ml/min and waste products begin to accumulate in the body.

Renal osteodystrophy Disease of the bone related to inadequate kidney functioning.

Renal threshold The capacity for reabsorption by the kidneys.

Residue The undigested material found in food.

Retinol equivalents (RE) A means of measuring the vitamin A content of food.

Retinopathy Disease of the eyes often found with uncontrolled diabetes; may include the growth of fragile blood vessels that can now be treated with laser surgery; a leading cause of blindness.

Rickets A bone disease that begins in childhood, is caused by a lack of vitamin D, and results in bowing of legs.

Salivary gland The glands in the mouth that secrete saliva.

Salmonella A rod-shaped bacteria that can cause gastroenteritis; often associated with dairy products.

Satiety The feeling of being satisfied or satiated; used to describe the point at which a person feels satisfied after eating a meal.

Saturated fat Solid fats; found in most animal fats in association with cholesterol and in hydrogenated fats.

Schizophrenia A large group of mental disorders characterized by mental deterioration, delusions, and withdrawal from the external world.

Self-monitoring of blood glucose (SMBG) The use of a personal blood glucose meter to monitor glucose levels.

Sepsis The presence in the blood or other tissues of harmful microorganisms or their toxins.

Sickle cell disease A serious hereditary disease that causes red blood cells to have a sickle shape and to be rigid; found mainly in persons of African ancestry, but also occurs in those with Mediterranean, Middle Eastern, and Asian Indian ancestry.

Sigmoid region A part of the intestinal tract.

Sodium The chief cation of extracellular body fluids.

Soluble fiber Forms of dietary fiber that dissolve in water and the digestive tract. Oat bran and legumes are high in soluble fiber.

Somogyi effect The condition in which blood glucose levels rise after hypoglycemia; related to the release of counterregulatory hormones that allow the breakdown of liver glycogen into blood glucose; named after Dr. Somogyi who first gave credence to this phenomenon.

Spastic Implying muscle spasms.

Specific dynamic action The increase in metabolism related to the process of digesting food.

Spina bifida Also known as neural tube defect; a developmental birth defect in which the spinal cord is not completely enclosed.

Sports anemia Anemia of athletes unrelated to iron intake.

Staphylococcus aureus A form of bacteria present on the skin and in the upper respiratory tract; often associated with a form of food poisoning when safe food handling procedures are not followed.

Starch Another term for digestible polysaccharides as found in grain products.

Steatorrhea Diarrhea characterized by excess fat in the stools.

Steroids An important group of body compounds that includes sex and adrenal hormones.

Sterols Lipid-like substances such as cholesterol found in animal fats.

Sugar The monosaccharide and disaccharide form of carbohydrate.

Sugar alcohols A form of sugar found in sugar substitutes that do not promote dental caries.

Systemic Implying involvement with interconnected systems of the body.

Tetany A condition with steady contraction of a muscle without distinct twitching caused by abnormal calcium metabolism.

Thalassemia A hereditary form of anemia.

Therapeutic lifestyle changes (TLC) A diet aimed at lowering serum cholesterol levels with the goals of 7% saturated fat, 30% total fat, less than 200 mg cholesterol, less than 2400 mg sodium, and kilocaloric intake aimed at achieving or maintaining a healthy weight; guidelines also advocate increased soluble fiber and up to 35% fat chiefly from monounsaturated fats for persons with the metabolic syndrome or the insulin resistance syndrome.

Thrifty food plan A meal plan that can provide all necessary nutrients at the most minimal cost; the current basis for Food Stamp allotments.

Thrifty gene The theory related to the historical survival of groups of people or populations who withstood cycles of famine.

Thrombosis The formation of a thrombus or clot formed from platelets and other blood substances, which may partially or totally obstruct blood flow.

Thrush A bacterial infection often manifested with white blotches on the tongue and in the oral cavity.

Thyroxine A hormone produced by the thyroid gland that increases the rate of metabolism.

Tolerable upper intake levels (ULs) A new term developed to state the upper level of intake of vitamins and minerals that appear to pose no health threat.

Tongue thrust A condition usually related to having a small oral cavity that cannot fully contain the tongue.

Total parenteral nutrition (TPN) Administration of nutrients through the superior vena cava.

Toxemia General intoxication sometimes resulting from absorption of bacterial products formed at an infection site. Also a condition in late pregnancy characterized by elevated blood pressure, edema, and proteinuria; in reference to pregnancy the current terminology is pregnancy-induced hypertension.

Trans fatty acids The form of fat found in hydrogenated fats.

Transferrin A serum globulin or protein that binds and transports iron.

Tricep skinfold An anthropometric measure in which calipers measure the fat on the back of the arm; such measuring requires training for accuracy.

Triglycerides The form of food fat found in the blood and body tissues.

Tube feeding A form of delivery of nutrients through a tube that may be placed through the nose or abdominal opening into the stomach or small intestine.

Type 1 diabetes The form of diabetes in which the pancreas loses its insulin production because of autoimmune destruction by GAD antibodies.

Type 2 diabetes The common form of diabetes generally related to insulin resistance; the general term used to describe all nonautoimmune forms of diabetes.

Tyramine Related to tyrosine and found in ripe cheese; closely related structurally to epinephrine (a hormone), which has a similar, but weaker, effect.

Ulcerative colitis A chronic condition manifested by abdominal pain and rectal bleeding; long-standing ulcerative colitis is a high-risk factor for the development of colon cancer.

Underweight A body mass index less than 19.

Unsaturated fats The form of fat with low levels of hydrogen; liquid or soft forms of fat.

Uremia The final stage of renal disease associated with severe azotemia; includes symptoms of headache, muscular twitching, mental disturbances, nausea, and vomiting.

U.S. dietary guidelines Guidelines aimed at reducing the mortality and morbidity of several diseases such as cardiovascular disease, hypertension, cancer, and diabetes mellitus. The guidelines recommend increased amounts of complex carbohydrates and dietary fiber, with reduced amounts of fat, sugar, salt, and alcohol. Maintaining or achieving desirable weight and including a variety of foods are also recommended.

Vegan A person who does not eat animal products. Protein is derived from plant sources such as legumes, nuts, and seeds.

Vegetarian A person who avoids eating meat for health or spiritual reasons. Some vegetarians avoid only red meat.

Videofluoroscopy A test done to determine a person's ability to swallow.

Villi The hairlike projections inside the intestinal tract; involved in absorption of digested food matter.

Vitamin B complex The term used to describe all of the B vitamins.

Waist-to-hip ratio (WHR) A measure in which the waist size is divided by the hip size; large WHR is related to a variety of chronic illnesses as found in the insulin resistance syndrome

Water-soluble vitamins The B vitamins and vitamin C; vitamins that are easily lost in cooking water or destroyed from overcooking or exposure to air.

Weaning To discontinue breast-feeding and substitute other forms of feeding; may also relate to weaning off of nutrition support or other life-support measures.

Wernicke-Korsakoff syndrome A disorder of the central nervous system related to depletion of vitamin B_1 or thiamin.

Women, Infants, and Children (WIC) Supplemental Food Program A federal program that began in the 1970s with the initial chief goal of eradication of iron-deficiency anemia. The program is aimed at lower-income women, infants, and children up to age 5 years that provides nutrition education, breast-feeding support, and food vouchers for foods that are high in iron, vitamin C, calcium, and protein.

Xerophthalmia Dryness and thickening of the membrane lining of the eyelid, eyeball, and cornea; results from vitamin A deficiency.

Xerostomia Dryness of the mouth caused by dysfunctional salivary glands; often induced with radiation treatment for cancer near the oral cavity; can result in severe dental decay because of the absence of the neutralizing effect of saliva.

Index

NOTES

NOTES

NOTES

DIETARY REFERENCE INTAKES (DRIs): RECOMMENDED INTAKES FOR INDIVIDUALS, VITAMINS

FOOD AND NUTRITION BOARD, THE INSTITUTE OF MEDICINE, NATIONAL ACADEMIES

LIFE STAGE GROUP	VITAMIN A (µg/d)[a]	VITAMIN C (mg/d)	VITAMIN D (µg/d)[b,c]	VITAMIN E (mg/d)[d]	VITAMIN K (µg/d)	THIAMIN (mg/d)	RIBOFLAVIN (mg/d)	NIACIN (mg/d)[e]	VITAMIN B6 (mg/d)	FOLATE (µg/d)[f]	VITAMIN B12 (µg/d)	PANTOTHENIC ACID (mg/d)	BIOTIN (µg/d)	CHOLINE[g] (mg/d)
INFANTS														
0-6 mo	400*	40*	5*	4*	2.0*	0.2*	0.3*	2*	0.1*	65*	0.4*	1.7*	5*	125*
7-12 mo	500*	50*	5*	5*	2.5*	0.3*	0.4*	4*	0.3*	80*	0.5*	1.8*	6*	150*
CHILDREN														
1-3 y	300	15	5*	6	30*	0.5	0.5	6	0.5	150	0.9	2*	8*	200*
4-8 y	400	25	5*	7	55*	0.6	0.6	8	0.6	200	1.2	3*	12*	250*
MALES														
9-13 y	600	45	5*	11	60*	0.9	0.9	12	1.0	300	1.8	4*	20*	375*
14-18 y	900	75	5*	15	75*	1.2	1.3	16	1.3	400	2.4	5*	25*	550*
19-30 y	900	90	5*	15	120*	1.2	1.3	16	1.3	400	2.4	5*	30*	550*
31-50 y	900	90	5*	15	120*	1.2	1.3	16	1.3	400	2.4	5*	30*	550*
51-70 y	900	90	10*	15	120*	1.2	1.3	16	1.7	400	2.4[h]	5*	30*	550*
>70 y	900	90	15*	15	120*	1.2	1.3	16	1.7	400	2.4[h]	5*	30*	550*
FEMALES														
9-13 y	600	45	5*	11	60*	0.9	0.9	12	1.0	300	1.8	4*	20*	375*
14-18 y	700	65	5*	15	75*	1.0	1.0	14	1.2	400[i]	2.4	5*	25*	400*
19-30 y	700	75	5*	15	90*	1.1	1.1	14	1.3	400[i]	2.4	5*	30*	425*
31-50 y	700	75	5*	15	90*	1.1	1.1	14	1.3	400[i]	2.4	5*	30*	425*
51-70 y	700	75	10*	15	90*	1.1	1.1	14	1.5	400	2.4[h]	5*	30*	425*
>70 y	700	75	15*	15	90*	1.1	1.1	14	1.5	400	2.4[h]	5*	30*	425*
PREGNANCY														
≤18 y	750	80	5*	15	75*	1.4	1.4	18	1.9	600[j]	2.6	6*	30*	450*
19-30 y	770	85	5*	15	90*	1.4	1.4	18	1.9	600[j]	2.6	6*	30*	450*
31-50 y	770	85	5*	15	90*	1.4	1.4	18	1.9	600[j]	2.6	6*	30*	450*
LACTATION														
≤18 y	1200	115	5*	19	75*	1.4	1.6	17	2.0	500	2.8	7*	35*	550*
19-30 y	1300	120	5*	19	90*	1.4	1.6	17	2.0	500	2.8	7*	35*	550*
31-50 y	1300	120	5*	19	90*	1.4	1.6	17	2.0	500	2.8	7*	35*	550*

Note: This table (taken from the DRI reports, see www.nap.edu) presents Recommended Dietary Allowances (RDAs) in **bold type** and Adequate Intakes (AIs) in ordinary type followed by an asterisk (*). RDAs and AIs may both be used as goals for individual intake. RDAs are set to meet the needs of almost all (97%-98%) individuals in a group. For healthy breast-fed infants, the AI is the mean intake. The AI for other life stage and gender groups is believed to cover needs of all individuals in the group, but lack of data or uncertainty in the data prevent being able to specify with confidence the percentage of individuals covered by this intake.

[a]As retinol activity equivalents (RAEs). 1 RAE = 1 µg retinol, 12 µg β-carotene, 24 µg α-carotene, or 24 µg β-cryptoxanthin in foods. To calculate RAEs from REs of provitamin A carotenoids in foods, divide the REs by 2. For preformed vitamin A in foods or supplements and for provitamin A carotenoids in supplements, 1 RE = 1 RAE.

[b]Cholecalciferol. 1 µg cholecalciferol = 40 IU vitamin D.

[c]In the absence of adequate exposure to sunlight.

[d]As α-tocopherol. α-Tocopherol includes RRR-α-tocopherol, the only form of α-tocopherol that occurs naturally in foods, and the 2R-stereoisomeric forms of α-tocopherol (RRR-, RSR-, RRS-, and RSS-α-tocopherol) that occur in fortified foods and supplements. It does not include the 2S-stereoisomeric forms of α-tocopherol (SRR-, SSR-, SRS-, and SSS-α-tocopherol), also found in fortified foods and supplements.

[e]As niacin equivalents (NE). 1 mg of niacin = 60 mg of tryptophan; 0-6 months = preformed niacin (not NE).

[f]As dietary folate equivalents (DFE). 1 DFE = 1 µg food folate = 0.6 µg of folic acid from fortified food or as a supplement consumed with food = 0.5 µg of a supplement taken on an empty stomach.

[g]Although AIs have been set for choline, there are few data to assess whether a dietary supply of choline is needed at all stages of the life style, and it may be that the choline requirement can be met by endogenous synthesis at some of these stages.

[h]Because 10%-30% of older people may malabsorb food-bound B₁₂, it is advisable for those older than 50 years to meet their RDA mainly by consuming foods fortified with B₁₂ or a supplement containing B₁₂.

[i]In view of evidence linking folate intake with neural tube defects in the fetus, it is recommended that all women capable of becoming pregnant consume 400 µg from supplements or fortified foods in addition to intake of food folate from a varied diet.

[j]It is assumed that women will continue consuming 400 µg from supplements or fortified food until their pregnancy is confirmed and they enter prenatal care, which ordinarily occurs after the end of the periconceptional period—the critical time for formation of the neural tube.

DIETARY REFERENCE INTAKES (DRIs): TOLERABLE UPPER INTAKE LEVELS (UL[a]), VITAMINS
FOOD AND NUTRITION BOARD, THE INSTITUTE OF MEDICINE, NATIONAL ACADEMIES

LIFE STAGE GROUP	VITAMIN A (μg/d)[b]	VITAMIN C (mg/d)	VITAMIN D (μg/d)	VITAMIN E (mg/d)[c,d]	VITAMIN K	THIAMIN	RIBO-FLAVIN	NIACIN (mg/d)[d]	VITAMIN B6 (mg/d)	FOLATE (μg/d)[d]	VITAMIN B12	PANTOTHENIC ACID	BIOTIN	CHOLINE (g/d)	CAROTE-NOIDS[e]
INFANTS															
0-6 mo	600	ND[f]	25	ND	ND	ND	ND	ND	ND	ND	ND	ND	ND	ND	ND
7-12 mo	600	ND	25	ND	ND	ND	ND	ND	ND	ND	ND	ND	ND	ND	ND
CHILDREN															
1-3 y	600	400	50	200	ND	ND	ND	10	30	300	ND	ND	ND	1.0	ND
4-8 y	900	650	50	300	ND	ND	ND	15	40	400	ND	ND	ND	1.0	ND
MALES, FEMALES															
9-13 y	1700	1200	50	600	ND	ND	ND	20	60	600	ND	ND	ND	2.0	ND
14-18 y	2800	1800	50	800	ND	ND	ND	30	80	800	ND	ND	ND	3.0	ND
19-70 y	3000	2000	50	1000	ND	ND	ND	35	100	1000	ND	ND	ND	3.5	ND
>70 y	3000	2000	50	1000	ND	ND	ND	35	100	1000	ND	ND	ND	3.5	ND
PREGNANCY															
≤18 y	2800	1800	50	800	ND	ND	ND	30	80	800	ND	ND	ND	3.0	ND
19-50 y	3000	2000	50	1000	ND	ND	ND	35	100	1000	ND	ND	ND	3.5	ND
LACTATION															
≤18 y	2800	1800	50	800	ND	ND	ND	30	80	800	ND	ND	ND	3.0	ND
19-50 y	3000	2000	50	1000	ND	ND	ND	35	100	1000	ND	ND	ND	3.5	ND

Sources: Dietary Reference Intakes for Calcium, Phosphorus, Magnesium, Vitamin D, and Fluoride (1997); Dietary Reference Intakes for Thiamin, Riboflavin, Niacin, Vitamin B6, Folate, Vitamin B12, Pantothenic Acid, Biotin, and Choline (1998); Dietary Reference Intakes for Vitamin C, Vitamin E, Selenium, and Carotenoids (2000); and Dietary Reference Intakes for Vitamin A, Vitamin K, Arsenic, Boron, Chromium, Copper, Iodine, Iron, Manganese, Molybdenum, Nickel, Silicon, Vanadium, and Zinc (2001). These reports may be accessed via www.nap.edu.

[a] UL = The maximum level of daily nutrient intake that is likely to pose no risk of adverse effects. Unless otherwise specified, the UL represents total intake from food, water, and supplements. Due to lack of suitable data, ULs could not be established for vitamin K, thiamin, riboflavin, vitamin B12, pantothenic acid, biotin, or carotenoids. In the absence of ULs, extra caution may be warranted in consuming levels above recommended intakes.

[b] As preformed vitamin A only.

[c] As α-tocopherol; applies to any form of supplemental α-tocopherol.

[d] The ULs for vitamin E, niacin, and folate apply to synthetic forms obtained from supplements, fortified foods, or a combination of the two.

[e] β-Carotene supplements are advised only to serve as a provitamin A source for individuals at risk of vitamin A deficiency.

[f] ND = Not determinable due to lack of data of adverse effects in this age group and concern with regard to lack of ability to handle excess amounts. Source of intake should be from food only to prevent high levels of intake.